AF544749

Neurobiology of Brain Tumors

VOLUME 4: CONCEPTS IN NEUROSURGERY

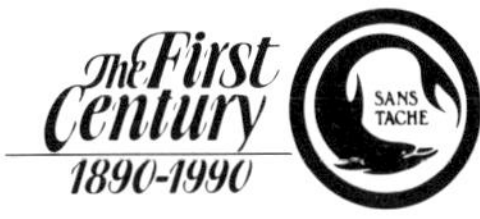

Neurobiology of Brain Tumors

VOLUME 4: CONCEPTS IN NEUROSURGERY

EDITOR

MICHAEL SALCMAN, M.D.

Professor and Chairman, Division of Neurosurgery
University of Maryland School of Medicine
Baltimore, Maryland

SERIES EDITORS

Fremont P. Wirth, M.D.
Robert A. Ratcheson, M.D.

SERIES ASSOCIATE EDITORS

Robert L. Grubb, Jr., M.D.
Julian T. Hoff, M.D.
Martin H. Weiss, M.D.

Sponsored by the
Congress of Neurological Surgeons

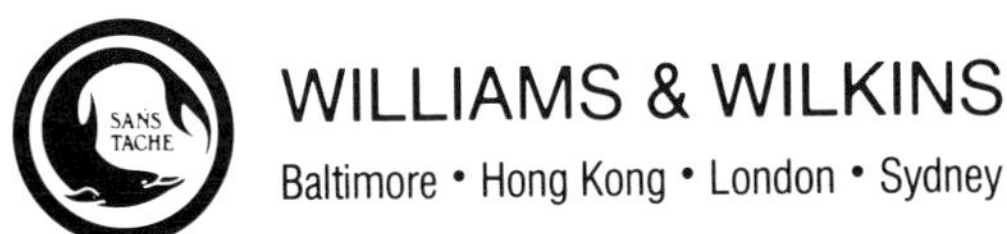

WILLIAMS & WILKINS
Baltimore • Hong Kong • London • Sydney

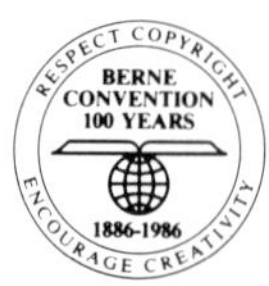

Accurate indications, adverse reactions, and dosage schedules for drugs are provided in this book, but it is possible that they may change. The reader is urged to review the package information data of the manufacturers of the medications mentioned.

Printed in the United States of America

Library of Congress cataloged this serial as follows:

Library of Congress Cataloging-in-Publication Data

Neurobiology of brain tumors/editor, Michael Salcman ; sponsored by the Congress of Neurological Surgeons.
p. cm.—(Concepts in neurosurgery ; v. 4)
Includes bibliographical references.
ISBN 0-683-07496-2
1. Brain—Cancer. 2. Brain—Tumors—Pathophysiology.
I. Salcman, Michael. II. Congress of Neurological Surgeons.
III. Series.
[DNLM: 1. Brain Neoplasms. W1 CO459RK v. 4/WL 358 N4935]
RC280.B7N49 1991
616.99'48107—dc20
DNLM/DLC
for Library of Congress 90-12320
CIP

90 91 92 93
10 9 8 7 6 5 4 3 2 1

Series Foreword

The Congress of Neurological Surgeons was founded in 1951 with the prime purposes being to maintain high standards of neurosurgery and to promote continuing education. While the emphasis has been on the needs of the resident in training and the younger neurosurgeon, the programs of the Congress have benefited not only neurosurgery but also the neuroscience fields in general.

To help provide for the continuing education needs of its members, the Congress began publication in 1953 of an annual volume entitled *Clinical Neurosurgery,* which presents in detail the invited presentations made at the annual meeting of the organization. This volume has become an important reference source for neurosurgeons. Then in 1977, after several years of planning, the Congress began publication of a monthly journal entitled *Neurosurgery,* which proved to be an outstanding addition to the medical literature.

Now, under the direction of Doctors Fremont P. Wirth and Robert A. Ratcheson, the Congress is embarking on another publication series entitled *Concepts in Neurosurgery.* The goals of this publication, as proposed by Dr. Ratcheson during his term as President of the Congress, are to provide a monograph that will cover a specific area in depth with basic scientific knowledge and theory applied to practical neurosurgical issues. For the resident in training this publication can supplement the educational program or provide knowledge in an area that might not be covered in depth in a training program. For the trained neurosurgeon, each monograph will provide the opportunity to review recent knowledge about a practical subject and supply up-to-date information in an important area of neurosurgery.

The Congress has selected Doctors Wirth and Ratcheson as editors, two individuals who have been members of the Executive Committee for several years and have recently been officers, who have also had considerable experience with educational programs. They will be aided by associate editors, Doctors Robert L. Grubb, Julian T. Hoff, and Martin Weiss, who also have had broad experience with publications and continuing education endeavors.

The Congress is again providing a leadership role in an important area that will benefit all of neurosurgery.

Robert G. Ojemann, M.D.

Foreword

This, the fourth volume of the *Concepts in Neurosurgery* series, represents the continuing commitment of the Congress of Neurological Surgeons to neurosurgical education. The neurobiology of brain tumors is a topic of fundamental importance to the neurosurgeon. For this volume, Dr. Michael Salcman has selected a group of authors uniquely qualified to discuss brain tumor biology. Epidemiology, oncogenesis, cell biology, the blood-brain barrier and immunology as factors affecting tumor growth and behavior are discussed in detail. The rationale underlying the various treatment modalities is presented. Cytoreduction, radiation, chemotherapy and immunotherapy are examined carefully, as are photoradiation and hyperthermia.

It is anticipated that the publication of this volume by the Congress of Neurological Surgeons will improve the care of our patients and serve as a valuable resource for the neurosurgeon in training and in practice. It should accomplish the aims of *Concepts in Neurosurgery,* as have the preceding three volumes.

Fremont P. Wirth, M.D., F.A.C.S.
Robert M. Ratcheson, M.D.

Preface

During the five years that this book has been in preparation, explosive growth has occurred in our knowledge of the pathogenesis and biological behavior of brain tumors. This wealth of new information and technology is certain to be the foundation upon which improved concepts and modes of therapy will be based. I have always felt that the contemporary perspective of general oncology in regard to mutations, cellular differentiation, and biological markers needed to be applied to important issues in neuro-oncology and that such information should be conveyed in a straightforward fashion to practicing clinicians as well as to those with a special interest in the study and treatment of brain tumors.

This book is organized so as to proceed from questions of oncogenesis and molecular biology through the development and growth of the tumor mass, its interaction with the host, and finally the consequences of biologic and clinical behavior in treatment planning. We are honored that the book begins with what are likely to have been the final scientific contributions written by Bruce Schoenberg, perhaps the preeminent neuroepidemiologist of our time, and by Lucien Rubinstein, a great friend of neurosurgery and our most outstanding neuropathologist. Schoenberg's chapter and that of Dr. Garcia cover the incidence and classification of all brain tumors, in accordance with an important theme of this volume, namely that the topics discussed are of general importance for all brain tumors and not just for malignant glioma. Hence, the frequent references throughout the text to the manner in which particular issues relate to a wide variety of neoplasms, including meningioma, medulloblastoma, acoustic schwannoma, and astrocytoma.

The masterly contribution by Dr. Rubinstein elaborates a theory by which one can explain the relative incidence and age of occurrence of nearly all brain tumors. The chromosomal alterations and base-pair mutations required by this theory are clearly discussed by Martuza, Berger, and Ali-Osman. External stimuli may interact with such genetic predispositions or accidents in the oncogenesis of neoplasms so as to produce a second "hit." Morantz discusses trauma and demyelination as two examples of such contributing etiologic agents. Once tumor growth has been initiated, it can take on any number of patterns as described by Schiffer and further elaborated by Kornblith, Merrill, and Hoshino in their discussions of the kinetics of growth and other manifestations of phenotypic expression.

The cellular properties of brain tumors are at least as fascinating as their origin and of at least as much potential importance in their treatment. These subjects are the focus of the next section of the book. Much of what we know about the behavior of brain tumor cells has come from in vitro work. Many of these studies have been carried out by Dr. Bigner and his colleagues, who review the topic for us. Modern immunostaining of pathological specimens, critical to both clinical and experimental analysis, is based on recent achievements in molecular biology and furthers our knowledge of the cellular properties of tumors, as Molenaar and Trojanowski indicate. Contemporary imaging techniques permit us to make in vivo correlations of these in vitro findings, as Paul Kornblith and David Thomas discuss in regard to the metabolism, tissue typing, and growth of tumors. Finally, we consider the cell biology of the tumor's host and three special issues are addressed: the immunological status of the patient, the nature and significance of the blood-brain barrier, and the importance of other biological and demographic factors in prognosis. As Young, Merchant, Apuzzo, and Packer clearly indicate, the biology of the tumor, the biology of the patient, and the success of therapy are inextricably bound together.

The book concludes with a discussion of the biologic rationale for a variety of therapeutic modalities of current interest. The topic of immunotherapy is covered in the chapter on immunocompetence. Drs. James Marks and Stuart Grossman bring us up to date on the two most widely applied adjuvant treatments, radiation and chemotherapy, while Wharen and colleagues discuss photoirradiation. A chapter on hyperthermia brings the book to a close and exemplifies the principle of multimodality therapy as a strategy for dealing with tumor heterogeneity.

Of course, there is no appropriate close to the story itself. The biology of brain tumors and the development of new modes of tumor therapy are among the most intellectually challenging and rapidly changing fields in all of neuroscience. In some ways, a book such as this one is out of date as soon as it appears. Nevertheless, because it is devoted to the application of basic principles from such disciplines as epidemiology, molecular biology, tissue culture, cell kinetics, and other subjects to the general problem of brain tumors, it may provide some useful service to the non-specialist audience for which it was intended and inspire a new generation of investigators to meet the challenges posed by an old and formidable adversary.

Michael Salcman, M.D.

Acknowledgments

I am deeply grateful to my very patient authors and to the Congress of Neurological Surgeons for making this book a reality. I was ably assisted by the excellent editorial and general support provided by Deborah Rudacille and Brenda Smith, two individuals without whom much would be impossible.

Contributors

SERIES EDITORS

Fremont P. Wirth, M.D.
Neurological Institute of Savannah
Director, Neurosurgical and Neurological Intensive Care Unit
St. Joseph's Hospital
Savannah, Georgia

Robert A. Ratcheson, M.D.
Professor and Chief
Division of Neurological Surgery
Case Western Reserve University
University Hospitals of Cleveland
Cleveland, Ohio

SERIES ASSOCIATE EDITORS

Robert L. Grubb, Jr., M.D.
Professor of Neurological Surgery
Washington University School of Medicine
St. Louis, Missouri

Julian T. Hoff, M.D.
Professor of Surgery
Head, Section of Neurosurgery
University of Michigan Hospital
Ann Arbor, Michigan

Martin H. Weiss, M.D.
Professor and Chairman
Department of Neurosurgery
LAC/USC Medical Center
Los Angeles, California

VOLUME EDITOR

Michael Salcman, M.D.
Professor and Chairman, Division of Neurological Surgery
University of Maryland School of Medicine
Baltimore, Maryland

CONTRIBUTORS

Francis Ali-Osman, D.Sc.
Neuro-Oncology Research and Therapy Section
Department of Neurological Surgery
University of Washington
Seattle, Washington

Robert E. Anderson, B.S.
Department of Neurosurgery
Mayo Clinic
Rochester, Minnesota

Michael L. J. Apuzzo, M.D.
Department of Neurological Surgery
University of Southern California School of Medicine
Los Angeles, California

Mitchel S. Berger, M.D.
Neuro-Oncology Research and Therapy Section
Department of Neurological Surgery
University of Washington
Seattle, Washington

Darell D. Bigner, M.D., Ph.D.
Department of Pathology
Preuss Laboratory for Brain Tumor Research
Duke University Medical Center
Durham, North Carolina

Sandra H. Bigner, M.D.
Department of Pathology
Duke University Medical Center
Durham, North Carolina

Richard D. Broadwell, Ph.D.
Division of Neurological Surgery
University of Maryland School of Medicine
Baltimore, Maryland

Henry S. Friedman, M.D.
Department of Pediatrics
Duke University Medical Center
Durham, North Carolina

Julio H. Garcia, M.D.
Professor of Pathology
Director
Division of Anatomic Pathology/Neuropathology
University of Alabama at Birmingham
Birmingham, Alabama

Stuart A. Grossman, M.D.
Assistant Professor of Oncology, Medicine, and Neurosurgery
The Johns Hopkins Oncology Center
The Johns Hopkins Medical Institutions
Baltimore, Maryland

Takao Hoshino, M.D., D.M.Sc.
Professor of Neurosurgery
Brain Tumor Research Center
Department of Neurological Surgery
University of California School of Medicine
San Francisco, California

Peter A. Humphrey, M.D., Ph.D.
Department of Pathology
Duke University Medical Center
Durham, North Carolina

Paul L. Kornblith, M.D.
Professor and Chairman
Department of Neurosurgery
Montefiore Medical Center and Albert Einstein College of Medicine
Bronx, New York

Edward R. Laws, Jr., M.D.
Department of Neurosurgery
George Washington University
Washington, D.C.

Yisheng Lee, M.D., Ph.D.
Department of Pediatrics
Duke University Medical Center
Durham, North Carolina

James E. Marks, M.D.
Chairman
Loyola-Hines Department of Radiotherapy
Loyola University of Chicago
Stritch School of Medicine
Maywood, Illinois

Robert L. Martuza, M.D.
Director, Neurofibromatosis Clinic
Massachusetts General Hospital
Associate Professor of Surgery (Neurosurgery)
Harvard Medical School and Massachusetts General Hospital
Boston, Massachusetts

Randall E. Merchant, Ph.D.
Associate Professor
Division of Neurosurgery
Department of Surgery
Medical College of Virginia/Virginia Commonwealth University
Richmond, Virginia

Marsha J. Merrill, Ph.D.
Staff Fellow
Surgical Neurology Branch
National Institute of Neurological and Communication Disorders and Stroke
National Institutes of Health
Bethesda, Maryland

Willemina M. Molenaar, M.D.
Associate Professor of Pathology
University of Groningen
Groningen, The Netherlands

Robert A. Morantz, M.D.
Clinical Professor of Neurological Surgery and Radiation Oncology
The University of Kansas School of Medicine
Director, The Brain Tumor Institute of Kansas City
Kansas City, Missouri

Roger J. Packer, M.D.
Professor of Neurology and Pediatrics
University of Pennsylvania
Director, Neuro-Oncology Program
Senior Attending Physician
The Children's Hospital of Philadelphia
Philadelphia, Pennsylvania

Lucien J. Rubinstein, M.D.
Professor of Pathology
Director, Division of Neuropathology
University of Virginia School of Medicine
Charlottesville, Virginia

Michael Salcman, M.D.
Professor and Chairman, Division of Neurological Surgery
University of Maryland School of Medicine
Baltimore, Maryland

Davide Schiffer, M.D.
II Department of Neurology
University of Turin
Turin, Italy

Bruce S. Schoenberg, M.D., M.S., Dr.P.H., F.A.C.P.
Chief, Neuroepidemiology Branch
Intramural Research Program
National Institute of Neurological and Communicative Disorders and Stroke
Bethesda, Maryland
Clinical Professor of Neurology
Georgetown University School of Medicine
Washington, D.C.

David G. T. Thomas, F.R.C.P.(G.), F.R.C.S.Ed.
Consultant Neurosurgeon and Senior Lecturer
The National Hospitals for Nervous Diseases
London, England

John Q. Trojanowski, M.D., Ph.D.
Associate Professor of Pathology and Laboratory Medicine
Division of Medical Pathology
University of Pennsylvania School of Medicine
Philadelphia, Pennsylvania

Fotios D. Vrionis, M.D., M.P.H.
Department of Pathology
Duke University Medical Center
Durham, North Carolina

Robert E. Wharen, Jr., M.D.
Department of Neurosurgery
Mayo Clinic
Jacksonville, Florida

Carol J. Wikstrand, Ph.D.
Department of Pathology
Duke University Medical Center
Durham, North Carolina

Harold F. Young, M.D.
Professor and Chairman
Division of Neurosurgery
Department of Surgery
Medical College of Virginia/Virginia Commonwealth University
Richmond, Virginia

Contents

Series Foreword v
Foreword vii
Preface ix
Acknowledgments xi
Contributors xiii

PART ONE
Epidemiology and Classification

CHAPTER **1**
Epidemiology of Primary Intracranial Neoplasms: Disease Distribution and Risk Factors 3
Bruce S. Schoenberg, M.D., M.S., Dr.P.H., F.A.C.P.

CHAPTER **2**
Classification of Brain Tumors 19
Julio H. Garcia, M.D.

PART TWO
Oncogenesis and Growth

CHAPTER **3**
Glioma Cytogeny and Differentiation Viewed through the Window of Neoplastic Vulnerability 35
Lucien J. Rubinstein, M.D.

CHAPTER **4**
Neurofibromatosis as a Model for Tumor Formation in the Human Nervous System 53
Robert L. Martuza, M.D.

CHAPTER **5**
Mutagenesis and DNA Repair Mechanisms 63
Mitchel S. Berger, M.D., and Francis Ali-Osman, D.Sc.

CHAPTER **6**
Trauma and Demyelination as Etiologic Factors in the Development of Brain Tumor 73
Robert A. Morantz, M.D.

CHAPTER **7**
Patterns of Tumor Growth 85
Davide Schiffer, M.D.

CHAPTER **8**
Differentiation and Phenotypic Expression in Human Gliomas **137**
Paul L. Kornblith, M.D., and Marsha J. Merrill, Ph.D.

CHAPTER **9**
Cell Kinetics of Brain Tumors **145**
Takao Hoshino, M.D., D.M.Sc.

PART THREE
The Cell Biology of Brain Tumors

CHAPTER **10**
In Vitro Growth of Brain Tumors **163**
Yisheng Lee, M.D., Ph.D., Carol J. Wikstrand, Ph.D.,
Peter A. Humphrey, M.D., Ph.D., Sandra H. Bigner, M.D., Ph.D.,
Henry S. Friedman, M.D., Fotios D. Vrionis, M.D., M.P.H., and
Darell D. Bigner, M.D., Ph.D.

CHAPTER **11**
Biological Markers of Glial and Primitive Tumors **185**
Willemina M. Molenaar, M.D., Ph.D., and John Q. Trojanowski, M.D., Ph.D.

CHAPTER **12**
Immunocompetence of Patients with Malignant Glioma **211**
Harold F. Young, M.D., Randall E. Merchant, Ph.D., and
Michael L. J. Apuzzo, M.D.

CHAPTER **13**
The Blood-Brain Barrier **229**
Michael Salcman, M.D., and Richard D. Broadwell, Ph.D.

CHAPTER **14**
Metabolic Studies of Brain Tumors in Vivo **251**
Paul L. Kornblith, M.D.

CHAPTER **15**
In Vivo Estimates of Kinetic Parameters **259**
David G. T. Thomas, M.A., and Michael Salcman, M.D.

CHAPTER **16**
Prognostic Factors in Patients with Brain Tumors **275**
Roger J. Packer, M.D.

PART FOUR
Therapeutic Rationale and Modes of Treatment

CHAPTER **17**
Ionizing Radiation **299**
James E. Marks, M.D.

CHAPTER **18**
Chemotherapy of Brain Tumors **321**
Stuart A. Grossman, M.D.

CHAPTER **19**
Photoradiation Therapy of Brain Tumors **341**
Robert E Wharen, Jr., M.D., Robert E. Anderson, B.S., and
Edward R. Laws, Jr., M.D.

CHAPTER **20**
Hyperthermia **359**
Michael Salcman, M.D.

Index **375**

PART I

Epidemiology and Classification

CHAPTER 1

Epidemiology of Primary Intracranial Neoplasms: Disease Distribution and Risk Factors

BRUCE S. SCHOENBERG,[a] M.D., M.S., DR.P.H., F.A.C.P.

GENERAL CONSIDERATIONS

Despite the fact that neuroepidemiology is a relatively new field, contributions to clinical neurology have already been many. Neuroepidemiologic research requires neither expensive nor sophisticated equipment, and the basic skills to implement investigations successfully (i.e., knowledge of clinical neurology and the methods of epidemiology) are present worldwide. Neuroepidemiology may be defined as the study of the distribution and dynamics of neurologic diseases in human populations and the factors that affect those characteristics (120). Whereas the clinician is concerned with disease in the individual patient, the neuroepidemiologist is concerned with the occurrence of neurologic disease in the entire community. Studies of the distribution of disease involve identifying the particular segments of the population affected. For example, does the disease occur more often in men or in a particular age group? Investigations of the dynamics of disease address the question of whether the disease is changing over time. Is it increasing or decreasing? Are the clinical manifestations changing?

The patterns of disease in the community, as derived from descriptive epidemiologic studies, provide important information for formulating etiologic hypotheses. Thus, if the incidence of a given disease has remained stable over several decades, one must search for a cause that has been present in the environment of the community for a considerable period of time.

The two most important considerations for the neuroepidemiologist in the design of studies are the representativeness of the population selected for investigation and the accuracy of the diagnoses in that population.

On the basis of their experience, clinicians review patients' signs and symptoms, establish a diagnosis and a prognosis, and institute appropriate forms of therapy. But how representative is the physician's personal experience? This is a critical concern for the epidemiologist. Certain physicians practicing in the community may specialize in brain tumors, whereas other clinicians in the same community may rarely treat patients with this problem. Because of a lack of financial resources and limited access to neurologic expertise, some individuals with the disease of interest may never seek medical care or may never be correctly diagnosed. The situation is analogous to blindfolded men examining different parts of an elephant, with each coming to an entirely different conclusion as to the characteristics of the beast. To avoid this problem, the neuroepidemiologist attempts to identify all cases of a particular neurologic disease in a well-defined population. In

[a]Deceased.

drawing conclusions from investigating disease occurrence in a population, one must know the characteristics of that population. One might arrive at very different conclusions by examining residents of a retirement community, as contrasted with inhabitants of a military base. One must therefore be certain that the community which has been studied is *representative* of the larger population to which one wishes to generalize the results.

Of equal importance is the problem of diagnostic accuracy. The results of the most sophisticated analysis are no better than the quality of the original data. The greater the accuracy and completeness of the physician's data, the greater the validity of the epidemiologic information concerning the spectrum of disease in the community under investigation. If residents of a community have little or no access to physicians with neurologic expertise, then it may be necessary to have a neurologist review all suspected cases. In comparing the results of several different studies, it is important to consider the criteria for making a diagnosis. Some investigations simply accept the diagnosis made by a physician, while other surveys set up strict criteria.

The magnitude of the disease burden in the community is usually expressed in terms of the population at risk. To say how many people had or died of a particular disease has little meaning unless one also states how many people were at risk of having or dying from that specific disease. To adjust for this, the epidemiologist usually expresses disease magnitude as a rate or ratio, in which the frequency of disease (numerator) is related to the population at risk of having disease (denominator). The magnitude of the disease burden in the population is usually defined in terms of certain epidemiologic indices, such as mortality, prevalence, and incidence. These are briefly defined in Table 1.1.

Epidemiologic studies of primary intracranial neoplasms pose some special problems. One must first decide which specific disease entities are to be included in the investigation. For central nervous system (CNS) neoplasms, different investigators have used a variety of terms to refer to the same tumor type. This has resulted in confusing and overlapping systems of nomenclature. This report will follow the classification scheme outlined in Table 1.2. It is adapted from the suggestions of Kernohan and Sayre (65) and Rubinstein (111) and is derived from the presumed cell type of origin of the tumor. Because of structural proximity, tumors of the pituitary gland and craniopharyngeal duct are included in the consideration of CNS neoplasms. The optic nerve and retina have their origin in the primary cerebral vesicle; therefore tumors of these sites are also discussed. The term "astrocytoma" will be used to designate Grade 1 and 2 gliomas of the astrocytic series, while the term "glioblastoma" designates Grade 3 and 4 gliomas of this series.

Unlike tumors of other sites, the clinical pattern of CNS neoplasms may not correlate with the histologic malignancy. For example, the same histologic tumor type can produce very different symptoms, depending on its anatomic location. A histologically benign, slow-growing tumor may produce devastating effects in a relatively short time because of its critical location,

TABLE 1.1.
Common Epidemiologic Indices[a]

Mortality measures the frequency of deaths within a specific population and is calculated for a given time interval and given place. It is often expressed as a death rate: deaths from a given disease per 100,000 persons at risk of dying of the disease per year.

Prevalence[b] measures the frequency of all current cases of disease within a specific population and is calculated for a given time and given place. It is usually expressed as a prevalence ratio: the number of persons with a given disease at a specified time per 100,000 persons capable of having the disease at the same specified time.

Incidence[b] measures the rapidity with which a disease occurs or the frequency of addition of new cases of a disease within a specific population. It is calculated for a given time interval and given place and is often expressed as an incidence rate: the number of new cases of a given disease during a specified period (usually 1 year) per 100,000 persons at risk of having the disease for the first time per year.

[a]Reprinted with permission from B.S. Schoenberg. Neurologic disease in the elderly: epidemiologic considerations. Semin. Neurol., *1*:5–12, 1981.

[b]Prevalence and incidence are related to each other as follows: prevalence approximately equals incidence multiplied by the average duration of the disease.

TABLE 1.2.
Classification of Central Nervous System Neoplasms[a]

Tumors of neuroglial origin (gliomas)
- Astrocytic series
  - Astrocytoma (grades 1 and 2)
  - Glioblastoma (grades 3 and 4)
- Oligodendroglioma
- Ependymoma

Tumors of neuronal cells and primitive bipotential precursors
- Medulloblastoma
- Ganglioneuroma
- Ganglioglioma
- Neuroblastoma

Tumors of mesodermal tissues
- Meningioma
- Sarcoma

Tumors of nerve roots (neurilemoma is used here as a general term to refer to nerve sheath tumors)
- Neurofibroma
- Schwannoma

Tumors of lymphoreticular system
- Reticulum cell sarcoma—microglioma

Tumors of blood vessel origin
- Hemangioblastoma

Tumors of pituitary gland
- Chromophobe adenoma
- Acidophilic adenoma
- Basophilic adenoma

Tumors of choroid plexus
- Choroid plexus papilloma

Tumors of pineal region
- Germ cell origin
  - Germinoma (pinealoma)

Tumors of pineal parenchyma
- Pineocytoma
- Pineoblastoma

Tumors of maldevelopmental origin
- Teratoma
- Craniopharyngioma

[a]Reprinted with permission from B.S. Schoenberg. Multiple primary neoplasms and the nervous system. Cancer, *40*:1961–1967, 1977.

while a histologically malignant CNS tumor may not produce any overt clinical manifestations for several months. Because of this difficulty, the terms "benign" and "malignant" do not have the same connotation for CNS neoplasms as they do for tumors elsewhere in the body. Hence, these terms are generally not used in epidemiologic investigations of CNS neoplasms.

Tumors of the CNS rarely metastasize to extracranial or extraspinal sites, although seeding within the CNS can often occur. The brain, however, is a common site for the metastatic lesions of malignancies arising elsewhere in the body. Bronchogenic carcinoma in men and breast cancer in women are the two most common origins of cerebral metastases (109, 111). Other tumor types that often metastasize to the brain include malignant melanoma and carcinoma of the kidney and gastrointestinal tract (36, 111). Metastatic tumors involving the skull and spine can cause neurologic symptoms by affecting underlying CNS tissue. Primary cancers of the breast, prostate, thyroid, kidney, and lung may metastasize to the cranium and vertebrae (37). Malignant tumors of the nasal sinuses or nasopharynx may spread intracranially by direct extension. Because of the frequent occurrence of metastatic lesions of the CNS, it is essential to microscopically examine an intracranial mass in a patient with a known primary malignancy outside the nervous system. Although not a problem in developed countries, one must use caution in many parts of the world in distinguishing neoplasms from intracranial masses due to tuberculosis or parasitic disease.

In deciding whether a particular patient is to be included as a case in an epidemiologic investigation of primary brain tumors, it is necessary to consider three levels of diagnosis. The first level involves a decision of whether an intracranial mass is present. The introduction of new neuroimaging techniques (e.g., computerized tomography and magnetic resonance imaging) have greatly improved the accuracy of diagnosing an intracranial mass. The second level involves determining whether the mass represents a primary neoplasm, a metastatic lesion, or is the result of some other disease process. Modern imaging procedures may provide additional clues to aid in this determination. Hence, the availability of these procedures may affect the level of case ascertainment and the ability to detect such lesions at an earlier time. The third level of diagnosis involves the delineation of the specific histologic type of an identified primary intracranial neoplasm. Diagnostic certainty must rely on the histologic examination of tissue or cells, however. One must exercise some degree of caution in this regard since different parts of the tumor may present somewhat different histologic pictures. Despite these many problems, epidemiologic investigations of primary intracranial neoplasms have been extremely valuable. With descriptive epidemiologic studies, the magnitude and distribution of neurologic disease can be documented, and misconceptions concerning disease frequency can be corrected. The patterns of disease in the community suggest etiologic hypotheses. These can be formally tested using the approaches of analytic epidemiology.

The remainder of this chapter describes the application of these techniques to our understanding of the patterns of primary intracranial neoplasms in different populations and the identification of factors associated with an increased risk of developing such tumors.

DESCRIPTIVE STUDIES: DISEASE MAGNITUDE AND DISTRIBUTION

Mortality Data

Mortality tabulations have a number of advantages. Many countries have routine systems for collecting such information in a centralized registry. Furthermore, such procedures have been in effect for many years. Thus, with mortality data, there is readily available information for many countries covering large populations over a long period of time (121). Despite these advantages, there are a number of important problems in using mortality tabulations. Most readers are familiar with the rather haphazard way in which the death certificate is often filled out. Furthermore, not all cases of brain tumor die of their disease and in mortality statistics there is a disproportionate representation of types of tumors with high case fatality ratios. Thus, glioblastoma accounts for a higher proportion of all fatal primary brain tumors than does meningioma. Another difficulty is that routine mortality statistics take into account only the *single, underlying* cause of death, even when other diseases are present and contribute to the patient's demise. Even if a primary brain tumor is listed on the death certificate, some other condition may be specified as the *single, underlying* cause of death. In fact, if we tabulate the number of times "benign brain tumor" appears anywhere on U.S. death certificates and compare it to the number of times it is listed as the *underlying* cause of death, the former figure is nearly 1.5 times greater than the latter figure (20). This is less of a problem with "malignant brain tumor"; this diagnosis is listed as the underlying cause of death for nearly all death certificates on which it appears (20). A further difficulty is the accuracy of the diagnoses appearing on the death certificate. This document may not be filled out by a physician. Even if a doctor has this responsibility, problems can arise. For example, a physician not previously involved in the care of a patient may be called on to pronounce that person dead. Lacking adequate medical records, he may get the required information from relatives and use these unconfirmed data in filling out the certificate.

Despite these deficiencies, interesting patterns emerge when analyzing data from the U.S. or from around the world. Bahemuka et al. (8) calculated average annual mortality rates (age-adjusted to the 1950 U.S. population) for primary nervous system neoplasms using data from 1967 through 1973 for 30 countries. Rates ranged from 4.2/100,000/year (for Chile) to 10.0/100,000/year (for the Federal Republic of Germany). Australia, New Zealand, and nations in Western Europe and North America had age-adjusted mortality rates between 6–8/100,000/year. Rates were generally higher for males. Compared to data available for 1951–1958 (45), most countries showed an increase in the death rates over time. This increase was thought to be the result of improvement in the diagnosis of these tumors, particularly among the elderly (8).

When U.S. primary nervous system neoplasm mortality rates for the years 1971 and 1972–1978 were analyzed, the age-specific curve was found to rise to a maximum in the 7th or 8th decade of life and then decline. The overall age-adjusted mortality rates were higher for males and for whites (20). Bharucha et al. (12) examined the trends in mortality from primary malignant nervous system neoplasms from 1940 through 1975 for U.S. whites. The results demonstrated a marked cohort effect among the elderly of either sex. For example, among white men aged 60 through 64 years, mortality rates increased steadily from 5.3/100,000/year for those born in 1880 to 16.1/100,000/year for the 1910 birth cohort. No definite cohort effect was observed in the young. The increase in mortality rates could be due to better diagnosis and more complete case ascertainment for deaths due to primary malignant nervous system neoplasms. The authors suggested, however, that additional studies are required to distinguish a real from an artifactual increase in mortality rates (12).

Morbidity Data

Despite the ready availability of mortality tabulations, their associated deficiencies as outlined earlier have prompted a number of investigations aimed at defining the morbidity of this group of diseases. Such data are much more difficult to obtain since most countries do not have established systems for collecting this information. Because of different procedures that are used to acquire such data, results must be compared with caution.

Some investigators have attempted to study a large number of patients coming to medical attention at particular medical institutions. However, these studies cannot precisely identify a population at risk; hence, it is not possible to calculate rates. Furthermore, patients coming to a particular medical institution may not be representative of all cases of the disease in the community. It is possible to minimize such bias by including only those cases derived from a well-defined population and being certain to obtain data from all medical facilities serving that population. This has been the strategy of special tumor registries. In other instances, special case-finding surveys have been carried out. These approaches have yielded more accurate measures of morbidity (9, 14, 17, 23, 25, 26, 34, 48, 49, 71, 75, 78, 100, 118, 128, 142). Even for population-based investigations there are differences that must be taken into account before making comparisons. For example, some registries include only CNS tumors specified as "malignant," while others restrict themselves to tumors of the brain (excluding other CNS sites).

Incidence data for primary nervous system neoplasms for 62 distinct population groups internationally were evaluated for various years between 1956 and 1967 (118). In general, males had higher rates than females. The median incidence rate (age-adjusted to the 1950 U.S. population) was between 4 and 5 cases/100,000/year. These figures probably underestimate the true rates, however. In addition, most data resources indicate the same age-specific pattern of incidence rates: a small peak in childhood, followed by a higher peak that reaches a maximum between ages 60 and 80 and then declines for the most elderly segment of the population.

Schoenberg et al. (126) analyzed Connecticut Tumor Registry data for primary intracranial neoplasms. This Connecticut resource serves as a model of large population-based tumor registries. A total of 3210 primary intracranial neoplasms diagnosed between 1935 and 1964 among Connecticut residents formed the basis for this investigation. Slightly more than three-fourths of the tumors were microscopically confirmed. Only those neoplasms with such confirmation were classified by histologic type. The most common tumor was glioblastoma, followed, in order, by meningioma and astrocytoma. Meningioma is the only relatively common primary intracranial neoplasm with a higher incidence rate among females.

The relative frequency of these various tumor types differs markedly in children compared to adults (127) (Table 1.3). Medulloblastoma is the most frequent tumor type in children, accounting for 24% of the histologically confirmed tumors, followed by astrocytoma (21%) and glioblastoma (20%). In contrast, glioblastoma accounts for more than half of the histologically confirmed tumors in adults. Meningioma and chromophobe adenoma, while common among adults, are rare in children.

In examining the age-specific incidence curves for the most common tumor types, each exhibits a distinctive pattern. Age-specific incidence rates for glioblastoma show a small childhood peak and a higher

TABLE 1.3.
Histologically Confirmed Primary Intracranial Neoplasms: Frequency Distribution, Connecticut, 1935–1964[a]

Children (0–14 years)			Adults (≥15 years)		
Type	No.	%	Type	No.	%
Medulloblastoma	74	24.2	Glioblastoma	1105	52.1
Astrocytoma	63	20.6	Meningioma	389	18.4
Glioblastoma	62	20.3	Astrocytoma	214	10.1
Ependymoma	20	6.5	Chromophobe adenoma	96	4.5
Craniopharyngioma	17	5.6	Neurilemoma	46	2.2
Meningioma	14	4.6	Hemangioma	41	1.9
Hemangioma	9	2.9	Craniopharyngioma	30	1.4
Neuroblastoma	8	2.6	Medulloblastoma	27	1.3
Teratoma	6	2.0	Ependymoma	27	1.3
Pinealoma	6	2.0	Acidophilic adenoma	26	1.2
Sarcoma	5	1.6	Oligodendroglioma	22	1.0
Oligodendroglioma	2	0.7	Sarcoma	19	0.9
Neurilemoma	2	0.7	Pinealoma	6	0.3
Others, specified	11	3.6	Others, specified	26	1.2
Others, unspecified	7	2.3	Others, unspecified	45	2.1
Total	306	100.2	Total	2119	99.9

[a]Reprinted with permission from B.S. Schoenberg, B.W. Christine, and J.P. Whisnant. The descriptive epidemiology of primary intracranial neoplasms—the Connecticut experience. Am. J. Epidemiol., *104:*499–510, 1976.

adult peak, similar to the pattern for all brain tumors analyzed together. The curve for astrocytoma also reveals a small peak among the young, but has a much smaller and flatter rise for the older age groups. The curve for meningioma shows, despite some fluctuations, a general increase in incidence rates with increasing age (126).

One notable exception to the age-specific incidence curve for all brain tumors analyzed together is provided by tabulations for Rochester, MN. With the unique circumstances that exist for residents of Rochester, it is possible to obtain accurate statistics by applying defined diagnostic criteria to information available in medical records. By means of a records-linkage system, data concerning all medical contacts (ie., outpatient records, inpatient records, physician house calls, emergency room visits, etc.) are kept together in a single, computerized file (73, 74). Furthermore, the population has easy access to expertise in neurologic diagnosis, and this access is not generally limited because of a lack of financial resources. Finally, the medical records contain sufficient details concerning the findings of the medical history, the physical examination, and the results of laboratory tests to allow retrospective review of the diagnosis.

When analyzed, the Rochester data show a small childhood peak, followed by a sustained rise in incidence rates with increasing age (122). In addition, the rates reported for Rochester are generally higher than those available from other data resources. Finally, the most common intracranial neoplasm among the Rochester population was meningioma, as contrasted with most other investigations, such as that based on Connecticut Tumor Registry data. These discrepancies were resolved by using the same criteria to compare the Rochester figures with those for Connecticut (128).

The relatively large number of cases first diagnosed at autopsy in Rochester (as contrasted with Connecticut) account, in large part, for the different age-specific incidence curves particularly among the elderly. Meningiomas make up most of the tumors first diagnosed at death. The results of comparisons between Rochester and Connecticut suggest that (*a*) a substantial number of asymptomatic tumors are missed among the elderly, and (*b*) as the autopsy rate increases, the age-specific incidence pattern will more closely resemble the Rochester curve (128).

Incidence rates for pituitary tumors taken as a single group increase with age.

The same pattern is true for chromophobe adenoma, the most frequently occurring of the histologically confirmed tumors of the pituitary gland (126). Incidence rates for pituitary tumors are approximately 1 new case/100,000/year (75). With regard to temporal trends, data for Olmsted County, MN indicate an increase in the number of cases of pituitary adenomas diagnosed in women of childbearing age, while there were no such increases for older women or for men of any age (3). The authors of that report explored the possibility of a relationship between the occurrence of these tumors and the use of oral contraceptives, but no association could be demonstrated. They attributed the observed increase to the use of new and improved diagnostic techniques for the detection of pituitary tumors in women of childbearing age who present with complaints of galactorrhea, amenorrhea, or infertility (3).

With regard to primary intraspinal neoplasms, the incidence rate for clinically apparent cases diagnosed before death in Rochester, MN is 0.9/100,000/year; the rate increases to 1.4/100,000/year if cases diagnosed at autopsy are included (115). Primary neoplasms of the peripheral nervous system have a similar incidence rate of about 1.5/100,000/year (78) as do optic nerve gliomas and retinoblastomas (Jordan and Schoenberg, personal communication).

Morbidity studies of the risk of primary intracranial neoplasms by race have been largely based on the analysis of a series of cases not derived from a defined population. Such investigations suggest that meningiomas and pituitary adenomas appear to occur more frequently among blacks than whites (37). This was confirmed in a population-based study of residents of the Washington, DC metropolitan area (55).

PROSPECTIVE STUDIES OF SURVIVAL

In attempting to analyze survival of patients with a primary intracranial neoplasm one must consider a multitude of factors that may influence the outcome. Such factors include the tumor type, tumor grade, tumor size, anatomic location(s) of the neoplasm, the patient's age, the presence of other diseases, the responsiveness of the neoplasm to chemotherapy or radiation, the surgeon's skill, the type of postoperative care, etc. Survival data for patients with brain tumors as well as for patients with tumors of other sites are collected through a special program operated by the National Cancer Institute (35). Data from 1950 through 1973 show a gradual increase in survival for those with a primary brain tumor. Such tabulations remain difficult to interpret, since they may reflect earlier diagnosis, a reduction of surgical mortality, improved methods of treatment, or some other factors.

Data from the Connecticut Tumor Registry reveal marked differences in survival as a function of tumor type. Patients with meningioma or hemangioma have the best outcome, while those with glioblastoma have the worst prognosis. The survival curves for patients with meningioma and hemangioma show a relatively linear decline over time, while those with other forms of primary brain tumor show a relatively rapid decrement within the first few years after diagnosis, followed by a more gradual decline (118).

IDENTIFYING THE PERSON AT HIGH RISK FOR A PRIMARY INTRACRANIAL NEOPLASM

Genetic Factors

No genetic factor has been shown to increase the risk of primary nervous system tumors taken as a single group. There is a known familial occurrence of bilateral retinoblastoma or chemodectoma (glomus tumors) with an autosomal dominant pattern of inheritance (72, 75, 118). However, such tumors account for only a small percentage of all primary nervous system neoplasms. With regard to more commonly occurring tumors, there are rare reports of glioma occurring in multiple members of the same family (118, 124). Some authors believe that a genetic factor may be involved in the occurrence of gliomas (6, 69, 84, 85, 140), while others have reported no evidence for such a factor (51, 52). Similarly for meningioma and medulloblastoma, although there have been isolated case reports of familial occurrence, no firm evidence for a genetic pattern has been reported (40, 64, 105, 107, 113).

Phakomatoses are associated with primary nervous system neoplasms. For example, glioblastoma (62), ependymoma (96), and ganglioneuroma (32) are seen in patients with tuberous sclerosis (119). The astrocytic tumors (the most common intracranial neoplasms seen in these patients) are thought to arise from foci of subependymal astrocytes that characterize tuberous sclerosis (111). Despite the well-documented relationship between tuberous sclerosis and primary intracranial neoplasms, such tumors are relatively rare when large series of tuberous sclerosis patients are evaluated (111).

Three distinct forms of von Recklinghausen's neurofibromatosis have been identified: a peripheral type, a central type, and a visceral type (111). The peripheral type is characterized by multiple peripheral nerve sheath tumors and cafe-au-lait skin pigmentation. The central form consists of multiple tumors of the cranial and spinal nerve roots. These tumors are usually schwannomas; they most commonly involve the eighth cranial nerve and are often bilateral (42, 89). Astrocytic gliomas (including those involving the optic nerve and retina) (32, 114) and multiple meningiomas and ependymomas (111) have been reported in this condition. Multiple primary neoplasms of the CNS (110), as well as syringomyelia (102, 110), have also been described in central neurofibromatosis.

Ganglioneuromas and nerve sheath tumors involving viscera and the autonomic nervous system and visceral neoplasms of neural crest origin are seen in the visceral type of von Recklinghausen's disease (111).

Those with von Hippel-Lindau disease have hemangioblastomas (often multiple and most commonly involving the cerebellum) of the CNS as well as angiomatosis of the retina (111). Occurrences of pheochromocytoma (21, 95), ependymoma (39), syringomyelia (102), and erythrocythemia (141) have all been documented in this condition.

Diffuse meningeal proliferation of melanocytes and large cutaneous nevi are the distinguishing features of neurocutaneous melanosis (58, 111, 134). Multiple neurofibromas of the peripheral nervous system are also observed in patients with this syndrome.

Besides the phakomatoses, there are several other genetically determined syndromes that are associated with primary nervous system neoplasms. These conditions are outlined in Table 1.4; more specific details concerning these syndromes have been reviewed by Schoenberg (119). Brain tumors have also been described in patients with ataxia-telangiectasia or in their family members (50, 66, 92).

Multicentric Primary Nervous System Neoplasms

The multifocal occurrence of primary nervous system tumors may alert the clinician to the presence of an hereditary syndrome or the presence of one of the phakomatoses. Among those nervous system tumors that have been reported to occur multicentrically are chemodectoma (2), ependymoma (112), ganglioneuroma (81, 135), glioblastoma (10, 16, 29, 88, 116), hemangioblastoma (105, 112), meningioma (91), neuroblastoma (112), neurofibroma (111), optic nerve glioma (31), pheochromocytoma (19, 30, 112, 137), retinoblastoma (2, 141), schwannoma (42, 89), and teratoma (59, 112). In addition different primary nervous system tumors occasionally occur together in the same individual. For example, ganglioneuroma may occur with neuroblastoma or pheochromocytoma (112), or meningioma has been described together with glioma in the same patient (1, 38, 67).

Analytic Studies: Documentation of Risk Factors

On the basis of descriptive studies of the distribution of primary intracranial neoplasms, it is possible to formulate hypotheses concerning causation. Such hypotheses can be formally tested using the techniques of analytic epidemiology, which is primarily aimed at identifying factors that are as-

TABLE 1.4.
Multiple Primary Tumors and Genetic Syndromes: Index Primary Neoplasms of the Nervous System

Condition	Nervous System Neoplasm	Nonnervous System Neoplasm	Author and Year
Wermer's syndrome (multiple endocrine adenomatosis I)	Anterior pituitary	Parathyroid; pancreatic islet cells; thyroid; adrenal cortex; carcinoid tumor (intestine, bronchus)	(Johnson *et al.*, 1967)
Sipple's syndrome (multiple endocrine adenomatosis II)	Pheochromocytoma; neurofibroma (multiple); submucosal neuromas	Medullary thyroid carcinoma; parathyroid neoplasm	(Schimke *et al.*, 1968; Mulvihill, 1975)
Turcot's syndrome	Brain tumor	Polyposis coli	(Turcot *et al.*, 1959; Baughman *et al.*, 1969)
Nevoid basal cell carcinoma syndrome	Medulloblastoma	Basal cell carcinomas; ovarian tumor	(Stout, 1947; Wiskemann, 1963; Meerkotter & Shear, 1964; Gorlin *et al.*, 1965; Hermans *et al.*, 1965; Graham *et al.*, 1968; Jackson and Gardere, 1971; Neblett *et al.*, 1971; Moynahan, 1973; Strong, 1977)
Cowden's disease (multiple hamartoma syndrome)	Meningioma	Lip and mouth papillomas; breast cancer; thyroid adenoma and carcinoma; lipoma; polyps; bone and liver cysts	(Mulvihill, 1975)

Reprinted with permission from B.S. Schoenberg. Multiple primary neoplasms and the nervous system. Cancer, *40:*1961–1967, 1977.

sociated with either a high or low risk of disease. The study of the occurrence of natural experiments is the domain of this area of epidemiology. During the course of our lives, different individuals are exposed to a variety of different factors or conditions, some of which may play an important role in the occurrence of disease. There are two general approaches to this type of study: case-control and prospective.

With a case-control investigation, one begins with a group of individuals who have the disease of interest (cases) and a group of individuals without the disease (controls). One then explores the present characteristics (in a cross-sectional study) or the history (in a retrospective study) of these two groups for the presence or absence of factors thought to be related to the occurrence of the disease. Obviously, one looks for factors that are distributed differentially among the cases as compared to the controls. In order to evaluate a possible association between a particular disease and a particular attribute, it is always necessary to have a control group against which to compare this association.

With the prospective approach, we begin with a group or cohort exposed to a particular factor(s) and a group not exposed to the specific factor(s). The two groups are observed over time to see how many in each group develop the disease under investigation. The frequency of disease in the cohort exposed to the factor is compared to the frequency in the unexposed cohort.

Since case-control investigations provide information relatively quickly and at much lower cost than the prospective approach, most analytic investigations of primary nervous system neoplasms have used the case-control design. In analyzing the results of analytic epidemiologic studies, we must always consider whether the results are artifactual (i.e., due to differences between the groups other than the factor(s) being studied) and whether the findings are statistically significant (i.e., the possibility that the findings occurred simply on the basis of chance). It is also important to remember that an association should *not* be equated with the cause of the disease. A particular characteristic may be only indirectly related to a biologically significant factor. However, there are a number of features of epidemiologic associations that suggest causal inferences. For example, one must decide whether the disease appears to follow exposure to a given agent after an appropriate period of time consistent with current knowledge concerning the latency of the agent's known effects. One must also consider the strength of the association and whether exposure to the given agent appears to lead to the specific neurologic disease of interest. If the link between a given factor and a specific disease is consistent with available knowledge of pathogenesis (i.e., there is a plausible biologic explanation as to how the factor can cause the disease), the possible etiologic role of the factor is more likely. Finally, one must examine the results of multiple studies to verify the consistency of a reported association. These principles have been applied in several analytic investigations of primary nervous system neoplasms.

Factors for possible study in analytic epidemiologic investigations have often been suggested by the results of laboratory investigations. For example, a variety of primary intracranial neoplasms can arise after the innoculation of viruses into animals. Tumor induction depends on several factors such as the host animals, the age of the animal, the site of innoculation, the particular virus, etc. Furthermore, there have been intriguing reports of "virus-like particles" observed on electron microscopic examination of human nervous system neoplasms (13). Similarly, in the area of chemical carcinogenesis it has been possible to induce brain tumors in animals following the intracranial or the systemic administration of a number of compounds (70).

In studies attempting to demonstrate the importance of a putative risk factor, one important methodologic problem has been that all brain tumors are often treated together as a single group. This is contrary to the evidence of descriptive epidemiologic data suggesting that each histologic type of primary nervous system neoplasm is a separate disease entity, with a specific incidence and survival pattern. Under these circumstances risk factors associated with specific tumor types could be obscured in studies that consider all brain tumors as a single disease.

There have been several investigations relating head trauma to the subsequent occurrence of brain tumors. Case reports have appeared that describe brain tumors, particularly meningiomas, arising at sites of previous trauma resulting from injuries or surgical procedures (108, 138). Others have found no such association (98). A case-control study of risk factors for meningiomas among women demonstrated a statistically significant relationship with head injury (103, 104). Similar positive results for head trauma were reported in a case-control study of glioblastoma (56, 57). Not all formal analytic investigations of the relationship between head trauma and brain tumors have been positive, however. An early case-control study of putative risk factors for all brain tumors taken as a single group found no association with head trauma (22). Using a prospective type of study design, Annegers et al. (4, 5) evaluated the subsequent brain tumor experience of Rochester, MN, residents who had suffered an episode of head trauma. There was no significant excess of observed brain tumors as compared to expectations. A population-based case-control study of neuroepithelial tumors was similarly negative with regard to head trauma (27, 28).

Investigations of the role of prenatal x-ray exposure as a putative risk factor for subsequent brain tumor occurrence have yielded conflicting results (22, 82). Several studies of the effects of scalp radiation in children as a treatment of tinea capitis have produced positive results (87, 133). Another investigation demonstrated a relationship between meningioma in women and medical or dental x-rays (103, 104).

Studies attempting to link smoking or alcohol consumption with brain tumors have been negative (22, 103). In an anecdotal report of urinary lead levels among a group of institutionalized children, two of the three with elevated levels subsequently developed astrocytic gliomas (129). Although there was no control group against which to compare this observation, the association with lead has some support from laboratory findings. Rats fed relatively large quantities of lead subacetate subsequently developed gliomas (97).

One case-control study focused on possible risk factors for primary brain tumors in children. Findings which attained statistical significance included living on a farm, a history of exposure to farm animals, and the patient's prior use of barbiturates (43, 44). Unfortunately, it was not possible to exclude with certainty whether some of the barbiturate use reflected treatment of seizure activity resulting from a brain tumor that had not yet been clinically detected. Other findings were suggestive of a heightened risk and appeared to the authors to have potential biological significance but did not reach statistical significance because of the relatively small number of subjects (44). Exposure to either insecticides or to sick pets fell into this equivocal category.

There have also been studies of the brain tumor experience of workers in particular industries or their relatives (15, 93, 101, 131). For example, some have reported that those involved in the manufacture and processing of rubber are at increased risk for brain tumors (76, 79). These findings require further confirmation and a more precise determination of the factors responsible for any increased risk. In another study, Waxweiler et al. (143) observed an excess of glioblastoma multiforme in workers exposed to vinyl chloride. Although a Texas petrochemical plant was found to have an elevated standardized mortality ratio for brain neoplasms, a case-control study was unable to document a specific exposure associated with an elevated risk of brain tumors, and no significant differences in duration of exposure to any of the suspected chemicals could be demonstrated between cases and controls (77).

Studies of a variety of possible risk factors have yielded equivocal results, including birth order (22, 44), ABO blood groups (18, 41, 44, 80, 132, 145), diabetes mellitus (7, 99), or epilepsy (25, 28, 57). Renal transplant patients receiving immunosuppressive therapy have an increased risk of reticulum cell sarcoma of the brain, an otherwise relatively uncommon tumor (94).

Analyses of the association between primary CNS neoplasms and primary tumors of other sites have been negative, with two exceptions: (*a*) the association between meningioma and breast cancer (125) and (*b*) the relationship between retinoblastoma and osteosarcoma (61, 68). Although not confirmed by a second study (104), the association between meningioma and breast cancer suggests etiologic possibilities when considered with other evidence. First, meningioma is the only common primary intracranial neoplasm with a higher incidence in women (126). Second, the abrupt clinical appearance or enlargement of this tumor during pregnancy has been described (86). A possible hormonal link between these two tumors is further supported by the finding of estrogen receptor protein in intracranial meningiomas (33).

Positive results have been reported for some other factors but await confirmation from other investigations. For example, toxoplasmosis was found to be linked to brain tumors in one study (130). In addition, there have been several reports of astrocytomas in multiple sclerosis plaques (106), but this relationship has not yet been documented in well-controlled investigations.

Future studies must address the issue of selective recall bias, in which family members of cases are more motivated to search for possible past exposures than family members of healthy controls. Furthermore, families of cases are more familiar with neurologic terms and symptoms and are more likely to recognize similar disorders in other family members. Strategies are being developed to address these methodologic problems. In the meantime, the recognition of persons at high risk for the development of a primary intracranial neoplasm remains an important goal. Detailed evaluation of such individuals will hopefully lead to a better understanding of the mechanisms involved in oncogenesis within the nervous system.

REFERENCES

1. Alexander, W.S. Multiple primary intracranial tumours—meningioma associated with a glioma—report of a case. J. Neuropathol. Exp. Neurol., *7:*81–88, 1948.
2. Anderson, D.E. Familial susceptibility. In: *Persons at High Risk of Cancer: An Approach to Cancer Etiology and Control,* edited by J.F. Fraumeni Jr, pp. 39–55. New York, Academic Press, 1975.
3. Annegers, J.F., Coulam, C.B., Abboud, C.F., *et al.* Pituitary adenoma in Olmsted County, Minnesota, 1935–1977: a report of an increasing incidence of diagnosis in women of childbearing age. Mayo Clin. Proc., *53:*641–643, 1978.
4. Annegers, J.F., Kurland, L.T., Grabow, J.D., *et al.* Abstract: the incidence of head trauma and subsequent risk of seizures and brain tumors. Neurology, *29:*578, 1979.
5. Annegers, J.F. and Kurland, L.T. Head trauma and sequelae in the Olmsted County, Minnesota, population. In: *Clinical Neuro-Epidemiology,* edited by F.C. Rose, pp. 361–365. Tunbridge, England, Pitman, 1980.
6. Armstrong, R.M. and Hanson, C.W. Familial gliomas. Neurology, *19:*1061–1063, 1969.
7. Aronson, S.M. and Aronson, B.E. Central nervous system in diabetes mellitus: lowered frequency of certain intracranial neoplasms. Arch. Neurol., *12:*390–398, 1965.
8. Bahemuka, M., Massey, E.W., and Schoenberg, B.S. International mortality from primary nervous system neoplasms: distribution and trends. Neuroepidemiology, *2:*196–205, 1983.
9. Barker, D.J.P., Weller, R.O., and Garfield, J.S. Epidemiology of primary tumours of the brain and spinal cord: a regional survey of southern England. J. Neurol. Neurosurg. Psychiatry, *39:*290–296, 1976.
10. Batzdorff, U. and Malamud, N. The problem of multicentric gliomas. J. Neurosurg., *20:*122–136, 1963.
11. Baughman, F.A. Jr, List, C.F., Williams, J.R., *et al.* The glioma—polyposis syndrome. N. Engl. J. Med., *281:*1345–1346, 1969.
12. Bharucha, N.E., Raven, R.H., and Schoenberg, B.S. Primary malignant nervous system neoplasms: birth cohort effect in the elderly. Arch. Neurol, *42:*1061–1062, 1985.
13. Bigner, D.D. Role of viruses in the causation of neural neoplasia. In: *Biology of Brain Tumors,* edited by O.D. Laerum, D.D. Bigner, and M.F. Rajewsky, pp. 85–111. Geneva, International Union Against Cancer, 1978.
14. Biometry Branch, National Cancer Institute. Third National Cancer Survey: Incidence Data. National Cancer Institute Monograph 41, DHEW Publication No. (NIH) 75–787, pp. 17, 21, 25. Bethesda, MD., National Cancer Institute, 1975.
15. Blair, A. and Hayes, H.M. Jr. Mortality patterns among US veterinarians, 1947–1977: an expanded study. Int. J. Epidemiol., *11:*391–397, 1982.
16. Borovich, B., Mayer, M., Gellei B., *et al.* Multifocal glioma of the brain: case report. J. Neurosurg., *45:*229–232, 1976.
17. Brewis, M., Poskanzer, D.C., Rolland, C., *et al.* Neurological disease in an English city. Acta Neurol. Scand. (Suppl. 24), *42:*21, 23, 41–46, 1966.
18. Buckwalter, J.A., Turner, J.H., Gamber, H.H., *et al.* Psychoses, intracranial neoplasms, and genetics. Arch. Neurol. Psychiatry, *81:*480–485, 1959.
19. Cahill, C.F. Pheochromocytomas. J.A.M.A., *138:*180–186, 1948.
20. Chandra, V., Bharucha, N.E., and Schoenberg, B.S. Mortality data for the U.S. for deaths due to and related to twenty neurologic diseases. Neuroepidemiology, *3:*149–168, 1984.
21. Chapman, R.C. and Diaz-Perez, R. Pheochromocytoma associated with cerebellar hemangioblastoma: familial occurrence. J.A.M.A., *182:*1014–1017, 1962.
22. Choi, N.W., Schuman, L.M., and Gullen, W.H. Epidemiology of primary central nervous system neoplasms. II. Case-control study. Am. J. Epidemiol., *91:*467–485, 1970.
23. Clemmesen, J. Statistical studies in the aetiology of malignant neoplasms. I. Review and results. Acta Pathol. Microbiol. Scand. (Suppl. 174), Part 1:422–424, 538–539, 542–543, 1965a.
24. Clemmesen, J. Statistical studies in the aetiology of malignant neoplasms. II. Basic tables: Denmark, 1943–1957. Acta Microbiol. Scand. (Suppl. 174), Part II:3, 8–9, 28–29, 68–69, 122–123, 194–195, 226–227, 252–253, 294–295, 308–309, 1965b.
25. Clemmesen, J. Statistical studies in the aetiology of malignant neoplasms. III. Testis cancer: basic tables, Denmark, 1958–1962. Acta Pathol. Microbiol. Scand. (Suppl. 209): lxv, 3, 14–15, 36–39, 44–47, 58–59, 91–92, 130–133, 142–143, 1969.
26. Cohen, A. and Modan, B. Some epidemiologic aspects of neoplastic diseases in Israeli immigrant population. III. Brain tumors. Cancer, *22:*1323–1328, 1968.
27. Codd, M.B. and Kurland, L.T. Head trauma

and seizures as risk factors in tumors of the glioma group. Neurology, *35:*1532–1533, 1985.
28. Codd, M.B., Kurland, L.T., O'Fallon, W.M., *et al.* Case-control study of neuroepithelial tumors in Rochester, MN, 1950–1970. Neuroepidemiology, in press, 1987.
29. Courville, C.B. Multiple primary tumors of the brain (review of the literature and report of 21 cases). Am. J. Cancer, *26:*703–731, 1936.
30. Cragg, R.W. Concurrent tumors of the left carotid body and both Zuckerkandl bodies. Arch. Pathol., *18:*635–645, 1934.
31. Davis, F.A. Primary tumors of the optic nerve (a phenomenon of Recklinghausen's disease)—a clinical and pathological study with a report of five cases and a review of the literature. Arch. Ophthalmol., *23:*735–827, 957–1022, 1940.
32. Davis, R.L. and Nelson, E. Unilateral ganglioglioma in a tuberosclerotic brain. J. Neuropathol. Exp. Neurol., *20:*571–581, 1961.
33. Donnell, M.S., Meyer, G.A., and Donegan, W.L. Estrogen-receptor protein in intracranial meningiomas. J. Neurosurg., *50:*499–502, 1979.
34. Dorn, H.F. and Cutler, S.J. Morbidity from Cancer in the United States. U.S. Dept. of Public Health Monograph No. 29. Washington, D.C., U.S. Government Printing Office, pp. 7–8, 11–12, 144–145, 151–159, 1955.
35. End Results Section, Biometry Branch, National Cancer Institute. Cancer Patient Survival, report number 5. DHEW Publication No. (NIH) 77–992, pp. 234–240. Bethesda, MD, National Institutes of Health.
36. Escourolle, R. and Poirier, J. *Manual of Basic Neuropathology,* translated by L.J. Rubinstein. Philadelphia, W.B. Saunders, 1973.
37. Fan, K.J., Kovi, J., and Earle, K.M. The ethnic distribution of primary central nervous system tumours: Armed Forces Institute of Pathology, 1958–1970. J. Neuropathol. Exp. Neurol., *36:*41–49, 1977.
38. Feiring, E.H. and Davidoff, L.M. Two tumors, meningioma and glioblastoma multiforme, in one patient. J. Neurosurg., *4:*282–289, 1947.
39. Fraumeni, J.F. Jr. Genetic factors. In: *Cancer Medicine,* edited by J.F. Holland and E. Frei III, pp. 7–15. Philadelphia, Lea & Febiger, 1973.
40. Gaist, G. and Piazza, G. Meningiomas in two members of the same family (with no evidence of neurofibromatosis). J. Neurosurg., *16:*110–113, 1959.
41. Garcia, J.H., Okazaki, H., and Aronson, S.M. Blood group frequencies and astrocytoma. J. Neurosurg., *20:*397–399, 1963.
42. Gardner, W.J. and Turner, O. Bilateral acoustic neurofibromas—further clinical and pathological data on hereditary deafness and Recklinghausen's disease. Arch. Neurol., *44:*76–99, 1940.
43. Gold, E., Gordis, L., Tanascia, J., *et al.* Increased risk of brain tumors in children exposed to barbiturates. J. Natl. Cancer Inst., *61:*1031–1034, 1978.
44. Gold, E., Gordis, L., Tanascia, J., *et al.* Risk factors for brain tumors in children. Am. J. Epidemiol., *109:*309–319, 1979.
45. Goldberg, I.D. and Kurland, L.T. Mortality in 33 countries from diseases of the nervous system. World Neurol., *3:*444–465, 1962.
46. Gorlin, R.J., Vickers, R.A., Kellen, E., *et al.* The multiple basal-cell nevi syndrome. Cancer, *18:*89–104, 1965.
47. Graham, J.K., McJimsey, B.A., and Hardin, J.C. Jr. Nevoid basal cell carcinoma syndrome. Arch. Otolaryngol., *87:*90–95, 1968.
48. Gudmundsson, K.R. A survey of tumours of the central nervous system in Iceland during the 10-year period 1954–1963. Acta Neurol. Scand., *46:*538–552, 1970.
49. Haenszel, W., Marcus, S.C., and Zimmerer, E.G. Cancer Morbidity in Urban and Rural Iowa. U.S. Dept. of Public Health Monograph No. 37, pp. 1–6, 55, 60, 63, 81. Washington, D.C., U.S. Government Printing Office, 1956.
50. Haerer, A.F., Jackson, J.F., and Evers, C.G. Ataxia-telangiectasia with gastric adenocarcinoma. J.A.M.A., *210:*1884–1897, 1969.
51. Harvald, B. and Hauge, M. On the heredity of glioblastoma. J. Natl. Cancer Inst., *17:*289–296, 1956.
52. Hauge, M. and Harvald, B. Genetics in intracranial tumours. Acta Genet., *7:*573–591, 1957.
53. Hermans, E.H., Grosfeld, J.C.M., and Spaas, J.A.J. The fifth phacomatosis. Dermatologica, *130:*446–476, 1965.
54. Herzberg, J.J. and Wiskemann, A. Die funfte phakomatose. Dermatologica, *126:*106–123, 1963.
55. Heshmat, M.Y., Kovi, J., Simpson, C., *et al.* Neoplasms of the central nervous system: incidence and population selectivity in the Washington, D.C. metropolitan area. Cancer, *38:*2135–2142, 1976.
56. Hochberg, F.H., Cole, P., Salcman, M., *et al.* Abstract: risk factors in glioblastoma development. Neurology, *32* (part *2*):A75, 1982.
57. Hochberg, F., Poniolo, P., and Cole, P. Head trauma and seizures as risk factors of glioblastoma. Neurology, *34:*1511–1514, 1984.
58. Hoffman, H.J. and Freeman, A. Primary malignant leptomeningeal melanoma in association with giant hairy nevi: report of two cases. J. Neurosurg., *26:*62–71, 1967.
59. Ingraham, F.D. and Bailey, O.T. Cystic teratomas and teratoid tumors of the central nervous system in infancy and childhood. J. Neurosurg., *3:*511–532, 1946.
60. Jackson, R. and Gardere, S. Nevoid basal cell carcinoma syndrome. Can. Med. Assoc. J., *105:*850–862, 1971.

61. Jensen, R.D. and Miller, R.W. Retinoblastoma—epidemiologic characteristics. N. Engl. J. Med., *285:*307–311, 1971.
62. Jervis, G.A. Spongioneuroblastoma and tuberous sclerosis. J. Neuropathol. Exp. Neurol., *13:*105–116, 1954.
63. Johnson, G.J., Summerskill, W.H.J., Anderson, V.E., *et al.* Clinical and genetic investigation of a large kindred with multiple endocrine adenomatosis. N. Engl. J. Med., *277:*1379–1385, 1967.
64. Joynt, R.J. and Perret, G.E. Meningiomas in a mother and daughter: cases without evidence of neurofibromatosis. Neurology, *11:*164–165, 1961.
65. Kernohan, J.W. and Sayre, G.P. Tumors of the central nervous system. In: *Atlas of Tumor Pathology,* Fascicle 35. Washington, D.C., Armed Forces Institute of Pathology, 1952.
66. Kersey, J.H. and Spector, B.D. Immune deficiency diseases. In: *Persons at High Risk of Cancer: An Approach to Cancer Etiology and Control,* edited by J.F. Fraumeni Jr., pp. 55–67. New York, Academic Press, 1975.
67. Kirschbaum, W.R. Intrasellar meningioma and multiple cerebral glioblastomas. J. Neuropathol. Exp. Neurol., *4:*370–378, 1945.
68. Kitchin, F.D. and Ellsworth, R.M. Pleiotropic effects of the gene for retinoblastoma. J. Med. Genet., *11:*244–246, 1974.
69. Kjellin, K., Muller, R., and Astrom, K.E. The occurrence of brain tumors in several members of a family. J. Neuropathol. Exp. Neurol., *19:*528–537, 1960.
70. Kleihues, P. Chemical carcinogenesis in the nervous system. In: *Biology of Brain Tumors,* edited by O.D. Laerum, D.D. Bigner, and M.F. Rajewsky, pp. 113–128. Geneva, International Union Against Cancer, 1978.
71. Kurland, L.T. The frequency of intracranial and intraspinal neoplasms in the resident population of Rochester, Minnesota. J. Neurosurg., *15:*627–641, 1958.
72. Kurland, L.T., Myrianthopoulos, N.C., and Lessell, S. Epidemiologic and genetic considerations of intracranial neoplasms. In: *The Biology and Treatment of Intracranial Tumors,* edited by W.S. Fields and P.C. Sharkey, pp. 5–47. Springfield, IL, Charles C Thomas, 1962.
73. Kurland, L.T. and Molgaard, C.A. The patient record in epidemiology. Sci. Am., *245:*54–63, 1981.
74. Kurland, L.T., Molgaard, C.A., and Schoenberg, B.S. Mayo Clinic records-linkage: contributions to neuroepidemiology. Neuroepidemiology, *1:*102–114, 1982.
75. Kurtzke, J.F. and Kurland, L.T. The epidemiology of neurologic disease. In: *Clinical Neurology,* edited by A.B. Baker and L.H. Baker, chapter 66, pp. 7–14. Hagerstown, MD, Harper & Row, 1983.
76. Lamperth-Seiler, E. Harnweg- und hirntumoren bei gummiarbeitern. Schweiz. Med. Wochenschr., *104:*1655–1659, 1974.
77. Leffingwell, S.S., Waxweiler, R., Alexander, V., *et al.* Case-control study of gliomas of the brain among workers employed by a Texas City, Texas chemical plant. Neuroepidemiology, *2:*179–195, 1983.
78. Leibowitz, U., Yablonski, M., and Alter, M. Tumors of the nervous system: incidence and population selectivity. J. Chronic Dis., *23:*707–721, 1971.
79. Mancuso, T.F. Tumors of the central nervous system: industrial considerations. Acta Unio. Internat. Contra. Cancrum, *19:*488–489, 1963.
80. Mayr, E., Diamond, L.K., Levine, R.P., *et al.* Suspected correlation between blood-group frequency and pituitary adenomas. Science, *124:*932–934, 1956.
81. McFarland, J. and Sappington, S.W. A ganglioneuroma in the neck of a child. Am. J. Pathol., *11:*429–448, 1935.
82. McMahon, B. Prenatal x-ray exposure and childhood cancer. J. Natl. Cancer Inst., *28:*1173–1191, 1962.
83. Meerkotter, V.A. and Shear, M. Multiple primordial cysts associated with bifid rib and ocular defects. Oral Surg., *18:*498–503, 1964.
84. Metzel, E. Betrachtungen zur genetik der familiaren gliome. Acta Genet. Med. Gemellol., *13:*124–131, 1964.
85. Metzel, E. and Mohadjer, M. Familial incidence of brain tumors. In: *Present Limits of Neurosurgery,* edited by I. Fusek and J. Kune, pp. 17–18. Prague, Avicenum, Czechoslovak Medical Press, 1974.
86. Michelson, J. and New, P.F.I. Brain tumour and pregnancy. J. Neurol. Neurosurg. Psychiatry, *32:*305–307, 1969.
87. Modan, B., Baidatz, D., Mart, H., *et al.* Radiation-induced head and neck tumours. Lancet, *1:*277–279, 1974.
88. Moertel, C.G., Dockerty, M.B., and Baggenstoss, A.H. Multiple primary malignant neoplasms. III. Tumors of multicentric origin. Cancer, *14:*238–248, 1961.
89. Moyes, P.D. Familial bilateral acoustic neuroma affecting 14 members from four generations: case report. J. Neurosurg., *29:*78–82, 1968.
90. Moynahan, E.J. Multiple basal cell naevus syndrome—successful treatment of basal cell tumours with 5-fluorouracil. Proc. R. Soc. Med., *66:*627–628, 1973.
91. Mufson, J.A. and Davidoff, L.M. Multiple meningiomas (report of two cases). J. Neurosurg., *1:*45–57, 1944.
92. Mulvihill, J.J. Congenital and genetic diseases. In: *Persons at High Risk of Cancer: An Approach to Cancer Etiology and Control,* edited by J.F. Fraumeni Jr., pp. 3–38. New York, Academic Press, 1975.
93. Musicco, M., Filippini, G., Bordo, B.M., *et al.* Gliomas and occupational exposure to car-

cinogens: case-control study. Am. J. Epidemiol., *116:*782–790, 1982.

94. Neblett, C.R., Waltz, T.A., and Anderson, D.A. Neurological involvement in the nevoid basal cell carcinoma syndrome. J. Neurosurg., *35:*577–584, 1971.
95. Nibbelink, D.W., Peters, B.H., and McCormick, W.F. On the association of pheochromocytoma and cerebellar hemangioblastoma. Neurology, *19:*455–460, 1969.
96. Norman, R.M. and Taylor, A.L. Congenital diverticulum of the left ventricle of the heart in a case of epiloia. J. Pathol. Bacteriol., *50:*61–68, 1940.
97. Oyasu, R., Battifora, H.A., Clasen, R.A., *et al.* Induction of cerebral gliomas in rats with dietary lead subacetate and 2-acetylaminofluorene. Cancer Res., *30:*1248–1261, 1970.
98. Parker, H.L. and Kernohan, J.W. The relation of injury and glioma of the brain. J.A.M.A., *97:*535–540, 1931.
99. Paton, A. and Petch, C.P. Association of diabetes mellitus with cerebral tumour. Br. Med. J., *1:*855–856, 1954.
100. Percy, A.K., Elveback, L.R., Okazaki, H., *et al.* Neoplasms of the nervous system: epidemiologic considerations. Neurology, *22:*40–48, 1972.
101. Peters, J.M., Preston-Martin, S., and Yu, M.C. Brain tumors in children and occupational exposure of parents. Science, *213:*235–237, 1981.
102. Poser, C.M. *The Relationship between Syringomyelia and Neoplasms.* Springfield, IL, Charles C Thomas, 1956.
103. Preston-Martin, S. Abstract: A case-control study of intracranial meningiomas in women. Am. J. Epidemiol., *108:*233–234, 1978.
104. Preston-Martin, S., Henderson, B.E., and Yu, M.C. Epidemiology of intracranial meningiomas: Los Angeles County, California. Neuroepidemiology, *2:*164–178, 1983.
105. Raney, R.B. and Courville, C.B. Multiple hemangioblastomas of the central nervous system. Bull. Los Angeles Neurol. Soc., *2:*104–114, 1937.
106. Reagan, T.J. and Freiman, I.S. Multiple cerebral gliomas in multiple sclerosis. J. Neurol. Neurosurg. Psychiatry, *36:*523–528, 1973.
107. Refsum, S. and Mohr, J. Genetic aspects of neurology. In: *Clinical Neurology,* edited by A.B. Baker and L.H. Baker, chapter 47, p. 40. New York, Harper & Row, 1971.
108. Reynolds, E.S. Trauma as a possible cause of brain tumor. Lancet, *ii:*13–14, 1923.
109. Richards, P. and McKissock, W. Intracranial metastases. Br. Med. J., *1:*15–18, 1963.
110. Rodriguez, H.A. and Berthrong, M. Multiple primary intracranial tumors in von Recklinghausen's neurofibromatosis. Arch. Neurol., *14:*467–475, 1966.
111. Rubinstein, L.J. Tumors of the central nervous system. In: *Atlas of Tumor Pathology,* Fascicle 6. Washington, D.C., Armed Forces Institute of Pathology, 1972.
112. Russell, D.S. and Rubinstein, L.J. *Pathology of Tumours of the Nervous System,* ed 3. Baltimore, Williams & Wilkins, 1971.
113. Sahar, A. Familial occurrence of meningiomas: case report. J. Neurosurg., *23:*444–445, 1965.
114. Saran, N. and Winter, F.C. Bilateral gliomas of the optic discs associated with neurofibromatosis. Am. J. Ophthalmol., *64:*607–612, 1967.
115. Sasanelli, F., Beghi, E., and Kurland, L.T. Primary intraspinal neoplasms in Rochester, Minnesota, 1935–1981. Neuroepidemiology, *2:*156–163, 1983.
116. Scherer, H.J. The forms of growth in gliomas and their practical significance. Brain, *63:*1–35, 1940.
117. Schimke, R.N., Hartmann, W.H., Prout, T.E., *et al.* Syndrome of bilateral pheochromocytoma, medullary thyroid carcinoma, and multiple neuromas. N. Engl. J. Med., *279:*1–7, 1968.
118. Schoenberg, B.S. Thesis—Primary Intracranial Neoplasms: A Study of Incidence, Epidemiological Trends, and the Association of These Neoplasms with Primary Malignancies of Other Sites. Rochester, MN, University of Minnesota, 1974.
119. Schoenberg, B.S. Multiple primary neoplasms and the nervous system. Cancer, *40:*1961–1967, 1977.
120. Schoenberg, B.S. General considerations. In: *Neurological Epidemiology: Principles and Clinical Applications,* edited by B.S. Schoenberg, pp. 11–16. New York, Raven Press, 1978a.
121. Schoenberg, B.S. Descriptive epidemiology. In: *Neurological Epidemiology: Principles and Clinical Applications,* edited by B.S. Schoenberg, pp. 17–42. New York, Raven Press, 1978b.
122. Schoenberg, B.S. Epidemiology of primary nervous system neoplasms. In: *Neurological Epidemiology: Principles and Clinical Applications,* edited by B.S. Schoenberg, pp. 475–493. New York, Raven Press, 1978c.
123. Schoenberg, B.S. Neurologic disease in the elderly: epidemiologic considerations. Semin. Neurol., *1:*5–12, 1981.
124. Schoenberg, B.S., Glista, G.G., and Reagan, T.J. The familial occurrence of glioma. Surg. Neurol., *3:*139–145, 1975.
125. Schoenberg, B.S., Christine, B.W., and Whisnant, J.P. Nervous system neoplasms and primary malignancies of other sites: the unique association between meningiomas and breast cancer. Neurology, *25:*705–712, 1975.
126. Schoenberg, B.S., Christine, B.W., and Whisnant, J.P. The descriptive epidemiology of primary intracranial neoplasms—the Connecticut experience. Am. J. Epidemiol., *104:*499–510, 1976a.

127. Schoenberg, B.S., Schoenberg, D.G., Christine, B.W., *et al.* The epidemiology of primary intracranial neoplasms of childhood: a population study. Mayo Clin. Proc., *51:*51–56, 1976b.
128. Schoenberg, B.S., Christine, B.W., and Whisnant, J.P. The resolution of discrepancies in the reported incidence of primary brain tumors. Neurology, *28:*817–823, 1978.
129. Schreier, H.A., Sherry, N., and Shaughnessy, E. Lead poisoning and brain tumors in children: a report of 2 cases. Ann. Neurol., *1:*599–600, 1977.
130. Schuman, L.M., Choi, N.W., and Gullen, W.H. Relationship of central nervous system neoplasms to toxoplasma gondii infection. Am. J. Publ. Health, *57:*848–856, 1967.
131. Selikoff, I.J. and Hammond, E.C. Brain tumors in the chemical industry. Ann. NY Acad. Sci., *381:*1–364, 1982.
132. Selverstone, B. and Cooper, D.R. Astrocytomas and ABO blood groups. J. Neurosurg., *18:*602–604, 1961.
133. Shore, R.E., Albert, R.E., and Pasternack, B.S. Follow-up study of patients treated by x-ray epilation for tinea capitis: resurvey of post-treatment illness and mortality experience. Arch. Environ. Health, *31:*21–28, 1976.
134. Slaughter, J.C., Hardman, J.M., Kempe, L.G., *et al.* Neurocutaneous melanosis and leptomeningeal melanomatosis in children. Arch. Pathol., *88:*298–304, 1969.
135. Stout, A.P. Ganglioneuroma of the sympathetic nervous system. Surg. Gynecol. Obstet., *84:*101–110, 1947.
136. Strong, L.C. Genetic and environmental interactions. Cancer, *40:*1861–1866, 1977.
137. Symington, T. and Goodall, A.L. Studies in phaeochromocytoma. I. Pathological aspects. Glasgow Med. J., *34:*75–96, 1953.
138. Tanaka, J., Garcia, J.H., Netsky, M.G., *et al.* Late appearance of meningioma at the site of partially removed oligodendroglioma. J. Neurosurg., *43:*80–85, 1975.
139. Turcot, J., Despres, J.P., and St Pierre, F. Malignant tumors of the central nervous system associated with familial polyposis of the colon—report of two cases. Dis. Colon Rectum, *2:*465–468, 1959.
140. van der Wiel, H.J. *Inheritance of Glioma: the Genetic Aspects of Cerebral Glioma and Its Relation to Status Dysraphicus,* pp. 249–252. Amsterdam, Elsevier Press, 1959.
141. Waldmann, T.A., Levin, E.H., and Baldwin, M. The association of polycythemia with a cerebellar hemangioblastoma: the production of an erythropoiesis stimulating factor by the tumor. Am. J. Med., *31:*318–324, 1964.
142. Walker, A.E., Robins, M., and Weinfeld, F.D. Epidemiology of brain tumors: the national survey of intracranial neoplasms. Neurology, *35:*219–226, 1985.
143. Waxweiler, R.J., Stringer, W., Wagoner, J.K., *et al.* Neoplastic risk among workers exposed to vinyl chloride. Ann. NY Acad. Sci., *271:*40–48, 1976.
144. Winston, K., Gilles, F.H., Leviton, A., *et al.* Cerebellar gliomas in children. J. Natl. Cancer Inst., *58:*833–838, 1977.
145. Yates, P.O. and Pearce, K.M. Recent change in blood-group distribution of astrocytomas. Lancet, *i:*194–195, 1960.

CHAPTER 2

Classification of Brain Tumors

JULIO H. GARCIA, M.D.

INTRODUCTION

The diagnosis of neoplasia whether in the central nervous system or other sites remains firmly based on the analysis of appropriate tissue samples by light microscopy and conventional histology. Likewise, the histologic classification of most neoplasms is based on pattern recognition that can be achieved best by the application of the appropriate methods of light microscopy. Electron microscopy has helped in this process primarily in cell identification; for example, the visualization of secretory granules in the tumor cells derived from the adenohypophysis, or the demonstration of intermediate filaments in the cytoplasm of cells of astrocytic derivation. Application of immunological techniques, such as the peroxidase antiperoxidase antisera, have helped in the identification of the constituent cells of lymphomas and in the specific demonstration of secretory products such as prolactin in the tumor cells of a pituitary microadenoma (62).

Classification, in biology, is a system whereby all items belonging to a common class (e.g., brain tumors) are subdivided into categories having features common to each subgroup. In the case of tumors (or neoplasms) the feature most commonly applied to the various classifications is the cytologic derivation of the tumor cell; accordingly, neoplasms derived from epithelia are called carcinomas, whereas the name sarcoma implies a mesenchymal derivation. The age group of patients among whom certain classes of tumors are more likely to occur and, most importantly, the presumed length of the patient's survival as it may be influenced by the tumor's expected biologic behavior, are additional features that may influence tumor classification.

A logical classification of brain tumors should be based on a system of *nomenclature* in which individual tumor types are named after the cell from which tumor cell(s) are thought to be derived. Accordingly, astrocytomas are presumed to be derived from the neoplastic transformation of astrocytes, while meningiomas are thought to be derived from meningothelial (or arachnoidal) cells. In practice tumor nomenclature, until now, has been based primarily on the microscopic characteristics of each tumor, as seen with light microscopy using conventional staining techniques. A tumor is defined (or named), in general, by histologic criteria defining the normal adult cell that the predominant neoplastic cell resembles most (62). Adoption of this method of naming most tumors avoids controversies concerning disputed histogenesis of specific cell types.

This system of tumor nomenclature is based on two assumptions:

(*a*) All tumors are derived from a single cell type; indeed, since most neoplastic cells express only a single isoenzyme, this strongly suggests that they are monoclonal in origin. In a minority of instances malignant neoplasms appear to be polyclonal and sometimes they may originate at multiple separate sites. Furthermore, some investigators have cautioned that the presence of a single clonal marker does not prove that the tumor started with the transformation of a single cell (20).

(*b*) The second premise assumes that identification of the cell from which the tumor may originate can be clearly established in all cases. However, because the definition of cell type(s) is based on identification of phenotypic features that become apparent only after the cell is fully differentiated, identifying the presumed cell of origin cannot be achieved with confidence in a significant number of cases. This is particularly true of tumors whose cellular differentiation is either incomplete or absent; these tumors are referred to as being *embryonal* to signify that the constituent cells retain features characteristic of the embryo (45).

Additional difficulties with cell typing and tumor nomenclature could arise in cases where a single cell type gives rise to cells having more than one phenotypic expression (57, 59), as is thought to be the case with teratomas or tumors in which germ cells are believed to simultaneously differentiate into epithelial, mesenchymal, and neuroepithelial elements.

Even when the phenotypic expression is easily recognized there may be a need to subdivide (or grade) a group of neoplasms belonging to a single class or family. This need was well exemplified by Bailey and Cushing (2) who were among the first to attempt to tailor the treatment of a brain tumor to its histological features. These authors remarked: "We were at loss to know how it could be that a patient from whose cerebellum a large ... "glioma" was removed . . . might prove to be living and well (several years later) whereas another patient from whom a "glioma" was removed in like fashion . . . might survive for a scant six months. . . ." Since that time the need to subdivide (or grade) tumors, such as "gliomas," has become increasingly more apparent and such subdivisions have been tied into factors like location (as in the case of cerebellar astrocytomas), gross features (such as cavitation in some gliomas), and specific histological qualities (e.g., presence/absence of coagulative necrosis). Cerebellar location, cavitation or "cyst" formation, and absence of necrosis are all features that have been associated with favorable prognosis among astrocytomas.

HISTORICAL NOTE ON TUMOR CLASSIFICATION

Zülch (70) has written a concise account of the historical developments that have taken place in the classification of brain tumors, both in Europe and in America. Müller suggested in 1838 (46) that "the essential criteria for a classification of tumors according to the intrinsic properties can be found only in the study of their chemical nature, the microscopic structure, and the manner and sequence of their development. . . ."

Systematic classification of neoplasms started with Virchow (67) who described the neuroglia (or neural glue) and separated gliomas from other "sarcomas" of the nervous system. Further refinements in understanding the cytology of the nervous system, through the work of German (9) and Spanish (26, 52) workers, resulted in a comprehensive classification of brain tumors into 14 separate categories (26, 50).

Attempts to incorporate the histologic characteristics of certain tumors with clinical features such as most common age of occurrence and preferential location were first undertaken by Bailey and Cushing (2). Subsequently, Kernohan *et al.* (41) introduced a simplified brain tumor classification in which histologic "grading" (or evaluation of the extent of cellular differentiation, and absence/presence of atypical mitosis) would be indicated by a roman numeral inserted after the name of the tumor. According to his proposal (adapted from Broders (14)) an astrocytoma grade I would have a much better prognosis than an astrocytoma grade IV. This subdivision or grading of astrocytomas into "low-grade" and "high-grade" would discriminate at least two subgroups of patients with astrocytoma for the purposes of postoperative management and would explain, in part, the reason for the puzzlement alluded to by Bailey and Cushing in their 1926 publication.

Zülch (70) was largely responsible for organizing at least two meetings of recognized experts on brain tumors, in Cologne, Germany (1961) and Santander, Spain (1955); these meetings were intended to seek an international and interdisciplinary consensus on both nomenclature and classification of brain tumors. Several years later an atlas with a histologic typing or definition of tumors of the central nervous system, reflecting international consensus, was published under the auspices of the World Health Organization (WHO) (71). More recently, Fields (28) edited the proceedings of a meeting held at M.D. Anderson Hospital (Houston, Tx) at which specific issues of controversy in the nomenclature and classification of brain tumors were discussed. Each of these controversial issues will be addressed succinctly in subsequent pages of this chapter.

DEFINITIONS

The word tumor is used in this chapter as a synonym of neoplasm. "A neoplasm is an abnormal mass of tissue, the growth of which exceeds and is uncoordinated with that of the normal tissues and persists in the same excessive manner after cessation of the stimuli which evoked the change" (69).

Differentiation refers to the process by which parenchymal cells resemble normal adult cells both morphologically and functionally.

"*Undifferentiated*" means that the tumor cells as evaluated by light and electron microscopy do not display any of the well known features of "mature" (or differentiated) normal cells.

Lack of differentiation is marked by a number of morphologic changes including: pleomorphism, cells that are many times larger than their neighbors, cells that may be extremely small and primitive appearing, nuclear hyperchromatism, abnormal nuclear: cytoplasmic ratio, and changes in nuclear features including chromatin granules that are coarsely clumped and distributed along the nuclear membrane. Large nucleoli, common in neoplastic cells, usually reflect a very active process of protein synthesis in these cells. More important than the number of mitotic figures is the presence of atypical and bizarre tripolar, quadripolar or multipolar spindles.

An important feature of *anaplasia* is the formation of giant tumor cells; in addition the orientation of anaplastic cells with respect to a basal lamina, for example, is markedly disturbed. Despite exceptions, the more rapidly growing and the more anaplastic a tumor, the less likely that there will be specialized functional activity (20).

"*Anaplasia*," in tumors of the central nervous system, indicates enough differentiation so as to allow cell typing accompanied by prominent pleomorphism, hypercellularity, and either lack or loss of differentiation. The typical example is *anaplastic astrocytoma*, a tumor in which the cytoplasmic or nuclear features of adult or mature astrocytes are clearly recognizable, but most cells show sufficient pleomorphism and there is enough hypercellularity to require the adjective of anaplastic.

GRADING (SUBTYPING) TUMORS

The ideal tumor nomenclature should incorporate into each tumor designation the name of the presumed cell of origin. The name of the tumor should also clearly denote the prognostic significance of each tumor type: benign or malignant. Only in this way can rational decisions be made about management of individual patients; hence, the need for attempting to develop reproducible, and reliable systems of tumor grading.

In general, *benign* tumors are well differentiated. *Malignant* neoplasms, in contrast, range from well differentiated to undifferentiated. Malignant neoplasms may lack differentiation or may be anaplastic. There is substantial evidence supporting the concept that many neoplasms arise from reserve or germ cells that are present in all specialized tissues; lack of neoplastic differentiation, then, is not necessarily the consequence of dedifferentiation.

Nearly all benign tumors grow as cohesive expansile masses that remain localized to their site of origin and do not infiltrate, invade or metastasize. Malignant neoplasms grow by progressive infiltration, invasion, and destruction of the surrounding tissue. Next to the development of metastases, invasiveness is the most reliable feature differentiating malignant from benign neoplasms. With few exceptions, all malignant neoplasms metastasize; major exceptions include malignant gliomas (seldom metastasize), some meningiomas (may metastasize while retaining benign features), and basal cell carcinomas (almost never metastasize.) In the central nervous system, the location of a tumor may take precedence as a factor determining malignancy; a very benign (histologically speaking) tumor located in the Sylvian aqueduct may prove lethal because its location makes it inaccessible to known forms of treatment.

The separation of tumor subtypes, as initially proposed by Kernohan for some primary tumors of the central nervous system, can be justified when analysis of large groups of patients shows different prognostic and epidemiological features for each tumor subtype (62). Analysis of large groups of patients with a diagnosis of astrocytoma, for example, and the collective experience of the past several decades have shown us that *astrocytoma* (pilocytic, juvenile, fibrillary or well-differentiated) has a favorable prognosis except when its location in the diencephalon or the base of the pons, makes its surgical resection impossible. In contrast, *astrocytoma* (anaplastic) and *glioblastoma* multiforme (or astrocytoma grade III and IV of Kernohan) are malignant tumors regardless of their location.

Traditional methods of *grading* brain tumors have been applied by several authors in attempts to identify subclasses of gliomas that may respond differently to diverse forms of treatment. Two recently published studies show that among gliomas of astrocytic derivation (or with astrocytic components) a single histologic feature, *necrosis*, separates two groups of patients having significantly different postoperative survival curves (17, 18, 48). Both of these studies aimed at establishing objective criteria by which *anaplastic astrocytoma* and *glioblastoma multiforme* could be clearly separated from one another.

A simple grading system was proposed in 1979 as a two-part classification scheme of gliomas; the two features being: (*a*) histologic "malignancy" (as defined above) and (*b*) histologic features of the tumor (58). Application of this system to a large number of patients has proved its reliability. A grading system for gliomas among a large group of patients who were studied at the same hospital has relied upon recognition of the presence/absence of four features: nuclear atypism, mitoses, coagulative necrosis, and endothelial proliferation. The method is binary and results in a summary score that can be translated into grades. Statistical analyses of studies conducted in a large series of patients, all of whom had cerebral astrocytomas, showed that this system of grading strongly correlates with survival ($p < 0.0001$). Double-blind grading conducted independently by two observers was concordant in 94% of ordinary astrocytomas. Reproducibility of the grading system was 81% in low grade and 96% in high grade tumors (21). Similar results have been reported by Davis (22) applying slightly different but comparable methods in the histologic evaluation of gliomas among adults.

Applying a uniform strategy in the grading of all primary neoplasms of the CNS does not result in the separation of meaningful subgroups. The highly variable biologic behavior of malignant ependymomas (44), and the absence of correlation between histologic features, location of the tumor or likelihood of tumor recurrence, contrasts with the clear-cut correlation that has been established in cerebral astrocytic gliomas. Similar discrepancies between the nature of histologic features and clinical behavior have been shown with respect to some of the oligodendrogliomas (61) and the subependymal giant cell astrocytomas (56).

Gilles (30) attempted to define the prognosis of brain tumors, among children, on the basis of a score derived from the evaluation of well-defined histologic features. As an example, among posterior fossa tumors the presence of *microcysts* correlates with a relatively good prognosis whereas the presence of *perivascular rosettes* is an ominous feature. This is based on analyses that avoid specific tumor names for the purpose of achieving a nonbiased appraisal of tumor subtypes.

Statistical methods to gain quantitative information about the prognosis associated with specific individual histologic features, clusters of histologic features and, as a separate entity, clusters of children with a specific distribution of histologic features have been applied to the study of brain tumors. When all the pertinent clinical information about each of the children included in a large population and their tumor localization is available, one can assign to each child with brain tumor a value for each of 13 individual clusters. The clustering algorithm may then separate groups of children on the basis of individual features, histologic or otherwise. The objective of this analysis is to provide *quantitative* information about tumor prognosis derived from the association with each of many in a constellation of histologic features (30).

In addition to the traditional histologic methods described above, definition or *typing* and *grading* of brain tumors can be achieved by immunohistochemical methods aimed at demonstrating proteins that are specifically expressed by selected cell types even after these cells become neoplastic. Because of their strong antigenicity, the methods of preparing sera rich in antibodies against specific proteins are relatively straight forward. Histologic demonstration of the antigen in a given tumor sample can be achieved by co-localization with a "brown" peroxidase. The proteins that are specific for certain cell types have been traditionally known as *markers*; several dozen tumor markers have been identified to date.

The markers with which most workers are primarily concerned are those regarded as being specific to the nervous system or as playing an important role in nervous system functions. They are conventionally divided into: *structural* proteins, i.e., proteins implicated in cytoskeletal structures or organelles or related to cell membranes, and *soluble* proteins that may function as enzymes, as local or systemic endocrine carriers, or even as neurotransmitters (56).

Intermediate filaments: these form a class of insoluble cytoplasmic structures measuring 7–11 nm in diameter that are intermediate in size between microtubules (22–25 nm in diameter) and microfilaments (5–7 nm). Five distinct groups are recognized: (*a*) *cytokeratins* of epithelial cells, (*b*) *neurofilaments* of most neurons, (*c*) *glial fibrillary acidic protein* characteristic of normal and pathologic astrocytes, (*d*) *desmin* of skeletal, cardiac and smooth muscle cells, and (*e*) *vimentin* of cells of mesenchymal derivation including fibroblasts and endothelial cells that are also found in the early stages of development of other cells. Observations derived from the application of immunohistochemical methods, including monoclonal antibodies, to the diagnosis and treatment of primary brain tumors have been published elsewhere (16, 19, 24, 25, 27, 32). Several other articles have dealt with markers specific for endothelial cells and basal laminae (12), astrocytic cells (24, 25, 49, 51), and for neurons (65, 66).

Current difficulties with tumor nomenclature, classification, and grading (discussed below) cannot be solved with the application of 100-year-old methods like light microscopy. The principal change that has occurred in the past 10 years in the field of tumor classification is the remarkable improvement in our ability to define phenotypic features by immunologic methods and chromosomal or DNA alterations and modifications; these methods have provided an increased understanding of the genetic and phenotypic definition of tumor cells. Although significant advances have been made, there are important limitations in the application of monoclonal antibodies to tissues embedded in paraffin. Many pathologists seem to be unaware of these limitations: (*a*) most monoclonal antibodies react with epitopes that are present only in living or frozen tissues; (*b*) intermediate filament proteins degrade very quickly, in a matter of 120 min; and (*c*) many monoclonal antibodies are not monospecific or epitope defined (10, 11).

The pathogenesis of spontaneously occurring tumors of the neuraxis remains essentially unknown; although radiation and local trauma have been frequently invoked as potential factors, conclusive evidence demonstrating their oncogenicity is still lacking. The only potential sources of tumors among dividing cells of the central nervous system are the glial elements and for all practical purposes the only cell type that actively divides is the astrocyte (56).

Tumors can be viewed as the result of altered gene expression and neoplasia can be equated with abnormal cell differentiation. In the process of neoplastic transformation, either repressed genes are derepressed or new DNA sequences are formed. In this context, neoplasia can be viewed as a result of cytogenetic alterations brought about by epigenetic phenomena. Up to 2 dozen genes (oncogenes) have been identified in the genome of RNA retroviruses; these oncogenes can transform other cells by transfection. Oncogenes have homologous counterparts in the DNA of normal cells, called proto-oncogenes, where they may play a significant role in normal cell biology; proto-oncogenes encode polypeptides acting as growth factors (56).

Molecular pathology methods have been applied in the study of neoplastic diseases for the purposes of detecting gene rearrangement, tissue-specific gene transcription, and oncogene activation (33). Forty to fifty percent of malignant gliomas demonstrate gene amplification, but this does not correlate with the clinical or morphological expression of the tumor. The most compelling evidence implicating oncogenes in tumorigenesis is related to n-myc which is overexpressed in neuroblastoma and retinoblastoma. Deletion of the long arm of chromosome 13 has been associated with retinoblastoma (56).

Increasing evidence suggests that chromosomal abnormalities may yield valuable clues to oncogene expression or other expressions in neoplastic transformation. The most common types of cytogenetic abnormalities found in tumor cells are: translocation, chromosomal deletions (or loss) and cytogenetic manifestations of gene amplification, i.e., extrachromosomal double-minute (DM) chromatin bodies and chromosomally integrated, homogeneously stained regions (HSR). The general concept is that the deleted genetic material has a suppressor, or regulatory function. At the cytogenetic level, such a functional loss may be manifested by chromosome deletion, or monosomy, whereas at the molecular level it may be manifested either by inactivation or by homozygosity for a defective gene (56).

The *cytogenetic abnormalities* of malignant human glioma, particularly glioblastoma multiforme, have now been well-defined. However, there are still technical obstacles to incorporating cytogenetic data into classification schemes because of the difficulties involved in obtaining satisfactory preparations from low grade tumors. It might be productive to launch a large prospective study to evaluate the diagnostic and classification significance of these cytogenetic abnormalities. Analysis of amplification of 4 genes and restriction fragment length polymorphism (RFLP) studies of chromosomes 10 and 17 can be carried out using standard recombinant DNA techniques. Although the same technical problems with low-grade tumors also apply to these molecular techniques, in situ hybridization may provide a means to circumvent these difficulties (11).

Immunostaining for Ki-67 (a marker for cells in the M phase of the cell cycle) represents a convenient and rapid method for the estimation of *growth fraction* in human central nervous system tumors. The future application of this technique would be meaningful only if the results obtained are of prognostic value and helpful in planning postoperative therapy. A correlation between clinical behavior and Ki-67 index is emerging in meningiomas. Significantly higher labeling indices are found in the hemangiopericytic variant, in anaplastic meningiomas and in recurrent lesions. A less convincing correlation seems to exist in pituitary adenomas. Gliomas represent a greater challenge for the prediction of biologic behavior and this is particularly true for glioblastoma in which changes in the total tumor mass may depend as much on cell loss as on the proliferative potential of viable tumor cells (42).

Until now tumor grading has been based solely on traditional morphologic criteria such as high cellularity, poor cellular differentiation, nuclear hyperchromatism, increased mitotic index, presence of atypical mitotic figures, pleomorphism, necrosis, and abnormal vascular proliferation. None of these criteria can be regarded as entirely dependable indicators of either anaplasia or speed of tumor growth. First steps toward quantifiable criteria for tumor grading are provided by immunohistochemical approaches such as the use of the Ki-67 antiserum. Supplementing and refining the traditional system of malignancy grading may lead to a better prognostication of the biologic behavior of brain tumors. However, the application of some of the immunohistochemical methods mentioned above, and of techniques such as DNA cytometry, requires the availability of fresh, unfixed tissues (68).

It seems inescapable that application of molecular biology methods to the understanding of neoplasia will find applications in tumor grading. In the glioblastomas, the presence in approximately one-half of the lesions of amplification for the erb B oncogene (epidermal growth factor) has been described. A clinical pathologic study suggested that there were no prognostic differences between patients who had glioblastomas with or without amplification. These results may reflect errors in the grading of glioblastomas; if so, the detection of gene amplification in malignant gliomas could become a prognostically useful means for grading gliomas (17).

DNA analysis by flow cytometry has shown a wide range of different ploidies in biopsy specimens ranging from diploid to strongly aneuploid nuclear DNA; a high proportion of glioblastomas are near-diploid, thus indicating that biological malignancy is not necessarily associated with aberration of DNA content. Chromosomal analysis of malignant gliomas has confirmed that most of these tumors have near-diploid DNA lines (56).

UNRESOLVED ISSUES IN BRAIN TUMOR

Nomenclature and Classification

The application of traditional histological methods and the observations collectively made over a span of about a century have resulted in a nomenclature for brain tumors that is fairly well standardized (Table 2.1) (71) but is not entirely acceptable to all experts; specific and current issues of controversy involve nomenclature of neuroectodermal embryonal tumors, grading of gliomas and meningiomas (38).

In 1990, more than 10 years after the publication of the original WHO classification one must decide whether this classification can be fine-tuned to take note of existing improvements and new entities that have come to light in the last few years, such as pleomorphic xanthoastrocytoma (31, 40) or whether a more radical realignment must take place in order that the system can be brought up to date and made more useful (3). Among the experts attending the 1989 Houston meeting there seemed to be a consensus that great progress has been made despite controversy on selected issues.

Embryonal Central Neuroepithelial Tumors

A modification of the WHO classification for brain tumors has been suggested, reflecting the views of neuropathologists dealing primarily with brain tumors in children. One of the suggestions made by that group was to introduce the term primitive neuroectodermal tumor (PNET) to designate multiple neoplasms in the brain that are primarily made up of small undifferentiated cells. The designation of primitive neuroectodermal tumor for this type of neoplasia has generated numerous editorials, personal letters, phone calls, rebuttals, and workshops (45). But, the proceedings of the Houston meeting suggest that some light has begun to emerge from the heated discussions.

Primitive neuroectodermal tumors occur most commonly in the vermis of the cerebellum but can also develop in the cerebrum, including the pineal region. These tumors characteristically spread through the subarachnoid space and can metastasize outside the nervous system. PNETs consist of primitive neuroectodermal cells containing small, round to oval nuclei within a narrow cytoplasmic rim. Sometimes these tumors contain large cells with round to oval nuclei and more prominent cytoplasm that may or may not be tapered to one side. Nuclei contain abundant chro-

TABLE 2.1.
WHO Histological Classification of Tumors of the Central Nervous System (71)

I. Tumors of Neuroepithelial Tissue
- A. *Astrocytic tumors*
  1. Astrocytoma
     a. Fibrillary
     b. Protoplasmic
     c. Gemistocytic
  2. Pilocytic astrocytoma
  3. Subependymal giant cell astrocytoma (ventricular, tumor of tuberous sclerosis)
  4. Astroblastoma
  5. Anaplastic (malignant) astrocytoma
- B. *Oligodendroglial tumors*
  1. Oligodendroglioma
  2. Mixed oligoastrocytoma
  3. Anaplastic (malignant) oligodendroglioma
- C. *Ependymal and choroid plexus tumors*
  1. Ependymoma
     a. Myxopapillary ependymoma
     b. Papillary ependymoma
     c. Subependymoma
  2. Anaplastic (malignant) ependymoma
  3. Choroid plexus papilloma
  4. Anaplastic (malignant) choroid plexus papilloma
- D. *Pineal cell tumors*
  1. Pineocytoma (pinealocytoma)
  2. Pineoblastoma (pinealoblastoma)
- E. *Neuronal tumors*
  1. Gangliocytoma
  2. Ganglioglioma
  3. Ganglioneuroblastoma
  4. Anaplastic (malignant) gangliocytoma and ganglioglioma
  5. Neuroblastoma
- F. *Poorly differentiated and embryonal tumors*
  1. Glioblastoma
     Variants
     a. Glioblastoma with sarcomatous component (mixed glioblastoma and sarcoma)
     b. Giant cell glioblastoma
  2. Medulloblastoma
     Variants
     a. Desmoplastic medulloblastoma
     b. Medullomyoblastoma
  3. Medulloepithelioma
  4. Primitive polar spongioblastoma
  5. Gliomatosis cerebri

II. Tumors of Nerve Sheath Cells
- A. *Neurilemoma* (schwannoma, neurinoma)
- B. *Anaplastic* (malignant) neurilemoma
- C. *Neurofibroma*
- D. *Anaplastic* (malignant) *neurofibroma* (neurofibrosarcoma, neurogenic sarcoma)

III. Tumors of the Meninges and Related Tissues
- A. *Meningioma*
  1. Meningotheliomatous (endotheliomatous, syncytial arachnotheliomatous)
  2. Fibrous (fibroblastic)
  3. Transitional (mixed)
  4. Psammomatous
  5. Angiomatous
  6. Hemangioblastic
  7. Hemangiopericytic
  8. Papillary
  9. Anaplastic (malignant) meningioma

TABLE 2.1—*continued*

B. *Meningeal sarcomas*
   1. Fibrosarcoma
   2. Polymorphic cell sarcoma
   3. Primary meningeal sarcomatosis
C. *Xanthomatous tumors*
   1. Fibroxanthoma
   2. Xanthosarcoma (malignant fibroxanthoma)
D. *Primary melanotic tumors*
   1. Melanoma
   2. Meningeal melanomatosis
E. *Others*

IV. Primary Malignant Lymphomas

V. Tumors of Blood Vessel Origin
   A. *Hemangioblastoma* (capillary hemangioblastoma)
   B. *Monstrocellular sarcoma*

VI. Germ Cell Tumors
   A. *Germinoma*
   B. *Embryonal carcinoma*
   C. *Choriocarcinoma*
   D. *Teratoma*

VII. Other Malformative Tumors and Tumor-like Lesions
   A. *Craniopharyngioma*
   B. *Rathke's cleft cyst*
   C. *Epidermoid cyst*
   D. *Dermoid cyst*
   E. *Colloid cyst of the third ventricle*
   F. *Enterogenous cyst*
   G. *Other cysts*
   H. *Lipoma*
   I. *Choristoma* (pituicytoma, granular cell "myoblastoma")
   J. *Hypothalamic neuronal hamartoma*
   K. *Nasal glial heterotopia* (nasal glioma)

VIII. Vascular Malformations
   A. *Capillary telangiectasia*
   B. *Cavernous angioma*
   C. *Arteriovenous malformation*
   D. *Venous malformation*
   E. *Sturge-Weber disease* (cerebrofacial or cerebrotrigeminal angiomatosis)

IX. Tumors of the Anterior Pituitary
   A. Pituitary Adenomas
      1. Acidophil
      2. Basophil (mucoid cell)
      3. Mixed acidophil-basophil
      4. Chromophobe

X. Local Extensions from Regional Tumors
   A. *Glomus jugular tumor* (chemodectoma, paraganglioma)
   B. *Chordoma*
   C. *Chondroma*
   D. *Chondrosarcoma*
   E. *Olfactory neuroblastoma* (esthesioneuroblastoma)
   F. *Adenoid cystic carcinoma* (cylindroma)
   G. *Others*

XI. Metastatic Tumors

XII. Unclassified Tumors

matin and usually one or more nucleoli; mitotic figures are readily identified. Ultrastructurally, the cells in PNETs are in close apposition to one another, often with interdigitation of cytoplasmic processes but without evidence of specialized intercellular junctions (4, 5).

Based on a review of the literature and her personal experience with a large number of brain tumors occurring in the pediatric age group, Rorke (54) has concluded that:

Tumors composed of primitive (undifferentiated) neuroepithelial cells occur most commonly but not exclusively in the cerebellar vermis of children.

Such tumors may contain, in addition to the embryonal elements, neoplastic cells with features characteristic of astrocytes, oligodendroglia, ependymal cells or neurons; even pigmented cells may be seen in exceptional examples.

The unique name assigned to a given tumor e.g., medulloblastoma, cannot be applied if the site of origin is not known.

Most of these tumors are biologically malignant and have a tendency to disseminate throughout the cerebrospinal fluid pathways.

The tumors have a variable connective tissue component and rarely may contain either smooth or striated muscle fibers.

Moreover, Rorke concluded that each tumor in this group is unique so that detailed investigation of one does not permit prediction of the biologic behavior of another. Evaluating a given specimen usually does not allow determination of either the ancestry or the differentiating potential of the tumor by any of the current available techniques. Thus, prudence dictates that for the central primitive neuroepithelial neoplasms a nomenclature be used that is based on the description of phenotypic characteristics (i.e., primitive neuroepithelial tumor) with a secondary notation as to the most likely site of origin. Specifically, Rorke suggested that such primitive neuroepithelial tumors (other than medulloblastoma of the cerebellum, retinoblastoma of the eye, and peripheral neuroblastoma) be reported as PNETs when they occur either in the cerebral hemispheres or in the area of the pineal body (54). Rorke (54) excluded from the category of primitive neuroectodermal tumors (PNET) olfactory neuroblastoma and retinoblastomas because these tumors can be easily identified on the basis of their location.

The concept of a single diagnostic term, primitive neuroectodermal tumor (PNET), as an independent entity from which several others derive has several flaws; these have had rather negative consequences in the establishment of therapeutic protocols (55). The concept of PNET, based on a paper published in 1973 and reporting a series of 23 brain tumors in children, is not a very convincing single entity. The criteria for its recognition lack precision and some of the tumors described under this name may have been anaplastic small cell gliomas, while others could represent cerebral neuroblastomas (55). The preservation of distinct tumor entities, based partly on their localization within the central neuraxis and partly on their differentiation capacities, is more likely to constitute a useful basis for future advances in the treatment of brain tumors (55).

Among undifferentiated brain tumors, advances in cell type identification by special neurohistologic, immunohistologic, and immunocytochemical techniques have permitted the discrimination of distinct cytomorphogenetic entities. The cerebral medulloepithelioma, the desmoplastic infantile ganglioglioma, the pineoblastoma, and the cerebellar medulloblastoma, are pluripotential in their capacity to exhibit divergent differentiation (7, 8). Growth factors and neurotransmitters could play a regulatory role in central neuroepithelial tumors, and thus the aberrant behavior of embryonal neoplasms could be modified by functional receptor responses or result from abnormal receptor responses to these substances (55).

Aside from the issue of nomenclature involving embryonal tumors, difficulties have not been surmounted in several attempts to grade medulloblastomas. There are two groups of patients with medulloblastoma, as classically defined and understood by most pathologists: one group does well in terms of survival whereas another group does not. These two groups cannot be separated by histologic criteria or by any other criterion that is known to date (17). There are tumors in the cerebellum that look like medulloblastoma and have astrocytic differentiation; there are also cerebellar astrocytomas in which the anaplastic components are indistinguishable from medulloblastoma. Treatment in these cases should be dictated by the presence of embryonal cells (55).

Several studies attempting phenotypic classification that have been undertaken with medulloblastoma biopsies have failed to show prognostic significance. This lack of success may reflect either inaccurate phenotyping or inadequate techniques in the preparation of the tissues. However, this kind of analysis may uncover significant correlations with ordinary light microscopic criteria with which a new classification scheme, based on molecular criteria, can be tested (11).

Tumors of the Pineal Region

The pineal region includes many cell types of both glial and nonglial derivation. The pineal body contains a wide range of cells, including pineocytes, astrocytes, oligodendrocytes, ependymocytes, ganglion cells and even Schwann cells from the conery nerve. The high frequency with which germinomas occur in this region, suggests that germ cells are another possible cell type of the human pineal body. The most frequent means of diagnosing tumors in the pineal region is the stereotactic biopsy, but the main disadvantage of this method is the small size of the biopsy specimen. More than immunohistochemistry, electron microscopy appears to be a useful tool in the diagnosis of small round cell tumors of the pineal region. Pinealomas (pineocytomas and pineoblastomas) offer a typical example of such a diagnostic process (34). Regardless of the histologic pattern of various pineal parenchymal tumors, numerous ultrastructural features consistently resemble those of mammalian pineocytes. The association of intermingled dark and clear cells, intra- or extracellular vacuolar spaces, pleomorphic cell processes, and the presence of some cytoplasmic organelles give these tumors a very specific pattern which can be distinguished from that of the neuronal and glial tumors developing in the same pineal region (35).

Astrocytomas

Among the cerebral hemispheric tumors of astrocytic derivation, the most significant remaining issue is defining the criterion for grading these tumors. Two independent studies, based on large series of patients, seem to agree on the conclusion that retrospective analysis of histologic preparations separates two groups with significantly different survival periods. The single, most reliable predictor of short survival among these patients was the presence of coagulative necrosis, whether pseudopalisading or not (18, 48). Thus, it has been proposed that, for the purposes of therapy, the designation glioblastoma multiforme be adopted for tumors with astrocytic components in which areas of necrosis are demonstrable either by microscopy or by in vivo imaging methods.

Kepes and associates (40) have identified, through the application of immunohistochemical methods, a variant of astrocytic tumors for which they suggested the designation pleomorphic xanthoastrocytoma. The importance of separating this subtype of astrocytoma is the observation that despite its ominous microscopic appearance, most patients have a long uneventful postoperative survival (31, 40).

Giant-cell astrocytoma of subependymal location, a tumor in most instances associated with the stigmata of tuberous sclerosis, is generally accepted as a variant of astrocytoma (64, 65). Several publications have dealt with the issue of tumor cell histogenesis based on the application of immunocytochemical and electron microscopic techniques (6, 13, 29, 47, 53, 60).

Meningiomas

The current WHO classification defines meningiomas as a "tumor originating from cellular elements of the meninges." This definition is too broad, as it cncompasses tumors derived from melanin-containing cells that are normal components of the leptomeninges. It would be more useful to restrict the term meningioma *only* to those tumors that can be shown to have their derivation from arachnoidal cap cells (39).

The term meningioma was introduced by Cushing more than 65 years ago and it has served us well. The WHO classification adhered to Cushing's concept in some instances as in the case of meningiomas called hemangioblastic. However, classical hemangioblastoma may involve the leptomeninges as it has been described in patients with the von Hippel-Lindau syndrome; these patients may have simultaneously cerebellar, brain stem and meningeal masses with identical histology to that of hemangioblastoma (37, 38, 63). It is erroneous to call the meningeal representative of this tumor group a meningioma when in another location the tumor is simply called a hemangioblastoma (39).

The psammomatous variant of hemangioma should not be classified independently but rather as a subtype of the meningotheliomatous type. Meningioma cells containing large numbers of cytoplasmic hyaline inclusions, or pseudopsammoma bodies, form an interesting group of tumors for which the name secretory meningioma should be retained (1). Certain meningiomas attract lymphocytic-plasma cell infiltrates that at times may overshadow the meningiomatous component of the intracranial mass. For these tumors a subgroup designated as meningiomas with massive lymphoplasma cell infiltrates would be a justifiable addition to the existing categories (39).

The biologic behavior of meningiomas can seldom be predicted from the histologic appearance alone, and application of ultrastructural or tissue culture methods has not added significantly to the solution of this problem. No obvious relationship seems to exist between the histologic subtype and the recurrence rate among meningiomas, except for the established intermediate anaplastic types (i.e., hemangiopericytic, papillary, and clearly anaplastic meningiomas) (36).

Cytokinetic studies utilizing both bromodeoxyuridine (BrdU) and Ki-67 labeling methods may increase the accuracy with which the proliferation potential of meningiomas can be predicted. Supplementing the histologic diagnosis, performed by routine methods, with these studies may improve the specificity of tumor prognosis among meningiomas (36). Current data do not allow definitive conclusions correlating the presence of either estrogen receptors or progesterone receptors with clinical behavior or with in vitro growth modulation of meningiomas. However, some promise in this area justifies continuing interest (15).

ACKNOWLEDGEMENT:

I am pleased to acknowledge the excellent collaboration of Ms. Marilynn Johnson in the preparation of this manuscript.

REFERENCES

1. Alguacil-Garcia, A., Pettigrew, N.M., and Sima, A.A.F. Secretory meningioma: A distinct subtype of meningioma. Am. J. Pathol., *10:*102–111, 1986.
2. Bailey, P. and Cushing, H. *Tumors of the Glioma Group.* Philadelphia, Lippincott, 1926.
3. Barnard, R. General discussion of Part One. In: *Primary Brain Tumors. A Review of Histologic Classification,* edited by W.S. Fields, pp. 91–97. New York, Springer Verlag, 1989.
4. Becker, L.E. Primitive neuroectodermal tumors: Views on a working classification. In: Primary Brain Tumors. A review of histologic classification, edited by W.S. Fields, pp. 59–69. New York, Springer Verlag, 1989.
5. Becker, L.E. and Hinton, D. Primitive neuroectodermal tumors of the central nervous system. Hum. Pathol., *14:*538–550, 1983.
6. Bender, B.L. and Yunis, E.J. Central nervous system pathology of tuberous sclerosis in children. Ultrastructural Pathology, *1:*287–299, 1980.
7. Bennett, J.P. Jr. and Rubinstein, L.J. The biological behavior of primary cerebral neuroblastoma: a reappraisal of the clinical course in a series of 70 cases. Ann. Neurol., *16:*21–27, 1984.
8. Berger, M.S., Edwards, M.S.B., Wara, W.M., *et al.* Primary cerebral neuroblastoma. Long-term follow-up review and therapeutic guidelines. J. Neurosurg., *59:*418–423, 1983.
9. Bergstrand, H. On gliomas in the cerebral hemispheres. Acta Pathol. Microbiol. Scand. Suppl., *11:*100–109, 1932.
10. Bigner, D. Phenotypic analysis of medulloblastoma with monoclonal antibodies. In: *Primary Brain Tumors. A Review of Histologic Classification,* edited by W.S. Fields, pp. 70–78. New York, Springer Verlag, 1989.
11. Bigner, D. Can cytogenetic and molecular genetic analysis of malignant human gliomas be used yet to supplement conventional classifi-

cation schemes? In: *Primary Brain Tumors. A Review of Histologic Classification*, edited by W.S. Fields, pp. 117–122. New York, Springer Verlag, 1989.

12. Bohling, T., Pateau, A., Ekblom, P., *et al.* Distribution of endothelial and basement membrane markers in angiogenic tumors of the nervous system. Acta Neuropathol. (Berl.), *62:*67–72, 1983.
13. Bonnin, J.M., Rubinstein, L.J., Papasozomenos, S.C.H., *et al.* Subependymal giant cell astrocytoma. Acta Neuropathol. (Berl.), *62:*185–193, 1984.
14. Broders, A.C. Carcinoma: grading and practical application. Arch. Pathol. Lab. Med., *2:*376–381, 1926.
15. Bruner, J.M. Meningiomas: immunocytochemistry and steroid hormone receptors. In: *Primary Brain Tumors: A Review of Histologic Classification*, edited by W.S. Fields, pp. 240–244. New York, Springer Verlag, 1989.
16. Bullard, D.E. and Bigner, D.D. Applications of monoclonal antibodies in the diagnosis and treatment of primary brain tumors. J. Neurosurg., *63:*2–16, 1985.
17. Burger, P.C. The grading of astrocytomas and oligodendrogliomas. In: *Primary Brain Tumors. A Review of Histologic Classification*, edited by W.S. Fields, pp. 171–180. New York, Springer Verlag, 1989.
18. Burger, P.C., Vogel, F.S., Green, S.P., Strike, T.A. Glioblastoma multiforme and anaplastic astrocytoma. Pathologic criteria and prognostic implications. Cancer, *59:*1106–1111, 1985.
19. Caccamo, D. and Rubinstein, L.J. Immunocytochemistry of neural tumors. In: *Diagnostic Neuropathology*, vol. 3 edited by J.H. Garcia, Philadelphia, Field & Wood, 1990.
20. Cotran, R.S., Kumar, V., and Robbins, S.L. *Robbins Pathologic Basis of Disease*, ed. 4 pp. 239–251. Philadelphia, 1989.
21. Daumas-Duport, C. A new uniform grading system (using Mayo Clinic material). In: *Primary Brain Tumors. A Review of Histologic Classification*, edited by W.S. Fields, pp. 159–170. New York, Springer Verlag, 1989.
22. Davis, R.L. Grading of gliomas. In: *Primary Brain Tumors. A Review of Histologic Classification*, edited by W.S. Fields, pp. 150–158. New York, Springer Verlag, 1989.
23. de Chadarèvian, J.P. and Hollenberg, G.R. Subependymal giant cell tumor of tuberous sclerosis: A light and ultrastructural study. J Neuropathol. Exp. Neurol., *38:*419–433, 1979.
24. Deck, J.H.N., Eng, L.F., Bigbee, J., *et al.* The role of glial fibrillary acidic protein in the diagnosis of central nervous system tumors. Acta Neuropathol (Berl.), *43:*183–190, 1978.
25. Deck, J.H.N. and Rubinstein, L.J. Glial fibrillary acidic protein in stromal cells of some capillary hemangioblastomas: significance and possible implications of an immunoperoxidase study. Acta Neuropathol. (Berl.), *54:*173–181, 1981.
26. del Río-Hortega, P: *Anatomía Microscópica de los Tumores del Sistema Nervioso Central y Periferico.* Madrid, Blass, 1934.
27. Eng, L.F. and Rubinstein, L.J. Contribution of immunohistochemistry to diagnostic problems of human cerebral tumors. J. Histochem. Cytochem., *26:*513–522, 1978.
28. Fields, W. *Primary Brain Tumors: a Review of Histologic Classification.* New York, Springer Verlag, 1989.
29. García-Bengochea, F. and Collins, G.H. Monstrocellular sarcoma of the brain: 6-year postoperative survival. Case report. J. Neurosurg., *31:*686–689, 1969.
30. Gilles, F. Classification of pediatric tumors. Alternative strategies. In: *Primary Brain Tumors. A Review of Histologic Classification*, edited by W.S. Fields, pp. 47–51. New York, Springer Verlag, 1989.
31. Gómez, J., García, J.H. and Colón, L.E. A variant of cerebral glioma called pleomorphic xanthoastrocytoma: Case report. Neurosurgery, *16:*703–706, 1984.
32. Graham, D.I., Thomas, D.G.T., and Brown, I. Nervous system antigens. Histopathology, *7:*1–21, 1983.
33. Grody, W.W., Gatti, R.A., and Naeim, F. Diagnostic molecular pathology. Mod. Pathol., *2:*533–562, 1989.
34. Hassoun, J. Pinealomas: need for an ultrastructural diagnosis. In: *Primary Brain Tumors. A Review of Histologic Classification*, edited by W.S. Fields, pp. 82–85. New York, Springer Verlag, 1989.
35. Hassoun, J., Gambarelli, D., Peragut, J.C., *et al.* Specific ultrastructural markers of human pinealomas. A study of four cases. Acta Neuropathol. (Berl.), *62:*31–40, 1983.
36. Jellinger, K.L. Biologic behavior of meningiomas. In: *Primary Brain Tumors. A Review of Histologic Classification*, edited by W.S. Fields, pp. 231–239. New York, Springer Verlag, 1989.
37. Jurco, S. III, Nadji, M., Harvey, D.G., *et al.* Hemangioblastoma: histogenesis of the stroma cells studied by immunocytochemistry. Hum. Pathol., *13:*13–18, 1982.
38. Kawamura, J., García, J.H., and Kamijyo, J. Cerebellar hemangioblastoma: histogenesis of stromal cells. Cancer, *31:*1528–1540, 1973.
39. Kepes, J.J. History and diagnosis of meningiomas. In: *Primary Brain Tumors. A Review of Histologic Classification*, edited by W.S. Fields, pp. 217–230. New York, Springer Verlag, 1989.
40. Kepes, J.J., Rubinstein, L.J. and Eng, L.F. Pleomorphic xanthoastrocytoma: a distinctive meningocerebral glioma of young subjects with relatively favorable prognosis. Cancer, *44:*1839–1852, 1979.
41. Kernohan, J.W., Mabon, R.F., Svien, J.H., *et al.* Symposium on a new and simplified concept of gliomas (a simplified classification of gliomas.) Proc. Staff Meet. Mayo Clin., *24:*71–75,

1949.
42. Kleihues, P., Aguzzi, A., Shibata, T., Wiestler, O.D. Immunohistochemical assessment of differentiation and DNA replication of brain tumors. In: *Primary Brain Tumors. A Review of Histologic Classification*, edited by W.S. Fields, pp. 123–132. New York, Springer Verlag, 1989.
43. McComb, R.D., Jones, T.R., Pizzo, S.V., *et al.* Localization of factor VIII/von Willebrand factor and glial fibrillary acidic protein in the hemangioblastoma: implications for stromal cell histogenesis. Acta Neuropathol (Berl.), *56:*207–213, 1982.
44. Mork, S.J. and Loken, A.C. Ependymoma. A follow-up study of 101 cases. Cancer, *40:*908–915, 1977.
45. Mork, S.J. and Rubinstein, L.J. Ependymoblastoma. A reappraisal of a rare embryonal tumor. Cancer, *55:*1536–1542, 1985.
46. Müller, J. *Uber den feineren Bau and die Formen der Krankhaften Geschwülste.* Berlin, Reimer, 1838.
47. Nakamura, Y. and Becker, L.E. Subependymal giant-cell tumor: astrocytic or neuronal. Acta Neuropathol (Berl.) *60:*271–277, 1983.
48. Nelson, J.S., Tsukada, Y., Schoenfeld, D., *et al.* Necrosis as a prognostic criterion in malignant supratentorial astrocytic gliomas. Cancer, *52:*550–554, 1983.
49. Osborn, M. and Weber, K. Tumor diagnosis by intermediate filament typing: a novel tool for surgical pathology. Lab Invest, *48:*372–394, 1983.
50. Penfield, W. A paper on the classification of brain tumors and its practical application. Br Med J *1:*337–342, 1932.
51. Raemaekers, F.S.C., Puts, J.J.G., Moesker, O., *et al.* Antibodies to intermediate filament proteins in the immunohistochemical identification of human tumors: An overview. Histochemistry, *15:*692–713, 1983.
52. Ramón y Cajal, S. Histologie du Systeme Nerveux de L'Homme et des Vertebres. Madrid, Consejo Superior de Investigaciones Científicas, 1972.
53. Ribadeau-Dumas, J.L., Poirier, J., and Escourelle, R. Etude ultrastructurale des lesions cérèbrales de la sclerose de Bourneveille, A propòs de deux cas. Acta Neuropathol (Berl.) *25:*259–270, 1983.
54. Rorke, L.B. Primitive neuroectodermal tumor—a concept requiring an apologia? In: *Primary Brain Tumors. A Review of Histologic Classification*, edited by W.S. Fields, pp. 6–15. New York, Springer Verlag, 1989.
55. Rubinstein, L.J. Justification for a cytogenetic scheme of embryonal central neuroepithelial tumors. In: *Primary Brain Tumors. A Review of Histologic Classification*, edited by W.S. Fields, pp. 16–27. New York, Springer Verlag, 1989.
56. Russell, D.S. and Rubinstein, L.J. *Pathology of Tumors of the Nervous System*, ed 5. Baltimore, Williams & Wilkins, 1989.
57. Sato, T., Shimoda, A., Takahashi, T., *et al.* Congenital cerebellar neuroepithelial tumor with multiple divergent differentiation. Acta Neuropathol, *50:*143–146, 1980.
58. Scanlon, P.W. and Taylor, W.F. Radiotherapy of intracranial astrocytomas: analysis of 417 cases treated from 1960 through 1969. Cancer, *5:*301–307, 1979.
59. Scheithauer, B.W. and Rubinstein, L.J. Cerebral Medulloepithelioma. Report of a case with multiple divergent neuroepithelial differentiation. Childs Brain, *5:*62–71, 1979.
60. Sima, A.A.F. and Robertson, D.M. Subependymal giant-cell astrocytoma. J Neurosurgery, *50:*250–245, 1979.
61. Smith, M.T., Ludwig, C.T., Godfrey, A.D., *et al.* Grading of oligodendrogliomas. Cancer, *52:*2107–2144, 1983.
62. Sobin, L.H. The international histologic classification of tumors. Bulletin WHO, *49:*813–819, 1981.
63. Spence, A.M. and Rubinstein, L.J. Cerebellar capillary hemangioblastomas: its histogenesis studies by organ culture and electron microscopy. Cancer, *35:*326–341, 1975.
64. Stefansson, K. and Wollman, R. Distribution of glial fibrillary acidic protein in central nervous system lesions of tuberous sclerosis. Acta Neuropathol (Berl.) *52:*135–140, 1980.
65. Stefansson, K. and Wollmann, R. Distribution of the neuronal specific protein, 14-3-2, in central nervous system lesions of tuberous sclerosis. Acta Neuropathol (Berl.) *53:*113–117, 1981.
66. Vinores, S.A., Bonnin, J.M., Rubinstein, L.J., *et al.* Immunohistochemical demonstration of neuron-specific enolase in neoplasms of the CNS and other tissues. Arch Pathol Lab Med, *108:*536–540, 1984.
67. Virchow, R. *Die Krankaften Geschwülste,* Vol 2, Berlin, Hischwald, pp. 343–378, 1864.
68. Wechsler, W. and Reifenberger, G. Application of immunohistochemistry for tumor grading in human neuro-oncology. In: *Primary Brain Tumors. A Review of Histologic Classification*, edited by W.S. Fields, pp. 133–141. New York, Springer Verlag, 1989.
69. Willis, R.A. *The Spread of Tumors in the Human Body.* London, Butterworth, 1952.
70. Zülch, K.J. *Brain Tumors. Their Biology and Pathology.* Third completely revised edition. Berlin, Springer Verlag, 1986.
71. Zülch, K.J. Histologic typing of tumors of the central nervous system. International classification of tumors, No. 21. Geneva, World Health Organization, 1979.

Part II

Oncogenesis and Growth

CHAPTER 3

Glioma Cytogeny and Differentiation Viewed through the Window of Neoplastic Vulnerability

LUCIEN J. RUBINSTEIN, M.D.[a]

The objective of this chapter is to review and, where necessary, update the concept of the window of neoplastic vulnerability in relation to the spontaneous incidence of different types of human glioma. The concept is, furthermore, useful for an understanding of the range of differentiation that may be expressed by the different cell populations which make up these tumors. It is based on the well-accepted premise that when one or more cells, or a cell clone, is the target of the first step that ultimately results in the phenotypic expression of malignant transformation, that cell or cell clone is either still replicating or capable of resuming replication. The size of the window results from the interaction of several factors: the existence of a reserve stem cell population, the capacity of differentiated cells to reenter the cycle, the number of replicating cells at risk at one particular time, the length of time during which a particular cell population remains in the cycle, the actual state of differentiation and the subsequent differentiation potential of that cell population, and the steps of differentiation through which successive cell generations are expected to progress. In so far as some of them are known or can be inferred from ontogenetic and experimental data, the incidence, cytogenesis and differentiating capabilities of central nervous system (CNS) tumors can be made intelligible through the operation of those events.

CENTRAL NEUROEPITHELIAL TUMORS: EMBRYONAL AND ADULT TYPES

A number of well-known distinctions should be recalled. The first of these is the difference between embryonal and adult-type tumors. Pathologists have long been familiar with this distinction, which can easily be made in organs that normally maintain a large population of cells of renewal and therefore are vulnerable to neoplastic transformation in adult life, i.e., the epidermis, the mucosal linings of the respiratory and gastrointestinal tracts, etc. The adult-type tumors are in this context distinct from the embryonal tumors, which are defined as those which arise during embryonal, fetal or early postnatal development from tissues that are still immature (122). Embryonal tumors display a capacity for differentiation similar to that of the parent developing tissue, but that capacity is usually less restricted than that of tumors originating from postnatal cells. In the CNS, a major problem exists in reference to this distinction because (*a*) the reserve neuroepithelial cell population—as estimated in the adult primate brain—is low and therefore the turnover of glial cells is slow (50, 87), and (*b*) the cells of renewal,

[a]Deceased.

which presumably are the target of neoplastic transformation, are by far the most numerous when the tissue is still undergoing morphogenesis, i.e., during development. The consequences in regard to the central neuraxial tumors are threefold. First, the conceptual distinction between adult-type and embryonal tumors may easily be perceived as becoming almost meaningless. Second, from the diagnostic point of view the cell forms and histological patterns encountered in both classes of tumor may be so closely alike that a more differentiated glioma showing foci of anaplasia may not be distinguishable from an embryonal neoplasm displaying areas of maturation. This is typically exemplified by those cases of cerebellar glioma that may equally well be interpreted as medulloblastomas showing astrocytic differentiation or as diffuse astrocytomas with anaplastic areas indistinguishable from medulloblastoma. The possible implications of such transitional examples on the question of medulloblastoma histogenesis and differentiation have recently been discussed by us (94). Third, it is evident that cytogenetic events in central neuroepithelial development will play a prominent role in defining the factors whose interactions will determine whether the window of vulnerability is wide or narrow.

DIVERGENT AND ABERRANT DIFFERENTIATION: METAPLASIA AND HETEROPLASIA

In nonneoplastic cells, the operation of divergent cellular differentiation is based on the understanding that the progeny of replicating stem cells mature along distinct lines and that the expressions of differentiation are in most instances mutually exclusive. In cell biology this rule entails relatively few exceptions. Such exceptions have, accordingly, been designated as "confused cells," e.g., when, in some experimental conditions, individual epidermal cells express mucin in their more superficial portion and filaments characteristic of young keratinizing cells in their deeper portion (29). The rule of mutual exclusivity also applies in large measure to tumor cells. In gangliogliomas, for example, cells will generally express either neuronal or glial features. However, the rule seems to break down more often in neoplastic than in normal development, and in the neoplastic state the exclusive nature of phenotypic expression seems to be more easily altered as a result of environmental changes. Thus in glioblastomas the synthesis of glial fibrillary acidic (GFA) protein and the secretion of fibronectin by the tumor cells are usually inversely related (47, 80), but in certain circumstances, i.e., after transplantation into nude mice, the cells appear capable of expressing both GFA protein and fibronectin (47). Simultaneous divergent intracellular differentiation may be seen in mixed neurogliogenic tumors, when both glial filaments and neurosecretory granules can sometimes be demonstrated within the same cell (91, 105), thus making their interpretation ambiguous.

Aberrant differentiation occurs when morphological features develop that are not found in the normal mature cell of the same lineage, or when the tumor synthesizes cell products that are not normally manufactured by that cell. An example is the expression of GFA protein in otherwise typical neoplastic oligodendroglia (94). Closely linked to this development is the existence of metaplasia, i.e., of legitimate modulations of differentiation within a range determined by the type of stem cell involved, e.g., the presence of cartilage, osteoid tissue and bone in the mesenchymal stroma of a gliosarcoma (8, 94). The term "heteroplasia" is sometimes employed when the expression of divergent differentiation is appreciably widened, as is often the case in embryonal tumors (122). Aberrant differentiation may also be expressed by the synthesis and secretion of extracellular products, e.g., matrix glycoproteins (laminin, fibronectin, various collagen types, and glycosaminoglycans), that are more commonly associated with mesenchymal cells and which, in the present context, may be induced in mature normal rat glial cells in vivo after injury (67), in the normal rat astrocyte in vitro (66), and in some human glioma cell lines both in vitro (1) and after xenogeneic transplantation (47). In particular, it should be noted that neoplastic, as opposed to normal, glial cells can produce an extracellular glioma-mesenchymal matrix glycoprotein (73) which may be involved in the modulation of cell adherence and migration and which has been identified with tenascin (60).

NEOPLASTIC DIFFERENTIATION IS LESS RESTRICTED THAN NORMAL DIFFERENTIATION

Two general principles operate in neoplastic differentiation. The first is that the range of the cellular differentiating potential of tumors is often less restricted than in the normal. This principle is not necessarily limited, as might be anticipated, to embryonal tumors or to tumors characterized primarily by their cellular heterogeneity or by the development of anaplastic populations. Choroid plexus papillomas, which are benign, nonembryonal and well-differentiated tumors of a single cell type that phenotypically expresses the characteristics of mature epithelial structures, contain variable numbers of epithelial cells which synthesize GFA protein (25, 58, 69, 94). The epithelium of the choroid plexus originates from a specialization of segments of primitive ventricular neuroepithelial cells at certain sites of the neural tube when these cells become apposed to intraventricular infoldings of the adjacent primitive mesenchyme. The fact that some of the epithelial tumor cells in choroid plexus papillomas contain GFA protein implies that they have retained the genetic information in their parental neuroepithelial precursors that will code for a glial phenotype in their progeny. In other words, in neoplastic development these transformed epithelial cells express a feature specific to glia that would have been demonstrable had these cells followed the alternative pathway of differentiating into ependymal cells. This is an example of aberrant differentiation expressing, so to speak, an ontogenetic memory.

Another example is provided by the occasional production, in an astrocytoma, of an intercellular chondroid matrix, thus resulting in the formation of tissue identical with cartilage. Concomitantly with this process, the astrocytes undergo progressive morphological changes into rounded cell forms with a vacuolated cytoplasm, thus becoming indistinguishable from chondrocytes (54). This form of metaplasia in neoplastic astrocytes no longer falls within our definition of legitimate metaplasia, but is presumably analogous to the formation of cartilage by epithelial cells in pleomorphic adenomas of the salivary glands. It is of interest that this type of metaplasia has now been reported to be occasionally displayed in cerebellar medulloblastoma (5).

A third example illustrates the principle that neoplastic cells possess a greater flexibility of adaptation to metabolic demands than normal cells. Neuron-specific or $\gamma\gamma$ enolase, a cytoplasmic enzyme that catalyzes one of the late steps of the glycolytic pathway (70), has been shown to be characteristic of normal neurons and neuroendocrine cells (70, 97). Its appearance correlates well with neuronal differentiation. As a marker, the enzyme was first found to be valuable in the identification of peripheral ganglion cell tumors (26, 78, 106) and neuroendocrine neoplasms (106, 121). However, in the CNS, using the polyvalent antiserum it is demonstrable also in tumor cells of nonneuronal origin (e.g., gliomas, meningiomas, schwannomas, etc.), presumably because it is needed to augment the rate of glycolysis required by the increased metabolic activity postulated to occur in neoplasia (114, 116, 118): this also seems to be the case in a number of extraneural tumors that do not belong to the endocrine or neuroendocrine systems (114, 121). The intracellular distribution of the enzyme in the neoplastic cell may also be different from that in the normal. Electron immunocytochemistry has shown it to be restricted to the cytoplasm of normal structures—thus, largely corresponding to the sites of ribosomes, granular endoplasmic reticulum and microtubules (117), whereas in neoplastic cells it is distributed more irregularly and is often localized on the cytoplasmic membranes (115, 116) and, in the case of glioma cells, on the intermediate filaments (115). Monoclonal antibodies to $\gamma\gamma$ enolase may, however, demonstrate a higher degree of neuronal and neuroendocrine cell specificity (99).

HETEROPLASTIC DIFFERENTIATION IS MORE OFTEN ENCOUNTERED IN EMBRYONAL TUMORS

The second general principle, namely, that divergent, or heteroplastic, differentiation is a feature met more often in embryonal than in adult-type tumors in the CNS, is illustrated by the occasional development of striated muscle fibers in medulloblastomas (102)—which have then been called medullomyoblastomas—as well as in another type of embryonal central neuroepithelial tumor, the cerebral medulloepithelioma (7). In the latter case, the phenomenon is susceptible of two interpretations: either as an extreme example of legitimate metaplasia in the mesenchymal stroma of a tumor already prone to display at times a prominent vascular and fibrous connective tissue stroma (51), or as an instance of heteroplastic metaplasia expressed in primitive central neuroepithelial cells, a phenomenon which can be aligned with tissue culture studies reported on nitrosourea-induced neuronal and glial cell lines, in which the progeny may display the phenotypic and neuropharmacological features of skeletal muscle cells (12, 61). A similar development has also been reported to occur in human glioma cell lines and to be further expressed in vivo after their xenogeneic transplantation (44). In any event, since the medulloepithelioma represents the most primitive of the embryonal CNS tumors and is endowed with the widest potential range of divergent neuroepithelial differentiation, the question may legitimately be raised as to whether such a range should not be widened even further so as to include also a myogenic differentiating capability. Further studies on the regulation of skeletal muscle genes in relation to neural cells (124) are needed to clarify to what extent this apparent development of "transdifferentiation" is applicable to this rare embryonal tumor.

An example of the phylo- and ontogenetic memory of an organ being expressed in its neoplastic development is provided by the presence of Flexner rosettes and of fleurettes, characteristic of retinoblastic differentiation, in pineoblastomas (94). In this embryonal tumor, therefore, morphological differentiation recalls both the function of the pineal gland as a photoreceptor organ in lower vertebrates and a transient stage of fetal and neonatal pinealocytes during which they exhibit the features of photoreceptor cells (23, 125). These features disappear soon after birth (2). The ontogenetic aspect of neoplastic differentiation in this instance may also be manifested by a different development, namely, by the occasional association of heritable retinoblastomas, usually bilateral, with a pineoblastoma in the same patient (81, 94). The term "trilateral retinoblastoma," which has been given to the association, is perhaps too inclusive as not all the pineoblastomas developing in this context have been shown to display retinoblastic differentiation. However, the strong genetic background of the condition suggests that in these embryonal tumors a germinal mutation specifically targets, for subsequent postzygotic mutation, intra- and extraocular cells that are phylogenetically of photoreceptor origin (39). This is confirmed by the demonstration of immunoreactive retinal S-antigen in both pineoblastoma and pineocytoma (94) as well as in the cerebrospinal fluid of a patient harboring such a pineal parenchymal tumor (57).

A third instance illustrating the widened range of heteroplastic differentiation that may be shown in embryonal CNS tumors is provided by an in vitro study of a cerebellar medulloblastoma which was maintained in an organ culture system for 6½ months and in which the tumor cells progressively demonstrated divergent differentiation into astrocytes and neuroblasts (37). The most notable feature was the appearance, in vitro only, of synaptic ribbons (also known as "vesicle-crowned rodlets" or "vesicle-crowned lamellae"), i.e., organelles characteristic of retinal photoreceptor cells, of sensory cochlear cells and, especially, of pinealocytes in a wide range of vertebrates (83, 123). Their development in vitro has been extensively documented in short- and long-term cultures of the mammalian pineal gland. In tumors, these structures have been noted in examples of human retinoblastoma (27) and pineocytomas (36, 38) and in an experimental pineocytoma induced in the hamster with the JC strain of human polyomavirus (112). Indeed, all the electron microscopic features categorized as neuronal in the example of medulloblastoma studied by us in vitro (37) have been encountered in human pineocytic tumors (36). This case may, therefore, represent an instance of heteroplastic differentiation in a cerebellar medulloblastoma, as a result of which both glial and pineocytic hallmarks have become divergently expressed. The link between cerebellar medulloblastoma and pineoblastoma has been strengthened by the demonstration of photoreceptor markers (retinal S-antigen and opsin) in some examples of cerebellar medulloblastomas (94) and by the reported occurrence of medulloblastoma in one and pineoblastoma in the other of monozygotic twins (94).

APPLICATION OF THE CONCEPT OF THE WINDOW OF VULNERABILITY TO THE INCIDENCE OF CNS TUMORS IN GENERAL

Two widely accepted facts characterize the incidence of CNS tumors as a whole. First, their general incidence is considerably lower than that of tumors arising in other organs or tissues. This is of course partly due to the protection of the central neuraxial structures from the different exogenous physical and chemical agents that are known to play such an important role in the development of cancer in the exposed epithelia of the body. However, it is also related to the fact that, throughout the span of postnatal life, the number of reserve stem cells at risk and of differentiated neuroepithelial cells (virtually entirely astrocytic) capable of reentering the kinetic cycle is appreciably lower than in those other organs and tissues in which there is a constant cycling population of cells of renewal. Secondly, one of the salient features of CNS tumors is their relatively high incidence in childhood. It is generally accepted that the CNS is the second most common site of neoplastic disease in the young. This fact must evidently be linked to our premise that the window of neoplastic vulnerability is at its widest in the course of neural development, cellular migration, and maturation. This, together with the experimentally demonstrated vulnerability of fetal and neonatal mammalian glial cells to the transplacental carcinogenicity of low doses of alkylating agents (56) and to the transforming action of intracerebrally injected oncogenic viruses (24, 126) points to the fetal and perinatal glial cells as being the most likely target of the first "hit" in neoplastic transformation. The inference is supported by a large statistical study of children with CNS tumors in whom age at diagnosis was correlated with the risk of later recurrence (103). It may therefore be instructive to examine the different types of CNS tumors in light of the factors which determine the width of the window of neoplastic vulnerability of their respective putative cell of origin.

EXAMPLES OF CNS TUMORS WITH A NARROW WINDOW OF NEOPLASTIC VULNERABILITY

The Cerebral Medulloepithelioma: Relationship of the Window to the Stages of Normal Neurocytogenesis in the Forebrain

The cerebral medulloepithelioma, which is the prototype of embryonal central neuraxial tumors, exhibits two hallmark features: (*a*) its histological pattern is similar to that of the primitive medullary epithelium, and (*b*) it displays a capacity for multiple divergent differentiation that may span the entire range of central neuroepithelial cytogenesis. Differentiation has been documented in almost 50 percent of the reported cases (94). Its characteristic histological pattern has only exceptionally been induced experimentally with an oncogenic virus (79), but it is often represented in the neuroepithelial cell populations derived from implants of the OTT-6050 transplantable mouse testicular teratoma line (110). Its rarity both as a spontaneous event and in its experimental production may be due to the fact that the replicating undifferentiated cells of the primitive medullary epithelium are for some reason resistant to transformation. Perhaps activated genes that might otherwise code for neoplastic change are then being selectively and almost fully utilized for organogenesis and, since they would then be temporarily released from some of the normal regulatory gene controls, carcinogenic interference with the structural integrity of those controlling regulatory genes might consequently become relatively ineffective. Alternatively, repair mechanisms depending on the enzymatic elimination of critical alkylation products from DNA, which are known to vary in different cell types, may likewise vary at different stages of individual cell maturation (86). It is also possible that, while these more primitive cells might be susceptible to the first neoplastic "hit," the experimental timetable simply does not permit the operation of the subsequent steps necessary for the phenotypic expression of neoplasia. It is well known that, in transplacental neurocarcinogenesis using a low dose of ethylnitrosourea (ENU) injected as a single pulse into the gravid rat, the nervous system of the offspring is maximally vulnerable to tumorigenesis in the last days of pregnancy and around birth, i.e., ENU has to be injected after the 14th day of gestation if it is to result in the production of neurogenic tumors in the offspring. It is also known that, by the 15th day of gestation, differentiation in the developing forebrain of the fetal rat has already proceeded in a large measure towards determined neuroblastic and glial cell lines. When ENU is given before the 13th day of gestation, no nervous system tumors are induced and the agent has solely toxic or life-incompatible teratogenic effects on the developing telencephalon (120). This would effectively preclude any of the later mutational changes needed for the development of tumors in the target cells or in their descendants.

Another factor may also play a role in determining the rarity of cerebral medulloepitheliomas. The classic neurocytogenetic sequence of events in the mammalian forebrain, as postulated in the last three decades (11, 31), is characterized by the development of three stages. In stage 1, undifferentiated and presumably uncommitted cells of the primitive neural tube undergo replication. In stage 2, the progeny of these cells undertake a first wave of migration: these migrating cells consist of committed neuroblasts. In the forebrain, the matrix layer is the only source of these cells which, once formed, no longer replicate. In stage 3, a second migration takes place, which consists of replicating glial precursor cells which are the committed, or uncommitted, progenitors of astrocytes and oligodendrocytes. At the onset of the third stage, the residual primitive ventricular cells begin to display the differentiating features of ependymocytes.

These neurocytogenetic stages do not, however, occupy an equal length of time and it is evident that a good deal of overlap must occur between the end of one stage and the beginning of the next. Stage 1, of which the cerebral medulloepithelioma represents the neoplastic equivalent (90), is, presumably, relatively brief. The evidence for this is indirect. In the chick embryo (from which, of necessity, many of our neurocytogenetic data are being extrapolated) the first neuroblasts withdraw from the cell cycle early in the third day of incubation and the first wave of migration is completed by the 8th day (42, 59). By the 8th day also, the residual cells lining the ventricular zone have begun to differentiate into ependymal cells (30, 34). Secondly, in the primate, well before neuroblasts have become postmitotic, the replicating ventricular cells already consist of a coexisting mixed population of glia-committed cells and neuroblasts (62, 63). Indeed the majority of the ventricular cells at the peak of neuroblast production, i.e., at midgestation, including those in mitosis, are GFA protein-positive and therefore glia-committed. The evidence therefore strongly suggests that commitment of neuroepithelial cells to alternative neuronal, glial, or ependymal lines is an early feature in normal forebrain development. Furthermore, there is immunohistochemical evidence that a similar early commitment to divergent differentiation may be demonstrated in the human cerebral medulloepithelioma (15). Thus the window of neoplastic vulnerability for uncommitted multipotential neuroepithelial cells in the telencephalon will be narrow, and tumors with the features of the primitive medullary tube will tend to be correspondingly rare. The situation, as will be discussed, is entirely different when the neurocytogenesis of the cerebellum is considered.

The Cerebral Neuroblastoma

Stage two, in the course of which neuron-committed cells migrate from the matrix layer and undergo progressive differentiation, begins at 7 to 9 weeks of embryonic life in the human fetal cerebrum (96). As these cells are normally postmitotic the window of neoplastic vulnerability should, by definition, be closed. Thus, neuronal tumors are hardly ever obtained after the transplacental injection of alkylating agents. In one example that seems to have been well-documented, i.e., a neuroblastoma of the spinal cord produced following the transplacental administration of methylnitrosourea (MNU) to a pregnant rat on the 16th day of gestation, the tumor was the only one induced among the 15 surviving offspring, all of which showed various forms of cerebral malformation (13). On the other hand, neuroblasts may be the target of transformation in the rat and hamster when the human adenovirus type 12 is injected locally in the neonate (76). Is there, therefore, at birth or shortly thereafter, still a turnover of cells whose differentiating potential is restricted to the neuronal line? Autoradiographic data on the rhesus monkey (87) indicate that, except for a few granule cells in the cerebellum and the hippocampal dentate gyrus (which seem to continue their genesis for several months after birth), almost all the neurons in the primate CNS are produced in the first half of gestation. Studies on the chick embryo neural tube may, however, give us an insight into the apparent paradox of neuroblastic vulnerability in the CNS. With the use of markers such as neurofilament protein (9, 107) and neuronal cell surface-specific antigens (72), it has been shown that there is a subset of replicating primitive matrix cells, probably in their last mitotic round, which are already neuron-committed. A narrow window of neoplastic vulnerability might therefore exist that would account for both the great rarity, and the occasional occurrence, of cerebral neuroblastomas in man (94). This is in contrast to the incidence of sympathetic and olfactory neuroblastomas: here, a considerably wider window may be postulated to exist, since the migration and maturation, and to some extent the proliferation, of cells of the sympathetic system extend from fetal life up to the time of puberty and since, in the nasal and accessory sinus mucosa, renewal of neurosensory olfactory cells is sustained throughout postnatal life.

The Desmoplastic Infantile Ganglioglioma

Such a narrow window of neuronal vulnerability in the CNS presumably also accounts for the rarity of gangliogliomas. Possibly the well-known prevalence of this tumor in the temporal lobe is related to the fact that the subgranular zone of the dentate gyrus may continue to function in the mammalian brain as a source of continuing cytogenesis for granular neurons in postnatal life (35). Some of the data on the primate brain, already mentioned, support such a hypothesis (87). Thus, the window of neuronal vulnerability for neoplastic transformation is, presumably, somewhat wider in the hippocampal region than in other areas of the central neuraxis.

Attention has been drawn to other sites in the supratentorial compartment in which neuroepithelial cells capable of differentiating along both neuronal and glial lines appear to be vulnerable to transformation in fetal or perinatal life and are the putative cells or origin of a highly characteristic form of neoplasia (111). The 11 examples of this type that we reported—and several others that we have subsequently studied—have been remarkably similar. The tumors present clinically as large cystic masses in infancy, often at 4 months of age, and most frequently involve the frontal and parietal regions. A feature common to all is the existence of an extensive desmoplastic component, which is associated with a predominantly leptomeningeal direction of growth. The fibroblastic elements are admixed with variable numbers of pleomorphic neuroepithelial cells among which divergent differentiation along astrocytic and neuronal lines is almost always demonstrable when immunohistochemical and special neurohistological techniques are employed. Astrocytic differentiation was confirmed in all by the presence of GFA protein. Immunoperoxidase preparations using a monoclonal antibody against the 200-kD neurofilament triplet polypeptide established the presence of neuronal differentiation, which in some cases was further documented by silver impregnations for neurites. In a number of examples, mature ganglion cells are found. By electron microscopy the neoplastic glial cells frequently display a pericytoplasmic basal lamina which is characteristic of subpial cerebral astrocytes. This group of tumors is in all likelihood identical with those examples, also restricted to infants, that have been described as superficial cerebral astrocytomas and are characterized by a similarly intense desmoplasia (108).

From the cytogenetic viewpoint, it is tempting to speculate that these neoplasms may be linked to foci of potential continuing neurocytogenesis located in the subpial granular layer of the cerebral hemispheres (14). In man this layer has substantially disappeared by the 8th month of intrauterine life, but remnants have been found in the frontal lobes 6 months after birth. The massive size of these tumors, which may most conveniently be termed "desmoplastic infantile gangliogliomas," certainly points to their pre- or perinatal development. From the clinical viewpoint, their histological recognition as a distinct entity is of considerable prognostic significance because, as both series reported so far (108, 111) indicate, and as confirmed in subsequently studied new cases, successful complete or subtotal resection has, despite the voluminous size of the tumors, been followed by a favorable postoperative course: in all operated cases this has extended over several years of tumor-free survival, and several such patients are now considered to be cured. We therefore have here a type of mixed neurogliogenic tumor of early life whose biological behavior makes it much more akin to the gangliogliomas than to the less differentiated forms of embryonal CNS tumor, such as the cerebral neuroblastoma or the cerebellar medulloblastoma.

The Ependymoblastoma

This embryonal tumor (94), in which differentiation is primarily restricted to the ependymal line, is as rare as the cerebral medulloepithelioma. In the scheme of normal cytogenesis of the forebrain in the chick embryo, the period which precedes the acquisition, by the residual primitive ventricular cells, of the differentiating features characteristic of ependymocytes is about 8 days (30, 34), i.e., equal to the length of time postulated to exist for the replicating undifferentiated cells of the primitive neural tube. Thus the window of neoplastic vulnerability would be expected to be about equally narrow for the cells which give rise to the cerebral medulloepithelioma and to the ependymoblastoma, respectively.

The Astroblastoma

In its pure form, this is a very rare, unusually well-circumscribed glioma of young subjects, characterized by a perivascular arrangement of the tumor cells. We recently reported on the pathological features of 23 such examples, examined by us over the last three decades, with a postoperative follow-up being available in 13 patients (10). Two such tumors were studied by electron microscopy and immunohistochemistry, one of them having been maintained in vitro in an organ culture matrix system up to 8 months (92). This study revealed in the tumor cells fine structural characteristics intermediate between those of astrocytes and ependymocytes. They recapitulated the structure of the tanycyte, a glial precursor cell which is normally found scattered along the ependymal lining of the embryonal and neonatal mammalian brain, but is distinct from epithelial ependymocytes (82). The migratory path of cells derived from tanycytes, and their subsequent line of differentiation, are disputed, but, in any event, the tanycyte of higher mammals represents only a transitory phase in central nervous system ontogeny. The hypothesis of its being the cell of origin of some astroblastomas would account for a number of characteristics in this enigmatic form of glioma: the usual paraventricular and subcortical localization of the tumor; the presence of fine structural features that are intermediary between those of astrocytes and ependymocytes; and the frequency with which the tumor may be confused with an ependymoma. The great rarity of the astroblastoma could be explained by the fact that, since the tanycytes may only briefly be present in central neuroepithelial ontogeny, the number of such replicating cells vulnerable to neoplastic transformation must be very small (92).

EXAMPLES OF CNS TUMORS WITH A WIDE WINDOW OF NEOPLASTIC VULNERABILITY

The Cerebellar Medulloblastoma

The well-known fact that this tumor is by far the most common of the embryonal CNS neoplasms must reasonably be linked to the much longer period of time during which germinative precursor cells remain mitotically active in that part of the central neuraxis. Such a period extends from most of the time of fetal life up to the end of the first postnatal year, taking into account that the cells of the fetal external granular layer, especially those of its outer zone, continue to replicate as they migrate to help in the formation of the internal granular layer (32, 71, 88, 109). Some of the germinative cells at risk are presumably undifferentiated and still uncommitted; others are already committed to the glial or the neuronal line, and others again are potentially capable of expressing divergent differentiation if given enough time to do so. These differences in the maturation potential of phenotypically similar primitive cell populations easily explain the variability in differentiating potential of medulloblastomas in situ (89, 90) and the results obtained in tissue culture conditions that favor the development of differentiation features (37, 94).

The hypothesis that the cells of the fetal external granular layer are a possible source of origin of some cerebellar medulloblastomas is based partly on morphological similarities, partly on experimental inferences, and partly on the exceptional documentation of the neoplastic proliferation of these cells in man in association with a congenital medulloblastoma (49). Since the publication of that observation, we have seen two further examples in which an abnormal proliferation of the cells of that layer was associated with a neuroepithelial tumor of the cerebellum (94). Another congenital instance in a neonate has been reported (3). Other histogenetic sites, especially primitive germinative cells in the posterior medullary velum (85), are likely to be at least as important. Indeed, the respective mean ages of incidence of the two chief types of medulloblastoma—classical and desmoplastic (17, 52, 93)—suggest that in the developing cerebellum the width of the window may vary at different sites according to the cytogenetic timetable. The hemispheric, and often desmoplastic, medulloblastomas, which are found most frequently in adolescents and young adults, may preferentially have originated from a neoplastic transformation of the cells of the fetal granular layer, whereas the midline medulloblastomas (which are more apt to be seen in patients in the first decade of life) are more likely to have arisen from cells of the primitive germinal bud in the roof of the fourth ventricle, i.e., at an earlier stage of morphogenesis. Such a generalization linking the localization of cerebellar medulloblastomas, their histological patterns and their respective clinical ages of incidence, is not, however, invariable. It seems at any rate, that, as shown by their immunoreactivity to a series of well-characterized monoclonal antibodies, the reticulin-free structures of desmoplastic medulloblastomas constitute cellular foci which display predominantly neuroblastic and, to a lesser degree, astroglial differentiation (52).

One of the difficulties that impede the study of the medulloblastoma is the relative rarity of animal experimental models, especially the common failure to produce cerebellar medulloblastomas after the injection of alkylating agents. The most consistent results so far have been obtained with the inoculation at birth of Syrian hamsters with the JC strain of human polyomavirus (77, 126, 127). An important contribution of this model has been the observation that, whereas the transformed cells are presumably those of the still mitotically active cells of the fetal granular layer—as inferred from the detection of T antigen in these cells 5 days after viral inoculation (77)—the tumors themselves, when examined, appear to originate microscopically from the internal granular layer.

The bipotential differentiating capacity of the medulloblastoma, which is convincingly demonstrated in vitro (94), suggests that it may also have arisen from a primitive neuroepithelial cell capable of two-directional differentiation and therefore expressing an earlier stage of ontogeny than those cells of the external granular layer which are already committed to become internal granular neurons. This would be consistent with the postulate that the window of neoplastic vulnerability for this tumor may be open at almost any stage of fetal development. Such an assumption is supported by a study performed on two children, aged respectively 5 years and 4 months at the time of operation, in whom the respective growth rates of the tumors were measured by consecutive CT scans and the DNA of the neoplastic cells quantified by cytofluorometry (41). Extrapolation of the growth curves suggested—assuming that in both cases tumor growth was exponentially linear throughout—that the tumors had their inception between the 14th and 23rd week of intrauterine life. The mean of that range, i.e., shortly before midgestation, corresponds in man to the events occurring between the 3rd and 18th postnatal days in the developing cerebellum of rodents, therefore to the time of maximal activity in the migration and differentiation of the cells of the fetal external granular layer.

Astrocytomas, Oligodendrogliomas, and Mixed Astrocytomas and Oligodendrogliomas

Since gliomas of adult-cell type, in particular of the astrocytic series—including here their anaplastic forms up to and including glioblastomas—are the most frequent types of CNS tumor, the window of neoplastic vulnerability is widest in regard to the astroglia. It seems that a modest turnover of glial cells is to some extent maintained in postnatal life and it is apparent that mature astrocytes will reenter the cycle following the appropriate stimulus. Another factor is the relatively long span of time during which embryonal glial precursor cells in their almost terminal stage of differentiation—and in which the range of their differentiating potential has therefore become correspondingly restricted—may be exposed to the events which result in transformation. Reference has already been made to studies in the fetal primate brain according to which the window for glia-committed cells is already open before midgestation (62, 63). The window could be open even earlier in development in respect to the embryonal glia, since GFA protein-positive radial glia, which have been postulated to be responsible for guiding developing neurons in their migration, already make their appearance in the first third of intrauterine life (19, 22, 64). In the rhesus, the radial glia enter a period of amitosis in midgestation (98) and the window then becomes temporarily closed, but it reopens again in later fetal life, when these cells reenter the mitotic cycle and become converted into mature protoplasmic and fibrillary astrocytes (18). In the rodent brain there is abundant evidence, from the experimental transplacental injection of single low doses of ENU (84) and the intracerebral inoculation of RNA oncogenic viruses (113), that a highly susceptible target for transformation is the migrating subependymal glial precursor cells whose progeny are presumed to differentiate into astrocytes and oligodendrocytes. The subependymal layer remains the major postnatal source of proliferating glial cells and presumably of glial replacement, a situation that has been shown to persist throughout life in the rodent (65) and has been inferred to occur also in the adult primate (50).

Secondly, away from the subependymal layer, a massive turnover of glial cells takes place in early postnatal life corresponding to the time of myelinogenesis, thus resulting in a marked increase first of astrocytes and later oligodendrocytes (65). Here too, the embryonal radial glia may play a part at a relatively early stage of development, since there is evidence that they give rise to both astrocytes and oligodendroglia (40). At the time of myelinogenesis some of the radial glia convert into myelin-forming oligodendrocytes (21). The process perhaps continues, but to a greatly diminished extent, throughout life (65). If the neoplastic "hit" corresponds to the crucial period when glial precursor cells are about to give rise to divergently differentiating astrocytic and oligodendroglial populations, the frequency of mixed astrocytomas and oligodendrogliomas in both human and experimental CNS tumors then becomes readily understandable. Indeed it is our experience that mixed astrocytomas and oligodendrogliomas are far more common than the figures on the relative incidence of the different glioma types available up until now seem to indicate. The majority of the gliomas which for convenience are classified as oligodendrogliomas are admixed with neoplastic astrocytes, and an oligodendrogliomatous component is frequently present in both the cerebral and cerebellar forms of astrocytoma. In addition, as noted above, typical oligodendrocytic tumor cells have now been repeatedly demonstrated to contain GFA protein (94) and this may perhaps be correlated with the fact that, in man, immature oligodendrocytes may transiently express GFA protein immediately before myelinogenesis (20).

In later postnatal life, i.e., after puberty, labeling experiments in the rhesus monkey have shown that astrocytes are virtually the only neuroepithelial cell types in the CNS that remain in the mitotic cycle (87). Although there is evidence that in mice mature oligodendrocytes too are capable of proliferation after trauma (68) and demyelination (6), in the normal primate brain the proliferating capacity of oligodendrocytes has been demonstrated to be largely restricted to prepubertal animals, predominantly in the white matter of the forebrain and in the pyramidal tracts, i.e., at sites of active myelination (87). The evidence for an active role of oligodendrocytes in the remyelination of the CNS in man is still indirect (33). Thus the ontogenetic and kinetic data, when considered collectively, account for the considerably higher frequency of astrocytic over oligodendrocytic gliomas in man, for the large incidence of mixed gliomas composed of astrocytes, oligodendrocytes, and intermediate cell forms, for the apparently aberrant expression of astroglial protein in neoplastic oligodendroglia, and for the fact that these are the two cell types most often in question when diagnostic and prognostic problems are raised in a differentiated glioma of mixed composition.

In the context of the present discussion, the glioblastoma represents the progression, through a variable span of time, but usually with a fairly rapid course, of anaplasia from an astrocytoma, more rarely from an oligodendroglioma, and rather often from a mixed astrocytoma and oligodendroglioma. In kinetic terms, it results from the recruitment of tumor cells from the nonproliferating to the proliferating cell pool, with a consequent increase of the growth fraction, followed by the development of preferentially selected clonogenic subpopulations which emerge so as to constitute the dominant proliferating populations (94). In the course of this progression, abnormal cell products may be synthesized, as mentioned above, or structural cellular features may appear which may even be quite unrelated to normal gliocytogenesis. Thus, adenoid-like formations resembling ducts and glands of adenocarcinoma, but which are demonstrably of astrocytic origin, may be found in glioblastoma and especially in gliosarcoma (53); papillary formations, mimicking medulloepithelioma, may be seen in both glioblastoma and gliosarcoma (74), and even squamous differentiation, with the development of epithelial whorls, keratin pearls and immunopositivity for cytokeratin—thus representing an extreme form of epithelial metaplasia in a malignant glioma—have been demonstrated in both tumor types (75).

Analysis of astrocytomas and glioblastomas by restriction fragment length polymorphisms suggests that anaplastic progression may be the result of the clonal expression of a cell population that shows loss of constitutional heterozygosity for loci at a specific chromosome. Thus, loss of alleles on chromosome 17p has been found to be the most frequent chromosomal aberration associated with astrocytomas, irrespective of their grade of malignancy (46), whereas loss of chromosome 10 sequences seems to be restricted to the stage of glioblastoma (45).

NEOPLASTIC VULNERABILITY OF GLIAL CELLS IN RELATION TO EVENTS OCCURRING IN POSTNATAL LIFE

In contrast to the experimental production of neural tumors by transplacental carcinogenesis, no decisive information is available so far on any epigenetic event or events that would either initiate or precipitate, in prenatal life, the spontaneous development of central neuroepithelial tumors in man, although various suggestions have been made on the possible roles of parental occupation and of intrauterine exposure to barbiturates or nitrosamine-containing substances (94). Besides the sites and periods of CNS myelinogenesis that are normally associated with increased postnatal gliocytogenesis, the question also arises to what extent the concept of the window of neoplastic vulnerability should take into account some of the other postnatal events that may induce astrocytes in the G_0 phase to reenter the cycle. These postnatal events of an exogenous nature are few and their implications may have only relative significance.

Progressive Multifocal Leukoencephalopathy

The experimental neurooncogenic properties of the strains of human polyomavirus causing progressive multifocal leukoencephalopathy (PML) are well-known (94), and so are the characteristic cytological appearances of the "transformed" astrocytes in the human disease. Although the demonstration of polyomavirus-related nucleic acid sequences and tumor antigens has been reported in a number of human neural tumors (94), the actual development of gliomas in the centers of the demyelinating lesions of PML has so far been limited to two well-documented reports (16, 101). However, it is of significance that in both instances the astrocytomas were multiple. That the JC strain of human polyomavirus is potentially capable of transforming human astrocytes is likely, and has indeed been documented in long-term primary cultures from the brain tissue of two patients (95), but the hypothesis that human gliomas might be due to a nonpermissive infection of astrocytes by the virus of PML is weak. In view of the prevalence, in the adult population at large, of circulating antibodies against the JC virus, this hypothesis tells us, moreover, relatively little about the neoplastic vulnerability of the human astrocyte in the adult brain.

Trauma

The development of a malignant glioma following brain injury and in conditions in which a clear connection can be established between the astrocytic proliferation implicated in cerebral scarring and subsequent neoplastic transformation remains exceptional. Rare cases of this nature include the occurrence of glioblastomas in tracts of leukotomy performed several years previously, of gliomas at the precise sites of ancient shell- or gunshot injuries, and of oligodendrogliomas in the scars of old cerebral contusions (94). These extraordinary sequelae are probably more suggestive than truly significant, but they indicate that increased glial proliferation due to any cause will expose these cells to the risk of neoplastic change.

Gliomas and Multiple Sclerosis

A condition like multiple sclerosis, in which proliferation of reactive astrocytes is a chronic response that may extend over a period of many years, possibly provides stronger evidence that their window of neoplastic vulnerability will be widened as a result. The literature up to 1981 has recorded 22 examples of the concurrence of multiple sclerosis and gliomas (94). In five of the cases, the gliomas were multiple, and in one it was diffuse. Continuity of the plaque with tumor was reported in half of the cases. It should be added that failure to demonstrate such a topographical link does not necessarily exclude it, since any such relationship might easily be obscured in the evolution of a malignant glioma. The interpretation of neoplastic transformation of the glia in areas of demyelination was advanced in six of the cases and the descriptions suggest that it might have been made in several of the others. The relatively high frequency of glioma multiplicity occurring in association with multiple sclerosis, and the demonstration that the tumors appeared in several instances to originate in the borders of plaques may simply signify that in the course of this prolonged and remitting disease a significant number of astrocytes have reentered the mitotic cycle over a sufficiently sustained period of time to render them statistically more likely to undergo neoplastic transformation.

Radiation-induced Gliomas

Rapidly increasing numbers of human malignant gliomas are being reported following radiation of the CNS for therapeutic or, occasionally, diagnostic purposes (43, 55, 94). The latency period preceding such a development has ranged from 5 to 25 years, with a mean of 11 years. Most of the tumors have been anaplastic astrocytomas or glioblastomas. The dosages of radiation delivered have varied widely, from 150 to 6000 rads. Since in most instances radiation was administered for a neoplastic condition in childhood, the great majority of the reported gliomas have developed in patients in the first three decades of life. Primary conditions for which radiation was given include notably medulloblastoma, craniopharyngioma and, in a few cases, pituitary adenoma.

Especially noteworthy is an increasingly larger group of children with previous acute lymphoblastic or lymphocytic leukemia, in whom a subsequent CNS malignancy developed following the combination of prophylactic brain radiation of 2400 rads and intrathecal methotrexate (28, 100). Such a development, which has occurred from 3 to 9 years after apparently successful cure of the leukemia, has been confirmed by us in four cases referred to us for consultation, all in patients in their second decade (28). It is of significance that in three of these patients the malignant gliomas were multifocal, as was the case in two of the patients reported by others (4, 48). The occurrence of iatrogenic gliomas needs further study to assess its frequency, to identify more closely the risk factors involved in the prophylactic treatment of the CNS in acute lymphocytic leukemia, and to determine what modifications should be envisaged in the modalities of therapy.

SUMMARY

Neuroepithelial cells in the CNS are vulnerable to neoplastic transformation as a result of the interaction of several factors: the existence of a reserve stem cell population, the capability of differentiated cells to reenter the cycle, the number of replicating cells at risk at one particular time, the length of time during which a particular cell population remains in the cycle, the state of differentiation and the further differentiation potential of that population, and the steps of differentiation through which successive cell generations are expected to progress. This concept explains many aspects of cerebral glioma incidence and the relationship of central neuroepithelial embryonal tumors to tumors of adult-cell type. The incidence of different types of central neuroepithelial tumors can be correlated with the width of the window of neoplastic vulnerability. The existence of a narrow window is illustrated by the occurrence of rare tumors such as the medulloepithelioma, the cerebral neuroblastoma, the ganglioglioma, the ependymoblastoma, and the astroblastoma. By contrast, cerebellar medulloblastomas, astrocytomas, mixed astrocytomas and oligodendrogliomas, and glioblastomas exemplify instances in which a relatively wide window of vulnerability exists in the context of cellular neuroontogeny and because of the capacity of glial cells to undergo postnatal replication. The relationship that may occasionally be established between the development of a glioma and the production of cellular gliosis such as may follow brain injury or accompany multiple sclerosis may also be viewed in the light of that concept. There is increasing awareness of the development of postradiation gliomas, especially after the apparently successful treatment of acute lymphocytic leukemia of childhood.

ACKNOWLEDGMENT

The work by the author and his colleagues, cited in this chapter, is supported in part by Research Grant CA 31271 from the National Cancer Institute, U.S. Department of Health and Human Services.

REFERENCES

1. Alitalo, K., Bornstein, P., Vaheri, A., *et al.* Biosynthesis of an unusual collagen type of human astrocytoma cells in vitro. J. Biol. Chem., *258:*2653-2661, 1983.
2. Altar, A. Development of the mammalian pineal gland. Dev. Neurosci., *5:*166–180, 1982.
3. Amacher, A.L., Torres, Q.U., and Rittenhouse, S. Congenital medulloblastoma: an inquiry into origins. Child's Nerv. Syst., *2:*262–265, 1986.
4. Anderson, J.R. and Treip, C.S. Radiation-induced intracranial neoplasms. A report of three possible cases. Cancer, *53:*426–429, 1984.
5. Anwer, U.E., Smith, T. W., DeGirolami, U., *et al.* Medulloblastoma with cartilaginous differentiation. Arch. Pathol. Lab. Med., *113:*84–88, 1989.
6. Arenella, L.S. and Herndon, R.M. Mature oligodendrocytes. Division following experimental demyelination in adult animals. Arch. Neurol., *41:*1162–1165, 1984.
7. Auer, R.N. and Becker, L.E. Cerebral medulloepithelioma with bone, cartilage, and striated muscle. Light microscopic and immunohistochemical study. J. Neuropathol. Exp. Neurol., *42:*256–267, 1983.
8. Banerjee, A.K., Sharma, B.S., Kak, V.K., *et al.* Gliosarcoma with cartilage formation. Cancer, *63:*518–523, 1989.
9. Bennett, G.S. and DiLullo, C. Expression of a neurofilament protein by the precursors of a subpopulation of ventral spinal cord neurons. Dev. Biol., *107:*94–106, 1985.
10. Bonnin, J.M. and Rubinstein, L.J. Astroblastomas. A pathological study of 23 tumors, with a postoperative follow-up in 13 patients. Neurosurgery, *25:*6–13, 1989.
11. The Boulder Committee. Embryonic vertebrate central nervous system: revised terminology. Anat. Rec., *166:*257–261, 1970.
12. Brandt, B.L., Kimes, B.W., and Klier, F.G. Development of a clonal myogenic cell line with unusual biochemical properties. J. Cell Physiol., *88:*255–275, 1976.
13. Brucher, J.M. and Ermel, A.E. Central neuroblastoma induced by transplacental administration of methylnitrosourea in Wistar-R rats. An electron microscopic study. J. Neurol., *208:*1–16, 1974.
14. Brun, A. The Subpial Granular Layer of the Foetal Cerebral Cortex in Man. Its Ontogeny and Significance in Congenital Cortical Malformations. Acta Pathol. Microbiol. Scand., (Suppl., *179*):1–98, 1965.
15. Caccamo D.V., Herman, M.M., and Rubinstein, L.J. An immunohistochemical study of the primitive and maturing elements of human cerebral medulloepitheliomas. Acta Neuropathol., *79:*248–254, 1989.
16. Castaigne, P., Rondot, P., Escourolle, R., *et al.* Leucoencéphalopathie multifocale progressive et "gliomes" multiples. Rev. Neurol., *130:*379–392, 1974.
17. Chatty, E.M. and Earle, K.M. Medulloblastoma: a report of 201 cases with emphasis on the relationship of histologic variants to survival. Cancer, *28:*977–983, 1971.
18. Choi, B.H. Radial glia of developing human fetal spinal cord: Golgi, immunohistochemical and electron microscopic study. Dev. Brain Res., *1:*249–267, 1981.
19. Choi, B.H. Prenatal gliogenesis in the developing cerebrum of the mouse. Glia, *1:*308–316, 1988.
20. Choi, B.H. and Kim, R.C. Expression of glial fibrillary acidic protein by immature oligodendroglia and its implications. J. Neuroimmunol., *8:*215–235, 1985.
21. Choi, B.H., Kim, R.C., and Lapham, L.W. Do radial glia give rise to both astroglial and oligodendroglial cells? Dev. Brain Res., *8:*119–130, 1983.
22. Choi, B.H. and Lapham, L.W. Radial glia in the human fetal cerebrum: a combined Golgi, immunofluorescent and electron microscopic study. Brain Res., *148:*295–311, 1978.
23. Clabough, J.W. Cytological aspects of pineal development in rats and hamsters. Am. J. Anat., *137:*215–230, 1973.
24. Copeland, D.D., Vogel, F.S., and Bigner, D.D. The induction of intracranial neoplasms by the inoculation of avian sarcoma virus in perinatal and adult rats. J. Neuropathol. Exp. Neurol., *34:*340–358, 1975.
25. Cruz-Sanchez, F.F., Rossi, M.L., Hughes, J.T., *et al.* Choroid plexus papillomas: an immunohistological study of 16 cases. Histopathology, *15:*61–69, 1989.
26. Dhillon, A.P., Rode, J., and Leathem, A. Neurone specific enolase: an aid to the diagnosis of melanoma and neuroblastoma. Histopathology, *6:*81–92, 1982.
27. Dickson, D.H., Ramsey, M.S., and Tonus, J.G. Synapse formation in retinoblastoma tumours. Br. J. Ophthalmol., *60:*371–375, 1976.
28. Fontana, M., Stanton, C., Pompili, A., *et al.* Late multifocal gliomas in adolescents previously treated for acute lymphoblastic leukemia. Cancer, *60:*1510–1518, 1987.

29. Foulds, L. *Neoplastic Development, vol. 1,* pp. 328–329. New York, Academic Press, 1969.
30. Fujita, H. and Fujita, S. Electron microscopic studies on the differentiation of the ependymal cells and the glioblast in the spinal cord of domestic fowl. Z. Zellforsch., *64:*262–272, 1964.
31. Fujita, S. The matrix cell and cytogenesis in the developing central nervous system. J. Comp. Neurol., *120:*37–42, 1963.
32. Fujita, S., Shimada, M., and Nakamura, T. ^{3}H-thymidine autoradiographic studies on the cell proliferation and differentiation in the external and internal granular layers of the mouse cerebellum. J. Comp. Neurol., *128:*191–208, 1966.
33. Ghatak, N.R., Leshner, R.T., Price, A.C., *et al.* Remyelination in the human central nervous system. J. Neuropathol. Exp. Neurol., *48:*507–518, 1989.
34. Glees, P. and Le Vay, S. Some electron microscopical observations on the ependymal cells of the chick embryo spinal cord. J. Hirnforsch. *6:*355–360, 1964.
35. Guéneau, G., Privat, A., Drouet, J., *et al.* Subgranular zone of the dentate gyrus of young rabbits as a secondary matrix. Dev. Neurosci., *5:*345–358, 1982.
36. Hassoun, J., Gambarelli, D., Peragut, J.C., *et al.* Specific ultrastructural markers of human pinealomas. A study of four cases. Acta Neuropathol., *62:*31–40, 1983.
37. Herman, M.M. and Rubinstein, L.J. Divergent glial and neuronal differentiation in a cerebellar medulloblastoma in an organ culture system: in vitro occurrence of synaptic ribbons. Acta Neuropathol., *65:*10–24, 1984.
38. Herrick, M.K. and Rubinstein, L.J. The cytological differentiating potential of pineal parenchymal neoplasms (true pinealomas). A clinicopathological study of 28 tumours. Brain, *102:*289–320, 1979.
39. Hethcote, H.W. and Knudson, A.G. Jr. Model for the incidence of embryonal cancers: application to retinoblastoma. Proc. Natl. Acad. Sci. USA, *75:*2453–2457, 1978.
40. Hirano, M. and Goldman, J.E. Gliogenesis in rat spinal cord: evidence for origin of astrocytes and oligodendrocytes from radial precursors. J. Neurosci. Res., *21:*155–167, 1988.
41. Hirakawa, K., Suzuki, K., Ueda, S., *et al.* Fetal origin of medulloblastoma: evidence from growth analysis of two cases. Acta Neuropathol., *70:*227–234, 1986.
42. Hollyday, M. and Hamburger, V. An autoradiographic study of the formation of the lateral motor column in the chick embryo. Brain Res., *132:*197–208, 1977.
43. Hufnagel, T.J., Kim, J.H., Lesser, R., *et al.* Malignant glioma of the optic chiasm eight years after radiotherapy for prolactinoma. Arch. Ophthalmol., *106:*1701–1705, 1988.
44. Jacobsen, P.F. and Papadimitriou, J.M. Mesenchymal differentiation of cell lines obtained from human gliomas inoculated into nude mice. Cancer, *63:*682–692, 1989.
45. James, C.D., Carlbom, E., Dumanski, J.P., *et al.* Clonal genomic alterations in glioma malignancy stages. Cancer Res., *48:*5546–5551, 1988.
46. James, C.D., Carlbom, E., Nordenskjold, M., *et al.* Mitotic recombination of chromosome 17 in astrocytomas. Proc. Natl. Acad. Sci. USA, *86:*2858–2862, 1989.
47. Jones, T.R., Ruoslahti, E., Schold, S.C., *et al.* Fibronectin and glial fibrillary acidic protein expression in normal human brain and anaplastic human gliomas. Cancer Res., *42:*168–177, 1982.
48. Judge, M.R., Eden, O.B., and O'Neill, P. Cerebral glioma after cranial prophylaxis for acute lymphoblastic leukaemia. Br. Med. J., *289:* 1038–1039, 1984.
49. Kadin, M.E., Rubinstein, L.J., and Nelson, J.S. Neonatal cerebellar medulloblastoma originating from the fetal external granular layer. J. Neuropathol. Exp. Neurol., *29:*583–600, 1970.
50. Kaplan, M.S. Proliferation of subependymal cells in the adult primate CNS: differential uptake of DNA labelled precursors. J. Hirnforsch. *23:*23–33, 1982.
51. Karch, S.B. and Urich, H. Medulloepithelioma: definition of an entity. J. Neuropathol. Exp. Neurol., *31:*27–53, 1972.
52. Katsetos, C.D., Herman, M.M., Frankfurter, A., *et al.* Cerebellar desmoplastic medulloblastomas. A further immunohistochemical characterization of the reticulin-free pale islands. Arch. Pathol. Lab. Med., *113:*1019–1029, 1989.
53. Kepes, J.J., Fulling, K.H., and Garcia J.H. The clinical significance of "adenoid" formations of neoplastic astrocytes, imitating metastatic carcinoma, in gliosarcomas. A review of five cases. Clin. Neuropathol., *1:*139–150, 1982.
54. Kepes, J.J., Rubinstein, L.J., and Chiang, H. The role of astrocytes in the formation of cartilage in gliomas. An immunohistochemical study of four cases. Am. J. Pathol., *117:*471–483, 1984.
55. Kitanaka, C., Shitara, N., Nakagomi, T., *et al.* Postradiation astrocytoma. Report of two cases. J. Neurosurg., *70:*469–474, 1989.
56. Koestner, A., Swenberg, J.A., and Wechsler, W. Transplacental production with ethylnitrosourea of neoplasms of the nervous system in Sprague-Dawley rats. Am. J. Pathol., *63:*37–56, 1971.
57. Korf, H.W., Bruce, J.A., Vistica, B.A., *et al.* Immunoreactive S-antigen in cerebrospinal fluid: a marker of pineal parenchymal tumors? J. Neurosurg., *70:*682–687, 1989.
58. Kouno, M., Kumanishi, T., Washiyama, K., *et al.* An immunohistochemical study of cytokeratin and glial fibrillary acidic protein in choroid plexus papilloma. Acta Neuropathol., *75:*317–320, 1988.
59. Langman, J. and Haden, C. Formation and mi-

gration of neuroblasts in the spinal cord of the chick embryo. J. Comp. Neurol., *138:*419–432, 1970.
60. Lee, Y., Bullard, D.E., Humphrey, P.A., *et al.* Treatment of intracranial human glioma xenografts with ^{131}I-labeled anti-tenascin monoclonal antibody 81C6. Cancer Res., *48:*2904–2910, 1988.
61. Lennon, V.A., Peterson, S., and Schubert, D. Neurectoderm markers retained in phenotypical skeletal muscle cells arising from a glial cell line. Nature, *281:*586–588, 1979.
62. Levitt, P., Cooper, M.L., and Rakic, P. Coexistence of neuronal and glial precursor cells in the cerebral ventricular zone of the fetal monkey: an ultrastructural immunoperoxidase analysis. J. Neurosci., *1:*27–39, 1981.
63. Levitt, P., Cooper, M.L., and Rakic, P. Early divergence and changing proportions of neuronal and glial precursor cells in the primate cerebral ventricular zone. Dev. Biol., *96:*472–484, 1983.
64. Levitt, P. and Rakic, P. Immunoperoxidase localization of glial fibrillary acidic protein in radial glial cells and astrocytes of the developing rhesus monkey brain. J. Comp. Neurol., *193:* 815–840, 1980.
65. Lewis, P.D. Cell proliferation in the postnatal nervous system and its relationship to the origin of gliomas. Semin. Neurol., *1:*181–187, 1981.
66. Liesi, P., Dahl, D., and Vaheri, A. Laminin is produced by early rat astrocytes in primary culture. J. Cell Biol., *96:*920–924, 1983.
67. Liesi, P., Kaakkola, S., Dahl, D., *et al.* Laminin is induced in astrocytes of adult brain by injury. EMBO Journal, *3:*683–686, 1984.
68. Ludwin, S.K. Proliferation of mature oligodendrocytes after trauma to the central nervous system. Nature, *308:*274–275, 1984.
69. Mannoji, H. and Becker, L.E. Ependymal and choroid plexus tumors. Cytokeratin and GFAP expression. Cancer, *61:*1377–1385, 1988.
70. Marangos, P.J. and Schmechel, D. The neurobiology of the brain enolases. In: *Essays in Neurochemistry and Neuropharmacology, vol. 4,* edited by M.B.H. Youdim, D.F. Lovenberg, D.F. Sharman, *et al.* pp. 211–247. New York, John Wiley & Sons, 1980.
71. Mareš, V., Lodin, Z., and Šrajer, J. The cellular kinetics of the developing mouse cerebellum. I. The generation cycle, growth fraction and rate of proliferation of the external granular layer. Brain Res., *23:*323–342, 1970.
72. Masuko, S. and Shimada, Y. Neuronal cell-surface specific antigen(s) is expressed during the terminal mitosis of cells destined to become neuroblasts. Dev. Biol., *96:*396–404, 1983.
73. McComb, R.D., Moul, J.M., and Bigner, D.D. Distribution of type VI collagen in human gliomas: comparison with fibronectin and glioma-mesenchymal matrix glycoprotein. J. Neuropathol. Exp. Neurol., *46:*623–633, 1987.
74. Mørk, S.J., Rubinstein, L.J., and Kepes, J.J. Patterns of epithelial metaplasia in malignant gliomas. I. Papillary formations mimicking medulloepithelioma. J. Neuropathol. Exp. Neurol., *47:*93–100, 1988.
75. Mørk, S.J., Rubinstein, L.J., Kepes, J.J., *et al.* Patterns of epithelial metaplasia in malignant gliomas. II. Squamous differentiation of epithelial-like formations in gliosarcomas and glioblastomas. J. Neuropathol. Exp. Neurol., *47:*101–118, 1988.
76. Mukai, N. Human adenovirus-induced embryonic neuronal tumor phenotype in rodents. In: *Progress in Neuropathology,* edited by H.M. Zimmerman, *vol. 3,* pp. 89–128. New York, Grune & Stratton, 1976.
77. Nagashima, K., Yasui, K., Kimura, J., *et al.* Induction of brain tumors by a newly isolated JC virus (Tokyo-1 strain). Am. J. Pathol., *116:*455–463, 1984.
78. Odelstad, L., Pahlman, S., Nilsson, K., *et al.* Neuron-specific enolase in relation to differentiation in human neuroblastoma. Brain Res., *224:*69–82, 1981.
79. Ogawa, K. Embryonal neuroepithelial tumors induced by human adenovirus type 12 in rodents. 2. Tumor induction in the central nervous system. Acta Neuropathol., *78:*232–244, 1989.
80. Paetau, A., Mellström, K., Westermark, B., *et al.* Mutually exclusive expression of fibronectin and glial fibrillary acidic protein in cultured brain cells. Exp. Cell Res., *129:*337–344, 1980.
81. Pesin, S.R. and Shields, J.A. Seven cases of trilateral retinoblastoma. Am. J. Ophthalmol., *107:*121–126, 1989.
82. Peters, A., Palay, S.L., and Webster, H. deF. *The Fine Structure of the Nervous System. The Neurons and Supporting Cells.* pp. 270–274. Philadelphia, Saunders, 1976.
83. Pévet, P. Secretory processes in the mammalian pinealocyte under natural and experimental conditions. Prog. Brain Res., *52:*149–192, 1979.
84. Pilkington, G.J. and Lantos, P.L. The development of experimental brain tumours. A sequential light and electron microscopy study of the subependymal plate. II. Microtumours. Acta Neuropathol., *45:*177–185, 1979.
85. Raaf, J. and Kernohan, J.W. Relation of abnormal collections of cells in posterior medullary velum of cerebellum to origin of medulloblastoma. Arch. Neurol. Psychiatry, *52:*163–169, 1944.
86. Rajewsky, M.F. Chemical carcinogenesis in the developing nervous system. In: *Theories and Models in Cellular Transformation,* edited by L. Santi and L. Zardi, pp. 156–171. London, Academic Press, 1985.
87. Rakic, P. Limits of neurogenesis in primates. Science, *227:*1054–1056, 1985.
88. Rakic, P. and Sidman, R.L. Supravital DNA

synthesis in the developing human and mouse brain. J. Neuropathol. Exp. Neurol., *27*:246–276, 1968.

89. Rubinstein, L.J. The cerebellar medulloblastoma: its origin, differentiation, morphological variants, and biological behavior. In: *Tumours of the Brain and Skull, Part III. Handbook of Clinical Neurology,* edited by P.J. Vinken and G.W. Bruyn, *vol. 18,* pp. 167–193. Amsterdam, North-Holland, 1975.
90. Rubinstein, L.J. Embryonal central neuroepithelial tumors and their differentiating potential. A cytogenetic view of a complex neurooncological problem. J. Neurosurg., *62*:795–805, 1985.
91. Rubinstein, L.J. and Herman, M.M. A light- and electron-microscopic study of a temporal-lobe ganglioglioma. J. Neurol. Sci., *16*:27–48, 1972.
92. Rubinstein, L.J. and Herman, M.M. The astroblastoma and its possible cytogenic relationship to the tanycyte. Acta Neuropathol., *78*:472–483, 1989.
93. Rubinstein, L.J. and Northfield, D.W.C. The medulloblastoma and the so-called "arachnoidal cerebellar sarcoma." A critical reexamination of a nosological problem. Brain, *87*:379–412, 1964.
94. Russell, D.S. and Rubinstein, L.J. *Pathology of Tumours of the Nervous System,* ed. 5, pp. 19, 20–24, 69, 70, 100, 104, 119, 159, 177, 234, 240, 250, 252, 258–260, 267–271, 279–289, 357, 384, 386, 391, 397, 425. Baltimore, Williams & Wilkins, 1989.
95. Sangalang, V.E. and Embil, J.A. Emergence of papovavirus in long-term cultures of astrocytes from progressive multifocal leukoencephalopathy patients. J. Neuropathol. Exp. Neurol., *43*:553–567, 1984.
96. Sasaki, A., Hirato, J., Nakazato, Y., *et al.* Immunohistochemical study of the early human fetal brain. Acta Neuropathol., *76*:128–134, 1988.
97. Schmechel, D., Marangos, P.J., and Brightman, M. Neurone-specific enolase is a molecular marker for peripheral and central neuroendocrine cells. Nature, *276*:834–836, 1978.
98. Schmechel, D.E. and Rakic, P. Arrested proliferation of radial glial cells during midgestation in rhesus monkey. Nature, *277*:303–305, 1979.
99. Seshi, B., True, L., Carter, D., *et al.* Immunohistochemical characterization of a set of monoclonal antibodies to human neuron-specific enolase. Am. J. Pathol., *131*:258–269, 1988.
100. Shapiro, S., Mealey, J. Jr., and Sartorius, C. Radiation-induced intracranial malignant gliomas. J. Neurosurg., *71*:77–82, 1989.
101. Sima, A.A.F., Finkelstein, S.D., and McLachlan, D.R. Multiple malignant astrocytomas in a patient with spontaneous progressive multifocal leukoencephalopathy. Ann. Neurol., *14*:183–188, 1983.
102. Smith, T.W. and Davidson, R.I. Medullomyoblastoma. A histologic, immunohistochemical, and ultrastructural study. Cancer, *54*:323–332, 1984.
103. Stewart, A.M., Lennox, E.L., and Sanders, B.M. Group characteristics of children with cerebral and spinal tumours. Br. J. Cancer, *28*:568–574, 1973.
104. Tada, T., Katsuyama, T., Aoki, T., *et al.* Mixed glioblastoma and sarcoma with osteoid-chondral tissue. Clin. Neuropathol., *6*:160–163, 1987.
105. Tang, T.T., Harb, J.M., Mörk, S.J., *et al.* Composite cerebral neuroblastoma and astrocytoma. A mixed central neuroepithelial tumor. Cancer, *56*:1404–1412, 1985.
106. Tapia, F.J., Polak, J.M., Barbosa, A.J.A., *et al.* Neuron-specific enolase is produced by neuroendocrine tumours. Lancet, *1*:808–811, 1981.
107. Tapscott, S.J., Bennett, G.S., and Holtzer, H. Neuronal precursor cells in the chick neural tube express neurofilament proteins. Nature, *292*: 836–838, 1981.
108. Taratuto, A.L., Monges, J., Lylyk, P., *et al.* Superficial cerebral astrocytoma attached to dura. Report of six cases in infants. Cancer, *54*:2505–2512, 1984.
109. Uzman, L.L. The histogenesis of the mouse cerebellum as studied by its tritiated thymidine uptake. J. Comp. Neurol., *114*:137–159, 1960.
110. VandenBerg, S.R., Herman, M.M., Ludwin, S.K., *et al.* An experimental mouse testicular teratoma as a model for neuroepithelial neoplasia and differentiation. I. Light microscopic and tissue and organ culture observations. Am. J. Pathol., *79*:147–168, 1975.
111. VandenBerg, S.R., May, E.E., Rubinstein, L.J., *et al.* Desmoplastic supratentorial neuroepithelial tumors of infancy with divergent differentiation potential ("desmoplastic infantile gangliogliomas"). A report on 11 cases of a distinctive embryonal tumor with favorable prognosis. J. Neurosurg., *66*:58–71, 1987.
112. Varakis, J.N. and ZuRhein, G.M. Experimental pineocytoma of the Syrian hamster induced by a human papovavirus (JC). A light and electron microscopic study. Acta Neuropathol., *35*:243–264, 1976.
113. Vick, N.A., Lin, M.J., and Bigner, D.D. The role of the subependymal plate in glial tumorigenesis. Acta Neuropathol., *40*:63–71, 1977.
114. Vinores, S.A., Bonnin, J.M., Rubinstein, L.J., *et al.* Immunohistochemical demonstration of neuron-specific enolase in neoplasms of the central nervous system and other tissues. Arch. Pathol. Lab. Med., *108*:536–540, 1984.
115. Vinores, S.A., Herman, M.M., and Rubinstein, L.J. Electron-immunocytochemical localization of neuron-specific enolase in cytoplasm and on membranes of primary and metastatic cerebral tumors and on glial filaments of glioma cells. Histopathology, *10*:891–908, 1986.

116. Vinores, S.A., Herman, M.M., and Rubinstein, L.J. Localization of neuron-specific (γγ) enolase in proliferating (supportive and neoplastic) Schwann cells. An immunohisto- and electron-immunocytochemical study of ganglioneuroblastoma and schwannomas. Histochem. J., *19:*439–448, 1987.
117. Vinores, S.A., Herman, M.M., Rubinstein, L.J., *et al.* Electron microscopic localization of neuron-specific enolase in rat and mouse brain. J. Histochem. Cytochem., *32:*1295–1302, 1984.
118. Vinores, S.A., Marangos, P.J., Bonnin, J.M., *et al.* Immunoradiometric and immunohistochemical demonstration of neuron-specific enolase in experimental rat gliomas. Cancer Res., *44:*2595–2599, 1984.
119. Wargotz, E.S., Sidawy, M.K., and Jannotta, F.S. Thorotrast-associated gliosarcoma. Including comments on thorotrast use and review of sequelae with particular reference to lesions of the central nervous system. Cancer, *62:*58–66, 1988.
120. Wechsler, W. Old and new concepts of oncogenesis in the nervous system of man and animals. Prog. Exp. Tumor Res., *17:*219–278, 1972.
121. Wick, M.R., Scheithauer, B.W., and Kovacs, K. Neuron-specific enolase in neuroendocrine tumors of the thymus, bronchus, and skin. Am. J. Clin. Pathol., *79:*703–707, 1983.
122. Willis, R.A. *The Borderland of Embryology and Pathology,* pp. 410–411. London, Butterworths, 1985.
123. Wolfe, D.E. The epiphyseal cell: an electron-microscopic study of its intercellular relationships and intracellular morphology in the pineal body of the albino rat. Prog. Brain Res., *10:*332–386, 1965.
124. Wright, W.E. Induction of muscle genes in neural cells. J. Cell Biol., *98:*427–435, 1984.
125. Zimmerman, B.L. and Tso, M.O.M. Morphologic evidence of photoreceptor differentiation of pinealocytes in the neonatal rat. J. Cell Biol., *66:*60–75, 1975.
126. ZuRhein, G.M. Studies of JC virus-induced nervous system tumors in the Syrian hamster: a review. In: *Polyomaviruses and Human Neurological Diseases,* edited by J.L. Sever and D.L. Madden, pp. 205–221. New York, Alan R. Liss, 1983.
127. ZuRhein, G.M. and Varakis, J.N. Perinatal induction of medulloblastomas in Syrian golden hamsters by a human polyoma virus (JC). Natl. Cancer Inst. Monogr., *51:*205–208, 1979.

CHAPTER 4

Neurofibromatosis as a Model for Tumor Formation in the Human Nervous System

ROBERT L. MARTUZA, M.D.

Neurofibromatosis (NF) is one of the most frequent and clinically important Mendelian disorders in humans. NF displays autosomal dominant inheritance and is associated with several of the most common tumor types found in the human nervous system including neurofibromas, acoustic neuromas, meningiomas, and astrocytomas (24, 31). The relatively high incidence of NF in the population (8, 37) and the presence of multiple tumors of various histologic types makes NF a useful model to study mechanisms of tumorigenesis within the human nervous system.

Recent advances in cancer research suggest that many tumors contain detectable abnormalities in one or more genes. Two general classes of genes have been identified to be associated with the process of neoplasia (20). The first are termed "oncogenes" which are dominantly acting genes that can cause malignancy when activated in an appropriate cell. The second class of tumor-related genes is recessive at the cellular level and has been termed an "antioncogene" or "tumor suppressor gene." In general, neoplasia results when both copies of a tumor suppressor gene are lost or inactivated. Molecular genetic studies provide evidence that both types of genes play an important role in the development of some of the most common tumors of the nervous system. For the tumors associated with NF, both types of genes may be involved. Additionally, it appears that the mechanisms elucidated for the tumors associated with NF are also associated with tumors of the same histologic type that develop sporadically as solitary neoplasms in the general population. Therefore, the study of tumorigenesis in NF has much broader implications for tumorigenesis in the nervous system in the general population (34–36).

NEUROFIBROMATOSIS

Neurofibromatosis (NF) is not a single disorder. In the past, terms such as "peripheral NF," "central NF," "disseminated NF," "von Recklinghausen's disease with acoustic neuroma," and others have been used in the literature. This has lead to much confusion. At present, two distinct forms of NF are recognized and account for most of the cases of NF. The first is termed NF-1 (von Recklinghausen NF, peripheral NF) and the second is termed NF-2 (bilateral acoustic NF, central NF). Other forms of NF may exist and broader classifications have been suggested, but these two types, NF-1 and NF-2, represent more than 95% of NF patients. If other forms exist, they are less common and at present are not characterized well enough to allow detailed study.

Both forms of NF are transmitted in an autosomal dominant manner with high penetrance (8, 31, 41). This means that if the NF gene is present, it is usually expressed as skin stigmata, eye lesions, nervous system tumors, or other abnormalities. The high penetrance also implies that a carrier state (where the gene is present, but there is no physical evidence of the disorder) is rare. At present, NF is diagnosed using a combination of physical examination, radiologic imaging, and electrophysiologic testing. Recent advances have defined the loci of the genes for NF-1 and NF-2 (1, 32, 33). Using techniques of linkage analysis within families, prenatal and presymptomatic testing is currently being performed for NF-1 and for NF-2 in certain instances. Such tests are not presently available for the individual case where no other family members are available for study; however, the cloning of these genes will soon lead to the availability of such testing even in the case of a new mutation at the NF locus.

CLINICAL FEATURES OF NF-1

NF-1 is a relatively common disorder which occurs approximately once in every 4000 births (8). Thus, NF-1 is more prevalent than several other genetic disorders of the human nervous system such as Huntington's disease, myotonic dystrophy, Duchenne-type muscular dystrophy, or Tay-Sachs disease (11). Approximately half of NF-1 patients have inherited the disorder from a parent, but the others represent new mutations. NF-1 has been noted to have a high rate of spontaneous mutation in several studies (8, 37). The reason for this is uncertain but includes the possibility that this gene is more unstable than others, is very large, or is a complex of several genes. Studies to localize and clone the NF-1 gene will allow such questions to be answered. At the time of this writing, the NF-1 gene has been localized to the proximal long arm of chromosome 17 near the centromere.

Although NF-1 is common and is highly penetrant, the expression of the gene within an individual patient is highly variable (8, 31). Within the same family, the physician may encounter one patient with severe manifestations and another with minimal stigmata. Therefore, all members of a family should be examined and a routine examination, a Wood's lamp examination of the skin, and a slit lamp examination of the iris should be included.

The most common clinical manifestations of NF-1 are seen in the skin and represent abnormal regulation or growth of cells embryologically derived from the neural crest (Schwann cells, melanocytes). Multiple cutaneous neurofibromas are the hallmark of the disorder. Patients may have variable numbers of tumors from zero to thousands. The cutaneous neurofibroma is usually absent during early childhood. Small raised skin areas typically begin to appear at or just before puberty and are first noticeable on the anterior abdominal wall. With time these develop into lesions varying in size from a few millimeters to a few centimeters. Cutaneous neurofibromas may develop anywhere but are most common in the thoracoabdominal area. They are so typical in appearance and usually invaginate when pressed that biopsy is needed for diagnosis only in the most unusual circumstances. Histologically, the cutaneous neurofibroma is primarily composed of Schwann cells admixed with varying amounts of fibroblasts, axons, mast cells, and vascular and connective tissue. The cutaneous neurofibroma can be conceptualized as a Schwann cell tumor of the distal nerve ending in the skin, but the admixture of other cellular elements has confounded some of the cellular and molecular studies on this lesion. Because cutaneous neurofibromas are often both visible and numerous, concerns about malignant degeneration are often raised. Fortunately, this is an unusual occurrence in this particular lesion.

The second common diagnostic feature of NF-1 is seen as abnormal patches of skin pigmentation. Cafe-au-lait (CAL) marks are present at birth or appear soon thereafter and therefore usually represent the earliest detectable abnormality suggesting the presence of the NF-1 gene. However, the fact that 10% of people in the normal population have at least one CAL mark may confound early diagnosis. Therefore, criteria have been suggested for the diagnosis of NF-1 based on the age of the patient as well as the size and number of CAL marks (8, 39).

Another diagnostic dilemma presented by the CAL mark of NF-1 is that it may be indistinguishable from that of Albright's disease. Prior emphasis on the shapes of the marks in these two disorders ("coast of California" vs. "coast of Maine") has not proven useful in all cases. However, histologic examination of biopsies of CAL marks have identified an intracellular abnormality termed a melanin macroglobule (MMG) (2, 17, 26, 27). Previously considered a macromelanosome and thought to represent a derangement of melanogenesis, recent ultrastructural studies suggest that the MMG is a melanin-containing autophagosome. MMG are seen in the CAL biopsies of NF-1 but not in those of Albright's syndrome or NF-2, nor in CAL marks found in the general population (2, 18). Thus, in some cases, MMG may be a useful diagnostic marker for NF-1.

MMG may represent a cellular derangement which is the phenotypic expression of the NF-1 gene. Since no other cellular marker exists for NF-1, and since melanocytes are the earliest detectable abnormality in NF-1, can be easily obtained, and can be selectively grown in culture (9, 13), the melanocyte may prove to be a useful model in the study of this disorder. Melanin serves as an easy marker for the melanocyte and can be seen as a golden color under phase microscopy or it can be more definitively identified with a DOPA stain. In culture, the morphology of the melanocyte is easily distinguished from fibroblasts and other cells. Its elongated dendrites bespeak its neural crest origin.

CAL marks are not the only pigmentary abnormality seen in NF-1. Often, a generalized increase in pigmentation or generalized freckling is noted. However, since both of these features can be induced by sun exposure in people of fair-skinned race, they are generally of little differential diagnostic usefulness. In contrast, freckling of intertriginous areas which are not drenched by the sun occurs in the NF-1 patient but not in others. Therefore, the axilla, inguinal area, buttock, and submammary region (in females) should be examined for freckling.

One of the most common diagnostic abnormalities in adult NF-1 patients is the Lisch nodule of the iris (31). This pigmented iris hamartoma is rarely present before age 6, and is present in varying degrees in late childhood and early teens, but is present in more than 90% of postpubertal patients with NF-1. Its diagnostic usefulness is underscored by an incidence of multiple Lisch nodules in the general population approaching zero. An iris slit lamp examination is generally necessary to distinguish the Lisch nodule from other more common pigmented iris lesions.

Other diagnostic features of NF-1 include developmental abnormalities of the skeletal system. Especially diagnostic are sphenoid wing dysplasia and congenital pseudoarthrosis or thinning of the tibia or other long bones. When either of these are noted, a suspicion of NF-1 should be raised. Scoliosis is prevalent enough in the general population that its sole presence is not enough to make the diagnosis of NF-1, but it may be useful as a part of the entire diagnostic picture, and it is worth detecting early because of its potential progression.

Learning disorders, poor fine motor skills, and macrocephaly appear to be associated with NF-1 in a larger percentage than is present in the remaining population, but their underlying causation is uncertain in both situations.

BENIGN NEUROLOGIC TUMORS IN NF-1

While the cutaneous neurofibromas noted above are Schwann cell tumors of the distal nerve endings, they are not generally categorized as nervous system tumors. Functionally, this is probably appropriate since although in some patients they may cause pain or itching, in most patients, they are asymptomatic, and they are never the cause of serious neurologic dysfunction. In contrast, *plexiform neurofibromas* are Schwann cell tumors admixed with fibroblasts and connective tissue which form within the major nerve trunks and can be a source of pain as well as neurologic disability. Histologically, the plexiform neurofibroma differs from the schwannoma in that the former usually has a larger proliferation of connective tissue and encases multiple axons or nerve fascicles. A complete surgical resection may, in some cases, entail resection of the nerve as well as the tumor. In contrast, the schwannoma is usually eccentric on the nerve, contains few or no detectable axons, and may generally be removed sparing the bulk of the nerve trunk. It is important to recognize that all Schwann cell tumors do not readily fit into one of these two categories and that an NF-1 patient should not be denied a surgical exploration of a deep tumor out of concern that it might be unresectable. NF-1 patients often prove to have resectable Schwann cell tumors. Most neurofibrosarcomas in the NF-1 patient appear to arise from plexiform neurofibromas and only very rarely from the cutaneous lesions. Therefore, any enlarging lesion or any lesion associated with a new onset of pain or neurologic dysfunction should be biopsied to assess the possibility of malignant degeneration.

Spinal nerve root neurofibromas are common in NF-1. Most remain asymptomatic. Although they are more commonly found in the cervical and lumbar areas than in the thoracic region and on the dorsal (sensory) root than on the ventral (motor) root, this is not invariable. The advent of magnetic resonance imaging (MRI) has allowed the noninvasive screening of NF-1 patients and early intervention for expanding lesions. Most spinal neurofibromas never grow to produce symptoms, and therefore their mere presence does not require removal.

Low grade astrocytomas of the optic pathways or of the cerebellum or brainstem occur in NF-1 in higher numbers than in the general population. Approximately 10% of patients with NF-1 have a radiologically demonstrable optic glioma or abnormality of the optic pathway. The radiologic picture of an optic glioma is so typical that biopsy is rarely required for diagnosis in the NF-1 patient. Most do not cause symptoms and may behave as hamartomas not requiring any intervention. Others may progressively grow requiring surgery and/or radiation or chemotherapy. It is not possible to predict which of these two categories will apply to a particular lesion; sequential visual and MRI studies are often helpful.

To date, karyotypes and molecular genetic studies of the benign tumors of NF-1 have not convincingly demonstrated a consistent abnormality to propose a mechanism of tumor formation in this disorder. By comparison, the mechanism of tumor formation in NF-2 is currently better understood.

CLINICAL FEATURES OF NF-2

Although NF-2 is less common (less than 1 in 100,000 births) than NF-1 (11), the progression of multiple intracranial and spinal tumors can be more neurologically devastating for the individual patient or family. NF-2 is also important to our understanding of the biology of several of the most common nervous system tumors including acoustic neuroma, meningioma, neurofibroma, and possibly some astrocytomas.

The hallmark of NF-2 is the development of bilateral acoustic neuromas. These are Schwann cell tumors of the vestibular portion of the eighth cranial nerve. Isolated cases of bilateral acoustic tumors have been known to occur for over a hundred years but prior reports often grouped them with cases of NF-1. Only recently has it been realized that NF-2 is genetically distinct from NF-1. It is important to distinguish these two forms of NF because the natural history and diagnostic and therapeutic problems differ. It is also important to distinguish the patient with bilateral acoustic neuromas from the patient with the unilateral acoustic neuroma because the latter is not genetically transmitted, tends to develop later in life, and causes fewer management problems.

The possibility of NF-2 should be raised in any of the following situations: (*a*) any person with a first degree relative (parent, child, sibling) with documented NF-2; (*b*) any child with a meningioma or Schwannoma; (*c*) any patient with an acoustic neuroma (even if presenting unilaterally) before age 30; (*d*) a patient with multiple neurologic tumors of uncertain cause; (*e*) a person in whom the possibility of NF is raised but who does not fit the standard criteria for NF-1 (e.g., no family history of NF-1 and only a few skin neurofibromas or CAL marks and no Lisch nodules).

Although skin stigmata such as CAL marks or neurofibromas may be present in some patients with NF-2, they may be subtle or even nonexistent (11, 24, 25). Therefore, the diagnosis of NF-2 can not rest solely upon physical examination. The primary diagnostic tests in screening for NF-2 are audiologic and radiologic. Anyone suspected of having NF-2 and any NF-2 family member at risk should have an audiogram with determination of word discrimination and a brain stem auditory evoked response. If these are inconclusive or if there is additional suspicion of NF-2, a radiologic imaging study of the internal auditory canals and cerebellopontine angle should be performed. If available, MRI with intravenous gadolinium enhancement is the procedure of choice since it is noninvasive and provides good visualization of small intracanalicular tumors. As more experience becomes available, this study may eliminate the need for use of audiologic tests in screening for NF-2. Ultimately a blood-DNA screening test will be used but this is not currently available for all NF-2 patients.

Ophthalmologic evaluations are worthwhile in all suspected NF-2 patients. Lisch nodules are absent in NF-2; however, presenile lens opacities have been detected in as many as half of NF-2 patients, and this may serve as a useful supplemental diagnostic marker for the presence of the gene.

In any patient in whom NF-2 is documented via any of the above tests, an MRI of the entire head and of the spine is recommended to evaluate for the presence of other central nervous system tumors. The overall treatment planning of the NF-2 patient requires consideration of the various tumors such a patient may harbor.

NEUROLOGIC TUMORS IN NF-2

Multiple central nervous system tumors are common in NF-2. While Schwann cell tumors are the most frequent, tumors of meningeal, astrocytic, and ependymal origin may also be present. The *acoustic neuroma* is the hallmark of this disorder. Three biologic features are particularly noteworthy. The first is that this tumor generally arises from one of the two vestibular branches of the eighth cranial nerve (14). This is important because it allows complete removal of small tumors or partial removal of large tumors with preservation of hearing in some cases (28). The second feature is that the cells in this tumor are almost exclusively Schwann cells. The near absence of contaminating cell populations has allowed the initial molecular genetic studies to be more easily performed in these tumors than in the more heterogeneous neurofibromas of NF-1. The third is that many acoustic neuromas in NF-2 patients are multinodular in appearance (25). This is in contrast to the smooth round appearance of most nonhereditary unilateral acoustic neuromas. This multinodularity could represent a multiclonal origin of some of these tumors.

While the usual presentation of a patient with a unilateral acoustic neuroma is in the 30s or 40s, patients with NF-2 usually become symptomatic in their teens or soon thereafter. However, the growth rate is quite variable and some patients have been first diagnosed in their 60s. The newer audiologic and radiologic techniques should provide earlier diagnosis and afford a better chance that treatment will spare hearing and facial function.

Spinal nerve root neurofibromas occur in both NF-1 and in NF-2. They are often multiple and their diagnosis and indications for treatment are similar in both disorders. Although radiologically often termed neurofibromas in both disorders, those that occur in NF-2 should be classified histologically as schwannomas.

Meningiomas are often multiple in NF-2. It is not uncommon to find multiple meningiomas or en plaque meningioma involving large portions of the intracranial cavity in some patients. Meningiomas may occur in the cerebellopontine angle and meningioma tissue has even been found within an acoustic neuroma in NF-2 patients. There appears to be a larger proportion of intraventricular meningiomas than is present in routine series of solitary nonhereditary meningiomas; however all of the usual locations for meningioma are also noted with NF-2.

Although optic gliomas are rare in NF-2, low grade *astrocytomas* occur in the spinal cord, brainstem, or cerebellum. Radiologically, they appear as intinsic infiltrating masses. In some cases a cystic cavity or syrinx may be present, and in others, an ependymoma or an intramedullary spinal schwannoma has been found.

MOLECULAR GENETIC STUDIES OF NF-2 TUMORS

Since NF-2 is associated with tumors that are also the most common nervous system tumors found sporadically in the general population, this disorder serves as an excellent model for the formation of several histologically different tumor types. Thus far, molecular genetic studies of acoustic neuromas and meningiomas suggest that a similar mechanism is operable in both the multiple tumors which form in the NF-2 patient as well as in solitary tumors of similar histologic type which sporadically form in the general population (34–36). Similar mechanisms may also exist for spinal neurofibromas and astrocytomas.

Karyotypes of sporadic meningiomas in the general population had been shown to commonly be associated with loss of one copy of chromosome 22 (42). Since meningiomas commonly occur and are often multiple in patients with NF-2, we initially hypothesized that tumorigenesis in NF-2 might be associated with an abnormality on chromosome 22. For the intial tumor studies, acoustic neuromas were chosen because of their relatively pure histologic cell type, because they are the hallmark of the disorder NF-2, and because they occur at a reasonable frequency in the general population to allow comparison of molecular studies of inherited acoustic neuromas with studies of sporadic tumors. However, karyotypes of cell cultures of acoustic neuromas are difficult to consistently obtain due to the relatively low mitotic rate of the Schwann cells in these slow growing benign tumors. Therefore, methods were utilized which allow the evaluation of DNA directly from the tumor using recently developed techniques for analyzing polymorphic DNA loci (6).

Polymorphic loci are randomly spaced sites within the DNA molecule that contain small mutations which do not cause disease but which do alter the pattern of digestion of the DNA by enzymes known as restriction endonucleases. Many restriction endonucleases have been isolated and each cuts the DNA at a specific location which is dependent upon the sequence of DNA base pairs at that site. For example, the enzyme HindIII makes a cut in the DNA whenever the sequence AAGCTT is present. If a mutation is present in this sequence of DNA changing it to AACCTT, the enzyme will not cut the DNA at this locus. The lack of a cut can be detected because that particular DNA fragment will then be larger than it would have been were it cut into two smaller pieces. The many fragments generated by endonuclease digestion of human DNA can be separated by size using gel electrophoresis. They are then transferred to a solid matrix such as a nylon membrane using the Southern blot technique and the specific fragment in question can be detected by annealing the matrix with a DNA probe. Such probes are purified radioactively labeled DNA fragments whose chromosomal location is usually known.

It has been estimated that a polymorphic site occurs in the human genome approximately every 500 base pairs. Using multiple restriction enzymes, polymorphic sites have now been identified on all of the human chromosomes. Since a particular base sequence may differ on the maternal and paternal copies of a particular chromosome pair, such restriction fragment length polymorphisms (RFLPs) can be used to trace transmission of a specific chromosome through multiple generations of a large family. This technique has been utilized to show that the inherited gene for NF-1 is on chromosome 17 (1, 33) and the gene for NF-2 is on chromsome 22 (32). RFLPs can also be used to demonstrate that loss or alteration of a chromosomal copy is associated with tumor formation.

In order to search for gene abnormalities in acoustic neuromas, DNA was isolated from acoustic neuromas as well as from peripheral blood leukocytes from the same patients. The leukocytes provide the control (nontumor) DNA which is used to intially study polymorphic sites in the DNA of a particular patient. If, using enzymes and probes known to detect polymorphic sites on chromosome 22, the leukocyte DNA shows two different patterns of digestion allowing differentiation of the maternal and paternal copies of a particular DNA sequence, the patient is said to show constitutional heterozygosity for that locus. In other words, the chromosome 22 inherited from the mother has a slightly different DNA base sequence from the chromosome 22 that is inherited from the father. Since these can both be detected in the normal tissue (leukocytes), an absence or change of one of the patterns in the tumor potentially will be detectable and the patient is then said to be "informative" for studies done at that locus. In contrast, if the maternal and paternal copies of a gene cannot be differentiated in the normal tissue, then studies on the tumor tissue at that particular RFLP site will be difficult to interpret for gene loss and the patient is said to be "noninformative" for study at that site.

In the initial study of acoustic neuromas, DNA was isolated from 21 patients who required acoustic neuroma tumor surgery at the Massachusetts General Hospital (35). Sixteen patients were heterozygous in their normal tissue for at least one of the three polymorphic DNA markers used and therefore were informative for studying alterations in those loci in the corresponding acoustic neuroma tumor tissue. Seven of these 16 informative cases (44%) showed loss or marked reduction in intensity of one of the two copies of the chromosome 22 marker studied. In contrast, no losses were seen when probes were utilized for multiple other chromosomes. This suggested that the acoustic neuromas were associated with a specific loss of genetic material on chromosome 22 or loss of one entire copy of chromosome 22.

Similar results were found in a study of meningiomas (34). Blood and tumor DNA were studied from 51 patients with meningiomas; 40 were constitutionally heterozygous for at least one chromosome 22 DNA marker and thus were informative for the study. Seventeen of these 40 (43%) displayed loss or marked reduction of one or several of the chromosome 22 markers. Karyotypes were performed on 14 of these 40 tumors. Seven karyotypes were abnormal with 6 showing loss of one entire copy of chromosome 22. In contrast to the acoustic neuromas, abnormalities were detected on other chromosomes, but these were less consistent than those on chromosome 22. Nonetheless, these other abnormalities are worthy of additional study and may be related to tumor growth or progression.

Most of the acoustic neuromas and meningiomas in the first two studies were of the noninherited solitary type as occur in the general population without NF-2 (34, 35). A third study focused specifically on tumors from NF-2 patients (36). This study demonstrated that loss of genes on chromosome 22 was associated with acoustic neuroma, meningioma, and spinal neurofibromas (now known to be schwannomas) in NF-2. Two additional features were noteworthy. First, in two of the acoustic neuromas tested from NF-2 patients, loss of one chromosome marker (called D22S1) was noted but no loss was noted for another marker (D22S9). Both of these markers are located on the long arm of chromosome 22, with D22S9 being located closer to the centromere (19). This finding suggested that some acoustic neuromas may be associated not with loss of an entire copy of chromosome 22 but with a much smaller deletion with a breakpoint between these two probe sites. This narrows the location of the NF-2 gene. Second, in patients with multiple tumors, the gene loss was always on the same copy of chromosome 22 in each tumor. This suggests that the remaining copy probably contains the inherited defective NF-2 gene. Linkage analysis of a large family with NF-2 has since provided direct evidence that the inherited gene in NF-2 is on chromosome 22 (32) and the combination of both linkage data and tumor data further narrows the locus of the NF-2 gene.

These studies provide a unifying model for the development of acoustic neuromas, meningiomas, and possibly some neurofibromas. It may even apply to some astrocytomas and ependymomas. We have suggested that the long arm of chromosome 22 contains a gene (or genes) in the general class of "tumor suppressor genes" or "antioncogenes" which is important in the growth control of these cells (20). Loss or inactivation of both copies of this gene are necessary for tumor formation.

This mechanism is similar to the mechanism proposed for retinoblastoma (7, 12, 21), Wilms tumor (22, 29), and some other cancers (5, 38). Retinoblastoma may be used as a well-studied example, since this eye tumor is analogous to the acoustic neuroma in that both may occur as sporadic tumors in the general population in which case they are solitary. Both may also occur as inherited tumors in which case transmission is in an autosomal dominant fashion and the tumors are usually multiple. In familial retinoblastoma, a mutation is present on the long arm of chromosome 13. An affected individual transmits this to 50% of the offspring. However, by itself, this one abnormality is not sufficient to cause the tumor. A retinoblastoma forms only when a second mutation adversely affects the normal gene on the other copy of chromosome 13, thereby inactivating both copies of what is considered to be a "tumor suppressor gene" or "antioncogene" which is important for the growth control of the retinal cells. In an analogous fashion, it is proposed that acoustic neuromas form through inactivation of both copies of a tumor suppressor gene on the long arm of chromosome 22 which appears to be important in the normal growth control of neural crest-derived cells. Therefore, in a patient in the general population, each cell contains two normal copies of this gene on chromosome 22. The occasional mutation of one of these genes during the person's life does not lead to tumor formation. A tumor forms only when both of the gene copies are lost or inactivated. The chance that two separate mutations will occur in the same cell at the same gene locus on each of the two copies of chromosome 22 is so small that such tumors are relatively uncommon in the population at large and patients with an acoustic neuroma or meningioma generally have only one tumor. In contrast, the patient with NF-2 has one of these inactivating mutations in every cell of his or her body. Thus, in NF-2, a tumor can form in one step through a mutational event of the other gene copy. Therefore, tumors are common and multiple in NF-2 patients.

This mechanism of loss or inactivation of genes on chromosome 22 has clearly been shown for meningiomas and for acoustic neuromas in both NF-2 patients as well as in these two tumor types in the general population (34–36). The same mechanism has also been shown for spinal neurofibromas in NF-2 patients (36), but studies of adequate numbers of noninherited spinal neurofibromas remain to be done. However, it is clear that a second mechanism of neurofibroma production also exists since skin, nerve, and spinal neurofibromas are common in NF-1. Genetic linkage studies of multiple families have shown that the gene for NF-1 is on chromosome 17 (1, 33). The means by which the NF-1 gene causes the tumors associated with NF-1 (neurofibroma, astrocytoma) is not yet clear. Loss of part or all of one copy of chromosome 17 has not yet been demonstrated in NF-1 tumors. This may imply that the tumors have considerable contamination with nontumor cells, or that loss of large segments of chromosome 17 are not compatible with cell survival. Alternatively, it may be that neurofibromas in NF-1 are caused not only by a different gene than those in NF-2 but that this NF-1 gene induces tumorigenesis via an entirely different mechanism than the NF-2 gene.

Studies of the development of malignant tumors (neurofibrosarcomas) have demonstrated genetic losses on chromosome 17, however, these losses have not been in the NF-1 region on the long arm, rather they are on the short arm (Seizinger *et al.*, unpublished data). Mutations in this same region have also been shown in astrocytomas (10, 15, 16) and in both cases the abnormality is in the region of the p53 gene which is a known cancer-associated gene that has been shown to be involved in human colon cancer. Thus, the formation of nervous system tumors involving Schwann cells, astrocytes, and meningeal cells appears to follow a pattern of multistep carcinogenesis as has been proposed for several other forms of cancer and the NF-1 and NF-2 genes may be important regulators of cell growth that, when deranged, play a role in the formation of nervous system tumors both in NF patients and in the population at large.

The studies in NF-1 and NF-2 will soon allow isolation and cloning of these genes. The initial benefits will be in more accurate diagnosis, presymptomatic diagnosis, and prenatal testing for NF. Ultimately, the function of each of these genes will be discovered and possible new therapies will develop. Such information should prove useful not only for families with NF-1 and NF-2 but also for the general population. As explained above, approximately half of the acoustic neuromas and meningiomas which occur in the general population have been shown to be missing genes on chromosome 22. As more probes become available, this percentage may increase since tumors caused by very small deletions may not be detectable with the currently available techniques. Additionally, it should be recognized that the NF-2 gene on chromosome 22 (and possibly the NF-1 gene on chromosome 17) may also be important in the development of gliomas in the general population. Cytogenetic studies of human gliomas have shown multiple abnormalities with loss or alteration of chromosome 22 as one of the more common defects (4, 40). Other common abnormalities include genetic losses on regions of the short arm of chromosome 17 and on chromosome 10, multiple copies of chromosome 7 associated with amplification or mutation of the gene for the epidermal growth factor receptor, and other less common changes involving the short arm of chromosome 9, and the development of marker chromosomes, homogeneously staining regions, and double minute chromosomes (3).

In summary, similar mechanisms appear to be operable both in disorders with increased genetic susceptibility to neurologic tumors as well as in the general population. Thus, the genetic mechanisms discovered for neurofibromatosis and related disorders will likely have a much broader application to the general public. These studies should prove useful to neuroscientists and geneticists for exploring a multistep model of tumorigenesis in the human nervous system and to neurologists and neurosurgeons for developing new diagnostic and therapeutic modalities.

ACKNOWLEDGMENTS

This work was supported in part by grants from NF Inc., Mass. Bay Area, and the National Institutes of Health (NS20025; NS24279).

REFERENCES

1. Barker, D., Wright, E., Nguyen, K., *et al.* Gene for von Recklinghausen neurofibromatosis is in the pericentric region of chromosome 17. Science, *236:*1100–1102, 1987.
2. Benedict, P.H., Szabo, G., Fitzpatrick, T.B., *et al.* Melanotic macules in Albright's syndrome and in neurofibromatosis. J.A.M.A., *205:*618–626, 1968.
3. Bigner, S.H., Mark, J., Bullard, D.E., *et al.* Chromosomal evolution in malignant human gliomas starts with specific and usually numerical deviations. Cancer Genet. Cytogenet., *22:*121–135, 1986.
4. Bigner, S.H., Mark, J., Mahaley, M.S., *et al.* Patterns of the early, gross chromosomal changes in malignant human gliomas. Heriditas, *101:*103–113, 1984.
5. Bodmer, W.S., Bailey, C.J., Bodmer, J., *et al.* Localization of the gene for familial adenomatous polyposis on chromosome 5. Nature, *328:*614–616, 1987.
6. Botstein, D., White, R.L., Skolnick, M., *et al.* Construction of a genetic linkage map in man using restriction fragment length polymorphisms. Am. J. Hum. Genet., *32:*314–331, 1980.
7. Cavanee, W.K., Dryja, T.P., Phillips, R.A., *et al.* Expression of recessive alleles by chromosomal mechanisms in retinoblastoma. Nature, *305:*779–784, 1983.
8. Crowe, F.W., Schull, W.J., and Neill, J.W. *A Clinical, Pathological, and Genetic Study of Neurofibromatosis.* Springfield, IL, Charles C Thomas, 1956.
9. Eisenger, M. and Marko, O. Selective proliferation of normal human melanocytes in vitro in the presence of phorbol ester and cholera toxin. Proc. Natl. Acad. Sci. USA, *79:*2018–2022, 1982.
10. El-Azouzi, M., Chung, R.Y., Farmer, G.E., *et al.* Loss of distinct regions on the short arm of chromosome 17 associated with tumorigenesis of human astrocytomas. Proc. Natl. Acad. Sci. USA, *86:*7186–7190, 1989.
11. Eldridge, R. Central neurofibromatosis with bilateral acoustic neuroma. Adv. Neurol., *29:*57–65, 1981.

12. Friend, H.S., Bernards, R., Rogeli, S., *et al.* A human DNA segment with properties of the gene that predisposes to retinoblastoma and osteosarcoma. Nature, *323:*643–646, 1986.
13. Gilchrest, B.A., Vrabel, M.A., Flynn, E., *et al.* Selective cultivation of human melanocytes from newborn and adult epidermis. J. Invest. Dermatol., *83:*370–376, 1984.
14. Hardy, M. and Crowe, S.J. Early asymptomatic acoustic tumor. Report of six cases. Arch. Surg., *32:*292–301, 1936.
15. James, C.D., Carlbom, E., Dumanski J.P., *et al.* Clonal genomic alterations in glioma malignancy stages. Cancer Res., *48:*5546–5551, 1988.
16. James, C.D., Carlbom, E., Nordenskjold, M., *et al.* Mitotic recombination of chromosome 17 in astrocytomas. Proc. Natl. Acad. Sci. USA, *86:*2858–2862, 1989.
17. Jimbow, K., Szabo, G., and Fitzpatrick, T.B. Ultrastructure of giant pigment granules (macromelanosomes) in the cutaneous pigmented macules of neurofibromatosis. J. Invest. Dermatol., *61:*300–309, 1973.
18. Johnson, B.L. and Charneco, D.R. Cafe-au-lait spot in neurofibromatosis and in normal individuals. Arch. Dermatol., *102:*442–446, 1970.
19. Kaplan, J-C., Aurias, A., Julier, C., *et al.* Human chromosome 22. J. Med. Genet., *24:*65–78, 1987.
20. Knudson, A.G., Jr. Hereditary cancer, oncogenes, and antioncogenes. Cancer Res. *45:*1437–1443, 1985.
21. Knudson, A.G., Jr., Hethcote, H.W., and Brown, B.W. Mutation childhood cancer: a probabilistic model for the incidence of retinoblastoma. Proc. Natl. Acad. Sci. USA, *72:*5116–5120, 1975.
22. Koufos, A., Hansen, M.F., Lampkin, B.C., *et al.* Loss of alleles at loci on chromosome 11 during genesis of Wilm's tumor. Nature, *309:*170–172, 1984.
23. Martuza, R.L. Genetics in neuro-oncology. Clin. Neurosurg., *31:*417–440, 1984.
24. Martuza, R.L. Neurofibromatosis and other phakomatoses. In: *Neurosurgery,* edited by R.H. Wilkins and S.S. Rengachary, pp. 511–521. New York, McGraw-Hill, 1984.
25. Martuza, R.L. and Ojemann, R.G. Bilateral acoustic neuromas: clinical aspects, pathogenesis, and treatment. Neurosurgery, *10:*1–12, 1982.
26. Martuza, R.L., Phillippe, I., Fitzpatrick, T.B., *et al.* Melanin macroglobules as a cellular marker of neurofibromatosis: A quantitative study. J. Invest. Dermatol., *85:*347–350, 1985.
27. Nakagawa, H., Hori, Y., Sato, S., *et al.* The nature and origin of the melanin macroglobule. J. Invest. Dermatol., *83:*134–139, 1984.
28. Ojemann, R.G., Levine, R.A., Montgomery, W.M., *et al.* Use of intraoperative auditory evoked potentials to preserve hearing in unilateral acoustic neuroma removal. J. Neurosurg., *61:*938–948, 1984.
29. Orkin, S.H., Goldman, D.S., and Sallan, S.E. Development of homozygosity for chromosome 11p markers in Wilm's tumuor. Nature, *309:*172–174, 1984.
30. Pearson-Webb, M.A., Kaiser-Kupfer, M.I., and Eldridge, R. Eye findings in bilateral acoustic (central) neurofibromatosis: association with presenile lens opacities and cataracts but absence of Lisch nodules. N. Engl. J. Med., *315:*1553–1554, 1986.
31. Riccardi, V.M. Von Recklinghausen neurofibromatosis. N. Engl. J. Med., *305:*1617–1627, 1981.
32. Rouleau, G.A., Wertelecki, W., Haines, J.L., *et al.* Genetic linkage of bilateral acoustic neurofibromatosis to DNA markers on chromosome 22. Nature, *329:*246–248, 1987.
33. Seizinger, B.R., Rouleau, G.A., Ozelius, L.J., *et al.* Genetic linkage of von Recklinghausen neurofibromatosis to the nerve growth factor receptor gene. Cell, *49:*589–594, 1987.
34. Seizinger, B.R., de la Monte, S., Atkins, L., *et al.* Molecular genetic approach to human meningioma: loss of genes on chromosome 22. Proc. Natl. Acad. Sci. USA, *84:*5419–5423, 1987.
35. Seizinger, B.R., Martuza, R.L., and Gusella, J.F. Loss of genes on chromosome 22 in tumorigenesis of human acoustic neuroma. Nature, *322:*644–647, 1986.
36. Seizinger, B.R., Rouleau, G., Ozelius, L.J., *et al.* Common pathogenetic mechanism for three tumor types in bilateral acoustic neurofibromatosis. Science, *236:*317–319, 1987.
37. Sergeyev, A.S. On the mutation rate of neurofibromatosis. Humangenetik, *28:*129–138, 1975.
38. Solomon, E., Voss, R., Hall, V., *et al.* Chromosome 5 allele loss in human colorectal carcinomas. Nature, *328:*616–619, 1987.
39. Whitehouse, D. Diagnostic value of the cafe-au-lait spot in children. Arch. Dis. Child., *41:*316–319, 1966.
40. Yamada, K., Kondo, T., Yoshioka, M., *et al.* Cytogenetic studies in twenty human brain tumors: association of No. 22 chromosome abnormalities with tumors of the brain. Cancer Genet. Cytogenet., *2:*293–307, 1980.
41. Young, D.F., Eldridge, R., and Gardner, W.J. Bilateral acoustic neuroma in a large kindred. J.A.M.A., *214:*347–353, 1970.
42. Zang, K.D. Cytological and cytogenetical studies on human meningioma. Cancer Genet. Cytogenet., *6:*249–274, 1982.

CHAPTER 5

Mutagenesis and DNA Repair Mechanisms

MITCHEL S. BERGER, M.D., and FRANCIS ALI-OSMAN, D.Sc.

INTRODUCTION

Mutagenesis is a complex, multistage process resulting from the molecular alteration of cellular DNA and often, but not always, leading to the expression of this damage as an abnormal phenotype in the living cell (8). Mutations may be caused by exogenous and endogenous chemicals, by physical agents, or may occur through naturally occurring processes. Chemical mutagens react with DNA either directly or after metabolic conversion to active electrophilic intermediates that interact more readily with DNA. One or more nucleotides in a DNA sequence, or a larger segment of the cellular genome may be involved in the mutational event. The induced damage to DNA, if unrepaired, has the potential to result in a fixed alteration of the DNA, i.e., mutations. A wide variety of clinically useful anticancer agents are also known mutagens.

Although cellular DNA is constantly undergoing damage, both from intracellular processes, and from environmental toxins, the cell is equipped with several mechanisms that recognize and repair these lesions, thus preventing them from becoming frank mutations. However, errors in the repair process can also occur, leading to other types of mutations (3). Thus, whether or not a mutation results depends on the extent to which the damaged DNA remains unrepaired or misrepaired. Mutagenesis, therefore, may be viewed as the result of many different types of cellular DNA damage, and the effectiveness and fidelity of the repair of these lesions by the cell.

This chapter will deal with the fundamental concepts of DNA damage and repair, and how the fine balance between the two processes is significant to the action of any potential mutagen.

Although mutations may be associated with the induction of neoplasia, this review will not involve a detailed discussion of carcinogenesis in the central nervous system (CNS). There is ample experimental evidence, using techniques such as the short term mutagenicity assay (2) to demonstrate that carcinogens are often mutagens, and vice versa. As in mutagenesis, the important event in carcinogenesis involves DNA as the principle cellular target for the carcinogen (27). Many different classes of known chemical mutagens, e.g., aromatic hydrocarbons, N-nitroso compounds, hydrazines, etc., have been shown to be CNS carcinogens and can produce brain tumors in animals. The N-nitroso compounds, especially the N-alkylnitrosoureas, have been particularly well-studied for their neurooncogenic potential (14). Their mechanism of action involves, in part, the transfer of alkyl groups to DNA. In particular, DNA alkylation at the O^6 position of guanine or the O^4 position of thymine lead to mutations and subsequently to carcinogenesis, as will be discussed later.

DNA DAMAGE AND REPAIR

Spontaneous DNA Damage

Spontaneous mutations represent a variety of DNA damage that results from intracellular events. During the normal process of semiconservative DNA replication, a purine (adenine, guanine) separates from its pyrimidine (thymine, cytosine) counterpart resulting in unwinding of the DNA double helix. Each DNA strand then serves as a template (parental DNA strand) for the synthesis of a complementary daughter strand. Errors in this DNA replicative process or, simply, limited fidelity of the replicative machinery can result in mutations. Insertion of a wrong nucleotide during the process results in base pair mismatches which are potentially mutagenic. Poor fidelity of repair of these mismatched base pairs can, in turn, be a source of mutations. Mispairings may also result from spontaneous base tautomerizations and are influenced by changes in the cellular microenvironment such as pH, ionic concentrations, and temperature (51). Additional spontaneous mutagenic events include the loss of amino groups (deamination) from bases, as well as loss (deletion) or addition (insertion) of individual purines and pyrimidines (15). Although spontaneous premutagenic DNA lesions occur constantly in cells under normal physiologic conditions, inherent cellular enzyme systems can repair them effectively. This, however, requires a high level of "fidelity" in DNA repair or synthesis (32), which, in the case of repair of mismatched DNA is dependent upon several factors such as the site of the mismatch, and the ability to recognize the incorrectly inserted nucleotide on the daughter DNA strand. The repair of base pair mismatches may also involve recombinational events in which the information for the repair is provided by an intact DNA duplex.

DNA Damage by Physical Agents

Table 5.1 provides an overview of the types of DNA damage that may be induced by various physical and chemical agents. Alteration of DNA by physical agents may affect the purine and pyrimidine bases, the N-glycosidic bond, the deoxyribose moiety, or the phosphodiester linkage. The resulting damage may result in breakage of one or both DNA strands, or in the formation of DNA monoadducts, or of intra- or interstrand crosslinks (10).

TABLE 5.1.
Kinds of Mutagen-Induced Modification to DNA[a]

Nature of Damage	Representative Mutagens
Base damage	
Cyclobutane pyrimidine dimers	UV light
Alkylation (e.g., O^6-alkylguanine, 3-alkyladenine)	β-propiolactone Alkylnitrosourea Dialkylsulfate
Covalent adducts between a base and a mutagen	Benz(*a*)anthracene *N*-acetylaminofluorene Aflatoxin
Depurination	Alkylating agents Spontaneous hydrolysis
Strand breaks	
Breaks with sugar destruction and possible base loss	X-rays
Crosslinks	
Interstrand crosslinks	Sulfur mustard Mitomycin-C Methoxypsoralen
DNA-protein crosslinks	UV light Cyclohexylnitrosourea
Intercalation	Ethidium bromide

[a] Reprinted with permission from Cleaver, J.E. Methods for studying excision repair of DNA damaged by physical and chemical mutagens. In: *Handbook of Mutagenicity Test Procedures*, edited by B.J. Kilby, M. Legator, W. Nichols, *et al.*, pp. 19–48. New York, Elsevier Scientific, 1977.

Ultraviolet (UV) Photoradiation

One of the most widely investigated DNA damaging physical agents is UV radiation. The predominant molecular product formed by the action of UV light on DNA is a cyclobutane-type intrastrand dimer between adjacent pyrimidine bases (48). Although the pyrimidine dimers are the major lesions, other DNA adducts have also been identified (12, 25). Pyrimidine dimers exert their biological effect by blocking the binding of DNA polymerase at the site of DNA replication and thus stopping the DNA replication process. To counteract the ubiquitous presence of UV radiation in the environment, an enzymatic mechanism exists within cells which, in the presence of light, can reverse the dimerization product and restore the bases to their original structure without damaging the phosphodiester bonds in the DNA "backbone." The enzyme responsible for this "photoreactivation" repair is DNA photolyase (42).

Pyrimidine dimers can also be eliminated from DNA via the excision repair process, which, in human cells, may be the more important process by which these lesions are repaired (7, 23, 39, 54, 57). Excision repair is a more complex repair process and is involved in the repair of many types of light-independent DNA damage (57).

Excision repair of pyrimidine dimers is outlined in Figure 5.1. In the initial enzymatic step, the dimer is recognized by a specific DNA endonuclease which nicks the phosphodiester bond at or near the damaged base. An exonuclease then excises the dimer, or DNA adduct, along with adjacent nucleotides. The gap at the site of the damaged DNA strand is then replaced through synthesis of a complementary polynucleotide segment using the opposite intact DNA strand as a template. This step of the DNA repair process, also referred to as repair replication (repair synthesis), is catalyzed by a DNA polymerase, and can be studied by measuring unscheduled DNA synthesis, i.e., the synthesis of DNA by cells not in the "S" phase of their growth cycle (7). A polynucleotide ligase completes the repair process by joining the newly synthesized DNA segment with its parent strand. In some cell systems, prior to the initiation of excision repair, helical DNA has to partially unwind with the help of a topoisomerase (33a).

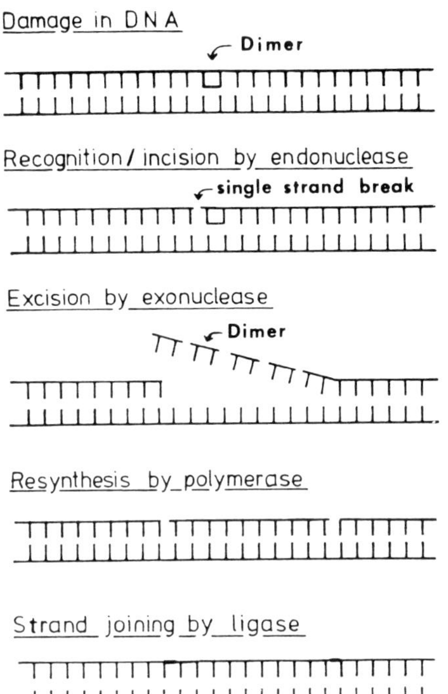

Figure 5.1. Repair process of UV-induced DNA damage. (Reprinted with permission from Anerson, D. Sub-mammalian tests other than the Ames test for mutagenesis. In: *Mutagenesis in Submammalian Systems*, edited by P.E. Paget, pp. 95–134. Baltimore, University Park Press, 1979.)

Regan and Setlow have characterized excision repair in prokaryotic cells on the basis of how many nucleotides are removed along with the lesion (40). So-called "short patch" repair refers to the removal of less than 10 nucleotides as opposed to a "long patch" in which up to 100 or more nucleotides may be excised. The long patch repair is typical of UV-induced damage and requires about 24 hours for removal of 70 to 90% of the dimers (53).

Ionizing Radiation

Ionizing radiation exerts its effect either directly on DNA or via the production of highly reactive chemical species, particularly hydroxyl radicals from water within the cell. The hydroxyl radicals and products, such as hydrogen peroxide, resulting from them, attack DNA (base, sugar, and phosphodiester), and other targets within the cell (58). The resulting DNA base modifications may be premutagenic, while DNA strand breakage can result in cell death. X-ray-induced DNA strand breaks are caused primarily by the disruption of the phosphodiester bonds of the polynucleotide chain of DNA, but may also occur through breakage of the deoxyribose ring. DNA strand breaks are easily detected with techniques such as alkaline sucrose gradient centrifugation or alkaline filter elution (21). The former exploits molecular weight differences between the fragmented DNA strands, while the latter estimates the number of strand breaks by measuring the rate at which the DNA fragments elute through a filter under alkaline, denaturing conditions.

DNA single strand breaks induced by ionizing radiation are readily repaired by DNA ligases. They may, but not always, lead to the formation of DNA double strand breaks, which are lethal if not repaired within a few hours (56). The extent and type of damage induced in cellular DNA depends upon the phase of the cell cycle the cell is in when the radiation exposure occurs. If exposure to X-rays occurs during the G^0 or G^1 part of the cell cycle, the likelihood of a chromosomal type aberration is great because of the relatively rapid DNA repair rate prior to DNA synthesis (S-phase). Preston (37) has shown that "misrepair" of the DNA damage under these conditions results in a high level of chromosomal aberrations. However, if repair of DNA damage is slow and persists into the S-phase of the cell cycle, the cell will attempt to replicate the damaged DNA, resulting in gaps in the daughter strand. Repair of these lesions is error-prone and, in turn, can lead to various mutations (17). This is in contrast to exposure of cells to ionizing radiation during the premitotic (G-2) cell cycle phase during which chromatin contains two molecules of DNA. Repair errors under these conditions result in aberrations of the chromatid structure. Both types of aberrations (chromosome and chromatid) would thus be expected to occur upon exposure of cells to x-rays during the DNA synthesis (S-phase) phase of the cell cycle.

The fact that DNA may be repaired during any stage of the cell cycle, may contribute to the radiotolerance (radioresistance) of normal cells. However, in cells with deficient DNA repair capacity, such as those of patients with ataxia telangiectasia (AT) or xeroderma pigmentosum, the repair of DNA lesions, including those induced by radiation, is impaired. Defects in genes coding for key DNA repair enzymes have been detected in cells of AT patients (35). The cells of these patients are more easily mutated than those of nonafflicted individuals, and they are more prone to developing neoplasms (24).

DNA Damage by Chemical Agents

When cells are exposed to chemical mutagens, structural alterations may develop in their DNA, RNA, proteins, and in cellular organelles such as mitochondria or the cell membrane. However, DNA represents the primary mutagenic target. Once inside the cell, the chemical compound either reacts directly with its target or is first converted to a reactive electrophile (13, 50). The subsequent reaction between the compound itself or its electrophilic intermediate with a nucleophilic site on DNA results in damaged bases. As mentioned earlier RNA, proteins and other cellular macromolecules also react with the electrophilic species. However, the resulting damaged molecules are subsequently eliminated by catabolism and are replenished by normal cellular DNA transcription and translation.

The postreplication repair referred to earlier can also be used to repair chemically induced DNA damage that has not been repaired by excision repair. In this process, the DNA strands containing the chemically damaged bases provide a faulty template for DNA replication (Fig. 5.2). The daughter strands synthesized on such templates have gaps at sites of the damaged bases in the parental strand. The gaps are then filled in with newly synthesized polynucleotide segments (23). This postreplication repair provides a mechanism by which the cell accommodates DNA damage and allows for normal DNA replication to occur regardless of the damaged bases. Post-replication repair is, however, error-prone and has mutagenic potential.

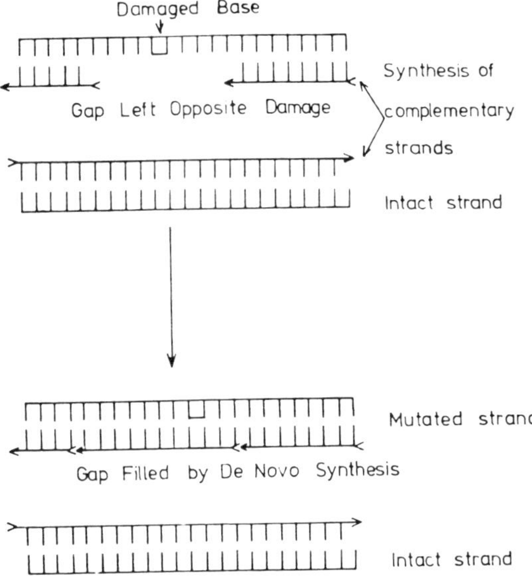

Figure 5.2. Steps involved with the postreplication repair mechanism. (Reprinted with permission from Anerson, D. Sub-mammalian tests other than the Ames test for mutagenesis. In: *Mutagenesis in Submammalian Systems*, edited by G.E. Paget, pp. 95–134. Baltimore, University Park Press, 1979.)

Alkylation, a process by which reactive alkyl groups (electrophiles) attack nucleophilic sites, particularly in DNA bases, consists of a number of events (Fig. 5.3). Alkylation of cellular proteins and RNA is not as crucial as DNA alkylation in determining the biological response of the cell, such as that expressed as mutations, chromosomal abnormalities, and malignant transformations. All four DNA bases, the deoxyribose, and the phosphodiester backbone are targets for alkylating electrophiles. The key nucleophilic sites on the bases are (41):

Adenine----N-1, N-3, N-6, N-7;
Guanine----N-1, N-2, N-3, N-7, O-6;
Cytosine----N-3, N-4, O-2; and,
Thymine----N-3, O-2, O-4.

Several factors influence which nucleophilic sites are attacked by a specific electrophile. These include the location of the site within the DNA double helix and the configuration of the DNA (20). Attack of the phosphodiester DNA "backbone" produces alkylphosphotriesters. Although these products comprise a significant amount of the entire alkylation (13), they have not been found to be mutagenic.

The alkylated bases (DNA alkyl adducts) may be lost from DNA under physiological conditions leaving base-free, apurinic or apyrimidinic (AP) sites. This results from the action of specific N-glycosylases which enzymatically hydrolyze the N-glycosidic bond between the deoxyribose sugar and the damaged purine or pyrimidine (18, 33). After formation of the AP sites, an AP en-

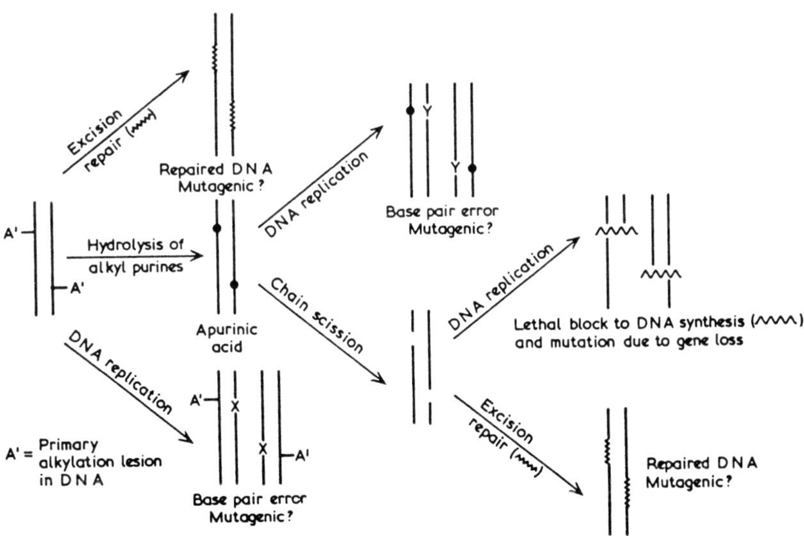

Figure 5.3. Alkylation-induced damage to DNA and its effect. (Reprinted with permission from Roberts, J.J. The repair of DNA modified by cytotoxic, mutagenic, and carcinogenic chemicals. Adv. Radiat. Biol., 7:269, 1978.)

donuclease (34) recognizes and nicks the DNA strand at that site, or, alternatively, a strand break may occur without the action of an endonuclease (30). In either case, the stages of excision repair that follow involve steps characterized by three enzymes, namely, an exonuclease, DNA polymerase, and DNA ligase (Fig. 5.4). An important component of the repair process at this point is regulation of the ligase by poly-ADP-ribose synthetase (38, 49). Although AP sites appear to be readily repaired, their persistence can result in a mutation (28).

Alkylation of the O^6-position of guanine is particularly mutagenic, since it can result in mispairing of guanine with thymine. Both eukaryotic and prokaryotic cells have a unique enzyme, O^6-alkylguanine-DNA-alkyltransferase (AT), for repairing this lesion. The AT enzyme has a cysteine at its active site and can accept the alkyl group from O^6-alkylguanine (6, 30, 36). The reaction is stoichiometric and results in irreversible loss of enzyme activity. The extent of the repair is therefore dependent upon the amount of AT protein available for acceptance of the alkyl group. If the concentration of the alkylated guanine is very high, extensive DNA damage could persist during the long time required for sufficient enzyme to be synthesized to accept the alkyl group (26). Although typically referred to as a "methyl" transferase, the AT enzyme is also able to accept other alkyl groups, such as an ethyl or a chloroethyl group, from the O^6 position of guanine (44, 47). This is particularly important since O^6-chloroethylguanine is the monoadduct precursor of the lethal DNA interstrand cross-link induced in tumor cells by the clinically active chloroethylnitrosoureas, which currently are the clinically most active agents against primary brain tumors.

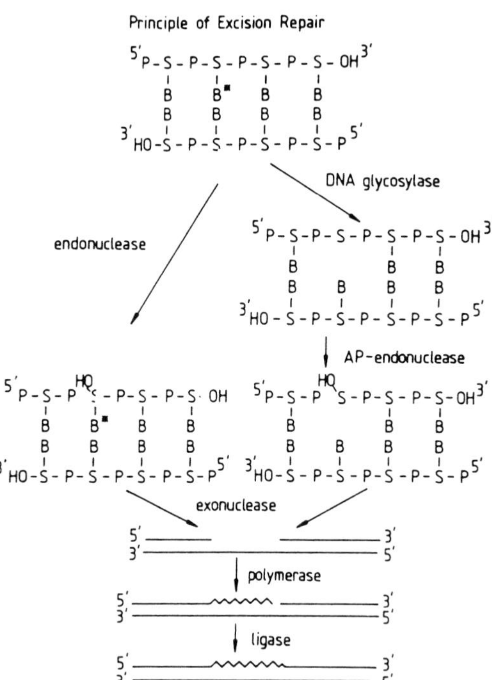

Figure 5.4. Enzymatic steps involved in the process of excision repair. (Reprinted with permission from Van Zeeland, A.A. DNA repair. In: *Mutations in Man*, edited by G. Obe, pp. 35–37. Berlin, Springer-Verlag, 1984.)

The discovery of brain tumor cells with varying ability to remove alkyl groups from the O^6-guanine positions of DNA has resulted in further investigations into this repair mechanism in the cells of CNS tumors. The MER(+) phenotype is expressed by those cells having the *M*ethyl *E*xcision *R*epair function, i.e., O^6-alkylguanine-DNA-alkyltransferase activity, as opposed to MER(−) cells which lack this activity (52, 59). Cells, however, readily adapt to the presence of O^6-alkylguanine lesions in their DNA, by generating increased amounts of the AT enzyme (46). This process of induction of the genes of repair enzymes following exposure to mutagens (9, 43) represents an important phenomenon in tumor cell drug resistance. Relative to other organ systems such as the liver, the normal brain has very little AT activity (19). Thus, normal glial cells cannot readily remove the O^6-alkylguanine DNA adducts which consequently persist for great lengths of time, after exposure of the cells to alkylating agents such as N-methylnitrosourea (22). This may explain, in part, why alkylnitrosoureas readily induce brain tumors in experimental animals. Furthermore, cells of some brain tumors that become resistant to alkylnitrosoureas would be expected to have increased alkyltransferase activity. Our laboratory (4) and those of Bodell et al. (5) have shown this to be the case in a subgroup of human brain tumors. Other non-CNS MER(−) and MER(+) tumor cell lines have also been identified (16, 45). We have also shown that pretreatment of MER(+) brain tumor cells with inhibitors of AT, such as O^6 methylguanine and streptozotocin, can result in sensitization of these cells to BCNU (4).

In the case of bifunctional alkylating agents, such as BCNU, if the first base adduct is not removed or quenched (1), it can subsequently react with DNA at an additional nucleophilic site, and a cross-link will result (13). This cross-link can occur between the two complementary DNA strands (interstrand), between adjacent bases in the same DNA strand (intrastrand), or may involve the DNA strand and a protein (DNA-protein). Bifunctional agents that have found use as anticancer agents include nitrogen mustard, melphalan, chloroethylnitrosoureas, platinum complexes, cyclophosphomide, mitomycin C, etc. Because of their cross-linking activity they are several times more cytotoxic than monofunctional alkylators (29). The cytotoxic effect of cross-linked DNA is due to its ability to block DNA replication by preventing the strands from separating and serving as templates for semiconservative DNA replication (23).

There is now increasing evidence that cells can repair DNA interstrand cross-links produced by a number of bifunctional alkylators. The process of DNA interstrand crosslink repair is, however, still not well understood, but may involve excision repair, as well as DNA recombinational events. DNA cross-link repair by recombination may be a key mechanism underlying sister chromatid exchanges observed in cells treated by alkylating agents such as BCNU (11). DNA replication proceeds in such a way that segments of intact DNA switch before and after the cross-link, resulting in an exchange between adjacent (sister) chromatids. It should also be mentioned that postreplicative mismatch repair can result in SCEs. Earlier, it was observed that, after BCNU treatment, fewer DNA interstrand crosslinks were present in BCNU resistant human glioma cells than in BCNU sensitive cells (45). This led to the conclusion that removal of the DNA monoadduct (via an alkyltransferase) *prior* to its conversion to a crosslink, rather than the repair of the cross-link itself, was the primary resistance mechanism in these tumors (31). However, most recently (55), we have provided evidence using the CAT gene transfection technique, as well as the direct assay of DNA interstrand crosslinks over time, to show that human malignant astrocytoma cells can and do repair DNA cross-links induced by BCNU.

SUMMARY

The understanding of the molecular aspects of DNA damage and the myriad types of repair mechanisms available to the cell make it apparent that the outcome of a DNA damaging event in the cell depends on the balance between these two processes.

Mutations can occur spontaneously, or be the result of DNA interactions with chemical or physical agents. Spontaneous mutations are the product of intracellular events, and range from errors of DNA synthesis and/or repair, to loss or gain of bases, and base pair mismatches. While UV light primarily causes cyclobutane dimers between adjacent bases, ionizing radiation can modify bases, or induce breakage of the DNA backbone. Chemical mutagens are generally electrophiles, or become electrophilic upon intracellular metabolism. The ability of cells to repair this wide variety of DNA damage is critical to the ultimate survival of the organism. If a cell survives DNA damage without proper repair, the resulting mutation could lead to neoplastic transformation. The upregulation of DNA repair enzymes in the resulting tumor cells can subsequently provide the cells with mechanisms with which they can become resistant to alkylating anticancer agents. These include increased activity of the enzyme, AT, in the case of cells exposed to N-alkylnitrosoureas. Most recently, the ability of brain tumor cells to repair DNA interstrand crosslinks induced by BCNU has been demonstrated. The core of all DNA damage is not only the ability or lack thereof of the cell to repair the lesions, but, most importantly, the fidelity with which these often error-prone repair processes are executed. Understanding the critical aspects of DNA damage and of the mechanisms involved in its repair is critical to understanding the fundamental processes underlying debilitating diseases such as cancer, and will provide the molecular basis to novel approaches of prevention and therapy of these diseases.

ACKNOWLEDGMENTS

This work was supported by NIH, NCI Grant CA 46410 (Dr. Ali-Osman), and NINCDS Grant NS01253-02 (Dr. Berger), and the American Cancer Society Career Development Award. The authors wish to thank Dr. Mark Rosenblum, Brain Tumor Research Center, University of California, San Francisco, for his critical comments in the preparation of this manuscript.

REFERENCES

1. Ali-Osman, F. Quenching of DNA Crosslink precursors of chloroethylnitrosoureas and attenuation of DNA interstrand crosslinking by glutathione. Cancer Res. *49:*5258–5261, 1989.
2. Ames, B.N., McCann, J., and Yamasaki, E. Methods for detecting carcinogens and mutagens with the Salmonella/mammalian-microsome mutagenicity test. Mutation Res., *31:*347–364, 1975.
3. Anderson, D. Submammalian tests other than the Ames test for mutagenesis. In: *Mutagenesis in Submammalian Systems,* edited by G.E. Paget. Baltimore, University Park Press, 1979.
4. Berger, M.S., Ali-Osman, F., and Mongan, P.J. Enhancement of DNA-DNA crosslinks and cytotoxicity induced by BCNU in a human glioblastoma cell line using a noncytotoxic O^6-alkylguanine-DNA alkyltransferase (AT) inhibitor. In: *Proceedings of the 8th Conference on Brain Tumor Research and Therapy.* Zermatt, Switzerland, 1989.
5. Bodell, W.J., Aida, T., Berger, M.S., *et al.* Increased repair of O^6-alkylguanine DNA adducts in glioma-derived human cells resistant to the cytotoxic and cytogenetic effects of 1,3-bis (2-chloroethyl)-1 nitrosourea. Carcinogenesis *7:*879–883, 1986.
6. Bogden, J.M., Eastman, A., and Bresnick, E. A system in mouse liver for the repair of O^6-methyl guanine lesions in methylated DNA. Nucleic Acids Res., *9:*3089–3103, 1981.
7. Bollum, F.J. Mammalian DNA polymerases. Prog. Nucleic Acids Res. Mol. Biol. *15:*109–144, 1975.
8. Bridges, B.A. Mutagenesis—the significance of DNA damage for man. In: *Mutagenesis in Submammalian Systems,* edited by G.E. Paget. Baltimore, University Park Press, 1979.
9. Cairns, J. Efficiency of the adaptive response of Escherichia coli to alkalating agents. Nature *286:*176–178, 1980.
10. Cleaver, J.E. Methods of staging excision repair of DNA damaged by physical and chemical mutagens. In: *Handbook of Mutagenicity Test Procedures,* edited by G.J. Kilby, M. Legator, W. Nichols, and C. Ramel. Amsterdam, Elsevier Scientific Publishing, 1977.
11. Cole, R.S. Repair of DNA containing interstrand crosslinks in Escherichia *coli:* sequential excision and recombination. Proc. Natl. Acad. Sci. USA, *70:*1064–1068.
12. Demple, B. and Linn, S. 5-6 Saturated thymine lesions in DNA: production by ultraviolet light or hydrogen peroxide. Nucleic Acids Res., *10:*3781–3789, 1982.
13. Doerjer, G., Bedell, M.A., and Oesch, F. DNA adducts and their biological relevance. In: *Mutations in Man,* edited by G. Obe, Springer-Verlag, 1984.
14. Drukrey, H. Specific carcinogenic and teratogenic effects of "indirect" alkylating methyl and ethyl compounds and their dependency on styles of ontogenic developments. Xenobiotica, *3:*271–303, 1973.
15. Duncan, B.K. and Miller, J.H. Mutagenic deamination of cytosine residues in DNA. Nature, *287:*560–561, 1980.
16. Erickson, L.C., Laurent, G., Sharkey, N.A., *et al.* DNA crosslinking and monoadduct repair in nitrosourea-treated human tumor cells. Nature, *288:*727–29, 1980.
17. Evans, H.J. Molecular mechanisms in the induction of chromosome aberrations. In: *Progress in Genetic Toxicology,* edited by D. Scott, B.A. Bridges, F.H. Sobels, Amsterdam, Elsevier Biomedical, 1977.
18. Evensen, G. and Seeberg, E. Adaptation to alkylation resistance involves the induction of a DNA glycosylase. Nature *296:*773–775, 1982.
19. Friedberg, E.C. DNA repair by reversal of damage. In: *DNA Repair.* New York, W.H. Freeman, 1985.
20. Friedberg, E.D. DNA damage. In: *DNA Repair,* pp. 1–77. New York, W.H. Freeman, 1985.
21. Friedby, E. and Hanawalt, P., eds. *Measurement of Strand Breaks and Crosslinks by Alkaline Elution. Part B,* pp. 329–401. New York, B.C. Decker, 1979.
22. Goth, R. and Rajewsky, M.F. Persistence of O^6 ethylguanine in rat brain DNA: correlation with nervous system specific carcinogenesis by ethylnitrosourea. Proc. Natl. Acad. Sci., *71:*639–643, 1974.
23. Hanawalt, P.C., Cooper, P.K., Ganesan, A.K., *et al.* DNA repair in bacteria and mammalian cells. Annu. Rev. Biochem., edited by E.E. Snell, *48:*783–836, 1979.
24. Harnden, D.G. and Taylor, A.M.R. The effects of radiation on the chromosomes of patients susceptible to cancer. In: *Mutagen Induced Chromosome Damage in Man,* edited by H.T. Evans, D.C. Lloyd, Edinburgh, Edinburgh University Press, 1978.

25. Kittler, L. and Lober, G. Photochemistry of the nucleic acids. Photochem. Photobiol. Rev., *2:*39–131, 1977.
26. Kleihues, P., Doerjer, G., Keefer, L.K., *et al.* Correlation of DNA methylation by methyl acetoxymethyl nitrosamine with organ-specific carcinogenicity in rats. Cancer Res., *39:*5136–5140, 1979.
27. Kleihues, P., Patzschike, K., and Doerjer, G. DNA modification and repair in the experimental induction of nervous system tumors by chemical carcinogens. Ann. NY Acad. Sci., *381:*1982.
28. Kunkel, T.A., Shearman, C.W., and Loeb, L.A. Mutagenesis in vitro by depurination of Phi-x 174 DNA. Nature *291:*349–351, 1981.
29. Lawley, P.D. and Brooke, P. Interstrand crosslinking of DNA by difunctional alkylating agents. J. Mol. Biol. *25:*143–160, 1967.
30. Lindahl, T. DNA repair enzymes. Ann. Rev. Biochem., *51:*61–87, 1982.
31. Lindahl, T., Sedgwick, B., Demple, B., *et al.* Enzymology and regulation of the adaptive response to alkylating agents. In: *Cellular Response to DNA Damage,* edited by E.C. Friedberg and B.A. Bridges, pp. 241–253. New York, Alan Liss, 1983.
32. Loeb, L.A. and Kunkel, T.A. Fidelity of DNA synthesis. Annu. Rev. Biochem., *51:*429–457, 1982.
33. Margison, G.P. and Pegg, A.E. Enzymatic release of 7-methyl guanine from methylated DNA by rodent liver extracts. Proc. Natl. Acad. Sci. USA, *78:*861–865, 1981.
33a. Mattern, M.A., Paone, R.F., and Day, R.S. III. Eukaryotic DNA repair is blocked at different steps by inhibitors of DNA topoisomerases and of DNA polymerases alpha and beta. Biochem. Biophys. Acta, *697:*6–13, 1982.
34. Mosbaugh, D.W. and Linn, S. Further characterization of human fibroblast apurinic/apyrimidinic DNA endonucleases: the definition of 2 mechanistic classes of enzymes. J. Biol. Chem., *255:*11743–11752, 1980.
35. Paterson, M.L., Smith, B.P., Lohman, P.H.M., *et al.* Defective excision repair of gamma-ray-damaged DNA in human (ataxia telangiectasia) fibroblasts. Nature, *260:*444–447, 1976.
36. Pegg, A.E., Roberfroid, M., Von Bahr, C., *et al.* Removal of O^6-methylguanine from DNA by human liver fractions. Proc. Natl. Acad. Sci., *79:*5162–5165, 1982.
37. Preston, R.J. DNA repair and chromosome aberrations: interactive effects of radiation and chemicals. In: *DNA Repair, Chromosome Alterations and Chromatin Structure,* edited by A.J. Natarajian, G. Obe, H. Altman. Amsterdam, Elsevier Biomedical, 1982.
38. Purnell, M.R. and Whish, W.J.D. Novel inhibitors of poly (ADP-ribose) synthetase. Biochem. J., *185:*775–777, 1980.
39. Rasmussen, R.E. and Painter, R.B. Evidence for repair of ultraviolet damaged DNA in cultured mammalian cells. Nature, *203:*1360–1362, 1964.
40. Regan, J.D. and Setlow, R.B. Two forms of repair in DNA of human cells damaged by chemical carcinogens and mutagens. Cancer Res., *34:*3318–3325, 1974.
41. Roberts, J.J. The repair of DNA modified by cytotoxic, mutagenic, and carcinogenic chemicals. Adv. Radiat. Biol., *7:*211–436, 1978.
42. Rupert, C.S. and Harm, W. Reactivation after photobiological damage. Adv. Radiat. Biol. *2:*1–81, 1966.
43. Samson, L. and Cairns, J. A new pathway for DNA repair in *Escherichia coli.* Nature, *267:*281–283, 1977.
44. Schendel, P.F., Robins, P.E. Repair of O^6-methyl guanine in adapted *Escherichia coli.* Proc. Natl. Acad. Sci., *75:*6017–6020, 1978.
45. Scudiero, D.A., Meyer, S.A., Clatterbuck, B.E., *et al.* Sensitivity of human cell strains having different abilities to repair O^6-methylguanine in DNA to inactivation by alkylating agents including chloroethylnitrosoureas. Cancer Res. *44:*2467–2474, 1984.
46. Sedgwick, B. Genetic mapping of ada and adc mutations affecting the adaptive response of *Escherichia coli* to alkylating agents. J. Bacteriol., *150:*984–988, 1982.
47. Sedgwick, B. and Lindahl, T. A common mechanism for repair of O^6-methylguanine and O^6 ethylguanine in DNA. J. Mol. Biol., *154:*169–175, 1982.
48. Setlow, R.B. Cyclobutane-type pyrimidine dimers in polynucleotides. Science *153:*379–386, 1966.
49. Shall, S., Durkacz, B., Ellis, D., *et al.* (ADP ribose) a new component in DNA repair. In: *Chromosome Damage and Repair,* edited by E. Seeberg and K. Kleppe. New York, Plenum Press, 1981.
50. Singer, B. The chemical effects of nucleic acid alkylation and their relation to mutagenesis and carcinogenesis. Prog. Nucleic Acid Res. Mol. Biol. *15:*219–284, 1975.
51. Singer, B. and Kresmierek, J.T. Chemical mutagenesis. Annu. Rev. Biochem. *51:*655–693, 1982.
52. Skler, R. and Strauss, B. Removal of O^6-methylguanine from DNA of normal and xeroderma pigmentosum derived lymphoblastoid lines. Nature, *289:*417–420, 1981.
53. Smith, C.A. Removal of T4 endonuclease V sensitive sites and repair replication in confluent human diploid fibroblasts. In: *DNA Repair Mechanisms,* edited by Hanawalt, Friedberg, and Fox. New York, Academic Press, 1978.
54. Soderhall, S. and Lindahl, T. DNA ligases of eukaryotes (FEBS) Lett. Fed. Europ. Biochem. Soc. *67:*1–8, 1976.
55. Sriram, R. and Ali-Osman, F. Repair of DNA interstrand crosslinks induced by 1,3-bis(2-chlorethyl)-1-nitrosourea in human brain tumor cells. Biochem Pharmacol., in press, 1990.
56. Van der Schans, G.P., Centen, H.B., and Lohman, P.H.M. DNA lesions induced by ionizing radiation. In: *DNA Repair, Chromosome Alteration and Chromatin Structure,* edited by

A.J. Natarajian, G. Obe, H. Altman. Amsterdam, Elsevier Biomedical, 1982.
57. Van Zeeland, A.A. DNA repair. In: *Mutations in Man*, edited by G. Obe. Berlin, Springer-Verlag, 1984.
58. Ward, J.F. Molecular mechanisms of radiation induced damage to nucleic acids. Adv. Radiat. Biol. *5*:181–239, 1975.
59. Yarosh, D.B., Foote, R.S., Mitra, S., *et al.* Repair of O[6]-methylguanine in DNA by demethylation is lacking in Mer(−)human tumor cell strains. Carcinogenesis, *4*:199–205, 1983.

CHAPTER 6

Trauma and Demyelination as Etiologic Factors in the Development of Brain Tumor

ROBERT A. MORANTZ, M.D.

Given mankind's inherent tendency to ascribe a causal role to memorable antecedent events, it is not at all surprising that both head trauma and demyelinating disease have been considered as etiologic agents in the development of brain tumor. In fact, the relationship between head trauma and brain tumor has been an area of controversy since the beginnings of neurology and neurosurgery. As early as 1888, Byron Bramwell (5) considered that "... amongst the more direct causes (of brain tumors) injury occupies an important place." During the ensuing century this topic has continued to surface at various times in the medical literature, and as yet no completely clear resolution of the issue is possible. In this chapter, we shall discuss both the clinical and experimental evidence for these two factors as etiologic agents and attempt to come to some tentative conclusions.

Before reviewing the clinical reports, however, we must first summarize some general concepts of carcinogenesis that may be relevant to the issue at hand. It is widely accepted that there are various factors or agents that can modify the tendency to form a neoplasm. Such modifying factors may cause inhibition or augmentation of carcinogenesis. Inhibition could be expressed as a reduction in the tumor yield or lengthening of the latency period between exposure to the carcinogenic agent and production of the tumor. Conversely, an augmenting or cocarcinogenic agent would be any agent that would enhance the response to the carcinogenic stimulus, so that tumors would arise earlier, or in greater numbers, or would be more likely to be malignant. More than 35 years ago the concept of carcinogenesis as a two-stage process was formulated. According to this view, "carcinogenesis is composed of an initiating process, responsible for the conversion of normal cells into latent tumor cells, and a promoting process whereby these latent tumor cells are made to develop into actual tumors" (18). More recently, our emphasis has shifted to the possible role of (viral) oncogenes as the cause of experimental and human neoplasia. Looked at in this manner, a promoting agent could be any factor that causes the activation or expression of these oncogenes at a particular time.

Most of the early experimental research on two-stage carcinogenesis was carried out using skin as the target organ (14). In general, if a promoting agent such as croton oil is repeatedly applied to mouse skin, the incidence of skin tumors will be significantly greater in animals receiving this treatment in conjunction with a carcinogen (such as benzypyrene or urethane) than in animals receiving the carcinogen alone. In addition, if the animals are treated with croton oil *be-*

fore they have been exposed to the carcinogen, there will be no demonstrable effect on tumor yield, whereas exposure to croton oil after the carcinogen will cause a dramatic increase in tumor incidence (45).

Many attempts have been made to apply the two-stage concept of carcinogenesis to other organs. In spite of the technical difficulties in carrying out these experiments, evidence in favor of a two-stage process of carcinogenesis has been reported in the liver (20), thyroid (27), mammary gland (31), as well as in other organs (23). Whether such a process can occur in the central nervous system (CNS) is unknown, although a similar schema has been proposed to explain the connection between trauma and brain neoplasia. According to this hypothesis, for brain tumors to arise, "There must be both a general carcinogenic factor and a local stimulus, such as trauma, that would produce a local alteration in brain tissue" (17). Based upon experience in other experimental systems, this local change would almost certainly become manifest as cellular hyperplasia, such as the reactive glial proliferation that occurs secondary to a cerebral traumatic injury or focus of demyelination.

There is a large body of experimental literature dealing with "foreign body tumorigenesis," which may in some instances be relevant to the situation under study. In these experiments, sarcomas are routinely produced in rodents by the subcutaneous implantation of a foreign material, such as plastic or glass (6). In this model, the induction of tumors is dependent upon cellular proliferation and infiltration, as well as on the presence of a fibrotic reaction around the foreign body. Experimental data has indicated that the progenitor cells are mesenchymal stem cells that are associated with the microvasculature. Such cells would appear to have neoplastic potential prior to the introduction of the foreign body, which in turn only creates the conditions necessary for the initiation of the neoplastic process.

Before we specifically study the situation relating to CNS trauma and brain tumors, we must briefly review the literature pertaining to the relationship of trauma to *non-CNS* carcinogenesis. Although trauma can be considered in many cases to be causally related to the aggravation of the symptoms of a *previously existing* malignancy, or may increase the metastatic potential of a primary neoplasm, in this discussion we are only concerned with the relationship of trauma to the *production* of a malignancy. In the early part of the twentieth century, Segond (54) proposed that specific criteria should be satisfied before a cancer could be considered to be traumatic in origin: (*a*) Proof must exist that the organ was traumatically impaired in a significant manner. (*b*) Evidence must exist that the part was normal before the injury. (*c*) Exact correspondence of the site of the injury with the cancer must be demonstrated. (*d*) A date of appearance of the tumor not too remote from the trauma must be present. (*e*) The diagnosis of cancer must be confirmed by pathological review.

In 1933 Coley and Higginbotham (10) reported 36 cases of bone sarcoma, of which approximately 50% had histories of local trauma. Many of these cases, however, did not satisfy even the minimal criteria listed above. In a 1943 study, Warren (62) introduced a criterion that many would agree with today and one that is especially important in the case of CNS neoplasia—i.e., that the trauma must be severe enough to have stimulated reparative tissue proliferation.

Although attempts have been made to link prior trauma with numerous malignancies, the relationship has been most commonly proposed for sarcomas of bone and soft tissue, for melanoma and for skin cancer. Ivins (30) has reported a history of trauma in many patients with sarcomas of the extremities. In 1965, Lea (34) reported 193 cases of malignant melanoma, of which 38% had a positive history of local trauma. Since its initial description in the first century and a more detailed account by Marjolin (38) in 1847, the occurrence of carcinomatous changes in long-standing scars has been well-documented. Reviews by Bowers and Young (4), Engler *et al.* (15) and Arons *et al.* (3) have extended the concept to include carcinoma arising in scars, burns, osteomyelitis, and chronic fistulas.

These authors agree that such cancers, which are almost always of the squamous cell type, arise in less than 2% of cases of chronic wounds. Although the pathogenesis of these conditions is unclear, most authors agree with the assertion of Engler that "the presence of scar tissue alone is unlikely to cause the degeneration into carcinoma. In most cases . . . more than one possible carcinogenic factor could be implicated" (15).

CNS TRAUMA AND BRAIN TUMOR

We must now turn to the clinical data linking head trauma specifically to CNS neoplasia. It is important here for us to distinguish between the putative connection of trauma to *intrinsic* malignant tumors of the glioma type and to benign tumors such as meningiomas, since the evidence would appear to be stronger in the case of the latter than in the former.

The literature on the relationship of neuroectodermal tumors and trauma is for the most part quite meager. There have been several case reports in the last 50 years, but in most of these adequate documentation is lacking. Thus, Marburg (36) found a 4.5 × 5 cm medulloblastoma in a child 6 weeks after he had fallen and struck his head. Although the author reported this as a causal connection, our current knowledge of the growth rate of such tumors would preclude our believing that this tumor was able to grow to this size in such a short period of time. Rather, it is more likely that the trauma served to uncover symptoms from a neoplasm that was already present. Hallevorden (22) reported on an oligodendroglioma that was intimately related to an area of previous trauma containing bone splinters. This case is, however, inadequately substantiated. More recent case reports by Wolf (64) and Noetzel (41) reported on a glioblastoma that developed in the scar of an old bullet wound. Finkemeyer and Behrend (16) have reported on a protoplasmic astrocytoma discovered in a 35-year-old man at the precise site of a missile injury of the brain that had been sustained 9 years earlier. This tumor was in direct continuity with the scar tissue that had been present on the dura and the superficial aspects of the brain.

At least three cases have been reported to follow documented *surgical* trauma. In 1954 Heyck (24) reported on finding a bifrontal butterfly glioblastoma at the site of a prefrontal leukotomy that had been carried out 5 years previously. Manuelides (35) reported on a 53-year-old woman who developed a glioblastoma 12 years after having a frontal lobotomy performed at the same site. Most recently, Prager *et al.* (46) described a 58-year-old male who developed a gliosarcoma at the site of an *Actinomyces* abscess that had been operated on 3 years earlier.

Perez-Diaz *et al.* (44) and associates described two patients who developed an oligodendroglioma 7 years and 8 years, respectively, after sustaining significant cerebral contusions. In each case pathological examination of the area around the tumor revealed microscopic evidence (e.g., gliosis, loss of myelin, hemosiderin deposits) of the previous cerebral contusion. Even more convincing is the recent case report by Troost and Tulleken (56), who described a patient who sustained a bombshell injury during World War II with the subsequent development of a brain abscess at the injury site. Thirty-seven years later he developed a contralateral hemiparesis and at surgery was found to have an anaplastic astrocytoma that was in direct continuity with the old abscess wall.

Aside from these anecdotal reports, there have been at least four retrospective studies that have attempted to determine if a statistical relationship exists between trauma and the development of brain tumors. In 1940 Globus *et al.* (21) studied the incidence of trauma in verified cases of brain tumor. Out of 423 verified tumor cases, 65 (or 15%) revealed a history of previous head trauma. The severity of the trauma in these cases was as follows: in 47 instances there were no neurological sequelae of the trauma, in 10 there was a brief period of unconsciousness, and in 8 there was prolonged unconsciousness and headache. Thus, a history of significant head trauma could be obtained in 18 of the 423 cases (or 4.2%). However, in a control group of 200 patients admitted with other diagnoses, 51 gave a history of head trauma, and in approximately ½ of these (i.e., 12.5%) the injury was followed by either a brief period of unconsciousness or a neurological deficit. Thus, the percentage of patients with brain tumors who had a positive history of significant head trauma was no greater than that found in the control population.

An excellent retrospective study was carried out by Parker and Kernohan in 1931 (43). These authors used the tumor registry at the Mayo Clinic to assemble a series of 431 cases of pathologically proven gliomas. A total of 58 patients (or 13.4%) gave a history of previous head injury, although only 14 (or 3.2%) of these patients had an injury which was sufficient to render them unconscious. In a control series of patients with other illnesses, the incidence of head trauma was 10.4%, and in a normal control group it was 35%. The authors concluded that the incidence of head trauma was not sufficiently high in the brain tumor group to suggest a causal relationship.

In 1970 Choi *et al.* (8) reported on interviews conducted with 126 patients or relatives of patients, who had brain tumors of various types, as well as a similar number of controls. He defined significant brain injury as "a fractured skull, unconsciousness, or bleeding from the head which required hospitalization." Using this criterion, he found that the group of patients with brain tumors did not differ from controls in the frequency of prior head injury. Hochberg and associates (25) carried out a case-control study of 231 patients with a diagnosis of glioblastoma who were seen in five participating hospitals over 4 years. There were 160 cases (68%) in whom questionnaires could be obtained and 125 controls who were matched for sex, age, and residence. They found that 18 brain tumor patients and 11 controls had a history of "mild" head injury, whereas 17 patients and 4 controls had a head injury that was classified as severe. The risk ratio (i.e., the ratio of the occurrence in the tumor population compared to the control population) for "mild head trauma" was 1.5, and for "severe head trauma" it was 3.8. The authors concluded that the "data suggests that severe head trauma in adults is a significant risk factor for glioblastoma" (25). This study, however, has been cogently critiqued by Codd and Kurland (9). They point out that the methodology of this study allowed for the inadvertent inclusion of several potential biases—most notably, the recall bias among the tumor patients. They argue that since only instances of *documented* head injury should have been included, and because the study was methodologically flawed in several other ways which are enumerated, its conclusion on the relationship between head trauma and brain tumor may be erroneous.

The most definitive statistical analysis of this issue to date, and the only *prospective* study reported thus far, was that of Anneger *et al.* (2) in 1979. Using the record system of the Mayo Clinic, they were able to follow sequentially—for almost 30,000 person-years—almost 3000 patients who experienced significant head trauma (defined as a head injury with brain involvement manifested by loss of consciousness, amnesia, or skull fracture). During the follow-up period, a total of four brain tumors (three meningiomas and one astrocytoma) were diagnosed, which according to the authors is almost exactly the incidence that would have been expected if the age-specific incidence rates for brain tumors in this same population were utilized.

The case for a causal relationship between head trauma and the subsequent development of a *meningioma* is somewhat more convincing. Attention was first drawn to this association by Harvey Cushing in his 1922 Cavendish Lecture (12). In this talk he presented 85 cases of meningioma and indicated that it was probably more than a coincidence that many of these patients developed a meningioma at the precise location of previous skull trauma. In his 1938 monograph with Dr. Eisenhart he elaborated upon his views (13). In this book he discussed 65 cases of meningioma, in whom a history of trauma could be established in approximately one-third. In addition, he described the celebrated case of General Leonard Wood, who developed a meningioma at the site of previous sharp trauma. Dr. Cushing concluded that "of all intracranial tumors in our experience, the incidence of trauma in meningiomas is particularly high. It was recorded in nearly one-third of the entire number . . . the direct relation of the blow to the locus of the ensuing growth is not infrequently so precise that the conclusion that an etiologic factor is involved is inescapable" (13).

Over the years there have been other reports of single cases or small series. In 1928 Reinhardt (49) reported the case of a 57-year-old male who at autopsy was found to have a large extracerebral meningioma of the floor of the frontal fossa. In the middle of the tumor lay a metal wire 1 cm × ⅓ cm that had been driven into the skull 20 years earlier by a boiler explosion. In more recent times Howath and Bunts (26) described a patient who developed a meningioma beneath a depressed skull fracture from an injury suffered 21 years previously. Walshe (61) reported on one of his patients who developed a meningioma following head injury. This was a middle-aged man, who 16 years before his death had a sharp piece of metal penetrate his skull. At the time of the second operation 16 years later a meningioma was seen precisely beneath the skull opening that had been made to remove the foreign body many years previously. In 1965 Lanigan (33) reported on two patients who experienced severe head trauma and were operated upon for meningiomas at the same site 2 and 13 years later. Walsh *et al.* (60) studied two patients who developed meningiomas 16 and 18 years after severe local injury. Turner and Laird (57) reported on a man with a penetrating gunshot wound who developed a meningioma at the same site 17 years later. Hung *et al.* (28) described a patient who was operated on for subdural hematoma and approximately 2 years later had removal of a meningioma located near the anterior border of the previous surgical site. Whatmore and Hitchcock (63) detailed the case of a man who suffered a bullet wound of the brain in World War II and 21 years later developed a meningioma directly beneath the fracture site.

Since the advent of computerized tomography, there have been two other case reports. Gardeur *et al.* (19) described two patients in whom the diagnosis of meningioma was made by computerized tomographic scanning. The first was a 60-year-old man who at age 20 suffered a skull fracture and an epidural hematoma that was surgically evacuated. Forty years later a meningioma was detected just anterior to the previous craniotomy site. In the second patient a meningioma developed at the site of a skull fracture that had been sustained 10 years previously. Most recently, Scheffer *et al.* (53) reported on three patients who developed meningiomas 8, 15, and 37 years after severe head injury. There have been only two large case-controlled studies of the relationship of trauma and meningioma. In these papers Preston-Martin *et al.* (47, 48) found that both men and women with meningioma had a significantly increased recall of prior head trauma than did corresponding control groups.

There has been a notable paucity of *experimental* data pertaining to the putative relationship between head trauma and the subsequent development of a brain tumor. The two main studies carried out to date have arrived at different conclusions. In the first, Mennel *et al.* (39) studied the effect of trauma on the offspring of pregnant rats who had been transplacentally exposed to the carcinogen ENU. In this experiment the pregnant mothers were injected with ENU at a dose of 40 mg/kg on day 20 of pregnancy, and the offspring were exposed to an intracerebral needle trauma at 12 days of age. The authors found no effect of the trauma on the number or localization of the tumors produced.

In a later study, Morantz and Shane (40) injected pregnant Fisher rats with ENU (20 mg/kg) on day 18 of gestation. The offspring were then randomly divided into two groups and one was exposed to a left cerebral stab wound at 30 days of age. In the traumatized group 62% of the tumors were gliomas, as compared to 47% in the control group. Survival curves indicated that the animals in the traumatized group died earlier than the controls. Finally, whereas the distribution of gliomas between the left and right side of the brain was equal in the control group (29 *vs.* 32%)

a greater percentage of gliomas was found on the traumatized side in the experimental group (43 *vs.* 19%). These data were interpreted to mean that under the highly artificial situation in which the rats had been exposed to a potent neurocarcinogen, intracerebral trauma *can* act as a co-carcinogen and enhance glioma formation.

DEMYELINATING DISEASE AND BRAIN TUMORS

It is extremely difficult to establish a causal relationship between two relatively uncommon conditions such as demyelinating disease and primary brain tumor. If one depends on the clinical examination alone, the diagnosis of brain tumor in a patient with demyelinating disease or the diagnosis of demyelinating disease in a patient with brain tumor is extremely difficult to make. Since physicians have been taught to search for a unitary diagnosis whenever possible, new symptoms and signs almost always are ascribed to a previously diagnosed condition. It is also true that relatively few patients with demyelinating disease come to autopsy, and it is conceivable that in some of these cases small gliomas may go unrecognized. Similarly, in patients dying with a known glioma, it is quite possible that the pathologist might overlook small areas of demyelination if he has not been alerted to their possible presence.

With the evermore widespread use of computerized tomography and magnetic resonance imaging, it has become clear that the plaque of multiple sclerosis may rarely present as a focal cerebral mass lesion with radiological features that are indistinguishable from a cerebral glioma (32, 37). In such cases the correct diagnosis will ultimately depend on the results of cerebral biopsy. As has been recently documented in the literature, even pathological examination of such multiple sclerosis biopsy specimens may lead to the erroneous diagnosis of a brain tumor. In this instance there is the possibility of erroneously diagnosing such a plaque as a brain tumor, since it may be characterized by monotonous sheets of gemistocytes interspersed with foamy macrophages (29). However, the use of special stains will allow the proper diagnosis to be made. The converse has also been reported by Roytta and Latvala (50), who described in detail two patients who had been followed for many years with a diagnosis of multiple sclerosis. At subsequent brain autopsy both patients were found to have diffusely infiltrating periventricular gliomas. This chapter will *not* review the numerous reports of multiple sclerosis plaques *simulating* a glioma or of glioma *simulating* multiple sclerosis on either radiologic or pathologic grounds.

Progressive multifocal leukoencephalopathy (PML) is a rare demyelinating disease which is now regarded as being caused by the replication of a papovavirus within glial cells. It is usually considered to be an opportunistic viral infection occurring in patients who are chronically debilitated or have an impaired immune response. The patient's death usually ensues within six months of onset. A few patients, however, have been described who lack demonstrable underlying disease, and in such patients, prolonged survival and spontaneous remissions have been described (58).

Pathological examination of affected areas of the brain in patients with this disease reveals that the astrocytes appear considerably enlarged, contain multiple and bizarre nuclei, and could on morphological grounds alone be considered neoplastic. In spite of this fact, the actual presence of neoplasia in this condition is extraordinarily rare, and has in fact been described on only two occasions. The first reported instance of glioma associated with PML is that of Castaigne *et al.* (7), who described the case of an 18-year-old man who had suffered a long-lasting immune deficiency syndrome. Pathologic examination 10 months after the onset of his neurologic deficit revealed PML as well as malignant glioma. The only other report of the association of PML and malignant glioma was that of Sima *et al.* (55), who described a 67-year-old male who presented with nystagmus and progressive cerebellar dysfunction. Four years later he entered hospital with profound dementia and died of pneumonia. Pathological examination revealed numerous active and inactive areas of demyelination secondary to PML. In addition, multiple malignant astrocytomas were found in the hippocampus, pons, and cerebellum. Virus particles consistent with the JC virus were found in the areas of PML, but not within the gliomas.

Experimentally, a variety of neural tumors, including astrocytomas, can be induced in laboratory animals by the intracerebral injection of papovaviruses (59). Consequently, the oncogenicity of papovaviruses in the *human* brain has long been suspected. What is notable, however, is the fact that of the many cases of PML that have been reported in the last 25 years, in only the above two cases has a possible association between PML and brain tumor been documented. It is also of interest that in both of these cases the PML was somewhat unusual in being rather indolent in its course. Thus, one possible explanation for the rare occurrence in these two patients would be that the protracted course and the partial immune unresponsiveness of these two patients may have been decisive in allowing sufficient time for the development of the virally associated malignant astrocytomas.

As of 1989 there have been approximately 23 cases reported of the concurrence of multiple sclerosis and brain tumor. The first report was that of Scherer (52), who described a 29-year-old woman with a diffuse periventricular glioblastoma, associated with numerous perivascular and periventricular foci of demyelination. In their textbook of neuropathology, Russell and Rubenstein (51) described three patients who on autopsy manifested both conditions, in two of whom the neoplasms were multiple. The first patient was a 36-year-old woman with multiple sclerosis who had two distinct neoplasms—a fibrillary astrocytoma and a glioblastoma—each of which arose on the border of plaques. The second case was that of a 66-year-old male who had both a left occipital glioblastoma and a right caudate subependymoma. Neither of these tumors was in continuity with a multiple sclerosis plaque. The third patient was a middle-aged man with multiple sclerosis who developed a gemistocytic astrocytoma. It is of interest that the cell type of the tumor was the same as that forming the majority of the reactive cells in the areas of demyelination.

Single cases have been reported in approximately 15 publications (see Table 6.1). In 1974 Currie and Urich (11) reported on three patients with multiple sclerosis who developed malignant glial tumors 7, 9, and 25 years after the onset of their demyelinating disease. In two of the cases there was continuity between the plaque and the tumor. These authors stated that there was suggestive but inconclusive evidence that the tumor arose from the astrocyte in the plaques. Anderson and coworkers (1) presented a detailed clinical and pathological study of three patients with demyelinating disease (two with multiple sclerosis and one with neuromyelitis optica) who developed neoplastic transformation of glia in areas of demyelination. Their careful pathological study demonstrated a gradual transition from areas of demyelination to gliosis to overt neoplasia. From this study they concluded that there was a causal relationship between the two conditions.

An analysis of the cases reported to date reveals several interesting facts. There is a slight female preponderance, which is in keeping with the increased incidence of multiple sclerosis in females. The most usual presentation is for a patient with a long history of multiple sclerosis to present with new and progressive symptoms, such as epilepsy or increased intracranial pressure. The development of a *brain* tumor in multiple sclerosis patients is especially interesting, since it has recently been reported that the incidence of *non-CNS* malignancy in these patients is, if anything, lower than in the general population. (42) In the vast majority of cases, the tumors that were discovered were astrocytomas or glioblastomas. In one case an oligodendroglioma was found, and in four cases there were mixed oligodendrogliomas-astrocytomas. This is in keeping with the fact that in the multiple sclerosis plaque the oligodendrocytes undergo degeneration, while it is the astrocytes that undergo proliferation.

In several of the cases reported, both the

TABLE 6.1
Reported Cases of Demyelinating Disease and Brain Tumor

Case	Author	Year	Reference	Age/Sex	Duration of MS	Glioma		Continuity of Plaque and Glioma
						Type	Location	
1	Scherer	1938	J Belge Neurol Psychiat 38:1–17, 1938	29/F	Not clinically diagnosed	GBM (diffuse)	Periventricular	Yes
2	Munch-Petersen	1949	Acta Psychiat Neurol Scand 24:599–605, 1949	49/F	9 yrs	GBM	R Cerebrum	No
3	Zimmerman Netsky	1950	Res Publ Assoc Ner Men Dis 28:271–312,1950	61/M	10 yrs	GBM	Cerebrum	—
4	Mathews	1962	Q J Med 31:141–155, 1962	51/F	28 yrs	Astro	L Frontal	—
5	Brihaye et al	1963	J Neuropath Exp Neurol 22:128–137, 1963	62/M	Not clinically diagnosed	Astro	R Temporo-occipital	Yes
6	Barnard Jellinek	1967	J Neurol Sci 5:441–455, 1967	43/F	16 yrs	Oligo	R Temporal R Cerebellar	Yes
7	Boyazis et al	1967	Rev Patol Nerv Ment 88:1–20, 1967	54/F	6 months	GBM	R Temporal	No
8	Aubert et al	1968	Rev Neurol 119:374–376, 1968	50/F	15 yrs	GBM	R Temporo-Parietal	No
9	Mathews, Moosay	1972	Arch Neurol 27:263–268, 1972	44/M	18 yrs	Mixed Oligo-Astro	L Fronto-Parietal	No
10	Reagan Freiman	1973	J Neurol Neurosurg Psychiat 36:523–28, 1973	45/F	5 yrs	GBM (multiple)	Cerebrum & cerebellum	Yes

TABLE 6.1 *continued*

Case	Author	Year	Reference	Age/Sex	Duration of MS	Glioma Type	Glioma Location	Continuity of Plaque and Glioma
11–13	Currie Urich	1974	J Neurol Neurosurg Psychiat 37:598–605, 1974	37/F	7 yrs	GBM	R Fronto-Temp	No
				63/M	9 yrs	GBM (multiple)	L Cerebral	Yes
				53/M	28 yrs	GBM	R Temporal	Yes
14–16	Russell Rubinstein	1959 1977	Pathology of the Tumors of the Nervous System Baltimore: Williams & Wilkins	36/D	—	Astro-GBM	R Frontal Corpus Callosum	Yes
				66/M	—	GBM Subependymoma	L Occipital R Caudate	No
				Middle Aged/M	—	Gemistocytic Astro	L Temporal	Yes
17	Palo Duchesne	1977	J Neurol 216:217–22, 1977	52/F	—	Astro	—	—
18	Scully, Galdabini	1978	NEJ of M 299:1060–1067, 1978	57/F	Not clinically diagnosed	Astro-Ependymoma	Spinal cord	No
19	Kalimo et al	1979	Acta Neuropath 46:231–234, 1979	36/F	18 yrs	Anaplastic Astro	L Fronto Temporal	No
20	Lahl	1980	Eur Neurol 19:192–197, 1980	50/M	Not clinically diagnosed	GBM	Diffuse	Yes
21–23	Anderson et al	1980	Brain 103:603–622, 1980	47/M	8 yrs	Mixed-GBM Oligo-Astro	R Frontal	Yes
				45/M	11 yrs	Oligo-Astro	L Frontal	Yes
				45/M	29 yrs	Oligo-Astro	R Gyrus Rectus	Yes
24	Ho Wolfe	1981	Cancer 47:2913–2919, 1981	63/F	25 yrs	Protopl Astro	R Cingulate Gyrus	No

areas of demyelination and the tumors have been located in the subependymal region. This is especially interesting in that this is a site of fetal and neonatal glial proliferation, and thus an area that has been shown to be particularly susceptible to the actions of neural carcinogens such as the N-nitroso compounds. (1) Finally, multiple tumors have been noted in approximately one-fourth of the cases reported. Since this percentage is considerably higher than the rate of approximately 5% that is accepted as the incidence of multicentricity in gliomas, this may be taken as evidence for a causal relationship between the two conditions.

SUMMARY AND CONCLUSIONS

It seems clear that if there is a potential relationship between trauma and brain tumors, we must restrict our definition of significant prior CNS trauma to injuries that by either direct CNS penetration or the presence of a foreign body could be reasonably certain to have led to reactive glial or arachnoidal cellular proliferation. Based upon our present concept of carcinogenesis, it is then conceivable that the stimulus to glial and arachnoidal cell proliferation that is produced by such significant traumas, the presence of a foreign body, or demyelination, could lead to the development of a brain tumor in patients whose CNS cells *already* harbored neoplastic potential. It is extremely unlikely that demyelination or trauma *alone* can lead to the growth of a CNS malignancy. The clinical evidence of the past century is least supportive of this hypothesis in the case of the production of a primary *glial* tumor secondary to head trauma. However, in certain situations of meningiomas arising secondary to penetrating cerebral injury or gliomas arising in conjunction with the reparative process caused by demyelination, it would appear that an association other than the mere coincidental occurrence of two rare conditions may indeed be operative.

REFERENCES

1. Anderson, J., Hughes, B., Jefferson, M., *et al.* Gliomatous transformation and demyelinating disease. Brain, *103:*603–622, 1980.
2. Anneger, J.A., Laws, E.R., Kurland, L.T., *et al.* Head trauma and subsequent brain tumors. Neurosurgery, *4:*203–205, 1979.
3. Arons, M.S., Lynch, J.B., Lewis, S.R., *et al.* Scar tissue carcinoma. Part I. A clinical study with special reference to burn scar carcinoma. Ann. Surg., *161:*170–188, 1965.
4. Bowers, R.F. and Young, J.M. Carcinoma arising in scars, osteomyelitis and fistulae. Arch. Surg., *80:*564–570, 1960.
5. Bramwell, B. Intracranial Tumors. Edinburgh, Young J. Pentland, 1888, p. 3.
6. Brand, K.G., Buoen, L.C., Johnson, K.H., *et al.* Etiological factors, stages, and the role of foreign body in foreign body tumorigenesis: a review. Cancer Res. *35:*279–286, 1975.
7. Castaigne, P., Roudot, P., Escourolle, R., *et al.* Leucoencephalopathie multifocale progressive et "gliomes" multiple. Rev. Neurol. (Paris), *130:*379–392, 1974.
8. Choi, N.W., Schuman, L.M., and Gullen, W.H. Epidemiology of primary central nervous system neoplasms. II. Case-controlled study. Am. J. Epidemiol., *91:*467–485, 1970.
9. Codd, M.B. and Kurland, L.T. Head trauma and seizures as risk factors in tumors of the glioma group. Neurology, *35:*1532–3, 1985.
10. Coley, W.B. and Higginbotham, N.L. Injury as a causative factor in the development of malignant tumors. Ann. Surg., *98:*991–1012, 1933.
11. Currie, S., Urich, H.: Concurrence of multiple sclerosis and glioma. J. Neurol. Neurosurg. Psychiatry, *37:*598–605, 1974.
12. Cushing, H.: The meningiomas (dural endotheliomas): their source and favored sites of origin. Brain, *45:*282–316, 1922.
13. Cushing, H. and Eisenhart, L.: *Meningiomas: Their Classification, Regional Behavior, Life History, and Surgical End Results.* Springfield, IL, Charles C Thomas, 1938, p 71.
14. Deelman, H.T.: The part played by injury and repair in the development of cancer with remarks on the growth of experimental cancers. Br. Med. J., *1:*872, 1927.
15. Engler, H.S., Fernandez, A., Bliven, F.E., *et al.* Cancer arising in scars of old burns and in chronic osteomyelitis, ulcers, and drainage sites. Surgery, *55:*654–664, 1964.
16. Finkemeyer, H. and Behrend, R.C.: Hirntrauma und gliomentstelung. Zentralbl Neurochir, *16:*318, 1956.
17. Fischer-Wasels, B.: Die traumlische entstehung der gliome und piatumoren nach r beneke. Monatsschr Unfallheilkd, *39:*489–527, 1932.
18. Friedwald, W. F. and Rous, P.: The initiating and promoting elements in tumor production. J. Exp. Med., *80:*101–126, 1944.
19. Gardeur, D., Allal, R., Sichez, J.P., *et al.* Posttraumatic intracranial meningiomas: recognition by computerized tomography in three cases. J. Comput. Assist. Tomogr., *3:*103–104, 1979.
20. Glinos, A.D., Bucher, N.L., Aub, J.C.: The effect of liver regeneration on tumor formation in

rats fed 4-dimethylaminoazabenzene. J. Exp. Med., *93*:313–324, 1951.

21. Globus, J.H., Zuchor, J., Saperstein, M., *et al.*: Tumor and head trauma. Trans. Am. Neurol. Assoc., *66*:165–168, 1940.
22. Hallevorden, J.: Oligodendrogliom nach hirntraume. Nervenarzt, *19*:163–167, 1948.
23. Haran-Ghera, N., Trainin, N., Fiore-Donati, L., *et al.*: A possible two-stage mechanism in rhabdomyosarcoma in rats. Br. J. Cancer, *16*:653–664, 1962.
24. Heyck, H.: Glioblastom nach leukotomie. Monatschr Psychiatr Neurol, 128–180, 1954.
25. Hochberg, F., Toniolo, P., and Cold, P. Head trauma and seizures as risk factors in glioblastoma. Neurology, *34*:1511–1514, 1984.
26. Howath, J.C. and Bunts, A.T.: Intracranial meningioma following trauma: report of a case. Cleve. Clin. Q., *17*:14–18, 1950.
27. Hall, W. H.: The role of initiating and promoting factors in the pathologenesis of tumors of the thyroid. Br. J. Cancer, *2*:273–280, 1948.
28. Hung, C.C., Change, W.Y., and Yao, Y.T.: Post-traumatic intracranial meningioma. J. Formosan Med. Assoc., *71*:214–219, 1972.
29. Hunter, S.B., Gallinger, W.E., and Rubin, J.J.: Multiple sclerosis mimicking primary brain tumor. Arch. Pathol. Lab. Med., *111*:464–468, 1987.
30. Ivins, J.C., Dockerty, M.B., and Ghormley, R.K.: Fibrosarcoma of the soft tissues of the extremities: a review of seventy-eight cases. Surgery, *28*:495–508, 1950.
31. Jull, J.W.: The effects of oestrogens and progesterone on the chemical induction of mammary cancer in mice of I.F. strain. J. Pathol. Bacteriol., *68*:547–559, 1954.
32. Kalyan-Raman, U.P., Garwacki, D.J., and Elwood, P.W.: Demyelinating disease of corpus callosum presenting as glioma on magnetic resonance scan: a case documented with pathological findings. Neurosurgery, *21*:247–250, 1987.
33. Lanigan, J.P.: Can a head injury cause a meningioma? J. Irish Med. Assoc., *56*:12–13, 1965.
34. Lea, A.J.: Malignant melanoma of the skin: the relationship to trauma. Ann. R. Coll. Surg. Engl., *37*:169–176, 1965.
35. Manuelides, F.E.: Glioma in trauma. In: *Pathology of the Nervous System*, edited by J. Minkler, vol. 2, pp. 2237–2240. New York, McGraw-Hill, 1971.
36. Marburg, P.: Unfull und hirngeschwulst. Vienna, Springer-Verlag, 1934.
37. Mastrostefano, R., Occhipinti, E., Bigotti, G., *et al.* Multiple sclerosis plaque simulating cerebral tumor: case report and review of the literature. Neurosurgery, *21*:244–246, 1987.
38. Marjolin, J.W.P.: Dictionnaire de Medicine Pratique, edited by M.F. Hoeffer. Paris: Firmen-Didot, 1847.
39. Mennel, H.D., Sato, K., and Zulch, K.T.: Traumatische Regeneration und resorptivkarzinogenese am Zentralnervensystem: I. Meteilulung. Acta Neurochir (Wien), *25*:197–206, 1971.
40. Morantz, R.A., Shain, W.: Trauma and brain tumors: an experimental study. Neurosurgery, *3*:181–186, 1978.
41. Noetzel, H.: Vortag Arbeitsgemeinschaft Hirntraumafragen. Mainz, 1953.
42. Palo, J., Duchesne, J., and Wilkstom, J. Malignant diseases among patients with multiple sclerosis. J. Neurol., *216*:217–222, 1977.
43. Parker, H.L. and Kernohan, J.W. The relation of an injury and glioma of the brain. J.A.M.A., *97*:535–540, 1931.
44. Perez-Diaz, C., Cabello, A., Lobato, R.D., *et al.* Oligodendrogliomas arising in the scar of a brain contusion. Surg. Neurol., *24*:581–586, 1985.
45. Pound, A.W. and Bell, J.R.: The influence of croton oil stimulation on tumor initiation by urethane in mice. Br. J. Cancer, *16*:690, 1962.
46. Prager, J., Zaret, B.S., Davidson, R., *et al.* Gliosarcoma at the site of a surgically treated actinomyces cerebral abscess. Neurosurgery, *15*:868–872, 1984.
47. Preston-Martin, S., Paganini-Hill, A., Henderson, B.E., *et al.* Case-control study of intracranial meningioma in women in Los Angeles County, California. J. Natl. Cancer Inst., *65(1)*:67–73, 1980.
48. Preston-Martin, S., Yu, M.C., Henderson, B.E., *et al.* Risk factors for meningiomas in men in Los Angeles County. J. Natl. Cancer Inst., *70*:863–886, 1983.
49. Reinhardt, G.: Trauma-Fremdkorper-Hirngeschwulst. Munch Med Wochenschschr, *75*: 399–401, 1928.
50. Roytta, M. and Latvala, M.: Diagnostic problems in multiple sclerosis. Eur. Neurol., *25*:197–207, 1986.
51. Russell, D.W. and Rubenstein, L.J.: Pathology of Tumors of the Nervous System, 4th ed, p. 179, Baltimore, Williams & Wilkins, 1977.
52. Scherer, J.J.: La "glioblastomatose en plaques." J. Belg. Neurol. Psychiatry, *38*:1–17, 1938.
53. Scheffer, J., Avidan, D., and Rapp, A.: Post-traumatic meningioma. Neurosurgery, *17*:84–87, 1985.
54. Segond, M.P.: Le cancer et les accidents du travail. Proc. Verb. Mem. Discuss. Assoc. Fr. Chir., *20*:745–782, 1907.
55. Sima, A., Finkelstein, A., and McLachlan, D.R.: Multiple malignant astrocytomas in a patient with spontaneous progressive multifocal leukoencephalopathy. Ann. Neurol., *14*:183–188, 1983.
56. Troost, D. and Tulleken, C.A.F.: Malignant glioma after bombshell injury. Clin. Neuropathol., *3(4)*:139–142, 1984.
57. Turner, O.A. and Laird, T.A.: Meningioma with traumatic etiology. J. Neurosurg., *24*:96–98, 1966.
58. Walker, D.L.: Progressive multifocal leukoencephalopathy. In *Handbook of Clinical Neurology*, vol. 35, edited by P.T. Vinken and G.W.

Bruyn, pp. 207–229. New York, North Holland, 1978.
59. Walker, D.L., Padgett, B.L., ZuRhein, G.M., *et al.* Human papovavirus (JC) induction of brain tumors in hamsters. Science, *181*:674–676, 1973.
60. Walsh, J., Gye, R., and Connelly, T.J. Meningioma: a late complication of head injury. Med. J. Aust., *1*:906–908, 1969.
61. Walshe, F.: Head injury as a factor in the etiology of intracranial meningioma. Lancet *7210*: 993–996, 1961.
62. Warren, S.: Minimal criteria required to prove causation of traumatic or occupational neoplasms. Ann. Surg., *117*:585–595, 1943.
63. Whatmore, W.J. and Hitchcock, E.R. Meningioma following trauma. Br. J. Surg., *60*:496–498, 1973.
64. Wolf, N.: Kriegsveretzungen des gehirns und hirntumorentwicklung. Z Unfallmed Berufskr, *44*:279–284, 1951.

CHAPTER 7

Patterns of Tumor Growth

DAVIDE SCHIFFER, M.D.

The diagnosis of tumors and establishment of a suitable strategy for their management are greatly assisted by an understanding of their natural history. Their origin, growth patterns and eventual transformation with the changes in morphology thus involved are all points that deserve closer study. The very early stages of human tumor development are unknown. There are, however, experimental models that enable the course of a tumor to be followed from the very start. An example of such diachronic monitoring of tumor development is provided by the transplacental induction of brain tumors with ethylnitrosourea (ENU).

THE TRANSPLACENTAL ENU MODEL

The Transformation Process

Nitrosourea derivatives have been employed systematically in the experimental induction of brain tumors by administration of carcinogens in sites distant from the brain itself (38). Such induction is possible both in utero and in newborn and adult animals, and relations have been established between carcinogen dose and site of administration, latency, and induction frequency (91). ENU and methylnitrosourea (MNU) are the compounds most commonly employed. ENU is effective transplacentally and in the first month of extrauterine life, MNU in the adult animal. A single dose of $\geqslant$ 20 mg ENU given I.V. to the rat on the 17th day of gestation produces brain tumors in almost 90% of the offspring. The number of tumors per rat increases and the latency period decreases with increasing doses (38).

The temporal and spatial development of such lesions can be followed in the hemispheres. The so-called "clinical" latency period, i.e., the interval between birth and the first neurological manifestations has been estimated at 5 to 6 months (14, 152), though lesions at different stages of development are observed in animals sacrificed at this age. Systematic sacrifice from the day of birth shows that early neoplastic lesions appear in the white matter on the 60th day, giving a histological latency period of 2 months. These lesions have been called "early neoplastic proliferations" (ENPs) (Fig. 7.1). Their histological picture is by no means distinct (96, 111, 200), since astrocytes, oligodendrocytes, and cells of uncertain nature are found (177), although the presence of abundant reactive astrocytes (see Fig. 7.16) is a striking feature (130, 172).

Microtumors 300 to 500 μm in diameter develop from ENPs between the 2nd and 3rd months. These have a higher cell density, more frequent mitoses, and proliferative centers consisting of densely packed cells with scanty cytoplasm and small, dark nuclei (Figs. 7.2 and 7.3). They continue to appear in the 4th and 5th months, whereas oligodendroglial foci (Fig. 7.4) develop in the cortex from the 3rd to the 6th months. The tumors that grow from these microtumors retain their morphology, including their proliferative centers (Fig. 7.5), but eventually become polymorphic. Isomorphic oligodendrogliomas in the cortex and white matter (Figs. 7.6 and 7.7) may be polymorphic later (Fig. 7.8). The cell kinetics show that malignancy is present at the microtumor stage, when mitosis is frequent and proliferative centers appear (96, 211).

Neurinomas are very common. They are

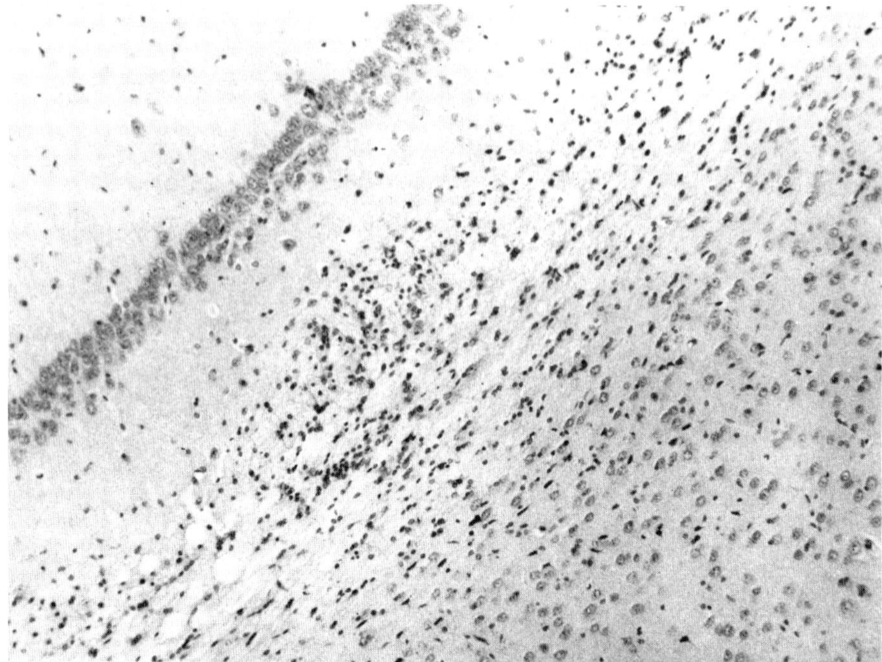

Figure 7.1. Transplacental ENU model (TEM). Early neoplastic proliferation (ENP) in the periventricular white matter. H&E ×100. (Reprinted with permission from D. Schiffer, M. T. Giordana, S. Pezzotta, *et al.*, Cerebral tumors induced by transplacental ENU: study of the different tumoral stages, particularly of early proliferations. Acta Neuropathol. [Berl.] *41*:27–31, 1978.)

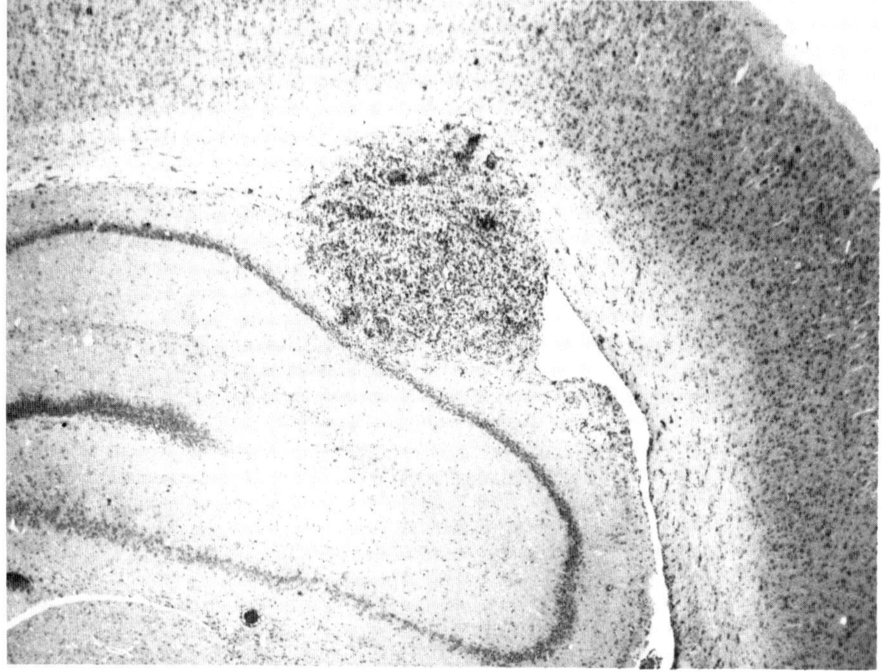

Figure 7.2. TEM. Microtumor in the periventricular white matter. H&E, ×50.

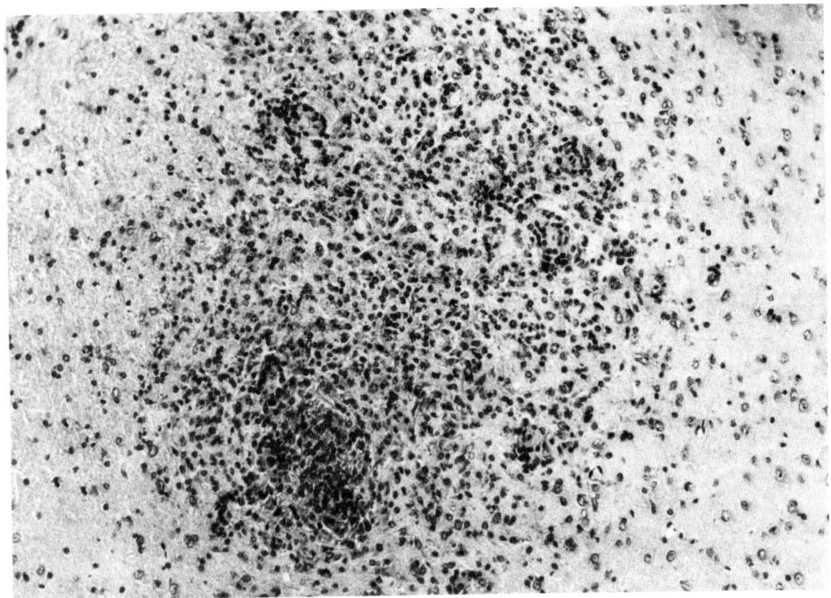

Figure 7.3. TEM. Microtumor with a proliferative center. H&E, ×100.

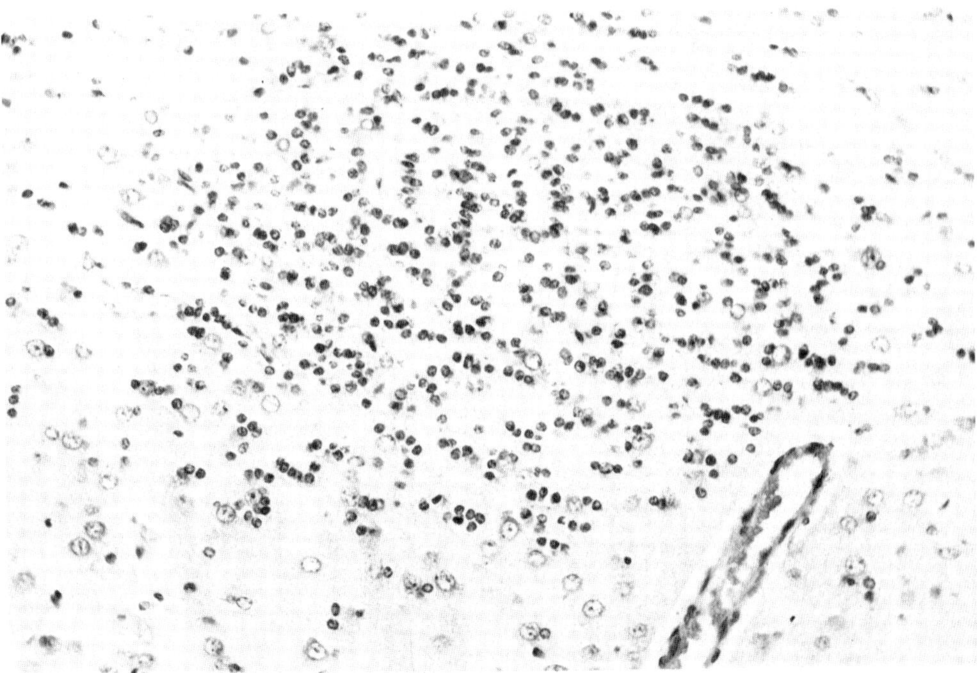

Figure 7.4. TEM. Oligodendroglial focus in the cerebral cortex. H&E, ×200.

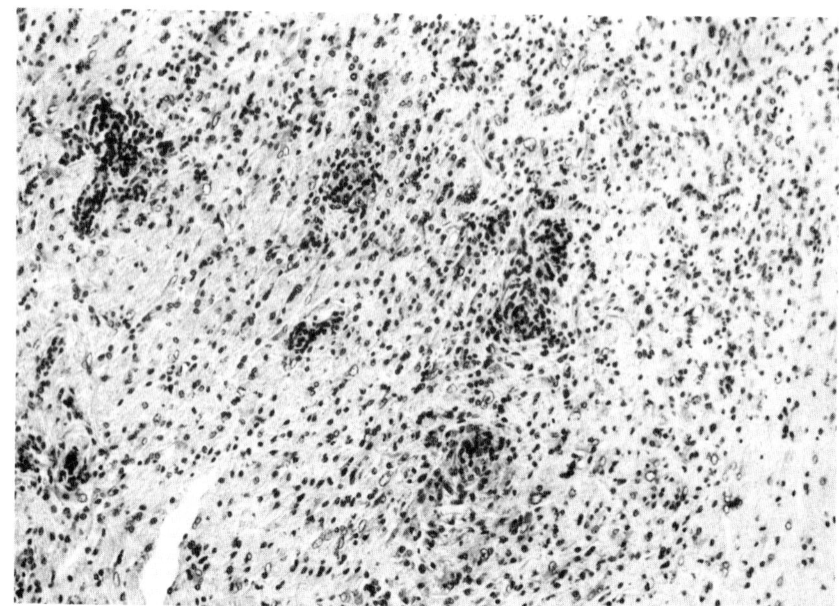

Figure 7.5. TEM. Proliferative centers in a large tumor. H&E, ×100.

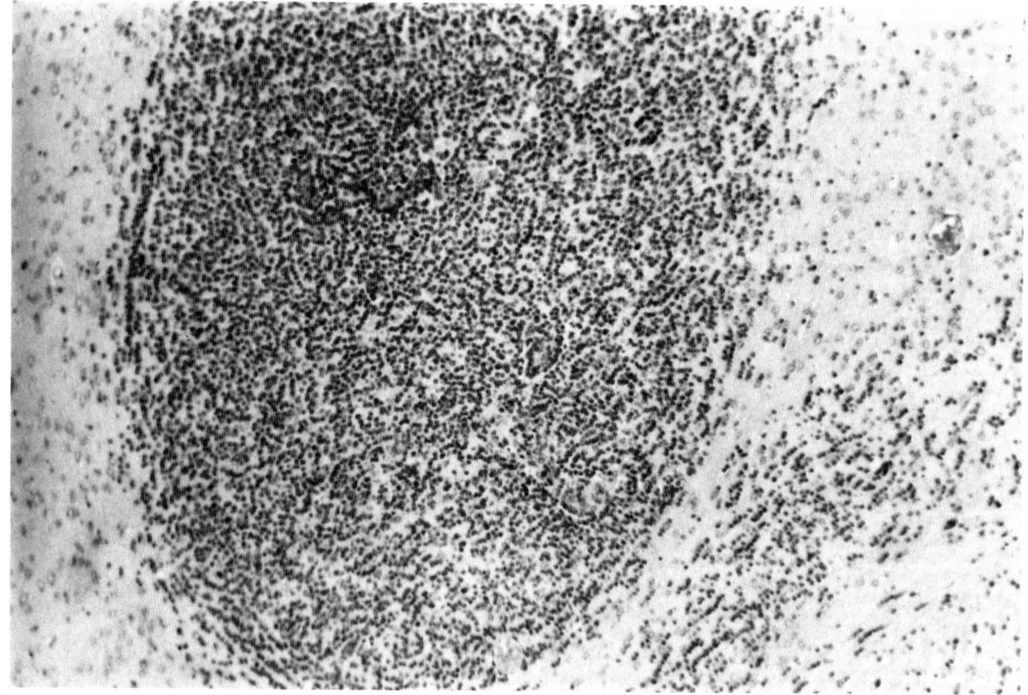

Figure 7.6. TEM. Isomorphic oligodendroglioma in the white matter. H&E, ×100.

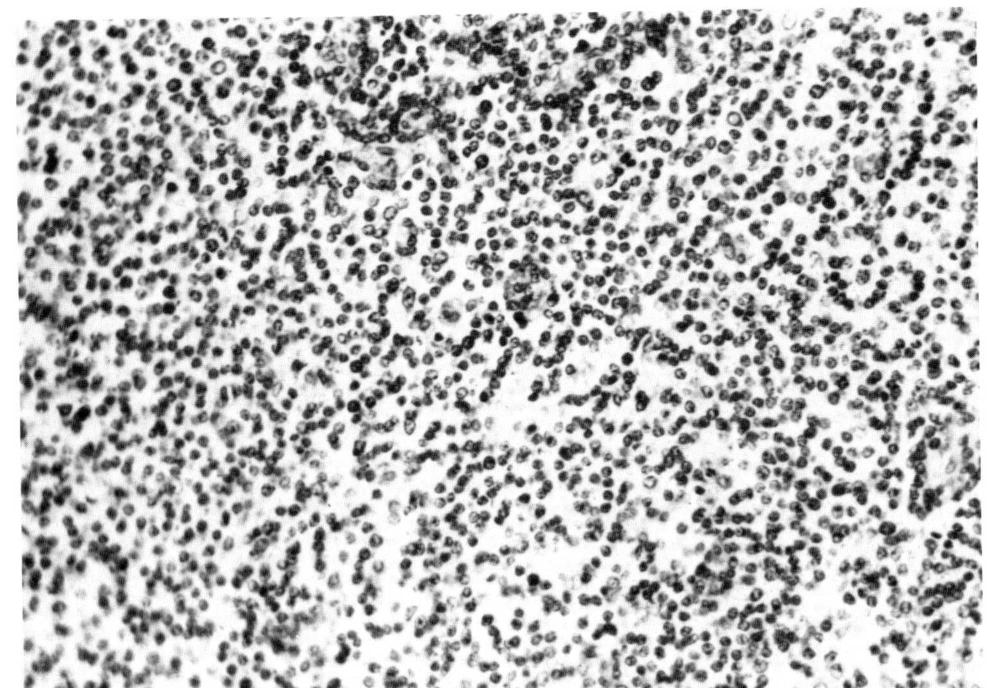

Figure 7.7. The same specimen as in Figure 7.6 showing the typical oligodendroglial aspect of the tumor cells. H&E, ×200.

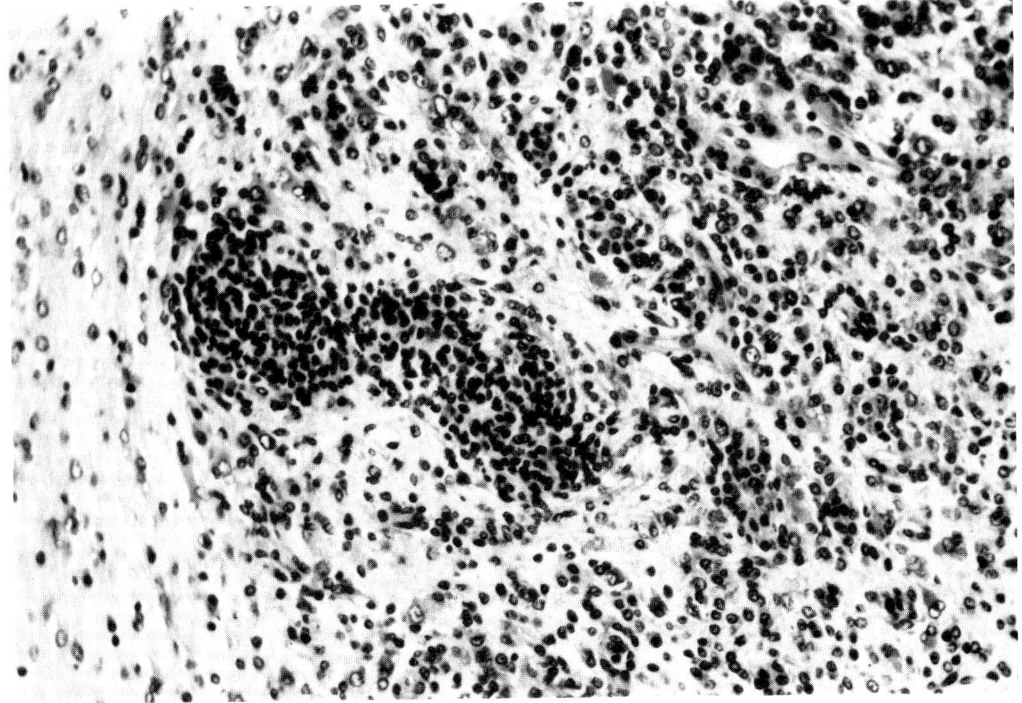

Figure 7.8. TEM. Polymorphic glioma of the hemisphere. H&E, ×100. (Reprinted with permission from D. Schiffer, M. T. Giordana, S. Pezzotta, *et al.*, Cerebral tumors induced by transplacental ENU: study of the different tumoral stages, particularly of early proliferations. Acta Neuropathol. [Berl.] *41*:27–31, 1978.)

mostly observed in the 5th cranial nerve and the dorsal roots, especially those of the lumbar and sacral nerves and constitute 41% of transplacentally and 53.2% of postnatally induced tumors (221). Their histological picture resembles that of human neurinomas, although with greater malignancy (Fig. 7.9), many mitoses and circumscribed areas of necrosis. They spread into the adventitial and subarachnoid spaces.

The cells of these neurinomas display rapid growth in primary cultures and closely resemble Schwann cells (27, 132). They also take on a tandem arrangement far from the explants (48). When transplanted subcutaneously or intracerebrally, they do not differ morphologically from the primary tumor cells (28).

Much pathogenetically useful information would emerge if the events that occur during the histological latency period could be clarified. Identification of the phenotypic changes in vivo of presumptive tumor cells, however, is an extremely difficult task (108). The nervous system has a polymorphic cell composition. In addition, only a minority of its cells undergo the changes that lead to malignant phenotypes. Furthermore, its architecture is substantially altered over the two months between the administration of ENU and the appearance of ENPs by the proliferation, migration, and differentiation of neuroepithelial cells moving from the germinal matrix to form the cortex and white matter.

Since the target of ENU is the paraventricular, subependymal germinal zone, which is directly derived from the germinal layer of the neural tube (92, 112), the causal and formal relation between its first effects on the matrix and the development of a tumor must be discussed with regard to cytogenesis, DNA modifications, and changes of phenotype.

In the early stages of development, the neural tube is composed of asynchronously proliferating germinal cells (Fig. 7.10). After a few days, cells enter the postmitotic phase and, as young neurons, migrate from the germinal to marginal zone, which eventually becomes the anlage of the pallium. Glial cells migrate later and continue to proliferate while doing so. The subventri-

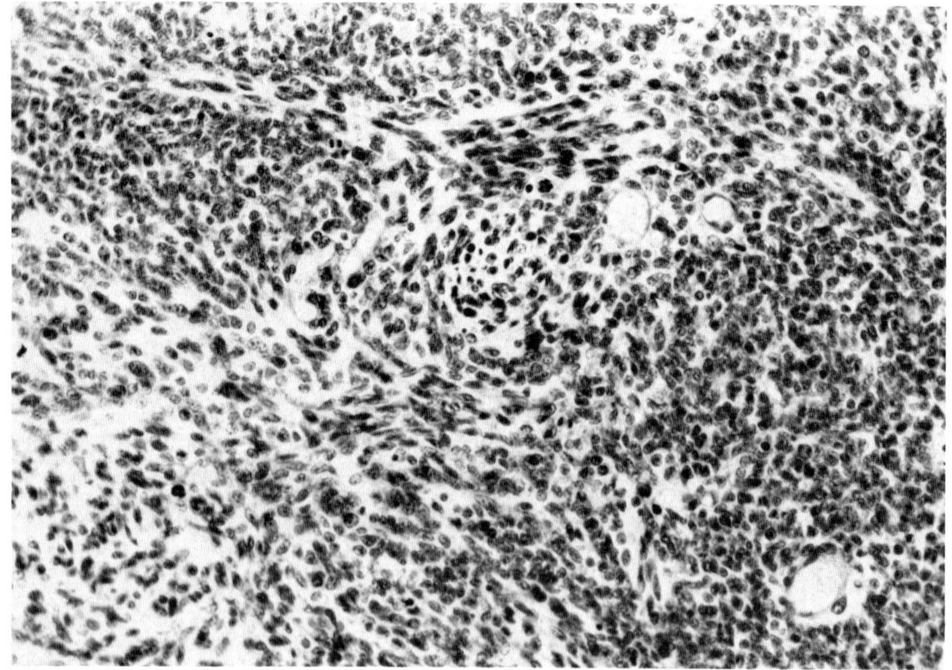

Figure 7.9. TEM. Neurinoma of the 5th cranial nerve. Many mitoses are present. H&E, ×200.

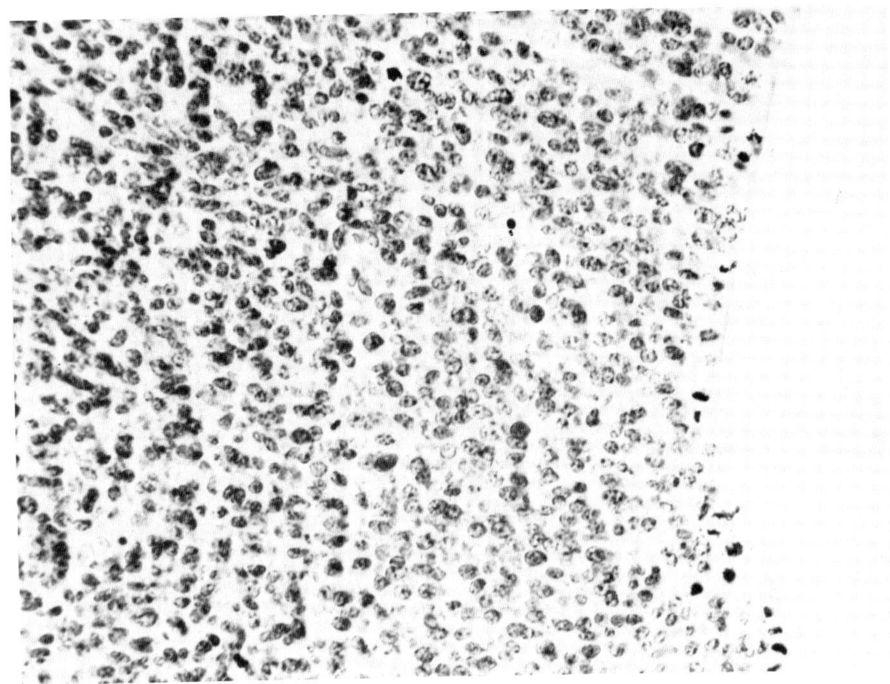

Figure 7.10. Four-day-old rat. Germinal cells of the paraventricular matrix with mitoses in the inner layer. H&E, ×100.

cular and intermediate zones will become the white matter and contain mitotic glial cells.

The question that has provoked the greatest discussion is whether neurons and glial cells are produced by the same germinal cells, by different, but histologically indistinguishable, cells (50), or from the same cells but consecutively (51, 52). Neurons originate in the germinal layer and cease to proliferate on migration, whereas glial cells continue to proliferate in the mantle layer, commissures, and fiber tracts (89).

The moment at which the neuronal and glial lines diverge is still a subject of discussion. His (77) regarded the germinal zone as composed of two cell lines, namely, the germinal cells ("Keimzellen") and the "spongioblasts," giving rise to neurons and glial cells, respectively. Schaper (162), on the other hand, postulated a single, mitotically active population producing "indifferent" cells that migrate into the mantle layer and give rise to both neurons and glial cells. Doubt, however, has recently been cast on these views by the observation in rodents of two populations with different generation times, and of the presence of radial glia and Bergmann's fibers as early as the final stages of neurocytogenesis (150, 151, 183). Similar findings have since been reported histochemically (6, 40) and in monkeys (117). Neuron and neuroglial precursors must thus coexist in the initial stages of development. It has been shown that the glia-committed matrix cells of the Macaca mulatta are GFAP-positive, whereas neuron-committed cells are not (116), indicating that the appearance of a specific phenotype is not rigidly linked to the final mitosis. Indeed, mitoses in GFAP-positive cells migrating from the matrix to the cortex can readily be demonstrated in the rat (Fig. 7.11). Account must be taken of these findings when interpreting the positive immunohistochemical staining of cell differentiation markers.

Glial cells are not produced until the production of neurons ceases (51) (Fig. 7.12) and this temporal dissociation may account for the absence of nerve cell tumors in ENU experiments, since the damage caused to neuroblasts by a carcinogen can only be transmitted for a few generations.

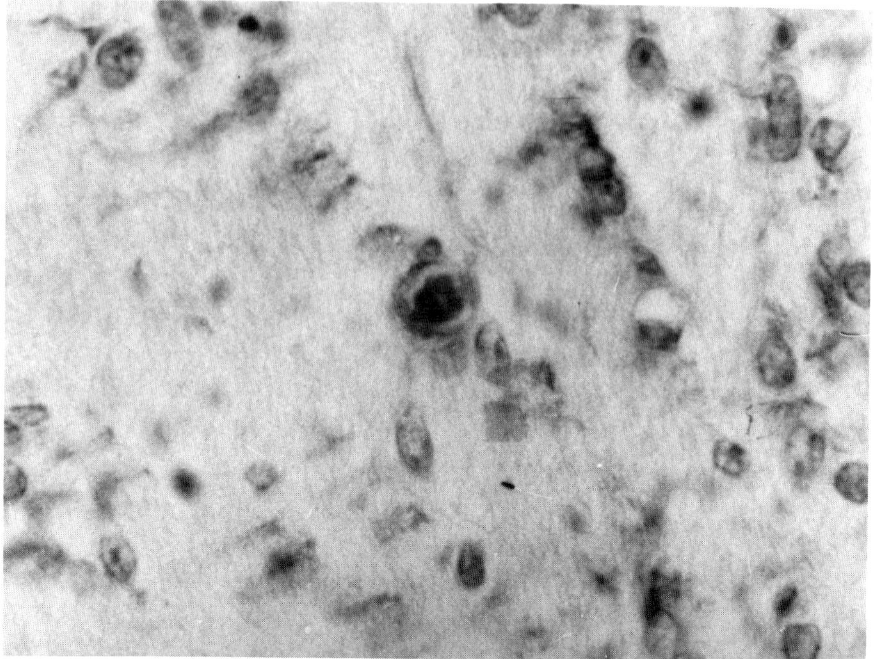

Figure 7.11. Two-day-old rat. GFAP-positive dividing cell during migration to the cortex. PAP method counterstained with hematoxylin, ×300.

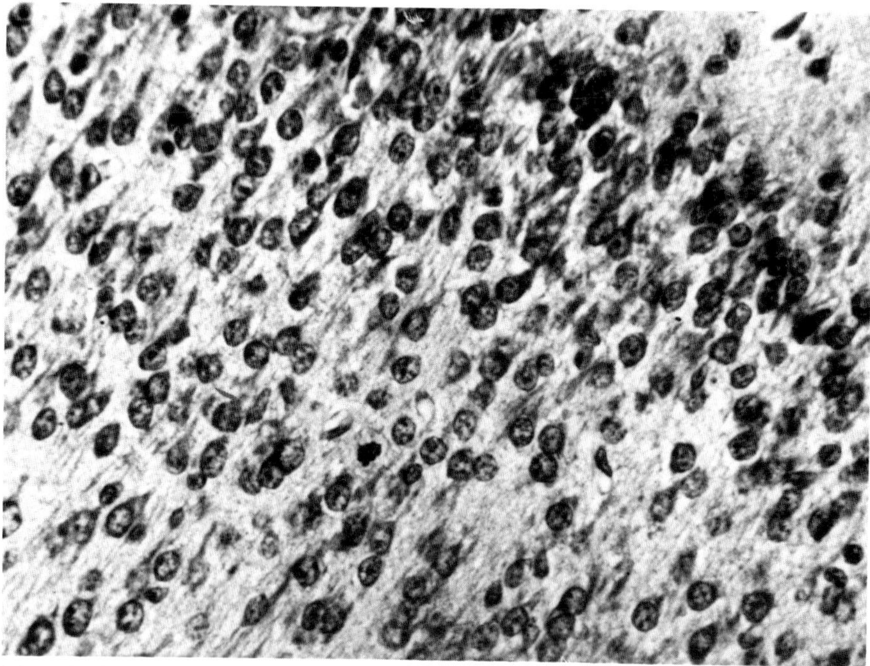

Figure 7.12. Four-day-old rat. Dividing glial cells among neurons in the cortex. H&E, ×200.

The vulnerability of the CNS to carcinogens is practically nil until the 11th day of intrauterine life, i.e., the peak of neuron production.

The histogenetic relationship between astrocytes and oligodendrocytes is still uncertain. The latter do not appear in the neocortex before birth (32, 198). The question is thus whether the two types arise simultaneously or consecutively, and from the same or different precursors. It should be stressed that they have a common origin (141, 148). Nonetheless, transitional forms are also observed (24).

A possible, although less likely eventuality, is the involvement of both glial precursors persisting in adult life and differentiated glial cells in the adult brain in neoplastic transformation (9). If the phenotype of malignant transformation is expressed by a sequence of mutations and the first hit is on glial precursors migrating from the germinal zone (157), not only cell displacement but also the turnover of adult glia must be taken into account as factors responsible for the origin of remote cortical tumors.

Gliogenesis in the adult animal has not yet been totally clarified. It is uncertain whether new glial cells originate from stem cells, or whether DNA is synthesized in terminally differentiated cells. A turnover of glial cells undoubtedly takes place (86). There is much evidence that the "subependymal plate" plays the main role (Fig. 7.13). It could contain the glial stem cells giving rise to glial cells (79, 118), those with a small, light nucleus being precursors of young astrocytes, and those with a small, dark nucleus being oligodendrocytes. Even so, it is not universally regarded as the only gliogenesis site (87, 102).

Stem cells are found in the adult myelination glia, outer granular layer of the cerebellar cortex, fascia dentata, and molecular layer (119). Glial proliferation could also occur in situ. It is thought to be much greater in the deep white matter than in the cortex (122). One-third of the subependymal plate cells, in fact, are in cycle, as opposed to only 1% of glial cells. A cautious approach must be taken, however, when seeking to interpret all these findings (197). Doubt has been cast on the reliability of in vivo experiments with

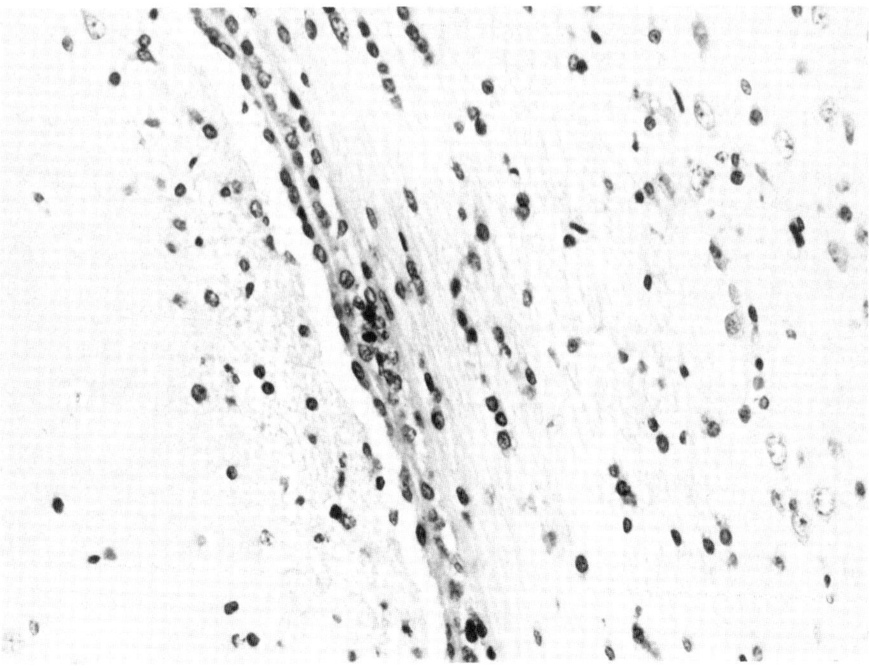

Figure 7.13. Adult rat. Subependymal plate with dividing cells. H&E, ×300.

[^{3}H]-thymidine. If they demonstrate the occurrence of cell division, the kind of glial cell involved must be established (133). Neuroglial mitosis certainly takes place in the adult. The cells should nonetheless be counted, and this is not an easy task for a number of reasons (22).

ENU's most important effect is *O*-alkylation with mispairing during transcription, due to substitution at 0-6 of guanine, 0-2 of cytosine, and 0-2 and 0-4 of thymine. Alkylation at the N-7 position of guanine and the N-3 position of adenine could be responsible for cytotoxic effects (95). A defective DNA repair capacity seems to be responsible for the susceptibility of the nervous system to the neurooncogenic effect of alkylating agents. The amount of 0-6-alkylguanine in cerebral DNA was 20 times that in hepatic DNA one week after administration of ENU to 10-day-old rats (62).

ENU's decreasing oncogenic effect during postnatal maturation has been attributed to reduction of the cell target mass (149). The opposite explanation can be proposed for its poor effect before the 15th day of intrauterine life (95). The target population comprises the germinal matrix, the subependymal plate and/or migrating or already migrated glia, and spinal subpial immature glial cells (138). ENU has both short-term and long-term effects (production of cerebral tumors) on the structures. The main short-term effects are cell death, nuclear pyknosis, and a temporary suspension of cell division in the germinal matrix (14). Enhanced proliferation is needed to secure genetic fixation of promutagenic structural changes (107), and the cytocidal effect of ENU is, in effect, followed by regenerative proliferation in the future tumor sites: subependymal zone of the lateral ventricle, peripheral nerve plexus, and proximal part of the cranial nerves, especially the 5th (199). The cranial nerve displays the peripheral and central parts very distinctly: the former with peripheral-type myelin and Schwann cells, the latter with central-type myelin and oligodendrocytes. Schwann cell proliferation has been demonstrated only 1 month after exposure to transplacental ENU (212). The eventual tumors may be peripheral neurinomas and central oligodendrogliomas that often intermingle (167).

In the period between ENU administration and the appearance of ENPs, there would appear to be no histologically detectable changes in the areas that progressively develop from the matrix. If fetal brain cells are cultured after exposure to ENU in vivo, however, they undergo phenotypic changes until tumors develop when transplanted into 5- to 10-day-old rats (108). It is worthy of note that when normal rat cells are cultured and when the transformation has reached the microtumor stage in vivo, the in vitro transformation can still be observed (155).

Transformation from fetal brain cells passes through four stages requiring a total of more than 100 days (107). Cell morphology changes precede the attainment of biological malignancy (i.e., tumorigenicity after transplantation into rats). In view of what will be said later, it is worth mentioning that GFAP is negative or only slightly positive in these cells. If glial maturation factor is added to the cultures, however, fetal glioblasts are quickly transformed into mature astrocytes (67, 121) and GFAP accumulates (69).

After 200 days, ENU-treated fetal brain cells produce tumors in isogenic hosts whose morphology is similar to that of the tumors induced by transplacental ENU (25, 109). If malignant cell aggregates are brought into contact with 9-day chick embryo heart fragments, heart cells are progressively replaced by tumor cells, showing that invasiveness is associated with in vivo tumorigenicity (34, 107).

As we have seen, no changes in tissue morphology can be discerned during the histological latency period. Cell counts in developing areas between the matrix and cortex of transplacentally ENU-treated rats showed that the picture is the same as in the controls until the 30th extrauterine day, after which cell numbers increase until glial hyperplasia is reached in the white matter. This can be seen as the earliest neoplastic lesion (172). The number of mitoses is the same as in the controls. DNA histograms after cytofluorimetry show that most cells are diploid with very few proceeding to tetraploid, as can also be found in the controls. Very few cells are in cycle, therefore, in both the paraventricular white matter and cell hyperplasia. This provided an ample explanation of the 1-month latency period. It will be recalled that the labeling index is <3% in ENPs (172).

Cell Characteristics of ENU-Induced Tumors

Recognition of the iso- and polymorphic oligodendroglial and astroglial nature of ENU-induced tumors has provided a clear picture of their cell composition and permitted a diachronic survey of their development. The transition from hyperplasia to ENPs is marked by the appearance of abundant reactive astrocytes (172).

Some histochemical and immunohistochemical aspects of ENU tumors have been used to gain a better understanding of their origin and diffusion. Accumulation of glycosoaminoglycans (GAGs) has been demonstrated by means of the Alcian blue technique (171) (Figs. 7.14 and 7.15) in ENPs and oligodendroglial foci, and in isomorphic (though not in dedifferentiated) oligodendrogliomas. It was thus supposed that oligodendroglia cells undergo neoplastic transformation after acquiring the ability to intervene in GAG metabolism, before and during myelinogenesis. The myelination and ENU-sensitivity periods overlap in the rat brain (172) and spinal cord (138). Involvement of oligodendroglia in neoplastic transformation, on the other hand, has also been confirmed by in vivo/in vitro investigation (15). The ability to accumulate GAGs could be lost in the process of dedifferentiation (58). Alcianophilia is observed in all human gliomas, including astrocytomas (11), and is not confined to oligodendroglioma and oligodendroglial areas of gliomas. Leaving the vessels aside, it is correlated with both tumor degeneration and the included normal nervous tissue (58). The same considerations can be applied to ENU-induced tumors as well (129).

Quantitative and qualitative biochemical analyses have revealed GAG accumulation in MNU-induced tumors prior to their appearance (42), but this does not happen in ENU-induced tumors. Interpretation of the presence of GAGs in the proliferative areas of tumors cannot be fully explained through the hypothesis mentioned earlier. A part of chondroitin sulfate may be related to cell proliferation (4).

Useful information has been gained by applying immunohistochemical procedures for cell differentiation markers, principally GFAP, to ENU tumors. This intermediate filament is found in normal rat astrocytes of the molecular layer, paraventricular white matter, hippocampus, and Bergmann's glia (5). Its distribution pattern is neither quantitatively nor qualitatively modified by the appearance of foci of cell hyperplasia in the paraventricular white matter on the 30th day of extrauterine life. By contrast, large GFAP-positive astrocytes are abundant in ENPs and in the ensuing tumors (Figs. 7.16 and 7.17). They have been interpreted as reactive, not tumoral, astrocytes, since they disappear within the tumor as it grows larger, being primarily confined to its periphery and the surrounding nervous tissue (130) (Fig. 7.18). It is not easy to distinguish tumoral from reactive astrocytes, even with the electron microscope (110). Reactive astrocytes, however, can be recognized by their general morphology and mainly from their distribution (39). There is no general agreement concerning the absence of GFAP-positive tumor astrocytes. Some workers maintain that a minor fraction can be detected (26, 142). What is more important is that many cells appearing to be astrocytes when stained with H & E do not express GFAP (142).

The lack or paucity of GFAP-positive astrocytes in tumors generally regarded as glial is surprising. One possibility is that tumor cells are astrocytes which are either too young, or dedifferentiated and too anaplastic to express GFAP (37). An alternative possibility is that they are really oligodendrocytes. The abundance of reactive astrocytes in ENPs may be attributed either to inapparent damage to the myelin sheaths (113), or to the location of ENPs in the paraventricular white matter, in other words, a site normally rich in stellate astro-

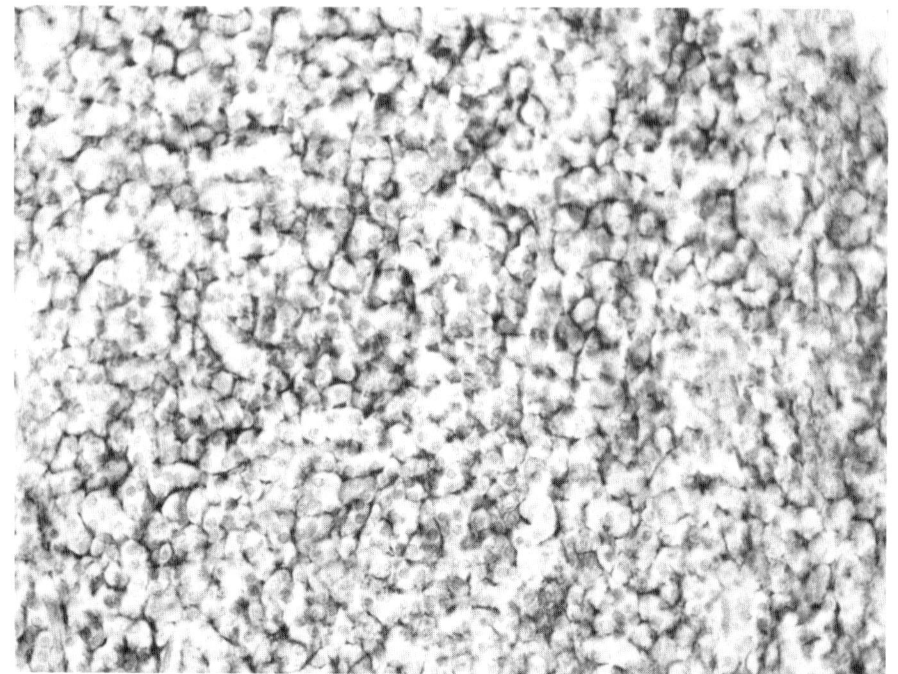

Figure 7.14. TEM. GAG accumulation in an oligodendroglioma. Alcian Blue, CEC 0.2 M $MgCL_2$, ×200.

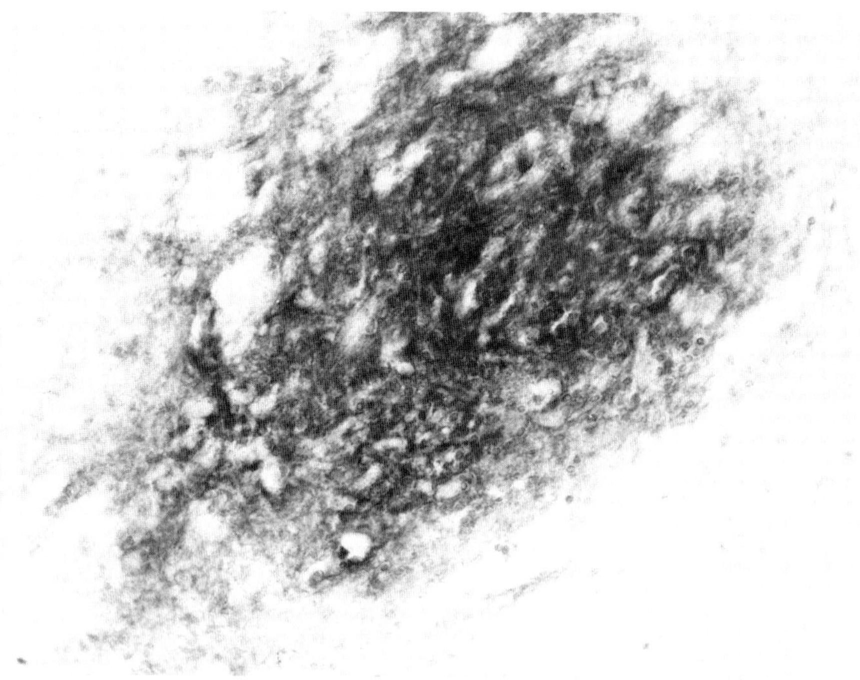

Figure 7.15. TEM. GAG accumulation in an oligodendroglial focus in the cerebral cortex. Alcian blue, CEC 0.2 M $MgCL_2$, ×200.

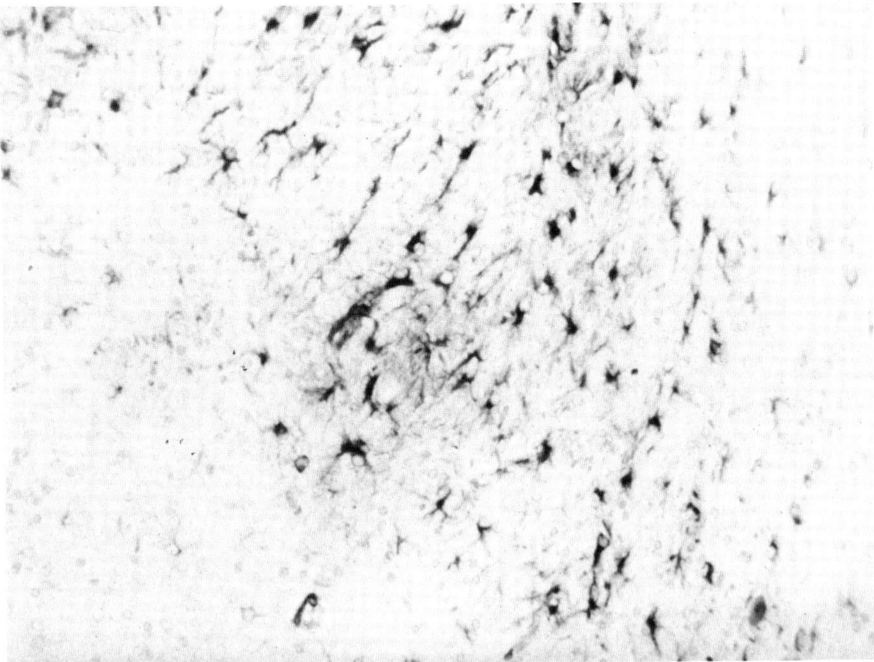

Figure 7.16. TEM. Large, intensely GFAP-positive reactive astrocytes in an ENP. PAP method, counterstained with hematoxylin, ×300.

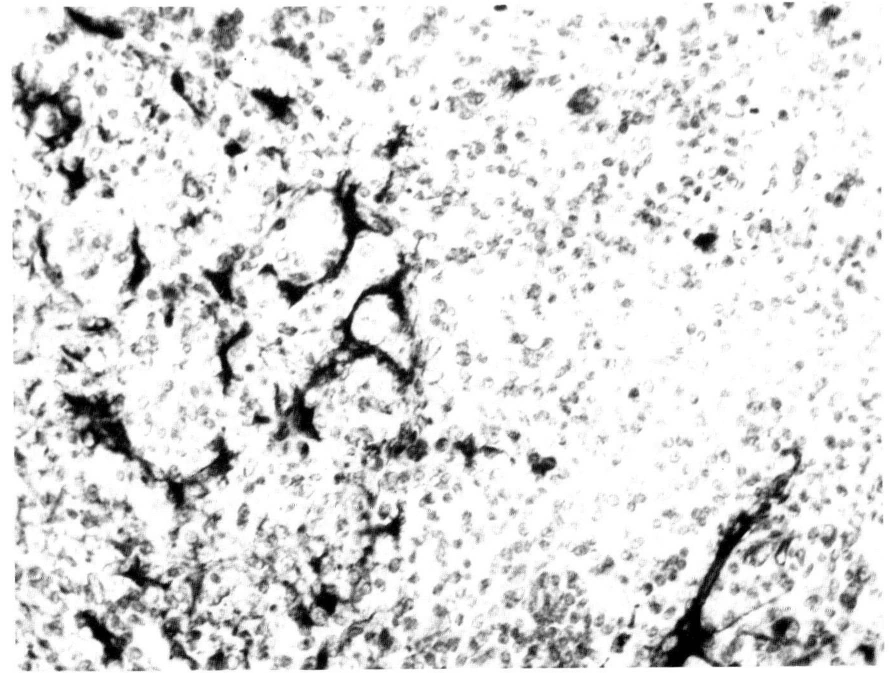

Figure 7.17. TEM. Large, GFAP-positive, reactive astrocytes in the peripheral parts of the tumor and in the surrounding normal nervous tissue. PAP method, counterstained with hematoxylin, ×300.

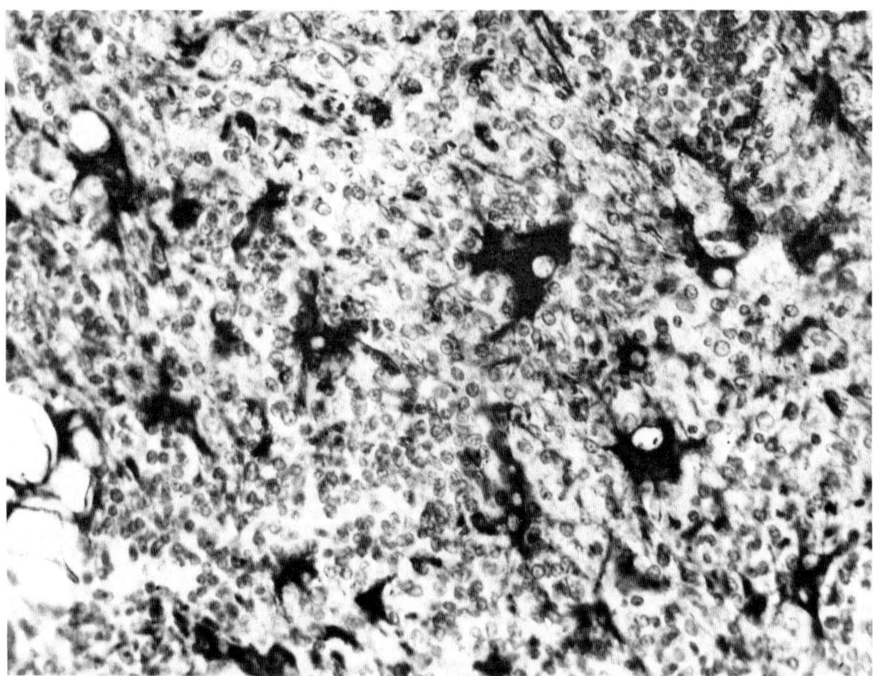

Figure 7.18. TEM. GFAP-positive reactive astrocytes in the tumor and GFAP-negative tumor cells. PAP method, counterstained with hematoxylin, ×200.

cytes in the rat. Lesions caused by other means in these areas are also rich in reactive astrocytes (175).

Immunohistochemical investigation of the distribution of vimentin in ENU tumors has also provided supplementary information concerning the nature of their cells. This intermediate filament is present in both mesenchymal and glial cells (23, 143) and coexists with GFAP in mature astrocytes (29) during development, though it is expressed earlier than GFAP (7, 43, 185). In the rat, it decorates some astrocytes of the white matter, granular layer and white matter of the cerebellum, hippocampus, cerebral cortex, and the ependyma in particular (185). In ENU tumors, vimentin evidences peritumoral GFAP-positive reactive astrocytes and the cells of proliferative centers (Figs. 7.19 and 7.20) found in microtumors and fully developed tumors (61, 168). Since the mesodermal nature of these cells is ruled out, for example, by their negative staining with Factor VIII/RAg, fibronectin and laminin, they can be regarded as immature astrocytes not yet expressing GFAP (37, 153). Little can be gathered from these findings with respect to the commencement of neoplastic transformation during neurocytogenesis. Fetal brain cells exposed to ENU in vivo display in vitro modification of the phenotypic expression preceding tumorigenicity. GFAP expression is poor unless glial maturation factor is added to the cultures (67, 107). The absence of GFAP expression in ENU tumor cells and the presence of vimentin may also be due to loss of the ability to express GFAP after transformation, since glial cells can express it even before the final mitosis during neurocytogenesis. Simultaneous expression of both GFAP and vimentin in reactive astrocytes has been reported on other occasions (29), as well as in human nervous tissue and tumors (174) and in electron microscopy studies (144).

Establishment of the nature of ENU tumor cells is complicated by the fact that carboanhydrase C (CA.C), a typical immunohistochemical marker of oligodendroglia (104), including human oligodendroglia

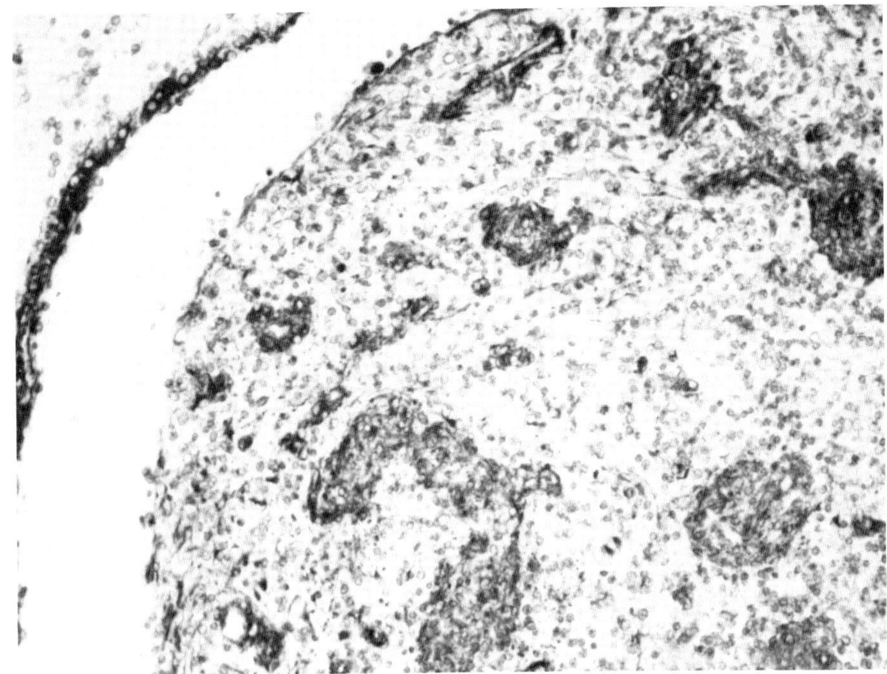

Figure 7.19. TEM. Vimentin-positive reactive ependymal cells and tumor cells of proliferative centers. PAP method, counterstained with hematoxylin, ×200.

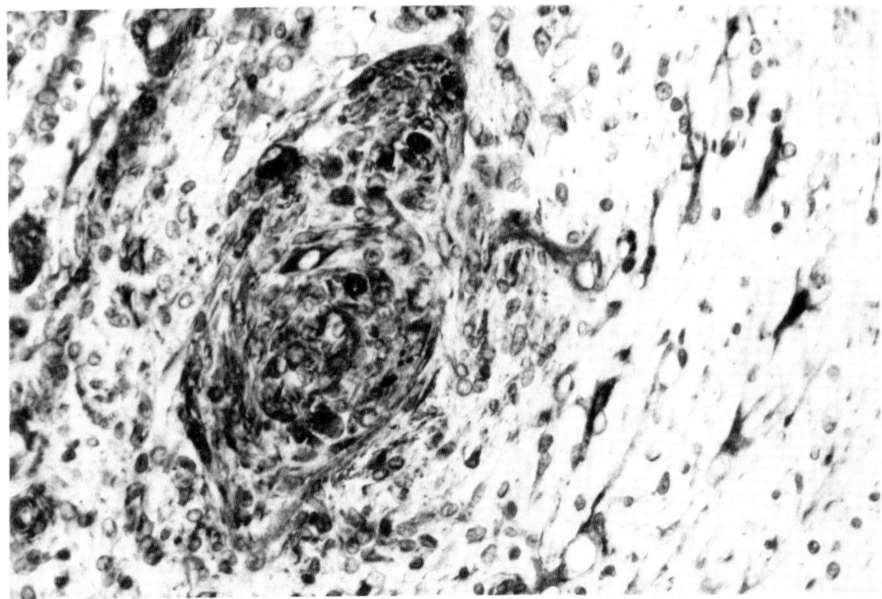

Figure 7.20. TEM. Vimentin-positive reactive astrocytes and tumor cells of proliferative centers. PAP method, counterstained with hematoxylin, ×400.

(105), is positive in normal rat cortex and white matter oligodendrocytes (Fig. 7.21), but not in tumoral oligodendrocytes (Fig. 7.22) (61, 168). This is surprising in tumors with an unequivocal oligodendroglial appearance. The failure of tumoral oligodendrocytes to express CA.C may perhaps reflect the fact that the typical distribution pattern is only attained after three weeks of extrauterine life.

The contribution of specific oncogenes to tumor progression has also been studied in cultured cells from ENU-treated animals. Transformed glioma cells contain a high level of c.sis transcripts compared with those not yet transformed, and then of functional platelet-derived growth factor (PDGF) (114). Autocrine stimulation has been suggested in view of the fact that glia cells have PDGF receptors (71). The neu gene has been detected in ENU-induced neuroblastomas (163). It is not yet known how many and which oncogenes are activated in the transformation process.

ENU Tumor Vasculature

In white matter cell hyperplasia and in ENPs, the vessels are those of the host tissue, whereas the formation of new vessels begins in microtumors and reaches its maximum in fully developed tumors. Endothelial buds and vascular glomeruli develop, and often constitute a wall against necrosis, tumor tissue, etc. (Fig. 7.23). The modality and moment of vessel formation have been investigated in tumors induced by intracerebral injection of cultured transplacental ENU tumor cells (33). An avascular stage is followed by the appearance of simple or complex capillary buds and immature capillaries in 1 to 4 mm tumors. Three zones can be distinguished in larger tumors: a central remnant of the vasculature stage, which eventually necroses; a peripheral angiogenesis zone; an intermediate zone with a population of polymorphic vessels displaying a variety of structural abnormalities. The buds are not dissimilar to normal embryonic buds, as in human tumors. Vessel density is higher in the peripheral zone, whereas endothelial hyperplasia is confined to the intermediate zone. There is an increase in the number of capillaries in the surrounding normal cortex, though their density is lower than that of the tumor.

Peritumoral angiogenesis proceeds from the host vessels (33). Their structural alterations have been the subject of particular

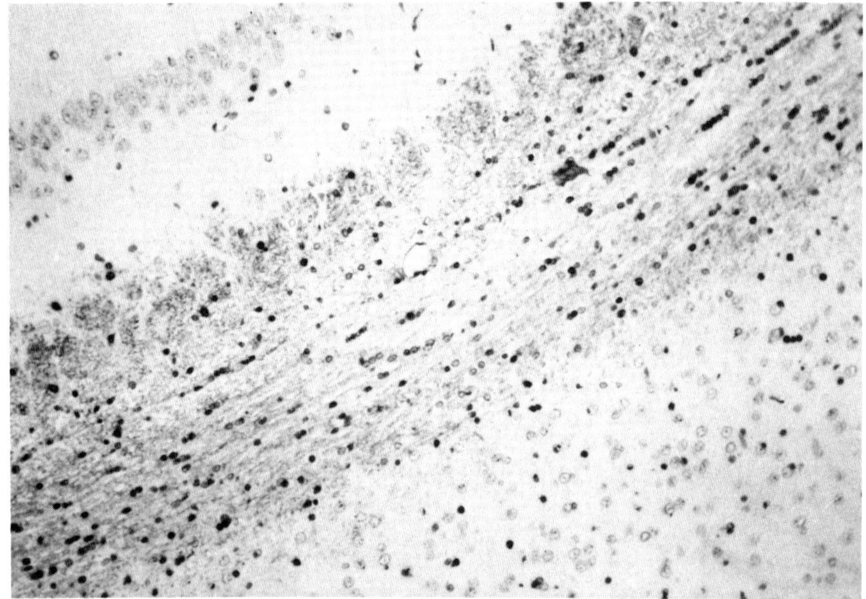

Figure 7.21. Adult rat. CAC-positive oligodendrocytes of the white and gray matter. PAP method, counterstained with hematoxylin, ×300.

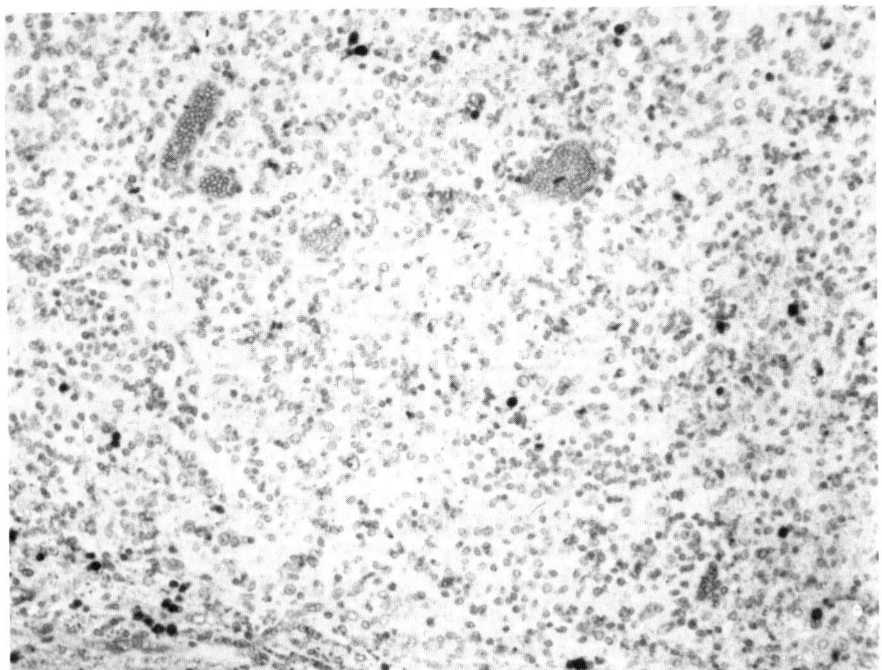

Figure 7.22. TEM. Oligodendroglioma. Most cells are CAC-negative. The positive ones are normal oligodendrocytes trapped in the tumor. PAP method, counterstained with hematoxylin, ×300.

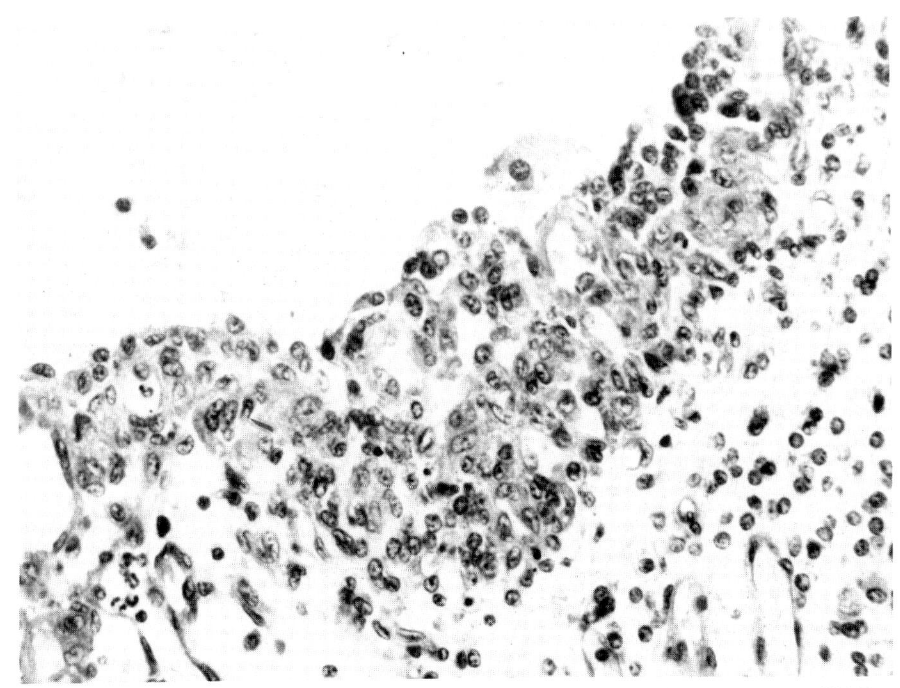

Figure 7.23. TEM. Wall of proliferated endothelial cells delimiting a cyst in a large tumor. H&E, ×400.

attention (139). The main change is the formation of large sinusoids or venous microvessels that act in the barrier function. It has been shown that blood flow is low in the central and peripheral zones and high in the intermediate zone (217).

Tumor Spreading

In their advanced stages, these tumors spread to the entire hemisphere (Fig. 7.24), the brainstem, and the subarachnoid space (Fig. 7.25). Total cancerization of the brain is a possible outcome. This picture is reached not only through actual diffusion of a given tumor, but also as the result of confluence of neoplastic lesions that may even be at different stages of development. Multiplicity, indeed, is a characteristic of transplacental ENU tumors and is related to the dose employed. The appearance of fresh neoplastic lesions when fully developed tumors are already present is naturally of great neuro-oncogenetic significance. Gliosarcomas are a later development. Their reticulin-producing sarcomatous component originates in the vessels of glial tumors and is often found in the center of the tumor (91).

The invasiveness of ENU tumors has been demonstrated in experiments simulating local growth. Normal rat brain fragments have been co-cultured with glioma cells derived from rat fetuses treated with ENU transplacentally. These cells progressively invade and replace the normal brain tissue (195). This is not the result of penetration nor phagocytosis, but of a postulated secretion of toxic substances (194).

Therapeutic Studies

Induction by transplacental ENU has been less frequently employed in radiotherapy and chemotherapy experiments than other models, e.g., induction of 9L gliosarcoma by MNU, and ASV astrocytoma (186). Radiotherapy of ENU tumors transplanted into the brain has been investigated (53, 193). A lower incidence of tumors is observed if neonatal administration of ENU is followed by x-irradiation (99). BCNU, CCNU, and other nitrosourea derivatives administered to rats prior to the appearance of tumors delay their development (178). NGF administered before or after ENU reduced the number of neurinomas observed on the 90th extrauterine day (207). The transplacental ENU model has been used for unilateral hyperosmotic blood-brain barrier disruption by intracarotid administration of mannitol, followed by A1B with 14C (209). Disruption had no significant effect on tumor permeability, nor on subsequent drug delivery.

THE DEVELOPMENT OF HUMAN GLIOMAS AND THEIR MALIGNANT PHENOTYPE

The Transformation Process

The early stages of human tumor development have not been identified. There are descriptions of different forms of initial proliferation noted casually during necroscopy (88), but systematic observations are lacking. General views of the pathogenesis of tumors have been advanced in the light of the relative frequency of individual oncotypes in children and adults and their growth modalities, and their comparison with known models of tumor induction with nitrosourea derivatives. Late fetal neuroepithelial cells are a putative target for neoplastic transformation (157, 159), together with the five sites in which neurocytogenesis continues after birth (119): the subependymal plate, astrocytes, and oligodendrocytes during myelinogenesis, the outer granular layer of the cerebellum, the gyrus dentatus, and the molecular layer of the cerebral cortex. Neoplastic transformation has also been regarded as a multistep process in human neuro-oncology. Great importance has been attached to shifting of the target cells between strikes, with the result that a tumor may arise elsewhere than in the site of the first strike, e.g., in the cerebral cortex (159).

When the first step occurs, the target cells are still capable of duplication or re-entering proliferation. A succinct idea of their susceptibility to transformation is offered by the concept of a "window of neoplastic vulnerability" (158), whose wideness depends on a variety of factors, such as the existence of a reservoir of stem cells, the ability of differentiated cells to re-enter the cycle, the number of duplicating cells at

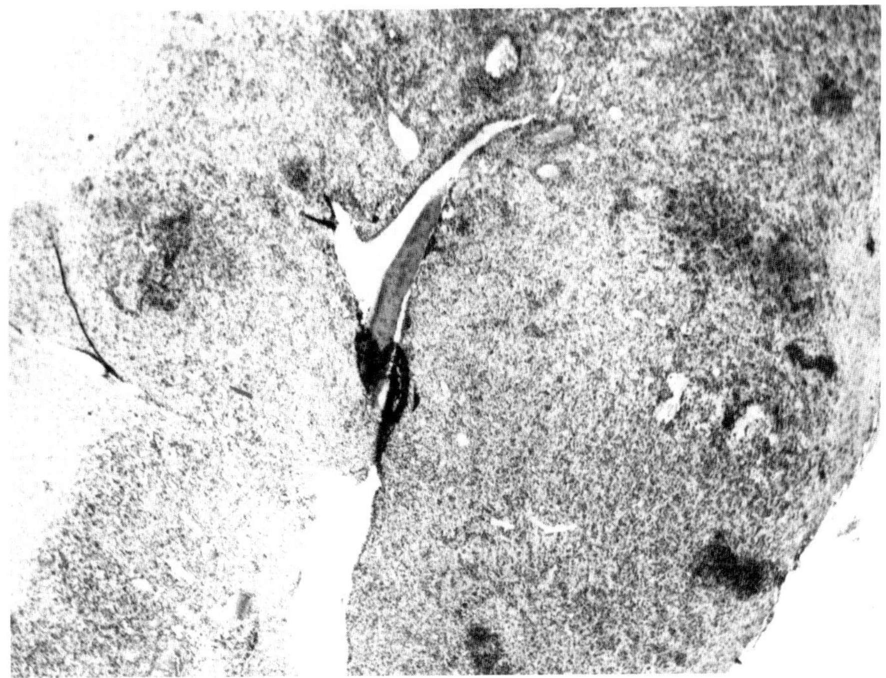

Figure 7.24. TEM. A polymorphic tumor spreading to the whole hemisphere. H&E, ×50.

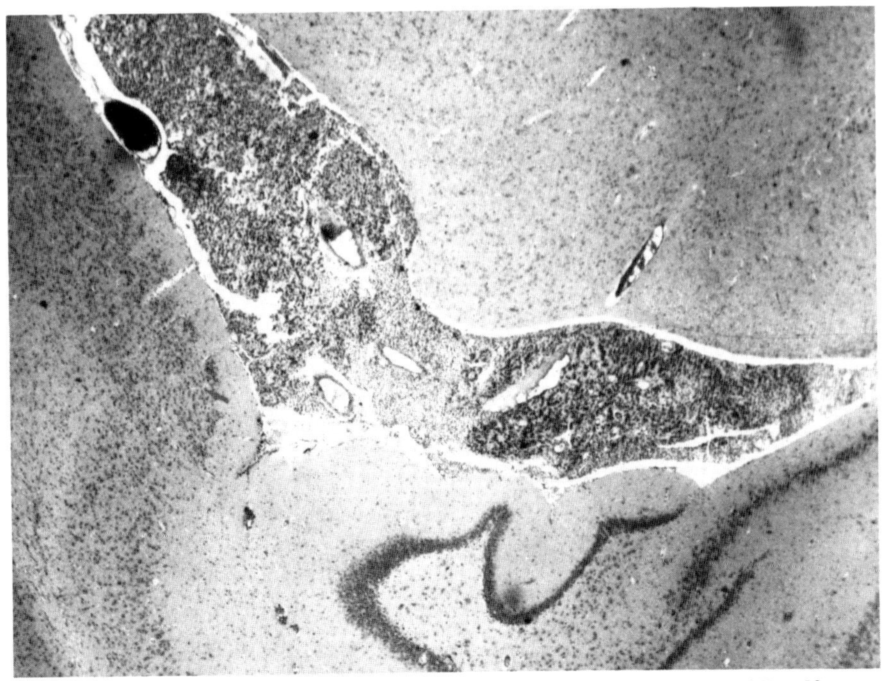

Figure 7.25. TEM. Spreading of a tumor in the subarachnoidal space. H&E, ×50.

risk at a given moment, the length of the period in which a cell population is in the cycle, and its differentiation status.

Since transformed neuroepithelial cells continue to differentiate and since differentiated tumors may undergo anaplasia, the pathogenesis of gliomas and their ability to proliferate must be examined with reference to the notion of differentiation and undifferentiation.

Very few CNS cells are susceptible to neoplastic transformation in the adult and their turnover is low. The possibility of a tumor arising in this way cannot, of course, be denied. It is more likely, however, that transformation during morphogenesis is almost always responsible. Cells continue to differentiate after transformation, but abnormally, and characteristics proper to cells with another differentiation pattern may appear (158). The earlier the cytogenetic stage at which transformation occurs, the greater the differentiating potential of the tumor (161, 164). Conversely, the smaller the vulnerability or the shorter its period, the lower the tumor frequency. The high frequency of medulloblastomas and gliomas, for example, is determined by the long mitotic activity of precursor cells, and by the persistence of a glial turnover in adulthood, respectively. From the neuropathological, diagnostic and clinical standpoints, the most important aspect of cerebral tumors is the relationship between benign and malignant forms, with particular reference to malignant transformation and the possibility of its morphological detection. A clear example is provided by the relationship between astrocytoma and its anaplastic variant. Irrespective of how it arises, an astrocytoma grows slowly, is composed of isomorphic cells, and has poor angiogenesis (Fig. 7.26). At a certain point in its biological course, however, it may change its rate of growth and become malignant. Cells pass from the nonproliferating to the proliferating pool and the growth fraction increases. This phenomenon is defined as anaplasia. Its morphological signs are an increase in cell density and mitosis (Fig. 7.27) and appearance of circumscribed necroses, and angiogenesis (Fig. 7.28). Some of these mechanisms have been clarified.

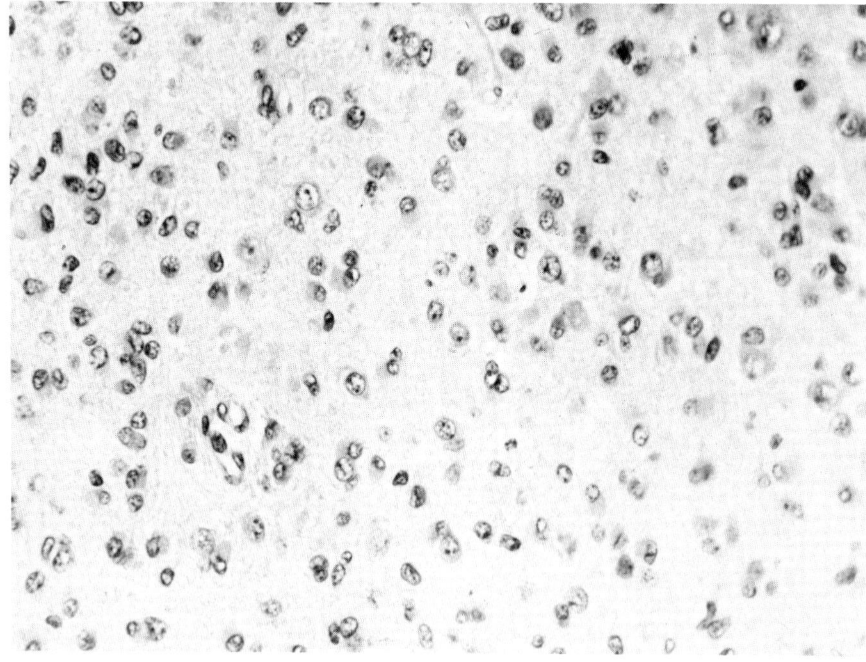

Figure 7.26. Astrocytoma in the cortex. Isomorphic nuclei, low cell density, very few small vessels are present. H&E, ×200.

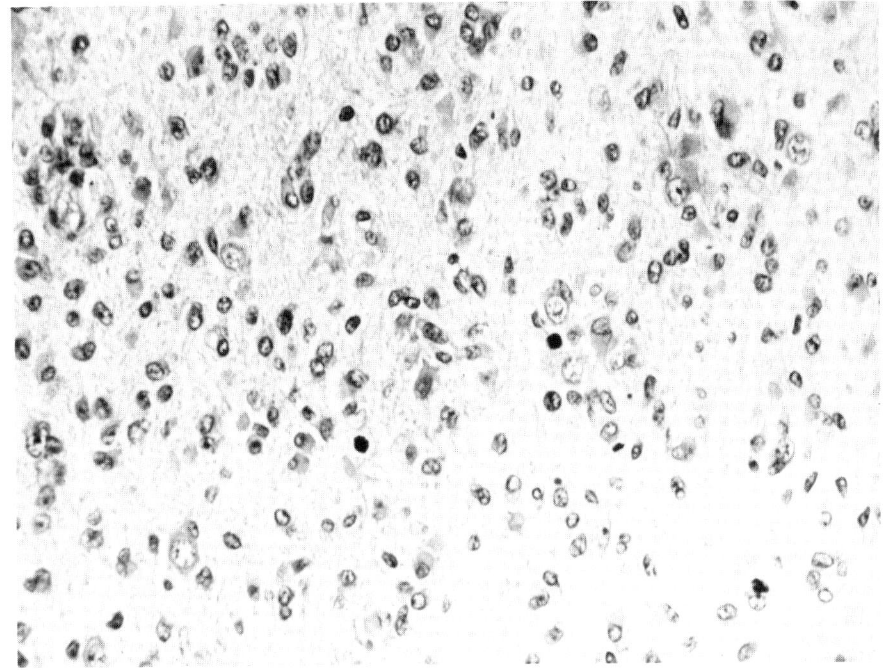

Figure 7.27. Astrocytoma. Early signs of anaplasia: increased cell density and mitoses. H&E, ×200.

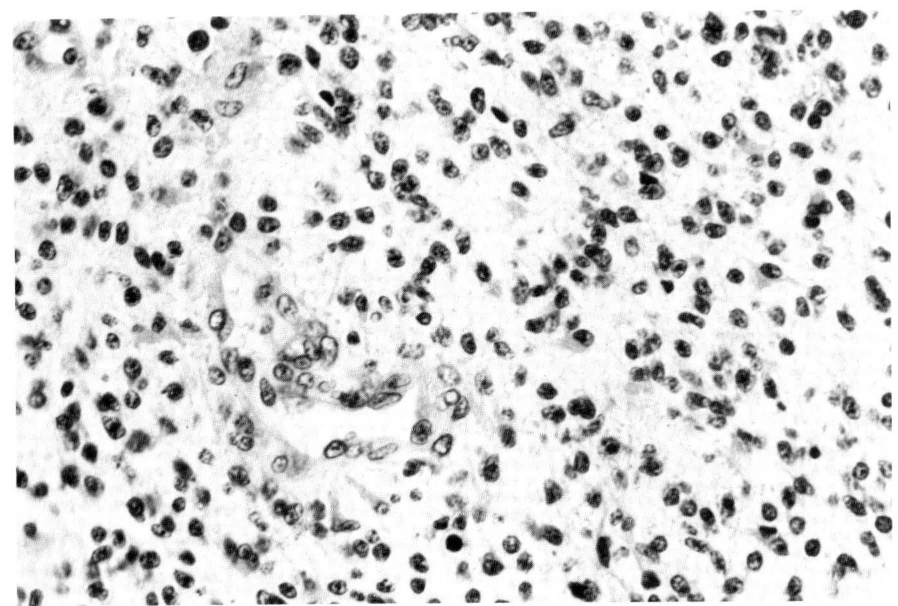

Figure 7.28. Astrocytoma. Anaplasia with increased cell density, mitoses and endothelial proliferations. H&E, ×200.

Anaplasia is classically regarded as a consequence of dedifferentiation, i.e., loss of morphological characteristics typical of a certain degree of differentiation, with regression to those of a more primitive stage. It can also be seen as a failure of differentiation whereby tumor cells do not reach morphological maturity (219).

This concept, however, has been the subject of profound rethinking in recent years. Anaplasia is now increasingly interpreted as an expression of the heterogeneity of the tumor cell population. Karyotype analysis (127, 189), cytophotometry and flow cytometry (81, 85), and comparisons of established human glioma cell lines (9) have provided evidence supporting this view. Whether such phenotype variations are genetic, i.e., the outcome of a progressive increase in maturation rates owing to the genetic instability of tumor cell populations, or depend on epigenetic factors, is still the subject of debate (8, 159).

The expression of GFAP, a characteristic marker of astrocyte differentiation (12, 36), is a phenotypic property that has been extensively studied in recent years and may be included among the manifestations of heterogeneity (93). GFAP is found in all glioma cells with gliofibrillogenetic capacity (Fig. 7.29), and the number of positive cells is inversely related to the degree of anaplasia (41, 204, 205). GFAP may be lacking in too primitive or too anaplastic cells. It must be stressed that the small, less mature cells that proliferate more rapidly (80) and are responsible for tumor invasiveness and growth (57) are GFAP-negative (205). The appearance of both anaplasia in mature astrocytomas (Fig. 7.30) and active proliferation in glioblastomas is supported by a cell population characterized by isomorphic nuclei, GFAP-negative cytoplasm, and many GFAP-negative mitoses (Fig. 7.31). Older, more differentiated cells are GFAP-positive and have fewer mitoses (176).

Irrespective of its mechanism, anaplasia involves a change in tumor cell kinetics. The growth fraction increases (80) and cells are recruited from the nonproliferating to the proliferating pool. Clonogenic populations will develop and be selected by competition (184). Tumor progression, in fact, can be thought of as a function of genetic instability and environmental selection

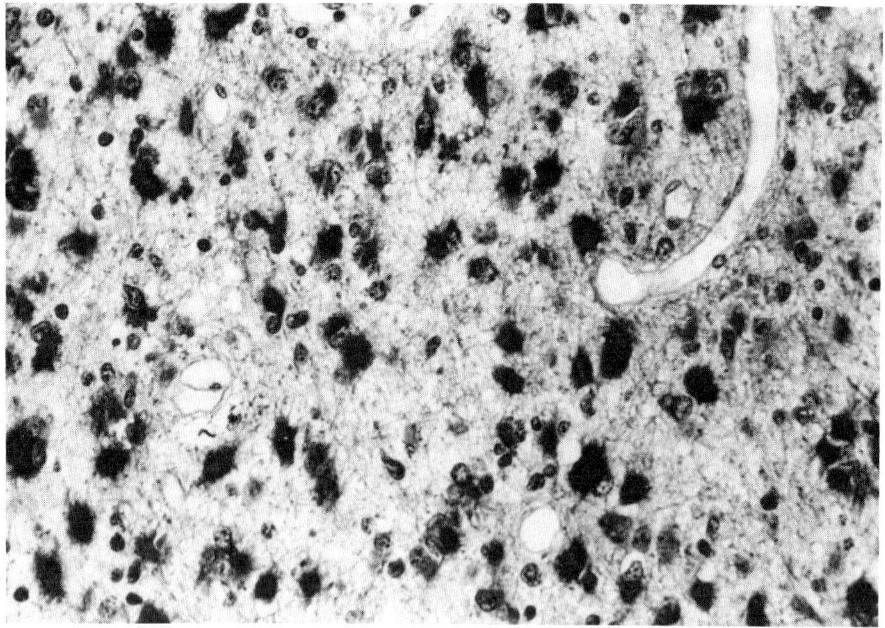

Figure 7.29. Astrocytoma. Most cells are GFAP-positive. PAP method, counterstained with hematoxylin, ×300.

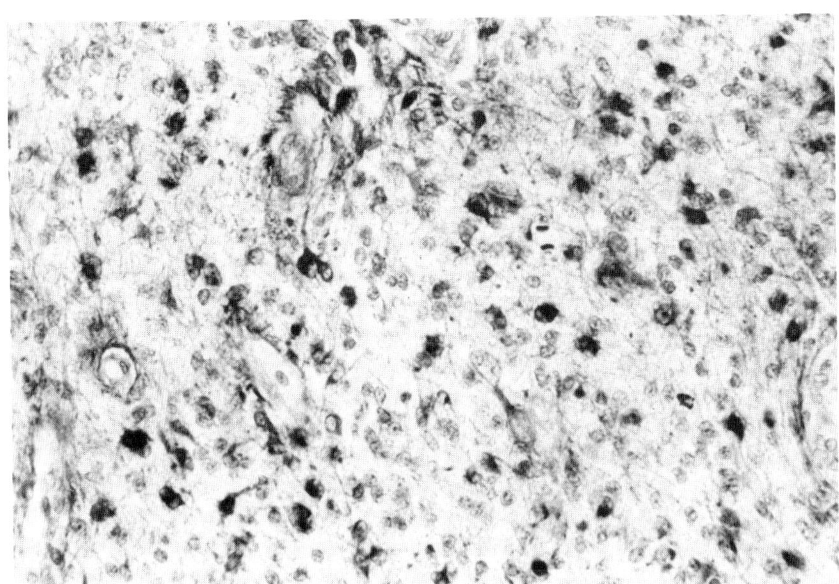

Figure 7.30. Anaplastic astrocytoma. Many cells with scanty cytoplasm and mitoses, GFAP-negative. PAP method, counterstained with hematoxylin, ×300.

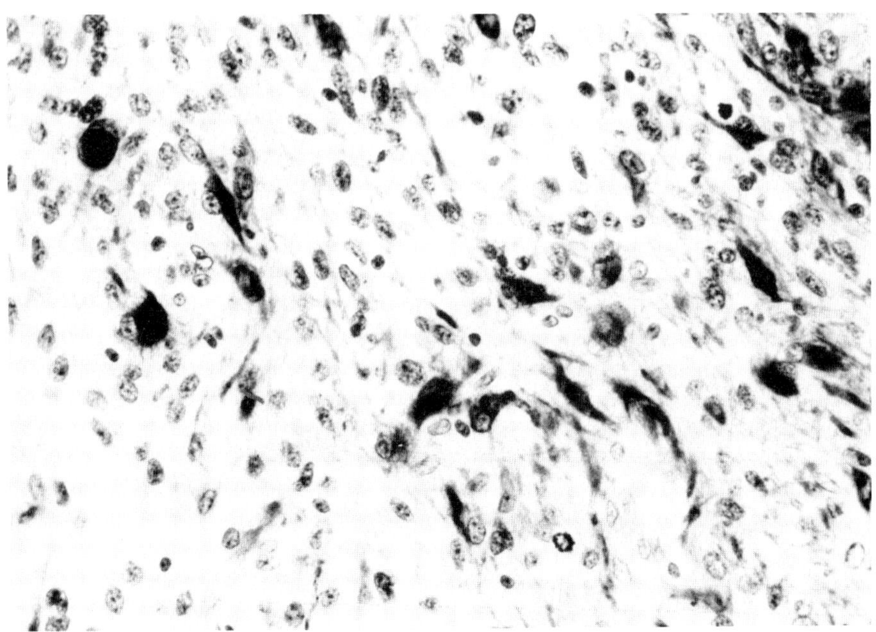

Figure 7.31. Glioblastoma. Area with GFAP-positive and negative cells. Mitoses are negative. PAP method, counterstained with hematoxylin, ×300.

(188), since the biochemical and cytogenetic evidence shows that tumor cell populations can further alter their genome.

Anaplasia can also be seen as the consequence of genetic modifications leading to the arrest of maturation, or an accelerated growth of already differentiating precursors (19). Tumor "stem" cells have long been postulated, but never demonstrated, and their identification is a matter of present concern. They could even be differentiated cells, provided they can reenter the cell cycle as has been suggested in the case of astrocytes and oligodendrocytes (123).

Typical histological findings follow the establishment of anaplasia: increasing cell density and frequency of mitoses, nuclear polymorphism, cell monstrosities, mitotic abnormalities, necrosis, and a new vasculature. All these signs are regarded as expressions of malignancy not only because they are directly or indirectly related to the new cell kinetics, but also because they are usually observed empirically in low-survival rate tumors. Even so, apart from cell density and frequency of mitoses, they cannot be taken as indicative of malignancy per se.

There are various ways of evaluating cell kinetics. The mitotic index is an approximately accurate and restrictive method. The labeling index (LI) after [^{3}H] thymidine correlates with prognosis (82, 85), though this method has not escaped criticism (13, 133). Administration of BUdR, revealed by a monoclonal antibody (137), to either patients or small fragments of tumor in culture (135), seems to be more precise as it labels cells in S-phase. Reaction of the monoclonal antibody Ki-67 with a nuclear antigen expressed by cells in cycle (54, 55), offers another method that appears to correlate with prognosis (18, 59, 154).

The transition from astrocytoma to glioblastoma through anaplasia also raises significant clinical issues. The main problem is the detection of anaplasia in vivo, since this aids decisions concerning therapy and prognosis. CT and MRI are of great assistance in this respect, and stereotaxic biopsy may even provide histological confirmation. There are several possibilitics for error; however, anaplasia may be a localized phenomenon in a benign glioma (160); a benign glioma may still become malignant after the histological or imaging diagnosis; the development of malignancy may affect the parenchyma only and, hence, escape detection by neuroimaging. Dynamics of this kind are reflected in Scherer's old distinction between primary and secondary glioblastomas (165). A secondary form should be recognized from the continued presence of astrocytomatous areas. However, anaplasia may be so extensive that all traces of the astrocytoma are destroyed and such recognition is impossible (90). It is also possible that astrocytomatous areas are the product of glioblastoma cell differentiation (179), which means that primary glioblastomas may be the only type (169). In effect, there is virtually no distinction between the two types (222). Nonetheless, the question of their occurrence is of particular theoretical interest (126).

If the development of malignancy is accompanied by changes in tumor cell kinetics, increased genetic lability, and new mutations, then GFAP, being an expression of astrocyte differentiation, should eventually disappear from a glioblastoma as the result of selection by competition (184). The short duration of glioblastoma, however, makes it impossible to determine the correctness of this supposition. By contrast, if GFAP expression is modulated by epigenetic factors, it might reappear in the cells (176). It is possible that stem cells in the tumor differentiate along the astrocytic line. Nonetheless, the possibility that astrocytomatous areas in a glioblastoma belong to a preceding astrocytoma cannot be ruled out (179).

As already mentioned, the development of brain tumors is a multistep process, like that of tumors in general (49, 98). Tumor "progression" has been defined through a series of stepwise changes in several unit characteristics: growth rate, ability to invade surrounding tissues and grow as freely dissociated cells in body fluids, and hormone independence (49). During such progression, subclones replace their predecessors. The pathology of tumors must therefore be seen as a continuous dynamic whose most outstanding feature is selection by competition (97).

Current thinking in the field of molecular genetics is that tumor development is promoted by oncogenes, activated by regulatory or structural changes, or opposed by suppressor genes or hemerogenes (203). Many oncogenes belonging to a variety of categories, such as growth factors, growth factor receptors, protein kinases, etc., are thought to be involved in brain tumors. Structural chromosome abnormalities described in malignant glioma include deletions, imbalanced translocations, and gene amplifications, especially of Epidermal Growth Factor Receptor (EGFR) (10). A self-stimulatory autocrine cycle has also been postulated for tumor cells expressing Platelet-derived Growth Factor (PDGF) and its receptor (70). Correlation of gene products and their mechanisms of action with the different aspects of glioma, particularly the development of malignant potential, must be one of the main goals of brain tumor pathology.

Particular Aspects

Necrosis and vasculature—two of the histological signs of malignancy well-known to the pathologist—are of particular significance in the case of brain tumors. Three types of necrosis are characteristic of glioblastomas: large, mainly centrally located coagulative necroses (Fig. 7.32); circumscribed necrosis with incomplete pseudopalisading, and small necrosis surrounded by complete pseudopalisading (Fig. 7.33). The second type is found on the periphery of the tumor, outside the central necrosis, in the direction of the meninges, vessel walls, etc., and must be regarded as the result of the crowding of tumor cells on an obstacle to their infiltration. The third type is particularly important, since it originates from highly proliferative areas (Fig. 7.33) with high cell density and many mitoses and is indicative of rapid growth. Necrosis of this type may be the outcome of mitotic imbalance (208), as the mean generation time of endothelial cells is longer than that of tumor cells (202). They disappear when proliferation is temporarily halted by radiotherapy and reappear when growth recommences (180). The proliferative areas are GFAP-negative, since their cells belong to the new population with its enhanced proliferative capacity.

There is no new vessel formation in well-differentiated astrocytoma of the cerebral hemisphere, since the tumor uses and alters the existing vessels. Massive vessel modification occurs in pilocytic astrocytomas of the midline, mainly in the cerebellum, but especially in glioblastoma, owing to endothelial proliferation leading to the formation of glomeruli. Three zones can be distinguished in glioblastomas: a periphery abounding in new vessels with endothelial proliferations; an intermediate zone with larger, dilated vessels; a central, necrotic zone, where the vessels are involved in the degenerative process (Fig. 7.32). The neovascularization cannot be regarded as a constant sign of malignancy. It has been shown, for example, that oligodendrogliomas are much more extensively vascularized than anaplastic astrocytomas. The presence of a dense vessel network may be just a characteristic of a tumor (187).

Most studies have been concerned with the differences between normal and tumor vessels. In normal capillaries endothelial cells are characterized by a basement membrane, tight junctions, few pinocytotic vesicles, and a narrow pericapillary space free from collagen and fibroblasts, since the basement membrane is in direct contact with that of the astrocytes (74, 208). Pericytes are occasionally observed (75). Fenestrated junctions are only found in certain special areas of the CNS, such as the area postrema and the choroid plexus. Tumor capillaries, on the other hand, display abnormalities of all kinds. Their lumen is larger. There are more endothelial cells and, hence, many junctions. Pinocytosis is more widespread, and the basement membrane is thicker. The pericapillary space is filled with collagen (208).

Malignant gliomas are characterized by thrombosis and endothelial proliferation. Endothelial cells increase in number, undergo mitoses and modify the vessel, mak-

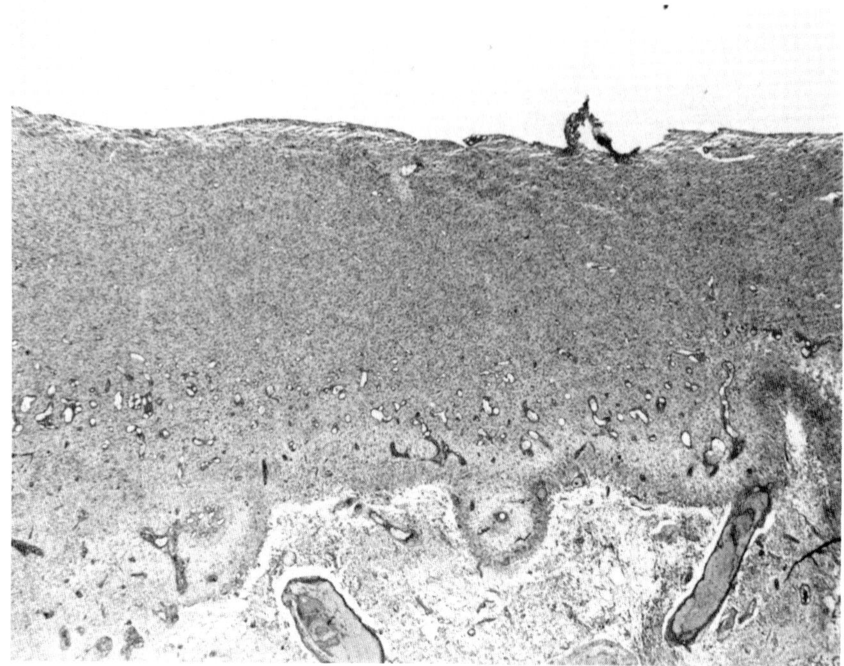

Figure 7.32. Glioblastoma. Large central necrosis and circumscribed necrosis in proliferative area. Vessels in the proliferative, intermediate and necrotic zones. H&E, ×50.

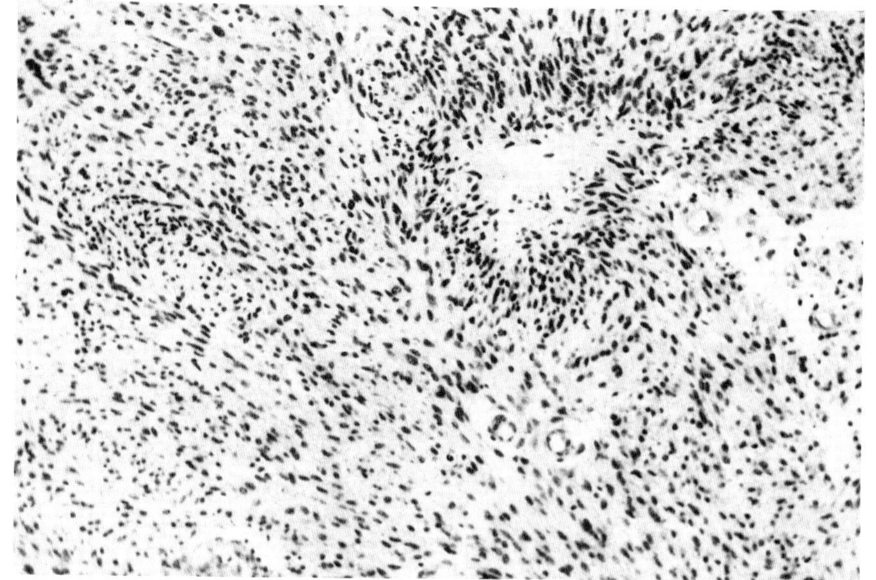

Figure 7.33. Glioblastoma. Circumscribed necrosis in an intensely proliferating area. H&E, ×200.

ing it tortuous, bumpy, and glomeruloid (Fig. 7.34). The transition from normal, peritumoral, and infiltration areas to a full proliferating tumor is accompanied by an increase in the number of endothelial cells and signs of their immaturity, such as few organelles and a high nucleus/cytoplasm ratio (213). Conglomerates of immature capillaries similar to normal capillaries during development (20) are formed in the transition areas, along with immature buds with slit-like lumina and a unique basement membrane (214) (Fig. 7.35).

Endothelial proliferation is regarded as either the source of new capillaries or dependent on thrombosis (21, 196). It is clearly related to the circumscribed necroses (Fig. 7.36), which are probably due to functional insufficiency of the vasculature, since endothelial and tumor cells have a different LI, as mentioned earlier (63, 84). Morphometric and computer-assisted three-dimensional reconstruction studies have shown that glomeruli represent the extreme degree of deformation by endothelial hyperplasia of the tree of the cortex, i.e., the meningeal vessels and their lateral branches (1, 2, 66), so that it can no longer supply oxygen to the tumor cells and necrosis takes place (170). New vessels are formed after cortical infiltration, which stimulates a hyperplastic response on the part of endothelial cells. However, the production of new capillaries by many sproutings (136) is not a constant consequence (Figs. 7.37–7.39). Usually, endothelial proliferation deforms the vascular tree through thickening, narrowing, and even obstruction. The endothelial cells are rich in Weibel-Palade bodies (103). Pericytes may be also involved in the process, although inconstantly and to a lesser extent (170).

Endothelial proliferation is necessary for angiogenesis, but the two conditions are not synonymous. Proliferation is a response to infiltration and often has the opposite effect through the development of necrosis. If infiltration proceeds from the white matter to the surface of the cortex, glomeruli and necrosis will be found in the deep layers, since endothelial proliferation and the formation of new vessels occur after infiltration, as already stated. When infiltration proceeds from below the pia mater to the white matter, glomeruli and necrosis will be found in the surface layers.

Reference is constantly made to angiogenetic factors when discussing the formation of new vessels, since it is assumed that solid tumors are angiogenesis-dependent (46). Many diffusible angiogenetic factors have been identified using a variety of methods (rabbit corneal pouch, chick embryo chorioallantoic membrane, endothelial cell cultures). They include: fibroblastic growth factor (FGF) and endothelial cell growth factor (ECGF) and their receptors, angiogenenin, transforming growth factor (TGF), factors regulating locomotion or proliferation of endothelial cells, heparin, copper, prostaglandins, etc. (47). Angiogenesis in brain tumors has been demonstrated in endothelial cell cultures (76, 94) and on chick embryo chorioallantoic membrane (124).

One very interesting finding is that the B chain gene of PDGF, the major serum growth factor for connective tissue- and glia-derived cells in culture (215), is the normal cell homologue to the *v-sis* oncogene of simian sarcoma virus (SSV) (210). Furthermore, SSV produces malignant glioma when administered to newborn marmosets (35). Human malignant glioma cell lines express PDGF. Some also express the receptor (140). This factor may thus play a part in the autocrine stimulation of tumor cells. In situ hybridization has demonstrated that endothelial cells also display the receptor and may therefore be involved in an autocrine mechanism (72). PDGF could be a member of the angiogenetic peptide family.

Neuroepithelial-mesodermal tumors are not uncommon. They may be derived from a gliomatous reaction to a sarcoma, or from a sarcomatous meningeal reaction to an infiltrating glioblastoma (45, 156). In most cases, however, they are true mixed tumors with a sarcomatous component generated by the vascular proliferation of a glioblastoma (64, 65, 125, 134, 182, 191). Overgrowth of the gliomatous by the sarcomatous component has been observed both in vivo (65) and in vitro (64).

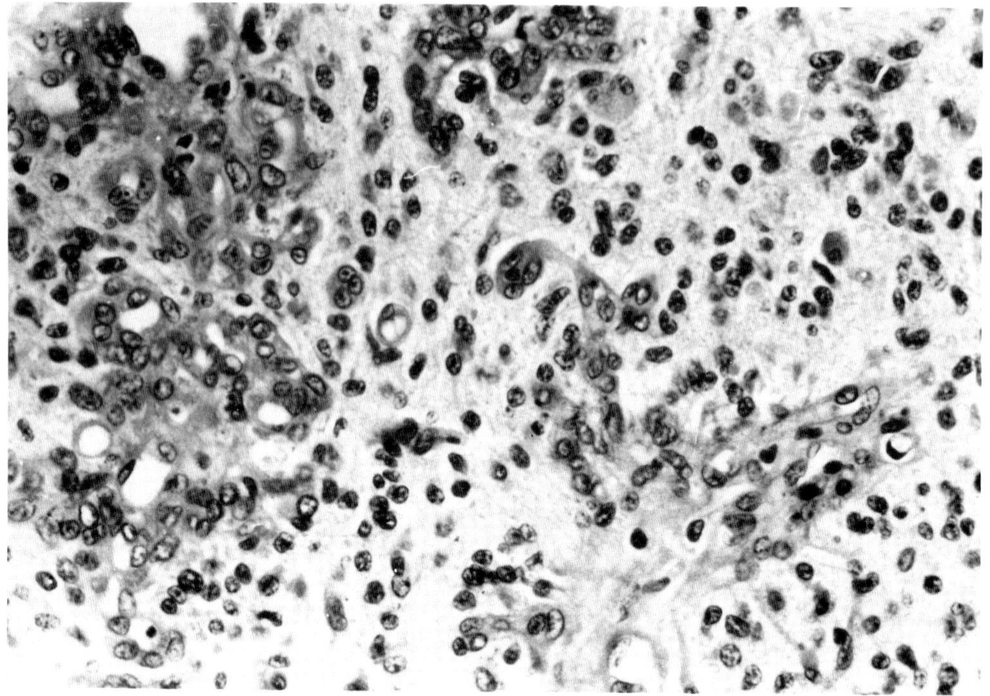

Figure 7.34. Glioblastoma. Endothelial proliferations with buds and sproutings. H&E, ×400.

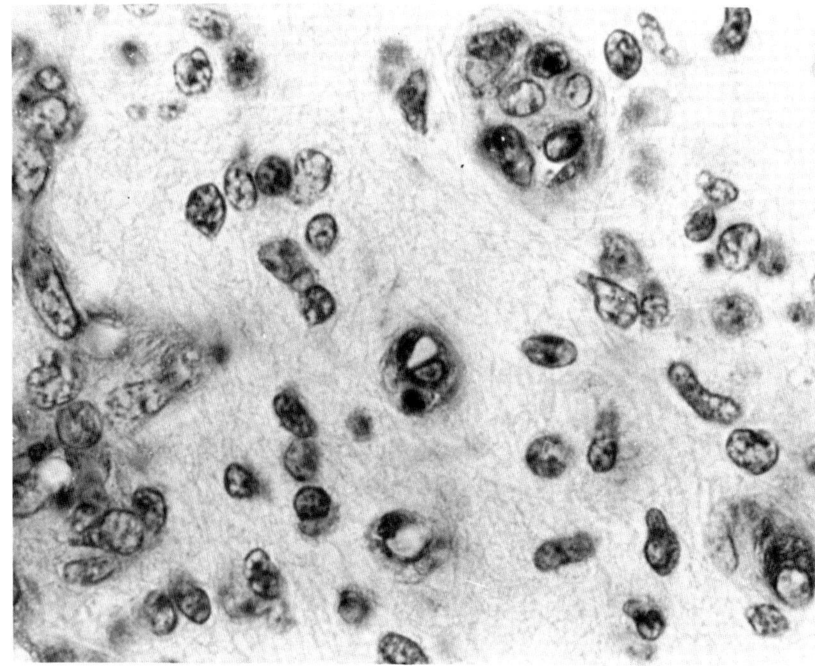

Figure 7.35. Glioblastoma. Endothelial buds with initial excavation. H&E, ×400.

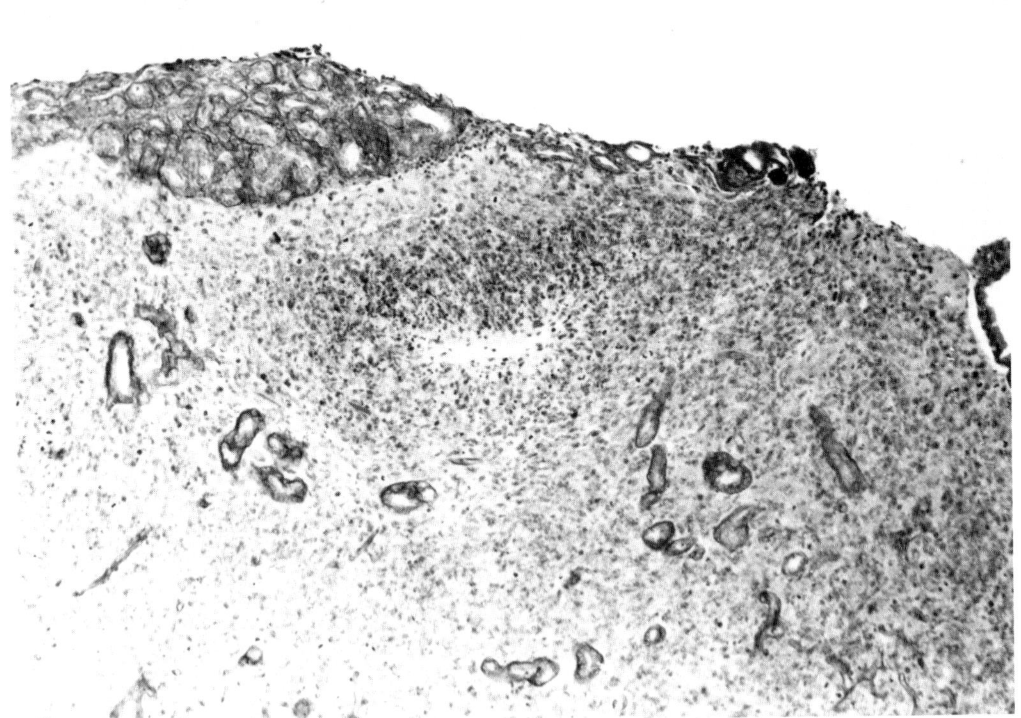

Figure 7.36. Glioblastoma. Circumscribed necrosis is associated with endothelial proliferation. H&E, ×200.

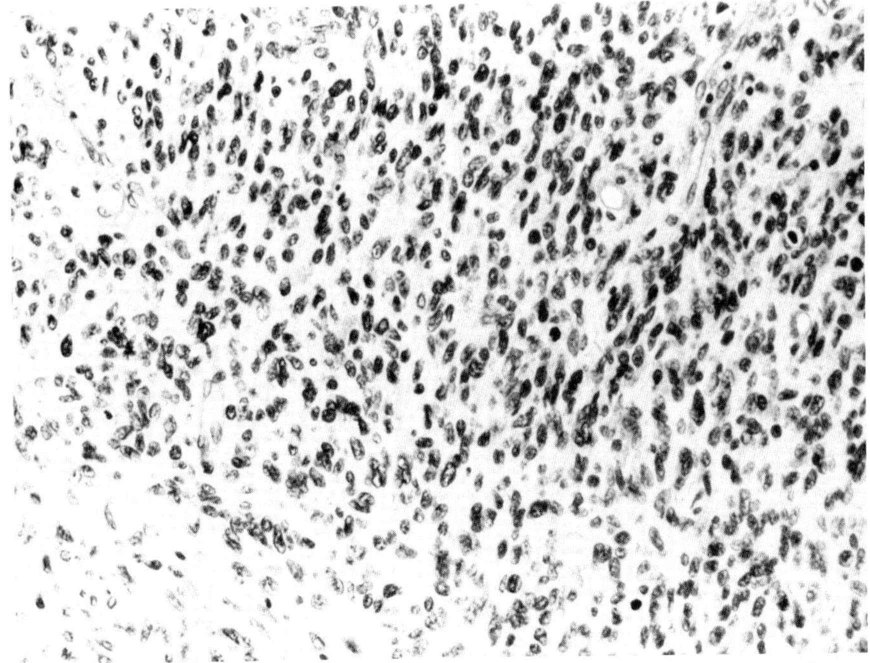

Figure 7.37. Glioblastoma. Infiltration area with very few small vessels. H&E, ×200.

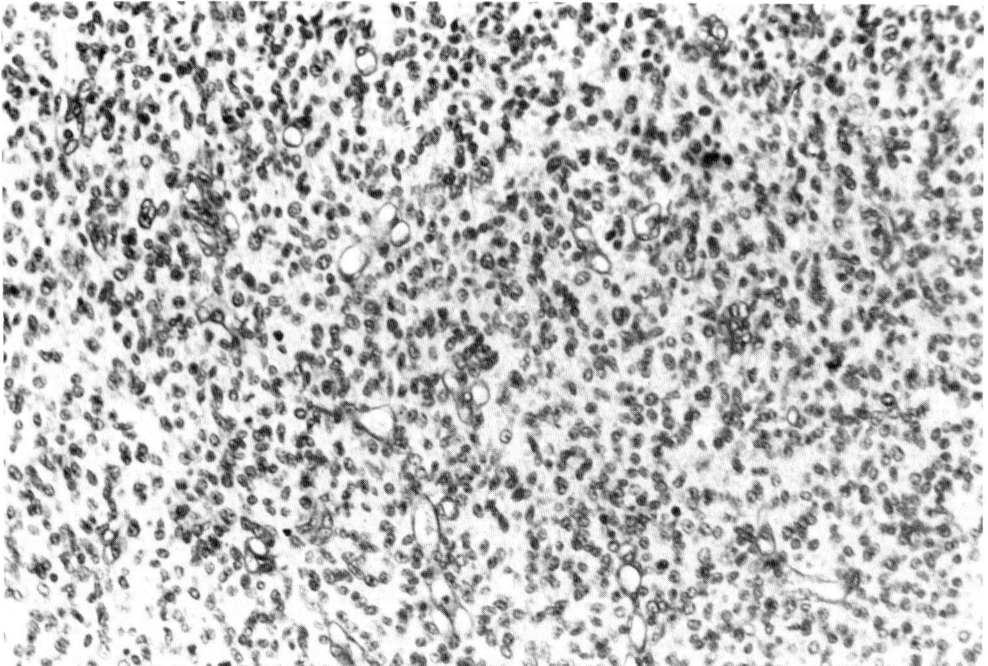

Figure 7.38. Glioblastoma. Infiltration area with many small vessels. H&E, ×200.

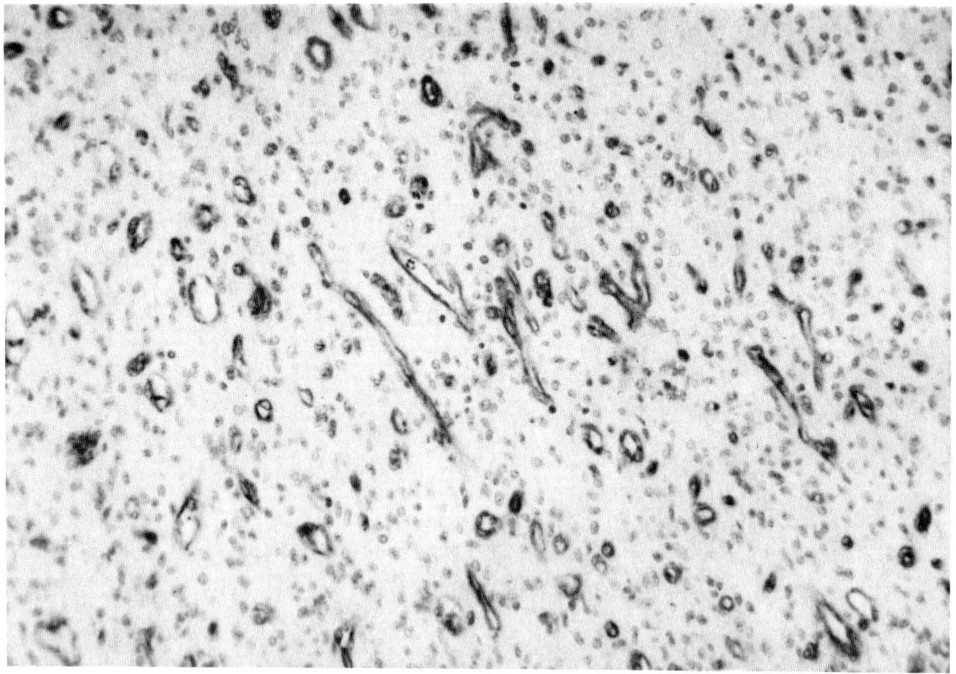

Figure 7.39. Glioblastoma. Neoformed capillaries and buds positive for Factor VIII/RAg in a proliferative area. PAP method, counterstained with hematoxylin, ×400.

The nosography of this tumor has been complicated by the presence of giant cells (Fig. 7.40). Some workers regarded these as glial and coined the term "giant-celled glioblastoma" (3, 78, 156), whereas others saw them as sarcomatous and spoke of "circumscribed monstrocellular sarcoma" of the vessels (16, 220). In point of fact, giant cells can be found in both the glial and/or the sarcomatous component and, hence, cannot be used to indicate the nature of the tumor. The existence of giant cell glioblastomas has been demonstrated immunohistochemically, and no uncertainty attaches to the existence of gliosarcomas, whether monstrocellular or otherwise. Immunohistochemical methods for GFAP and fibronectin can readily be used to demonstrate the neuroepithelial-mesodermal component (Fig. 7.41), delimited by basement membrane (60). Gliosarcomas are the result of sarcomatous transformation of the vasculature of glioblastomas, so that there is a continuum from one form to the other through a gradual increasing rate of mesodermic proliferation.

Since Factor VIII/RAg, a typical endothelial marker, is negative in the fibrosarcomatous proliferations of gliosarcoma, this tumor may originate from endothelial cells no longer capable of expressing the factor, from pericytes, or from perivascular fibroblasts (131). Factor VIII/RAg (Fig. 7.42) decreases in intensity from the lumen-lining to the peripheral cells of glioblastoma glomeruli. When glomeruli are in continuity with the fibrosarcomatous proliferations, a progressive loss of Factor VIII/RAg expression accompanies the transition from endothelial to spindle cells (173, 192). The endothelial origin of the mesenchymal component of gliosarcoma has been repeatedly suggested (44, 145).

Adventitial histiocytes have been put forward as an alternative source of fibrosarcomatous proliferation owing to their frequent a-1-antichymotrypsin, lysozyme and α-1-antitrypsin positivity (100). The mechanisms and factors, however, leading to the transition from normal proliferating endothelial cells to neoplasia are unknown.

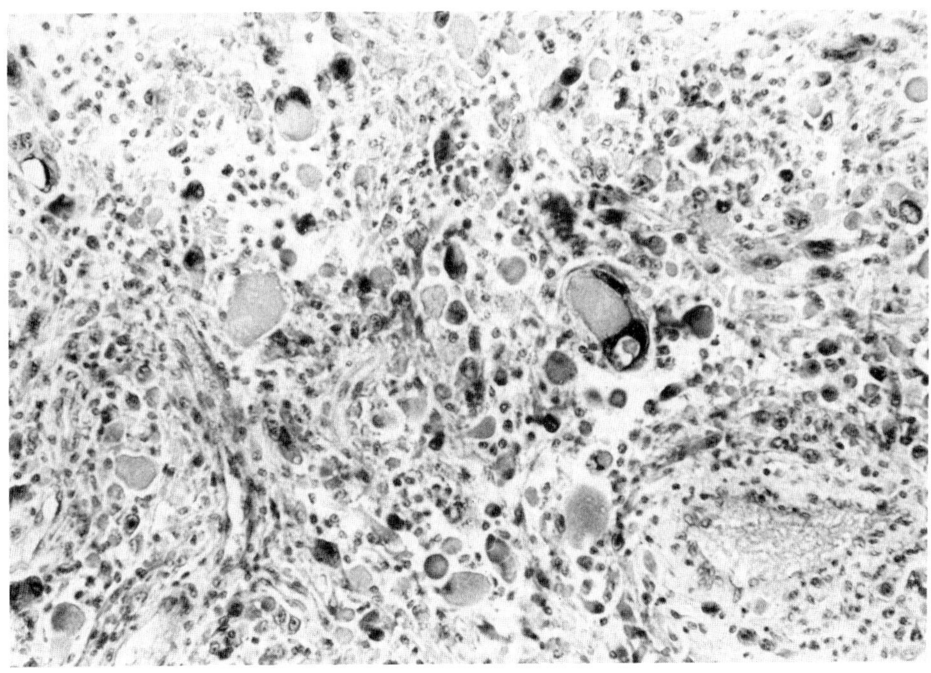

Figure 7.40. Giant cell in a glial area of a gliosarcoma. H&E, ×300.

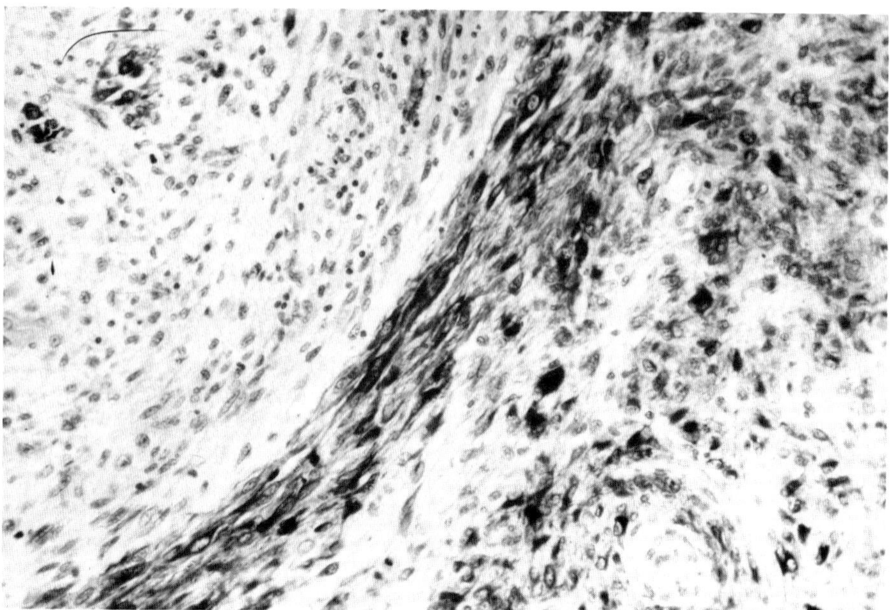

Figure 7.41. Gliosarcoma. The glial component is GFAP-positive. PAP method, counterstained with hematoxylin, ×400.

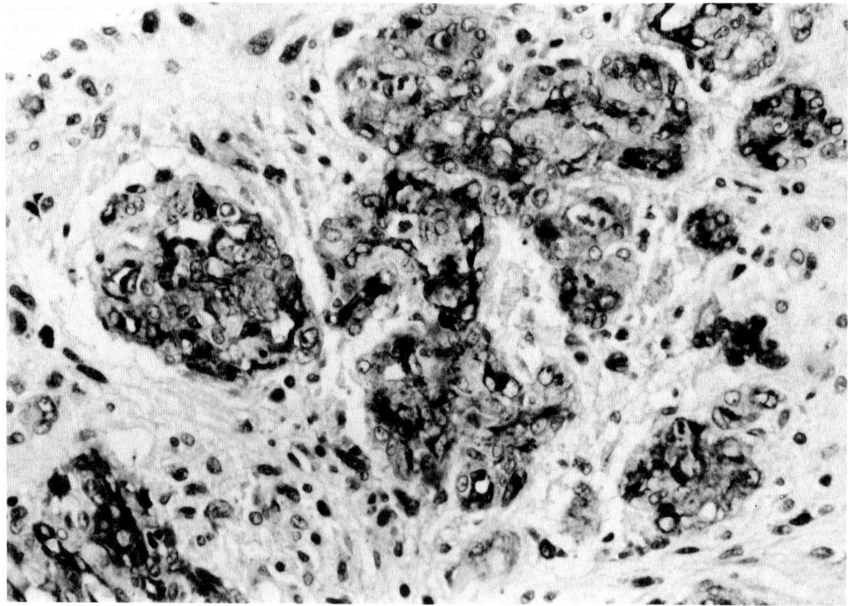

Figure 7.42. Glioblastoma. Vascular glomeruli with cells positive for Factor VIII/RAg. PAP method, counterstained with hematoxylin, ×400.

Growth Pattern, Spreading and Secondary Transformation of Cerebral Tumors

Cell proliferation and its supporting stroma confer a more or less specific general architecture on all brain tumors. Their final histological appearance, however, is greatly dependent on the pathoplastic influence of the normal nervous tissue and the occurrence of degenerative changes. A classic distinction is drawn between primary, secondary and tertiary architectures (165). Primary architectures are those spontaneously produced as a result of tumor cell atavism: true rosettes, pseudorosettes, ependymal canals, etc. Secondary architectures develop in response to the influence of normal nervous tissue. Tertiary architectures are the reactive response to regression. The existence of a relationship between growth pattern, proliferation rate, and architecture is the general rule for all the neoplasias. This determines both the imaging of a tumor and its susceptibility to treatment.

Brain tumors grow by expansion or infiltration. Expansion may or may not be accompanied by encapsulation. Neurinomas, meningiomas, pinealomas and teratomas are fully or partially encapsulated. Partial encapsulation is readily observable in meningioma. The capsule does not continue over the dura and fails to prevent invasion of the meninges.

Angioblastomas, choroid plexus papillomas, and ependymomas are not encapsulated. They push aside the nervous tissue, which may undergo atrophy and gliosis. In ependymomas, for example, there may be a distinct border between the tumor and the nervous tissue (Fig. 7.43). However, this does not preclude infiltration elsewhere. Pineal tumors, particularly germinomas and pinealblastomas, grow over the lamina quadrigemina, but eventually invade the posterior part of the third ventricle and reach the commissura intermedia, or even the foramina of Monro. The thalami are pushed aside, the posterior part of the corpus callosum upwards, and the vermis downwards and backwards. All these structures may be infiltrated as well.

Growth by infiltration is typical of gliomas but is also observed in other tumors.

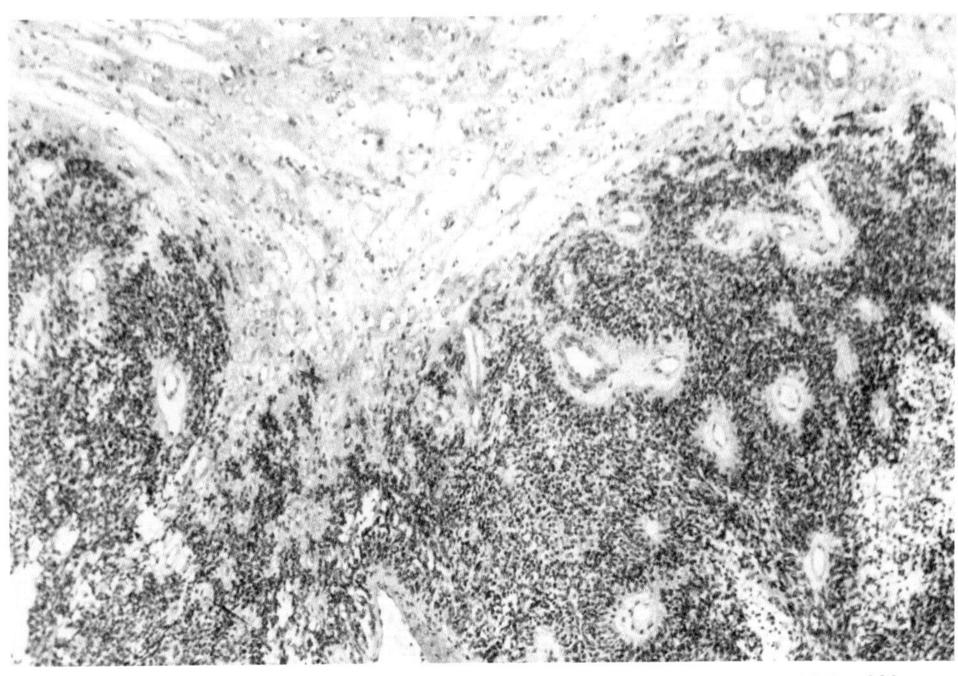

Figure 7.43. Ependymoma. Clearcut delimitation towards the normal tissue. H&E, ×200.

It may be circumscribed or diffuse (21). Circumscribed infiltration is typical of cerebellar and midline astrocytomas, oligodendrogliomas and glioblastomas, whereas diffuse infiltration is associated with astrocytomas, glioblastomas, medulloblastomas, oligodendrogliomas, and malignant lymphomas. The limits of the tumor cannot even be established histologically, since its cells are mixed with normal and reactive cells (Fig. 7.44). Sharp limits, however, may also be displayed by an infiltrating tumor (Fig. 7.45).

The spreading capacity of neuroepithelial tumors is largely due to their primary growth and invasive behavior. Invasiveness depends on many factors, among which are certain biological properties. In vitro studies have shown that fibrinolytic activity (73, 218), the phagocytic activity of glioma cells (142), and a high migratory capacity (68, 147) are important with regard to invasiveness; the invasiveness of tumor cells has been directly demonstrated (106). It is clear that invasiveness and infiltration are not synonymous, and that the latter is not a synonym for malignancy. In this connection, it should be pointed out that the idea that expansion is typical of benign and infiltration of malignant tumors meant that diffuse astrocytomas were once regarded as malignant (165). The main difference between the spreading of slowly growing hemispheric and malignant gliomas is that the former are often diffuse with no sharp delimitation, whereas the latter grow by both expansion and infiltration.

The way a tumor spreads is greatly influenced by the existing structures and by the general anatomy of the organ in which growth takes place. If a tumor grows in the ventricle, e.g., an ependymoma, choroid plexus papilloma or medulloblastoma, or if it reaches it from the parenchyma, as oligodendrogliomas, glioblastomas (Fig. 7.46) and germinomas often do, the cavity may be filled.

Growth out of a ventricle is exemplified by the passage of ependymoma from the fourth ventricle to the subarachnoid space through the foramina of Luschka. A tumor may also spread from one cavity to another. Pineal tumors, for example, pass from the third ventricle to the lateral ventricles

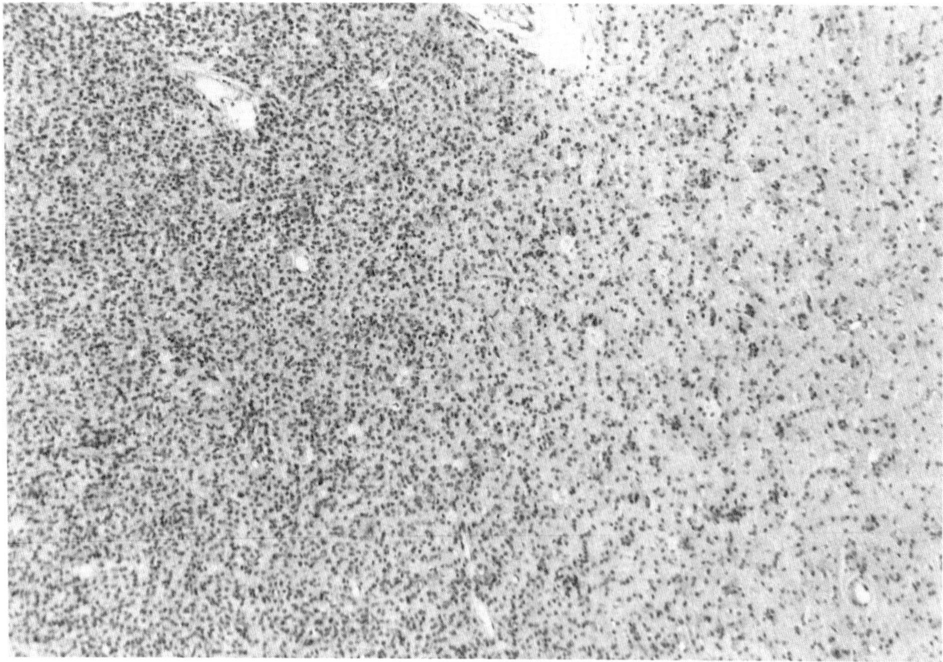

Figure 7.44. Oligodendroglioma. Progressive infiltration of the cortex. H&E, ×100.

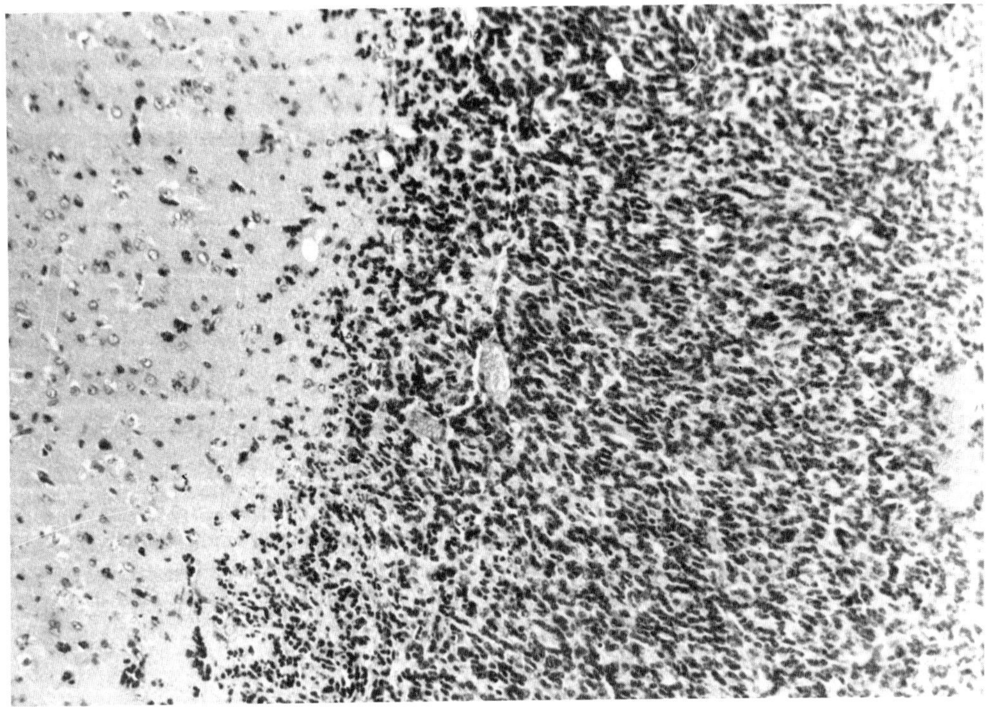

Figure 7.45. Oligodendroglioma. Clearcut delimitation of the tumor. H&E, ×100.

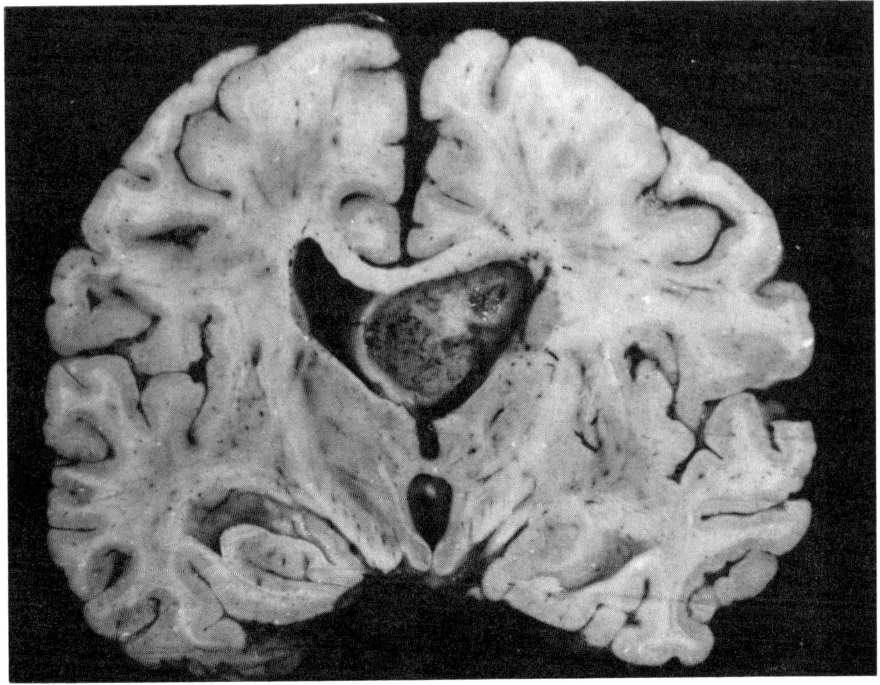

Figure 7.46. Glioblastoma filling the lateral ventricle.

through the foramina of Monro. A tumor can reach the subependymal layers and grow into them, with or without protrusion into the cavity (Fig. 7.47). It may also spread into the ventricular system and the subarachnoid space.

If tumor cells find their way into the CSF, metastatic spread can be retrograde as well as along the spinal cord. Medulloblastomas, ependymomas and glioblastomas are mainly responsible for this kind of colonization. Intradural metastases can be found on the arachnoid, among the posterior roots, and in the cauda region. These observations have guided the strategy of radiotherapy so that the entire neuraxis is treated in cases of medulloblastoma and ependymoma.

A tumor can also spread in the cortex and along its outer surfaces. A glioma growing from the white matter to the cortex has several courses open to it. It may invade the cortical layers, creating the pattern of satellitosis, though the neurons themselves may remain visible for a long time (Fig. 7.48). It may cross the pia and give rise to a subpial and leptomeningeal growth (Fig. 7.49), from which the cortex itself may be reinvaded. The cortex is often invaded from both sides. Expansion to the leptomeninges results in meningeal gliomatosis (146). The cerebral convolutions are either normal or invaded (Fig. 7.50). The same picture is created when oligodendrogliomas infiltrate convolutions and give them a "hypertrophic" appearance. As they pass from one convolution to another, tumors produce "garlands" by forcing a passage through the cortex in the same way as a fungus.

One of the main routes for the spread of hemispheric gliomas is along fiber tracts: corona radiata, capsula internal, corpus callosum, commissura anterior (128). The spreading pattern also depends on the tumor's initial location and is schematically predictable (21). Progress is in the ipsilateral hemisphere or by way of the corpus callosum to the opposite side, giving rise to the classic picture of a "butterfly" tumor (Fig. 7.51).

Histologically, elongated cells can be observed among the myelin fibers. They acquire a pilocytic or a spongioblastic appearance (Fig. 7.52), since their growth

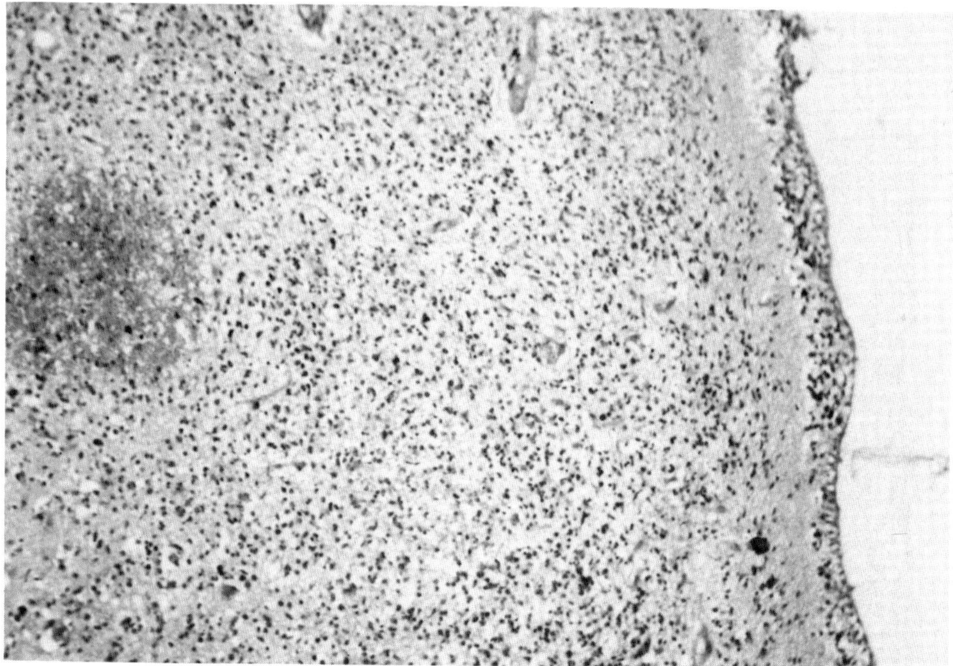

Figure 7.47. Tumor proliferation reaching the subependymal layers and lining the surface of the cavity. H&E, ×200.

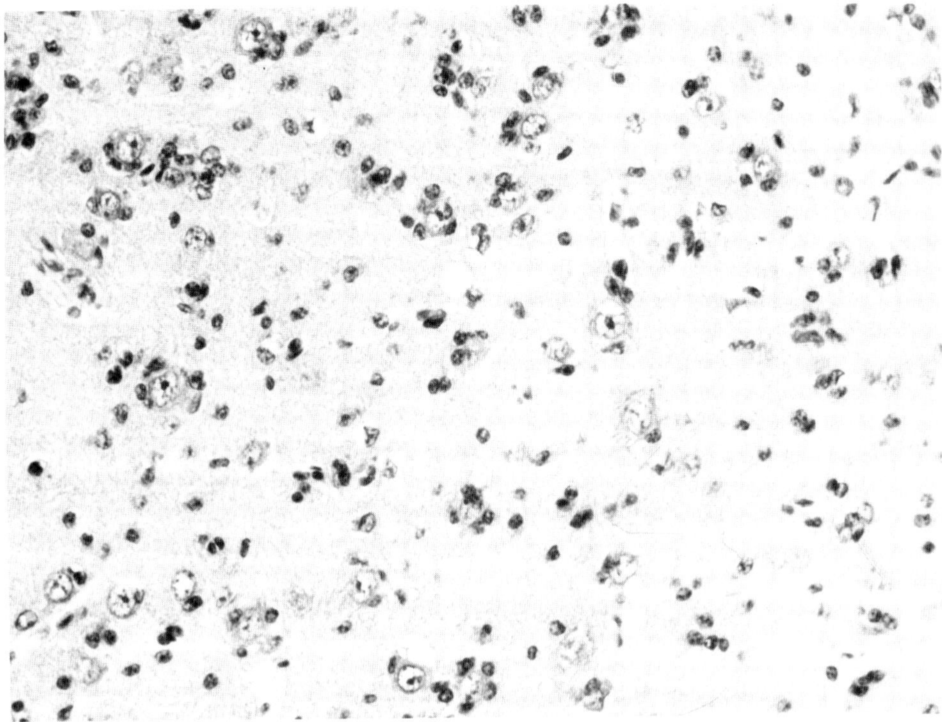

Figure 7.48. Oligodendroglioma. Perineuronal satellitosis. H&E, ×200.

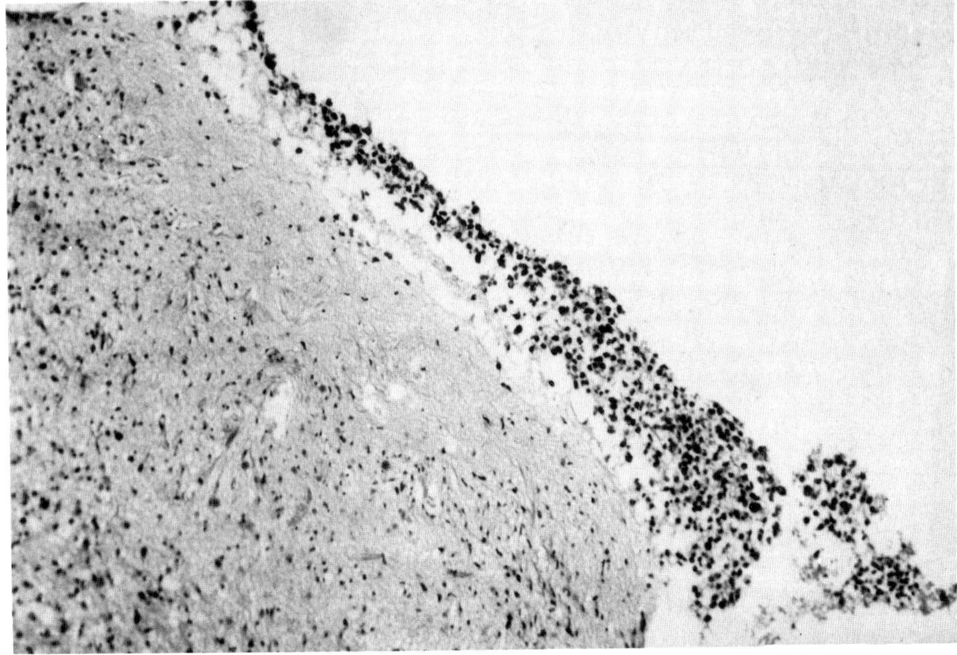

Figure 7.49. Oligodendroglioma. Tumor proliferation in the subarachnoid space. H&E, ×50.

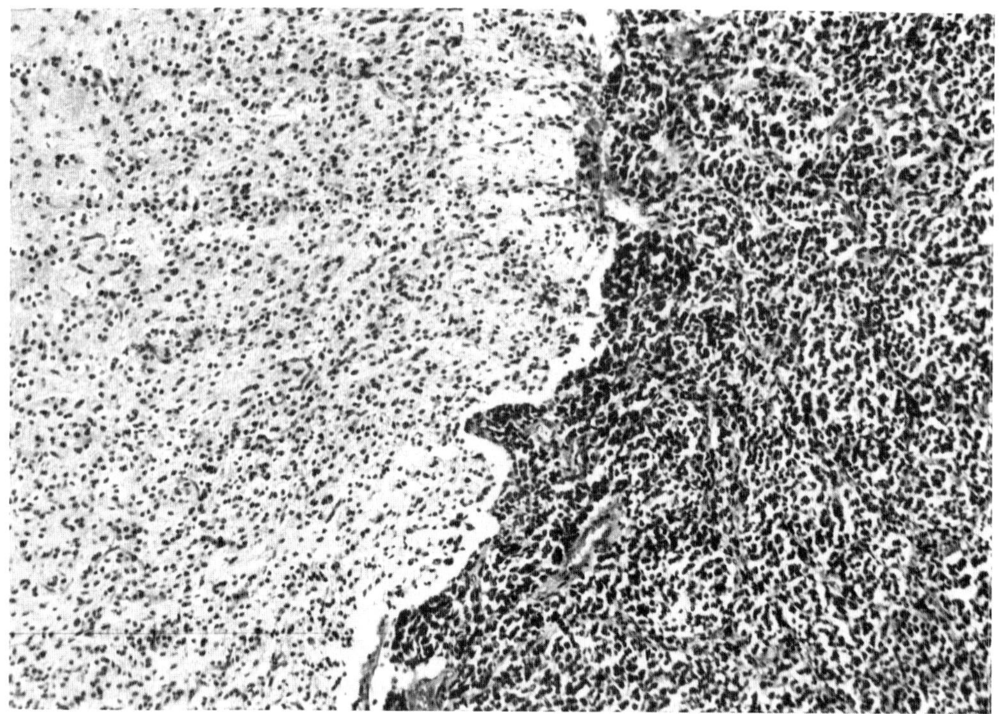

Figure 7.50. Oligodendroglioma. Tumor proliferation in the meninges over an infiltrated cortex. H&E, ×100.

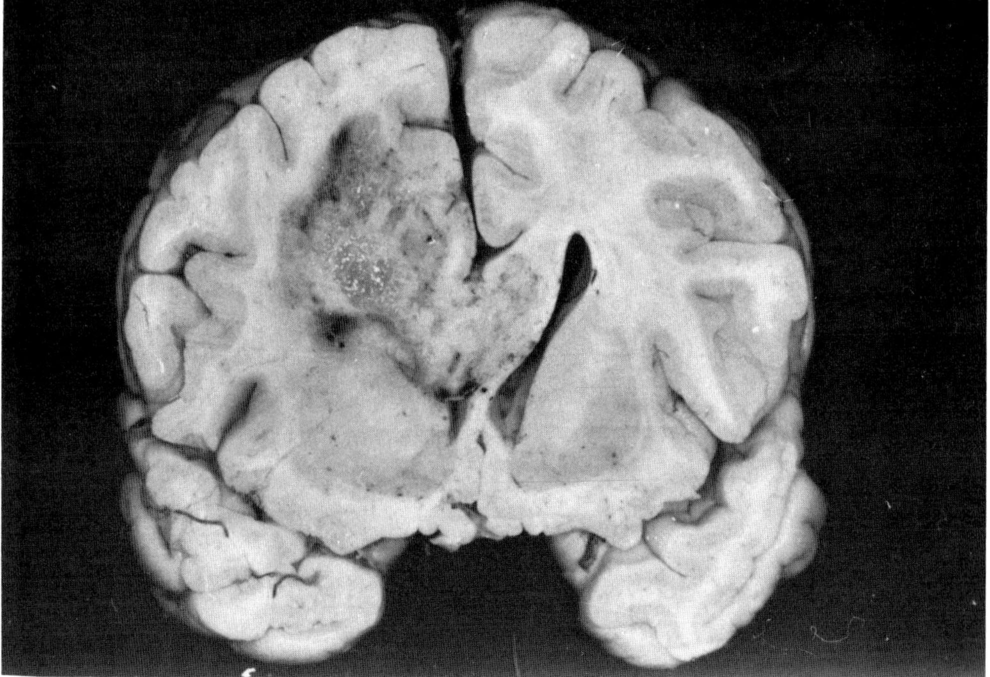

Figure 7.51. Glioblastoma invading the corpus callosum with butterfly aspect.

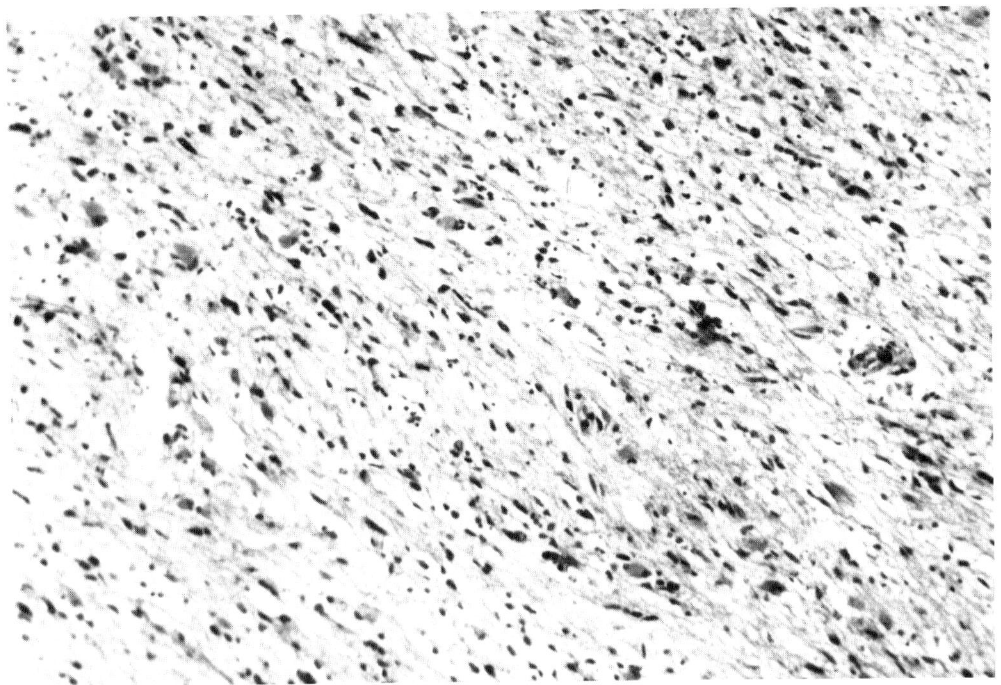

Figure 7.52. Tumor cells of pilocytic aspect infiltrating a fiber bundle. H&E, ×200.

pattern is greatly influenced by the existing fiber plane. It is often difficult to determine whether they have a primary or a secondary architecture. When the cell density is low, it is even difficult to recognize the advancing tumor. This growth pattern is shared by glioblastoma and different types of hemispheric and midline pilocytic astrocytomas.

Malignant gliomas very often present as multicentric growths or as multicentric malignant transformations of a diffuse astrocytoma. The first possibility raises serious difficulties in the differential diagnosis of metastases by CT. It is in any event difficult to prove the multifocality of a tumor, since in most cases it is merely apparent. Several sites may be connected by thin strips of proliferation involving commissurae or septa, such as the septum pellucidum (Figs. 7.53 and 7.54). In other cases, multifocality may be mimicked by diffusion through the CSF followed by reimplantation (Fig. 7.55).

The second possibility includes the eventuality of malignant change achieved over a period of time. In this case, astrocytomatous proliferation, not detectable by CT, may unite all the foci into a large, single tumor (120). This situation is of great importance when it is necessary to establish the extent of a tumor by CT so that an appropriate radiotherapy strategy can be devised (166).

Peritumoral Tissue

The tissue immediately adjacent to a tumor (BAT) is of special importance in tumor spreading on account of the many processes that occur in it. Infiltration is the work of small, GFAP-negative cells with hyperchromatic, isomorphic nuclei. They probably represent a new, fast-growing population (176). Mitoses, in fact, are numerous and mostly located around the vessels, as shown (inter alia) by autoradiography (83). Intense growth occurs after surgery, irradiation or chemotherapy (206). Vessels display endothelial proliferation as well as the other abnormalities already mentioned. Formation of vascular glomeruli is readily demonstrable in glioblastomas and metastases (Fig. 7.56). Edema is one of the main events in the BAT, along

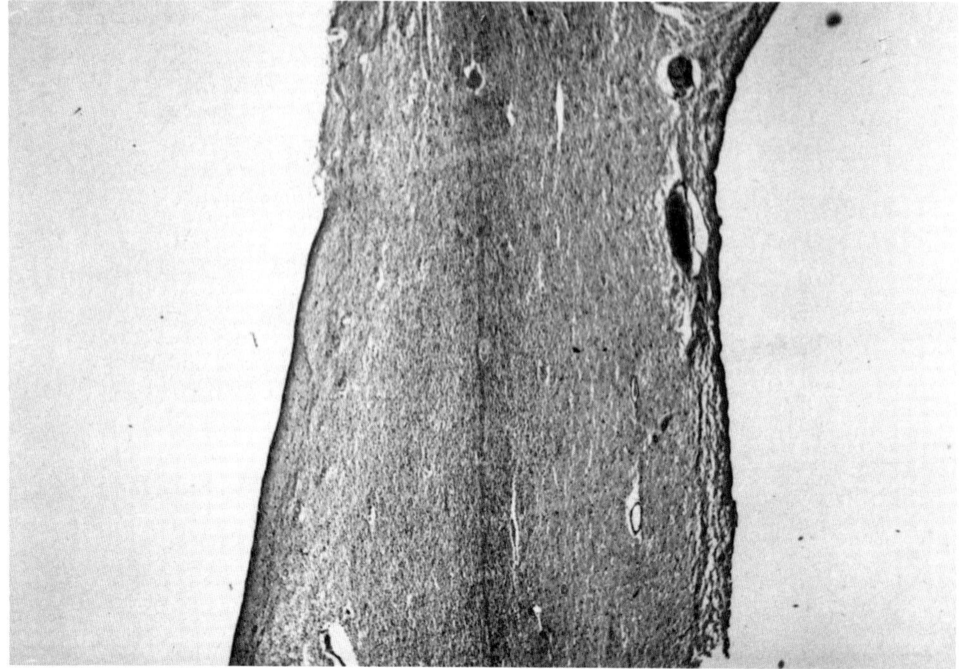

Figure 7.53. Septum pellucidum infiltrated by tumor cells. H&E, ×50.

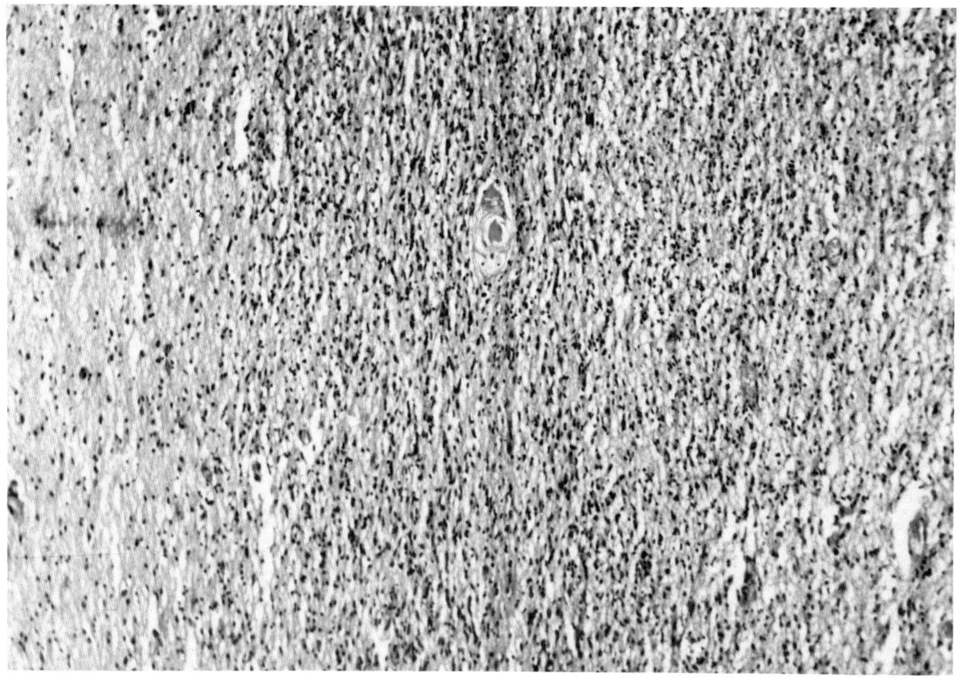

Figure 7.54. The same as in Figure 7.53 at higher magnification. H&E, ×200.

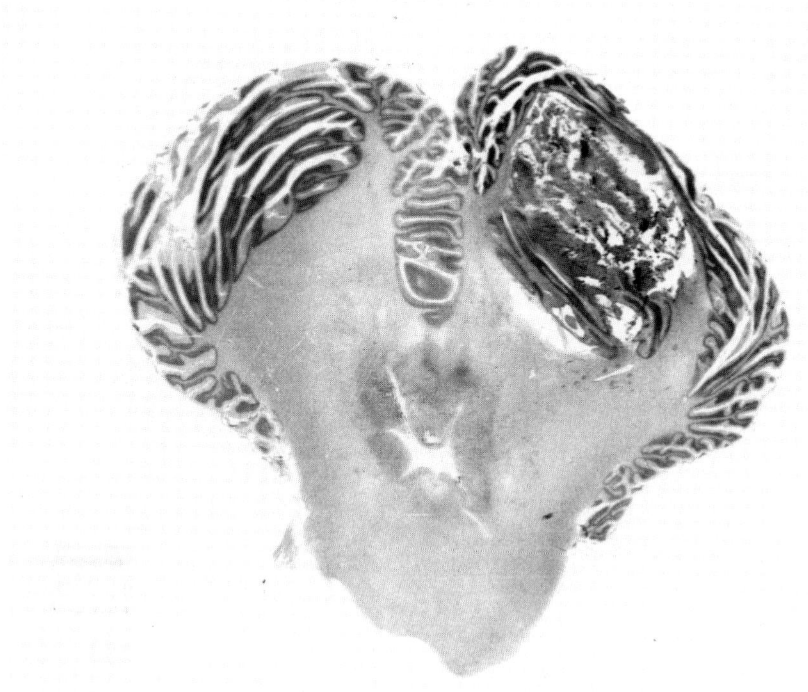

Figure 7.55. Tumor proliferation bordering the IV ventricle.

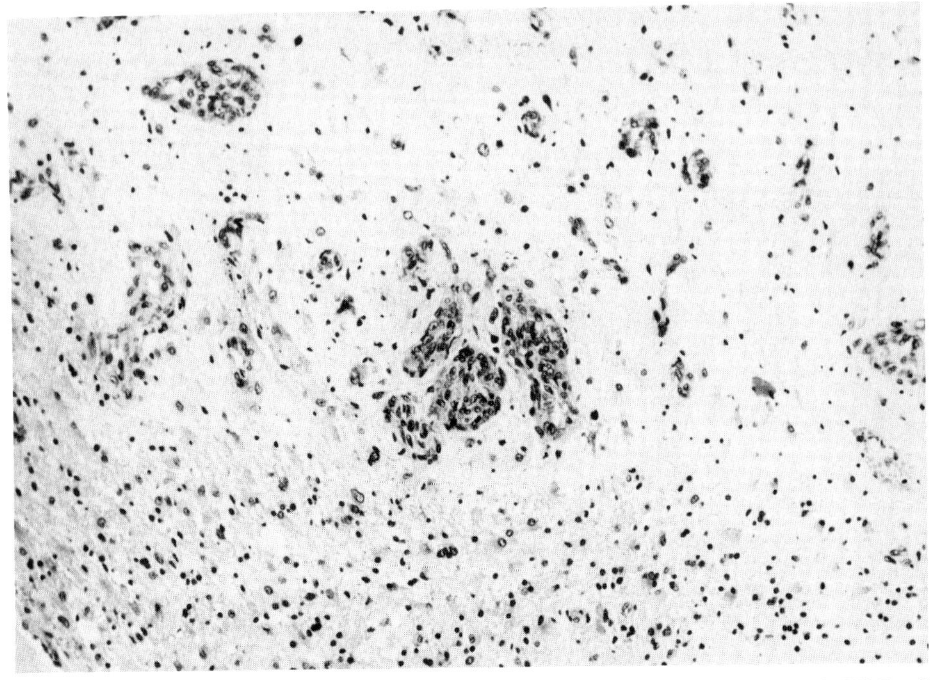

Figure 7.56. Vascular glomeruli and endothelial buds in the brain adjacent to tumor (BAT). H&E, ×200.

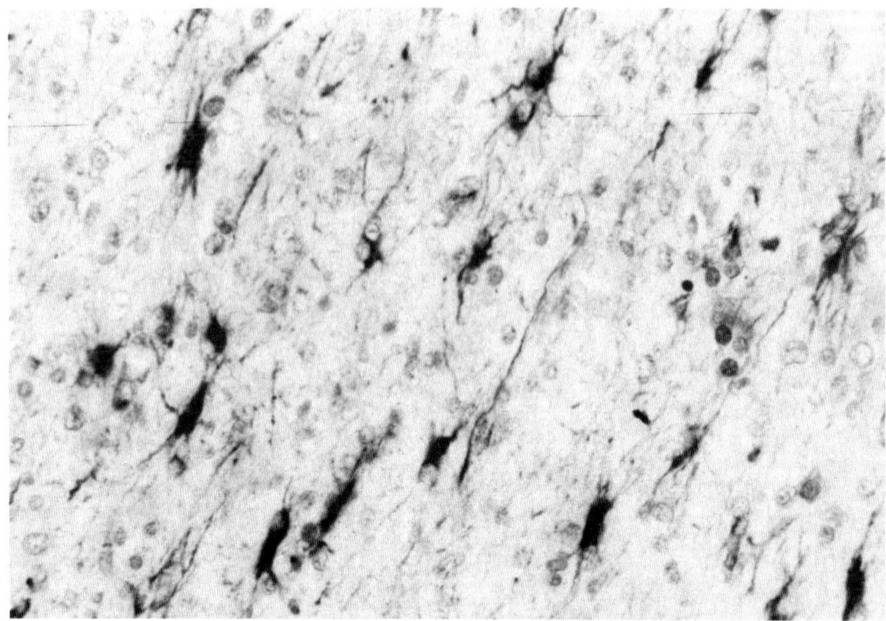

Figure 7.57. GFAP-positive reactive astrocytes in the BAT. PAP method, counterstained with hematoxylin, ×300.

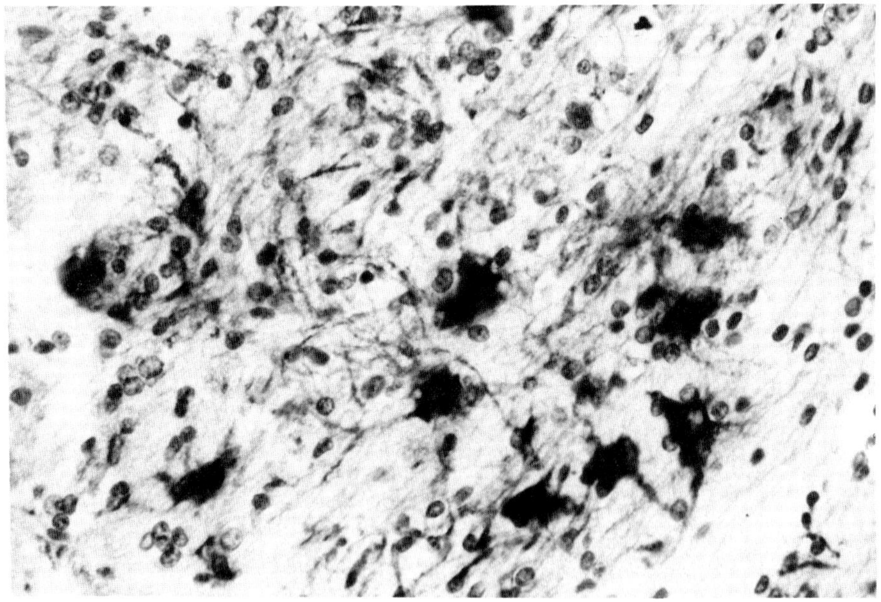

Figure 7.58. Reactive astrocytes in the advancing tumor infiltration. PAP method, counterstained with hematoxylin, ×400.

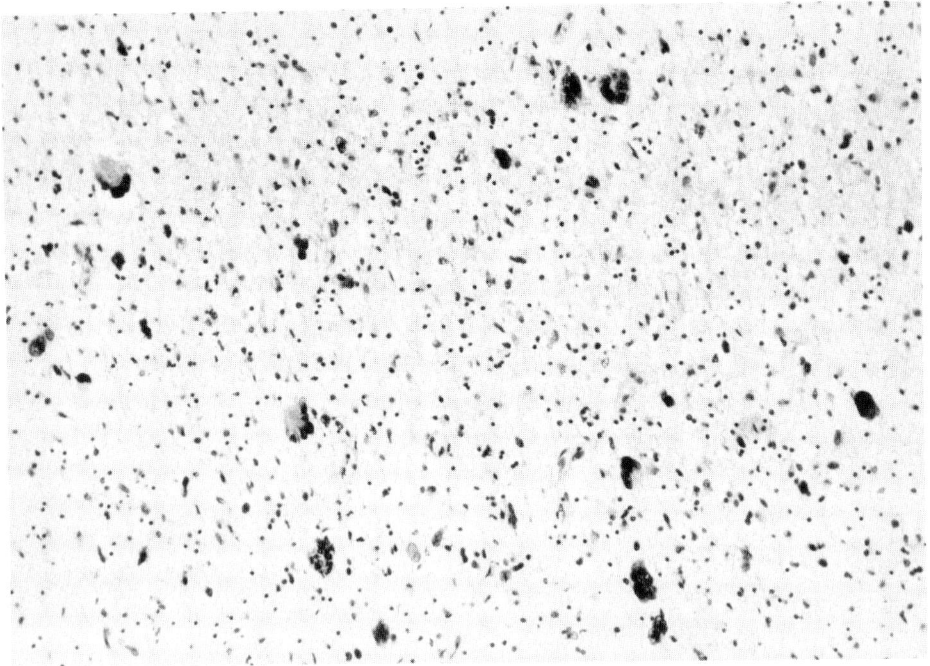

Figure 7.59. Astrocytes with bizarre nuclei in the BAT. H&E, ×200.

with vessel wall degeneration and the appearance of reactive astrocytes. In irradiated glioblastomas, radionecrotic changes occurring in the BAT (17, 181) must be taken into account when discussing the functional relationship between tumor and brain after radiotherapy (115, 216). The appearance of the BAT is not always the same. The BAT in the cortex is essentially characterized by tumor and endothelial cell proliferation, whereas that in the white matter is marked by changes in permeability with edema and vessel wall degeneration.

Two further aspects of the BAT in glioblastomas require consideration, namely the occurrence of reactive astrocytes, and the possible replacement of normal tissue by an astrocytomatous area. Reactive astrocytes are intensely GFAP-positive and may be trapped in the advancing proliferation, which is mostly composed of small, GFAP-negative, isomorphic cells. In this case, they gradually lose their processes and more deeply in the tumor become indistinguishable from GFAP-positive tumor astrocytes (Figs. 7.57 and 7.58). The occurrence of mitoses is not conclusive, since this is quite common in reactive astrocytes; the latter then play a role in the morphological composition of the proliferative areas of malignant gliomas. This factor must be taken into account when assessing the degree of malignancy of a tumor on small tissue fragments.

Astrocytes with bizarre nuclei (Fig. 7.59) are often observed, especially after radiotherapy and chemotherapy (56, 181, 190). It is impossible to determine whether these are nonneoplastic glial cells that have modified spontaneously or in response to the treatment (190), or neoplastic cells similarly transformed into monstrous cells. Differentiation of reactive and tumor astrocytes is of paramount importance in determining the limits of a tumor (201). Nuclear characteristics are the main guide (30, 31). Account may also be taken of the consideration that bizarre forms are indicative of neoplasia, whereas regular distribution in the tissue is a sign of reactive origin (39).

ACKNOWLEDGMENTS

Supported by a grant of the Italian National Research Council, Special Project "Oncology", contract number 88.00875.44 and by the Italian Association for Cancer Research (A.I.R.C.).

REFERENCES

1. Bãr, T. Patterns of vascularization in the developing cerebral cortex. In: *Development of Vascular System*. Ciba Foundation Symposium 100. London, Pitman, 1983, pp. 20–36.
2. Bãr, T. *The Vascular System of the Cerebral Cortex*. Berlin, Springer, 1980.
3. Becker, D.P., Benyo, R., and Roessman, U. Glial origin of monstrocellular tumor: case report of prolonged survival. J. Neurosurg., *26:*72–77, 1967.
4. Bertolotto, A., Giordana, M.T., Magrassi, M.L., *et al.* Glycosoaminoglycans in human cerebral tumors. Part I. Biochemical findings. Acta Neuropathol. (Berl.), *58:*115–119, 1982.
5. Bignami, A., Dahl, D., and Rueger D.C. Glial fibrillary acidic protein (GFAP) in normal neural cells and in pathological conditions. Adv. Cell Neurobiol., 285, 1980.
6. Bignami, A., Eng., L.F., Dahl, D., *et al.* Localization of the glial fibrillary acidic protein in astrocytes by immunofluorescence. Brain Res., *43:*429–438, 1972.
7. Bignami, A., Rajn, T., and Dahl, D. Localization of vimentin, the nonspecific intermediate filament protein in embryonal glia and in early differentiating neurons. Dev. Biol., *91:*286–295, 1982.
8. Bigner, D.D. Biology of gliomas: potential clinical implications of glioma cellular heterogeneity. Neurosurgery, *9:*320–326, 1981.
9. Bigner, D.D., Bigner, S.H., Pontén, J., *et al.* Heterogeneity of genotypic and phenotypic characteristics of fifteen permanent cell lines derived from human gliomas. J. Neuropathol. Exp. Neurol., *40:*201–229, 1981.
10. Bigner, S.H., Vogelstein, B., and Bigner, D.D. Chromosomal abnormalities and gene amplification in malignant gliomas. ISI Atlas Sci., *1:*333–336, 1988.
11. Bõck, P. and Jellinger, K. Detection of glycosoaminoglycans in human gliomas by histochemical methods. Acta Neuropathol. (Berl.), *57:*299–305, 1982.
12. Bonnin, J.M. and Rubinstein, L.J. Immunohistochemistry of central nervous system tumors. J. Neurosurg., *60:*1121–1133, 1984.
13. Bookwalter, III, J.W., Selker, R.G., Schiffer, L., *et al.* Brain-tumor cell kinetic correlated with survival. J. Neurosurg., *65:*795–798, 1986.
14. Bosch, D.A. Short and long term effects of methyl- and ethylnitrosourea (MNU & ENU) on the developing nervous system of the rat. II. Short term: concluding remarks on chemical neuro-oncogenesis. Acta Neurol. Scand., *55:*106–122, 1977.
15. Bressler, J.P., Cole, R., and De Vellis, J. Neoplastic transformation of newborn rat oligodendrocytes in culture. Cancer Res., *43:*709–715, 1983.
16. Brucher, J.M. Le sarcome monstrocellulaire du cerveau. Etude anatomoclinique de sept cas. Acta Neurol. Psychiatr. Belg., *62:*193–200, 1962.
17. Burger, P.C., Mahaley, M.S., Dudka, L., *et al.* The morphologic effects of radiation administered therapeutically for intracranial gliomas. A post mortem study of 25 cases. Cancer, *44:*1256–1272, 1979.
18. Burger, P.C., Shibata, T., and Kleihues, P. The use of the monoclonal antibody Ki-67 in the identification of proliferating cells: application to surgical neuropathology. Am. J. Surg. Pathol., *10:*611–617, 1986.
19. Cairncross, J.G. The biology of astrocytoma: lesions named from chronic myelogeneous leukemia-hypothesis. J. Neuro-oncol., *5:*99–104, 1987.
20. Caley, D.W. and Maxwell, D.S. Development of the blood vessels and extracellular spaces during postnatal maturation in the rat cerebral cortex. J. Comp. Neurol., *138:*31–48, 1970.
21. Calvo, W. Growth patterns of intracranial neoplasms. In: *Pathology of the Nervous System*, Vol. 2, edited by J. Minckler, New York, McGraw-Hill, 1971, pp. 1960–1976.
22. Cavanagh, J.B. and Lewis, P.D. Perfusion-fixation, colchicine and mitotic activity in the adult rat brain. J. Anat., *104:*341–350, 1969.
23. Chin, F.C., Norton, W.T., and Fields, K.L. The cytoskeleton of primary astrocytes in cultures contains actin, glial fibrillary acidic protein and the fibroblast-type filament protein vimentin. J. Neurochem., *37:*147–155, 1981.
24. Choi, B.H. and Kim, R.C. Expression of glial fibrillary acidic protein in immature oligodendroglia. Science, *223:*407–409, 1984.
25. Claisse, P.J., Lantos, P.L., and Roscoe J.P. Analysis of N-ethyl-N-nitrosourea-induced brain carcinogenesis by sequential culturing during the latent period. II. Morphology of the tumors induced by cell cultures. J. Natl. Cancer Inst., *61:*391–398, 1978.
26. Conley, F.K. The immunocytochemical localization of GFA protein in experimental murine tumors. Acta Neuropathol. (Berl.), *45:*9–16, 1979.
27. Cravioto, H., Palekar, L., Weiss, E., *et al.* Experimental neurinoma in tissue culture. Acta Neuropathol. (Berl.), *21:*154–164, 1972.
28. Cravioto, H., Weiss, J.F., Weiss, E., *et al.* Biological characteristics of peripheral nerve tumors induced with ethylnitrosourea. Acta Neuropathol. (Berl.), *23:*265–280, 1973.
29. Dahl, D., Bignami, A., Weber, K., *et al.* Filament proteins in rat optic nerves undergoing wallerian degeneration: localization of vi-

mentin, the fibroblastic 100-A filament protein, in normal and reactive astrocytes. Exp. Neurol., *13*:496–506, 1981.
30. Daumas-Duport, C., Scheithauer, P.W., and Kelly, P.J. A histologic and cytologic method for the spatial definition of gliomas. Mayo Clin. Proc., *62*:435–449, 1987.
31. Daumas-Duport, C., and Szikla, G. Delimitations et configuration spatiale des gliomes cérébraux: données histologiques, incidences thérapeutiques. Neurochirurgie, *27*:273–284, 1981.
32. Davison, A.M., Cuzner, M.L., Banik, H.L., *et al.* Myelinogenesis in the rat brain. Nature (Lond.), *212*:1373–1374, 1966.
33. Deane, B.R. and Lantos, L.P. The vasculature of experimental brain tumors. Part 1. A sequential light and electron microscope study of angiogenesis. Part 2. A quantitative assessment of morphological abnormalities. J. Neurol. Sci., *49*:55–77, 1981.
34. De Ridder, L. and Laerum, O.D. Invasion of rat neurogenic cell lines in embryonic chick heart fragments in vivo. J. Natl. Cancer Inst., *66*:723–728, 1981.
35. Deinhardt, F. In Klein G. (ed) *Viral Oncology.* Raven Press, New York, 1980, p. 357–398.
36. De Armond, S.J., and Eng, L.F. Immunohistochemistry: techniques and application to neurooncology. In Rosemblum, M.L., Wilson, C.B., (eds): *Brain Tumor Biology.* Progr. Exp. Tumor Res., Basel, Karger, V 27, 1984, p. 92–117.
37. De Armond, S.J., Eng, L.F., and Rubinstein, L.J. The application of glial fibrillary acidic (GFAP) protein immunohistochemistry in neurooncology. Pathol. Res. Pract., *168*: 374–379, 1980.
38. Druckrey, H., Ivankovic, S., Preussman, R., *et al.* Selective induction of malignant tumors of the nervous system by resorptive carcinogens. In: Kirsh, W.M., Grossi-Paoletti, E., Paoletti, P. (eds): *The Experimental Biology of Brain Tumors.* Springfield, Thomas, 1972, p. 85.
39. Duffy, P.E. *Astrocytes: normal, reactive, and neoplastic.* New York, Raven Press, 1983.
40. Eng, L.F. The glial fibrillary acidic (GFAP) protein. In: Bradshaw, R., Schneider, D., (eds) *Proteins of the Nervous System.* New York, Raven Press, 1980, p. 85.
41. Eng, L.F., and Rubinstein, L.J. Contribution of immunohistochemistry to diagnostic problems of human cerebral tumors. J. Histo-Cytochem., *26*:513–522, 1978.
42. Engelhardt, A. and Bannasch, P. Histochemie sâuer Mucopolysaccharide wãhrend der Genese Methylnitrosoharns-toffinduzierter Hirntumoren der Ratte. Acta Neuropathol. (Berl.), *42*:197–204, 1978.
43. Fedoroff, S., White, R., Neal, J., *et al.* Astrocyte cell lineage. II. Mouse fibrous astrocytes and reactive astrocytes in cultures have vimentin- and GFP-containing intermediate filaments. Dev. Brain Res., *7*:303–315, 1983.
44. Feigin, I., Allen, L.B., Lipkin, L., *et al.* The endothelial hyperplasia of cerebral blood vessels with brain tumors, and its sarcomatous transformation. Cancer, *11*:264–277, 1958.
45. Feigin, I. and Gross, S.W. Sarcoma arising in glioblastoma of the brain. Am. J. Pathol., *31*:633–653, 1955.
46. Folkman, J. Angiogenesis: initiation and control. Ann. NY Acad. Sci., *401*:212–227, 1982.
47. Folkman, J. and Klagsbun, M. Angiogenetic factors. Science, *235*:442–447, 1987.
48. Fornatto, L. and Schiffer, D. In vitro culture observations on neurinoma induced experimentally in the rat by ethylnitrosourea. Acta Neuropathol. (Berl.), *20*:199–206, 1972.
49. Foulds, L. The natural history of cancer. J. Chron. Dis., *8*:2–9, 1958.
50. Fujita, H. and Fujita, S. Electron microscopic studies on neuroblast differentiation in the central nervous system of domestic fowl. Z. Zellforsch. Mikrosk. Anat., *60*:463–478, 1963.
51. Fujita, S. An autoradiographic study on the origin and fate of the subpial glioblasts in the embryonic chick spinal cord. J. Comp. Neurol., *124*:51–60, 1965.
52. Fujita, S. Application of light and electron microscopic autoradiography to the study of cytogenesis of the forebrain. In: *Evolution of the Forebrain*, edited by R. Hassler and H. Stephan, New York, Plenum Press, 1966, p. 180.
53. Geraci, J.P. and Spence, A.M. RBE of cyclotron fast neutron for a rat brain tumor. Radiat. Res., *79*:579–590, 1979.
54. Gerdes, J. An immunohistological method for estimating cell growth fractions in rapid histopathological diagnosis during surgery. Int. J. Cancer, *35*:169–171, 1985.
55. Gerdes, J., Schwab, U., Lemke, H., *et al.* Production of a mouse monoclonal antibody reactive with a human nuclear antigen associated with cell proliferation. Int. J. Cancer, *31*:13–20, 1984.
56. Gerstner, L., Jellinger, K., Heiss, W.D., *et al.* Morphological changes in anaplastic gliomas treated with radiation and chemotherapy. Acta Neurochir., *36*:117–138, 1977.
57. Giangaspero, F. and Burger, P.C. Correlations between cytologic composition and biologic behavior in the glioblastoma multiforme. Cancer, *52*:2320–2333, 1983.
58. Giordana, M.T., Bertolotto, A., Mauro, A., *et al.* Glycosaminoglycans in human cerebral tumors. Part II. Histochemical findings and correlations. Acta Neuropathol. (Berl.), *57*: 299–305, 1982.
59. Giangaspero, F., Doglioni, C., Rivano, M.T., *et al.* Growth fraction in human brain tumors defined by the monoclonal antibody Ki-67. Acta Neuropathol. (Berl.), *74*:179–182, 1987.
60. Giordana, M.T., Germano, I., Giaccone, G., *et*

al. The distribution of laminin in human brain tumors: an immunohistochemical study. Acta Neuropathol. (Berl.), *67:*51–57, 1985.

61. Giordana, M.T., Mauro, A., Germano, I., *et al.* Transplacental ENU tumors of the rat: immunohistochemical contribution to the recognition of cell types. In: *Biology of Brain Tumors*, edited by M. D. Walker and D. G. T. Thomas, Boston, Martinus Nijoff, 1985, pp. 121–129.
62. Goth, R. and Rajewsky, M.F. Persistence of O^6-ethylguanine in rat brain DNA. Correlation with nervous system specific carcinogenesis by ethylnitrosourea. Proc. Natl. Acad. Sci. USA, *71:*639–653, 1974.
63. Groothuis, D.R., Fisher, J.M., Vick, N.A., *et al.* Experimental gliomas: an autoradiographic study of the endothelial component. Neurology, *30:*297–301, 1980.
64. Gullotta, F. Zur in vitro-Diagnostik gliõs-mesenchymaler Mischgeschwũlste. Dtsch Z. Nervenheilkd., *186:*323–335, 1964.
65. Hadfield, M.G. and Silverberg, S.G. Light and electron microscopy of giant-cell glioblastoma. Cancer, *14:*841–852, 1961.
66. Harnarine-Singh, D., Geddes, G., and Hyde, J.B. Size and number of arteries and veins in normal human neopallium. J. Anat., *11:*171–179, 1972.
67. Haugen Å. and Laerum, O.D. Induced glial differentiation of fetal rat brain cells in culture: an ultrastructural study. Brain Res., *150:* 225–238, 1978.
68. Haugen, Å. and Laerum, O.D. Scanning electron microscope of neoplastic neurogenic rat cell lines in culture. Acta Pathol. Microbiol. Scand. A., *86:*101–110, 1978.
69. Haugen, Å., Laerum, O.D., and Bock, E. Responsiveness of fetal rat brain cells to glia maturation factor during neoplastic transformation in cell culture. Acta Pathol. Microbiol. Scan. A. Pathol., *89:*393–402, 1981.
70. Heldin, C.H. and Westermark, B. Platelet-derived Growth Factor and its relation to oncogenes. ISI Atlas of Science, *1:*44–46, 1988.
71. Heldin, C.H., Westermark, B., and Wasteson, A. Specific receptors for platelet-derived growth factor on cells derived from connective tissue and glia. Proc. Natl. Acad. Sci., *78:*3664–3668, 1981.
72. Hermansson, M., Nister, M., Betscholz, C., *et al.* Endothelial cell hyperplasia in human glioblastoma: coexpression of mRNA and platelet-derived growth factor (PDGF) B chain and PDGF receptor suggests autocrine growth stimulation. Proc. Natl. Acad. Sci., *85:*7748–7752, 1988.
73. Hince, T.A. and Roscoe, J.P. Fibrinolytic activity of cultured cells derived during ethylnitrosourea induced carcinogenesis of rat brain. Br. J. Cancer, *37:*424–433, 1978.
74. Hirano, A. and Matsui, T. Vascular structure in brain tumors. Human Pathol., *6:*611–621, 1975.
75. Long, D.M. Capillary ultrastructure and the blood-brain barrier in human malignant brain tumors. J. Neurosurg., *32:*127–144, 1970.
76. Hirschberg, H. Endothelial growth factor production in cultures of human glioma cells. Neuropath. Appl. Neurobiol., *10:*33–42, 1984.
77. His, W. Die Neuroblasten und deren Entstehung in embryonal Marke. Abh. Math. Phys. Cl. Kgl. Sach. Ges. Wiss., *15:*313–372, 1889.
78. Hitselberger, W.E., Kernohan, J.W., and Uihlein, A. Giant cell fibrosarcoma of the brain. Cancer, *14:*841–852, 1961.
79. Hopewell, J.W. A quantitative study of the mitotic activity in the subependymal plate of adult rats. Cell and Tissue Kinetics, *4:*273–278, 1971.
80. Hoshino, T. Cellular aspects of human brain tumors (gliomas). In: *Advances in Cellular Neurobiology*, edited by S. Fedoroff and L. Hertz, New York, Academic Press, V 2, 1981, pp. 167–181.
81. Hoshino, T. Heterogeneity of tumor cell DNA content. In: *Brain Tumor Biology*, edited by M. L. Rosemblum and C. B. Wilson, Progr. Exp. Tumor Res., Basel, Karger, V 27, 1984, pp. 83–91.
82. Hoshino, T. The cell kinetics for gliomas: its prognostic value and therapeutic implications. Neurooncology, *1:*105–112, 1979.
83. Hoshino, T., Tonwsend, J.J., Muraoka, I., *et al.* An autoradiographic study of human gliomas: growth kinetics of anaplastic astrocytoma and glioblastoma. Brain, *103:*967–984, 1980.
84. Hoshino, T., Towsend, J.J., Muraoka, I., and Wilson, C.B. An autoradiographic study of human gliomas: growth kinetics of anaplastic astrocytoma and glioblastoma multiforme. Brain, *103:*967–984, 1980.
85. Hoshino, T. and Wilson C.B. Cell kinetic analyses of human malignant brain tumors (gliomas). Cancer, *44:*956–962, 1979.
86. Hubbard, B.M. and Hopewell, J.W. Changes in the neuroglial cell population of the rat spinal cord after local X-irradiation. British Journal of Radiology, *52:*816–821, 1979.
87. Hubbard, B.M. and Hopewell, J.W. Quantitative changes of the cellularity of the rat subependymal plate after X-irradiation. Cell and Tissue Kinetics, *13:*403–413, 1980.
88. Iglesias-Rozas, J.R. and Collia-Fernandez, F. Primeros estadios de los tumores del sistema nervioso en el hombre. Morf. Norm. Patol., *4:*511–525, 1980.
89. Jacobson, M. *Developmental Neurobiology.* New York, Plenum Press, 1978.
90. Jãnisch, W., Gũthert, H., and Schreiber, D. *Pathologie der Tumoren des Zentralnervensystems.* Jena, Fischer, 1976.
91. Jãnisch, W. and Schreiber D. Experimentelle Geschwũlste des Zentralnervensystems. Jena, Fisher, 1969. English edition, *Experimental tumors of the central nervous system,* edited by D. D. Bigner and J.A. Swenberg, Kalamazoo, Upjohn, 1977.

92. Jãnisch, W., Schreiber, D., Warzok, R., *et al.* Frũhstadien von Geschwũlsten des Zentralnervensystems. Experimentellmorphologische Untersuchung. Exp. Path., *4:*60–68, 1970.
93. Jones, T.R., Bigner, S.H., Shold, S.C., Jr., *et al.* Anaplastic human gliomas in athymic mice. Morphology and glial fibrillary acidic expression. Am. J. Pathol., *105:*316–327, 1981.
94. Kelly, P.J., Suddith, R.L., Hutchinson, H.T., *et al.* Endothelial growth factor present in tissue culture of CNS tumors. J. Neurosurg., *44:* 342–346, 1976.
95. Kleihues, P. and Rajewsky, M.F. Chemical neuorooncogenesis: role of structural DNA modifications, DNA repair and neuronal target cell populations. In: *Brain tumor biology,* edited by M. L. Rosemblum and C. B. Wilson. Progr. Exp. Tumor Res., Basel, Karger, V. 27, 1984, p. 1
96. Kleihues, P., Matsumoto, S., Wechsler, W., *et al.* Morphologie und Wachstum der mit Athylnitroso-Harnstoff transplacentar erzeugten Tumoren des Nervensystems. Vern. Dtsch. Ges. Path., *52:*372–388, 1968.
97. Klein, G. Oncogenes and tumor suppressor genes. Acta Oncologica, *27:*427–437, 1988.
98. Klein, G. and Klein, E. Evolution of tumors and the impact of molecular oncology. Nature (Lond.), *315:*190–195, 1985.
99. Knowles, J.F. The effect of X-radiation given after neonatal administration of ethylnitrosourea on incidence of induced nervous system tumors. Neuropath. Appl. Neurobiol., *8:*265–276, 1982.
100. Kochi, N. and Budka, H. Contribution of histiocytic cells to sarcomatous development of the gliosarcoma. An immunohistochemical study. Acta Neuropathol. (Berl.), *73:*124–130, 1987.
101. Koestner, A., Swenberg, J.A., and Wechsler, W. Transplacental production of neoplasms of the nervous system in Sprague-Dawley rats. Amer. J. Path., *63:*37–56, 1971.
102. Korr, H. Proliferation of different cell types in the brain. Adv. Anat. Embryol. Cell Biol., *61:*1–72, 1980.
103. Kumar, P., Kumar, S., Marsden, H.B., *et al.* Weibel-Palade bodies in endothelial cells as a marker for angiogenesis in brain tumors. Cancer Res., *40:*2010–2019, 1980.
104. Kumpulainen, T. and Korhonen, L.K. Immunohistochemical localization of carbonic anhydrase isoenzyme in the central and peripheral nervous system of the mouse. J. Histo-Cytochem., *30:*283–292, 1982.
105. Kumpulainen, T., Dahl, D., Korhonen, L.K., *et al.* Immunolabeling of carbonic anhydrase isoenzyme C and glial fibrillary acidic protein in paraffin-embedded tissue sections of human brain and retina. J. Histo-Cytochem., *31:*879–886, 1983.
106. Laerum, O.D., Bjerkvig, R., Sverre, K., *et al.* Invasiveness of primary brain tumors. Cancer Metast. Rev., *3:*223–236, 1984.
107. Laerum, O.D., Mørk, S.J., and De Ridder, L. The transformation process. In: *Brain Tumor Biology,* edited by M. L. Rosemblum and C. B. Wilson, Progr. Exp. Tumor Res., Basel, Karger, V. 27, 1984, p. 17.
108. Laerum, O.D. and Rajewsky, M.F. Neoplastic transformation of fetal rat brain cells in culture after exposure to ethylnitrosourea in vivo. J. Natl. Cancer Inst., *55:*1177–1187, 1975.
109. Laerum, O.D., Rajewsky, M.F., Schachner, M., *et al.* Phenotypic properties of neoplastic cell lines developed from fetal rat brain cells in culture after exposure to ethylnitrosourea in vivo. Z Krebsforsch, *82:*273–295, 1977.
110. Lantos, P.L. An electron microscope study of reacting astrocytes in gliomas induced by N-ethyl-N-nitrosourea in rats. Acta Neuropathol. (Berl.), *30:*175–181, 1974.
111. Lantos, P.L. The fine structure of the periventricular pleomorphic gliomas induced transplacentally by N-ethyl-nitrosourea in BD-IX rats. With a note on their origin. J. Neurol. Sci., *17:*443–460, 1972.
112. Lantos, P.L. and Cox, D.J. The origin of experimental brain tumors: a sequential study. Experientia, *32:*1457–1468, 1976.
113. Lantos, P.L. and Pilkington, G.J. The development of experimental brain tumors: a sequential light and electron microscope study of the subependymal plate. I. Early lesions (abnormal cell clusters) Acta Neuropathol. (Berl.), *45:*167–175, 1979.
114. Lens, P.F., Altena, B., and Nusse, R. Expression of c-sis and platelet-derived growth factor in in vitro-transformed glioma cells from rat brain tissue transplacentally treated with ethylnitrosourea. Molecular and Cellular Biology, *6:*3537–3540, 1986.
115. Levin, V.A., Freeman-Dove, M., and Landahe, H.D. Permeability characteristics of brain adjacent to tumors in rats. Arch. Neurol., *32:*785–791, 1975.
116. Levitt, P., Cooper, M.L., and Rakic, P. Coexistence of neuronal and glial precursor cells in the cerebral ventricular zone of the fetal monkey: an ultrastructural immunoperoxidase analysis. J. Neurosci., *1:*27–39, 1981.
117. Levitt, P. and Rakic, P. Immunoperoxidase localization of glial fibrillary acidic protein in radial glial cells and astrocytes of the developing rhesus monkey brain. J. Comp. Neurol., *193:*417–448, 1980.
118. Lewis, P.D. A quantitative study of cell proliferation in the subependymal layer of the adult in rat brain. Exp. Neurol., *20:*203–207, 1968.
119. Lewis, P.D. Cell proliferation in the postnatal nervous system and its relationship to the origin of gliomas. Semin. Neurol., *1:*27–39, 1981.
120. Lilja, A., Bergstrõm, K., Spãnnare B., *et al.* Reliability of computed tomography in assessing histopathological features of malignant supratentorial gliomas. J. Comput. Assist. Tomogr., *5:*625–636, 1981.
121. Lim, R. and Mitsonobu, K. Brain cells in culture: morphological transformation by a pro-

tein. Science, *185:*63–64, 1974.
122. Ludwin, S.K. An autoradiographic study of cellular proliferation in remyelination of the central nervous system. Am. J. Pathol., *95:*683–696, 1979.
123. Ludwin, S.K. Proliferation of mature oligodendrocytes after trauma to the central nervous system. Nature, *308:*274–275, 1984.
124. Lye, R.H., Elstow, S.F., and Weiss, J.B. Neurovascularization of intracranial tumors. In: *Biology of Brain Tumors*, edited by M. D. Walker and D. G. T. Thomas, Martinus Njihoff, Boston-Dordrecht-Lancaster, pp. 61–74, 1986.
125. Lynn, J.A., Panopio, I.I., Martin, J.H., *et al.* Ultrastructural evidence for astroglial histogenesis of the monstrocellular astrocytoma (so-called monstrocellular sarcoma of brain). Cancer, *30:*989–996, 1972.
126. Manuelidis, E.E. and Solitare, G.B. Glioblastoma multiforme. In: *Pathology of the Nervous System*, edited by J. Minckler, New York, McGraw-Hill, V 2, 1971, pp. 2026–2071.
127. Mark, J., Westermark, B., Ponten, J., *et al.* Banding patterns in human gliomas cell lines. Hereditas, *87:*243–260, 1977.
128. Matsukado, Y., MacCarty, C.S., and Kernohan, J.W. The growth of glioblastoma multiforme (astrocytomas grades 3 and 4) in neurosurgical practice. J. Neurosurg., *18:*636–644, 1981.
129. Mauro, A., Bertolotto, A., Giordana, M.T., *et al.* Biochemical and histochemical evaluation of glycosoaminoglicans in brain tumors induced in rats by nitrosourea derivatives. J. Neuro-oncol., *1:*299–306, 1983.
130. Mauro, A., Giordana, M.T., Migheli, A., *et al.* Glial fibrillary acidic protein (GFAP) in rat brain tumors transplacentally induced by ethylnitrosourea (ENU). J. Neurol. Sci., *61:* 349–355, 1983.
131. McComb, R.D., Jones, T.R., Pizzo, S.V., *et al.* Immunohistochemical detection of F VIII/ von Willebrand factor in hyperplastic endothelial cells in glioblastoma multiforme and mixed glioma-sarcoma. J. Neuropath. Exp. Neur., *41:*479–489, 1982.
132. Mennel, H.D. Gewebekulturuntersuchungen an experimentell erzeugten, transplantierten malignen Neurinomen. Z. Neurol., *201:*269–278, 1972.
133. Molnar, P., Groothuis, D., Blasberg, R., *et al.* Regional thymidine transport and incorporation in experimental brain and subcutaneous tumors. J. Neurochem., *43:*421–432, 1984.
134. Morantz, R.A., Feigin, I., and Ransohoff, J. Clinical and pathological study of 24 cases of gliosarcoma. J. Neurosurg., *45:*398–408, 1976.
135. Morimura, T., Kitz, K., and Budka, H. In situ analysis of cell kinetics in human brain tumors. Acta. Neuropathol. (Berl.), *77:*276–282, 1989.
136. Murray, K.J., White, J.G., and Douglas, S.D. Comparative biochemical and ultrastructural studies of capillaries from normal humans, normal mice, and human cerebral astrocytes. Surg. Neurol., *14:*53–58, 1980.
137. Nagashima, T., De Armoand, S.J., Murovic, J., *et al.* Immunocytochemical demonstration of S-phase cells by anti-bromodeoxyuridine monoclonal antibody in human brain tumor tissues. Acta. Neuropathol. (Berl.), *67:*155–159, 1985.
138. Naito, M., Naito, T., Ito, A., *et al.* Spinal cord tumors induced by N-Ethyl-N-nitrosourea in rats: presence of spinal subpial cells. J. Natl. Cancer Inst., *72:*715–724, 1984.
139. Nishio, S., Ohta, M., Abe, M., *et al.* Microvascular abnormalities in ethylnitrosourea (ENU)-induced rat brain tumors: structural basis for altered blood-brain barrier function. Acta Neuropathol. (Berl.), *59:*1–10, 1983.
140. Nister, M., Libermann, T., Betsnoltz, C., *et al.* Expression of messenger RNA_1 for platelet-derived growth factor and transforming factor-a and their receptors in human malignant glioma cell lines. Cancer Res., *48:*3910–3918, 1988.
141. Noble, M., Murray, K., Stroobant, P., *et al.* Platelet-derived growth factor promotes division and motility and inhibits premature differentiation of the oligodendrocyte / type-2 astrocyte progenitor cell. Nature, *333:*560–562, 1988.
142. Noske, W., Leutzen, H., Lange, K., *et al.* Phagocytotic activity of glial cells in culture. Exp. Cell Res., *142:*437–445, 1982.
143. Osborn, M., Ludwig-Festl, M., Weber, K., *et al.* Expression of glial fibrillary acidic protein and vimentin type intermediate filaments in cultures derived from human glial material. Differentiation, *19:*161–167, 1981.
144. Paulus, W. and Roggendorf, W. Vimentin and glial fibrillary acidic protein are codistributed in the same intermediate filament system of malignant glioma cells in vivo. Virchws. Archiv. B Cell Pathol., *56:*67–70, 1988.
145. Peña, L.E. and Felter, R. Ultrastructure of a composite glioma-sarcoma of the brain. Acta. Neuropathol. (Berl.), *23:*90–94, 1973.
146. Polmeteer, F.E. and Kernohan, J.W. Meningeal gliomatosis: study of 42 cases. Arch. Neurol., *57:*593–616, 1947.
147. Ponten, J. *Neoplastic Human Glia Cells in vitro.* New York, London, Plenum Press, 1975, pp. 175–206.
148. Raff, M.C., Lillien, L.E., Richardson, W.D., *et al.* Platelet-derived growth factor from astrocytes drives the clock that times oligodendrocyte development in culture. Nature, *333:* 562–565, 1988.
149. Rajewsky, M.F. Pulse-carcinogenesis by ethylnitrosourea in the developing rat nervous system: molecular and cellular mechanisms. In: *Chemical carcinogenesis.*, edited by Nicolini, New York, Plenum Press, 1982, p. 363.
150. Rakic, P. Mode of cell migration to the superfi-

cial layers of fetal monkey neocortex. J. Comp. Neurol., *145:*61–84, 1972.

151. Rakic, P. Neuron-glia relationship during granule cell migration in developing cerebellar cortex. A Golgi and electron microscopic study in macacus rhesus. J. Comp. Neurol., *141:*283–312, 1971.

152. Rath, F.W., Schneider, H., and Van Calker, H. Histochemische Untersuchungen an Frũhstadien experimenteller Hirntumoren. In: *Experimentelle Neuroonkologie*, edited by D. Schreiber and W. Jãnisch, Leipzig, Barth, 1974, p. 94.

153. Reifenberger, G., Bilzen, T., Seitz, R.J., *et al.* Expression of vimentin and glial fibrillary acidic protein in ethylnitrosourea-induced rat gliomas and glioma cell lines. Acta Neuropathol. (Berl.), *78:*270–282, 1989.

154. Roggendorf, W., Schuster, T., and Peiffer, J. Proliferative potential of meningiomas determined with the monoclonal antibody Ki-67. Acta Neuropathol. (Berl.), *73:*361–364.

155. Roscoe, F.P. and Claisse, P.J. A sequential in vivo-in vitro study of carcinogenesis induced in the rat brain by ethylnitrosourea. Nature, *262:*314–316, 1976.

156. Rubinstein, L.J. The development of contiguous sarcomatous and gliomatous tissue in intracranial tumors. J. Pathol., *71:*441–459, 1956.

157. Rubinstein, L.J. Embryonal central neuroepithelial tumors and their differentiating potential. A cytogenetic view of a complex neuro-oncological problem. J. Neurosurg., *62:* 795–805, 1985.

158. Rubinstein, L.J. The correlation of neoplastic vulnerability with central neuroepithelial cytogeny and glioma differentiation. J. Neuro-oncol., *5:*11–27, 1987.

159. Rubinstein, L.J., Herman, M.M., and Vanden-Berg S.R. Differentiation and anaplasia in central neuroepithelial tumors. In: *Brain Tumor Biology*, edited by M. L. Rosenblum and C. B. Wilson, Progr. Exp. Tumor. Res., Basel, Karger, V 27, 1984, p. 32.

160. Russell, D.S. and Rubinstein, L.J. *Pathology of tumours of the nervous system*. London, Arnold, Fifth Edition, 1989.

161. Sato, T., Himoda, A., Takahashi, R.T., *et al.* Congenital cerebellar neuroepithelial tumor with multiple divergent differentiations. Acta Neuropathol. (Berl.), *50:*143–146, 1980.

162. Schaper, A. The earliest differentiation in the central nervous system of vertebrates. Science, *5:*430–431, 1897.

163. Schechter, A.L., Stern, D.F., Vaidjanathan, L., *et al.* The neu oncogene: an erb-B-related gene encoding a 185.000-M_r tumour antigen. Nature (Lond.), *312:*513–516, 1984.

164. Scheithauer, B.W. and Rubinstein, L.J. Cerebral medulloblastoma. Report of a case with multiple divergent neuroepithelial differentiation. Child's Brain, *5:*62–71, 1979.

165. Scherer, H.J. The forms of growth in gliomas and their practical significance. Brain, *63:*1–112, 1940.

166. Schiffer, D. Neuropathology and imaging: the ways in which glioma spreads and varies in its histological aspect. In: *Biology of Brain Tumors*, edited by M. D. Walker and D. G. T. Thomas, Boston, Martinus Nijoff, 1986, pp. 163–172.

167. Schiffer, D. On the occurrence of oligodendroglia-like areas in neurinomas experimentally induced in the rat by nitrosourea derivatives. J. Neurol. Sci., *19:*45–52, 1973.

168. Schiffer, D., Bertolotto, A., Giordana, M.T., *et al.* Induction of brain tumors by transplacental ENU: correlation between neurocytogenesis and tumor development. In: *Developmental neuroscience: physiological, pharmacological and clinical aspects.*, edited by F. Caciagli, E. Giacobini, R. Paoletti, Amsterdam, Elsevier, 1984, p. 267.

169. Schiffer, D., Cavicchioli, D., Giordana, M.T., *et al.* Analysis of some factors effecting survival in malignant gliomas. Tumori, *65:*119–125, 1979.

170. Schiffer, D., Chiò, Giordana, M.T., *et al.* Vascular response to tumor infiltration in malignant gliomas. Morphometric and reconstruction study. Acta Neuropathol. (Berl.), *77:* 369–378, 1989.

171. Schiffer, D. and Giordana, M.T. On the occurrence and significance of acid mucopolysaccharides in oligodendrogliomas experimentally induced in the rat b nitrosourea derivatives. In: *Experimentelle Neuroonkologie*, edited by D. Schreiber and W. Jãnisch, Leipzig, Barth, 1974, p. 101.

172. Schiffer, D., Giordana, M.T., Mauro, A., *et al.* Experimental brain tumors by transplacental ENU. Multifactorial study of latency period. Acta Neuropathol. (Berl.), *49:*117–122, 1980.

173. Schiffer, D. Giordana, M.T., Mauro, A. *et al.* GFAP, Factor VIII/RAg, laminin and fibronectin in gliosarcomas: an immunohistochemical study. Acta Neuropathol. (Berl.), *67:*201–210, 1985.

174. Schiffer, D., Giordana, M.T., Mauro, A.. *et al.* Immunohistochemical demonstration of vimentin in human cerebral tumors. Acta Neuropathol. (Berl.), *70:*209–219, 1986.

175. Schiffer, D., Giordana, M.T., Migheli, A., *et al.* Glial fibrillary acidic protein (GFAP) and vimentin in the experimental glial reaction of the rat brain. Brain Res., *374:*110–118, 1986.

176. Schiffer, D., Giordana, M.T., Germano, I., *et al.* Anaplasia and heterogeneity of GFAP in gliomas. Tumori, *72:*163–170, 1986.

177. Schiffer, D., Giordana, M.T., Pezzotta, S., *et al.* Cerebral tumors induced by transplacental ENU: study of the different tumoral stages, particularly of early proliferations. Acta Neuropathol. (Berl.), *41:*27–31, 1978.

178. Schiffer, D., Giordana, M.T., Pezzotta, S., *et al.* Chemotherapeutic effects of some alkylating derivatives of nitrosourea on the develop-

ment of tumors transplacentally induced in rats by ENU. Acta Neuropathol. (Berl.), *34:*21–31, 1976.

179. Schiffer, D., Giordana, M.T., and Soffietti, R. Effects of radiotherapy on the astrocytomatous areas of malignant gliomas. J. Neurooncol., *2:*167–175, 1984.

180. Schiffer, D., Giordana, M.T., Soffietti, R., *et al.* Histological observations on the regrowth of malignant gliomas after radiotherapy and chemotherapy. Acta Neuropathol. (Berl.), *58:*291–299, 1982.

181. Schiffer, D., Giordana, M.T., Soffietti, R., *et al.* Radio- and chemotherapy of malignant gliomas. Pathological changes in the normal nervous tissue. Acta Neurochir., *58:*37–58, 1981.

182. Schiffer, D., Giordana, M.T., Soffietti, R., Tarenzi, L., *et al.* On the nature of the so-called monstrocellular sarcoma of the brain. Neurosurgery, *6:*391–397, 1984.

183. Schmechel, D.E. and Rakic, P. A Golgi study of radial glia cells in developing monkey telencephalon: morphogenesis and transformation into astrocytes. Anat Embryol (Berlin), *156:*115–152, 1979.

184. Schmitt, H.P. Rapid anaplastic transformation in gliomas of adulthood. Path. Res. Pract., *176:*313–323, 1983.

185. Schnitzer, J., Franke, W.W., and Schachner, M. Immunohistochemical demonstration of vimentin in astrocytes and ependymal cells of developing and adult nervous system. J. Cell Biol., *90:*435–447, 1981.

186. Schold, S.C., and Bigner, D.D. A review of animal brain tumor models that have been used for therapeutic studies. In: *Oncology of the nervous system*, edited by M. D. Walker, Boston, Martinus Nijhoff, 1983, p. 31.

187. Seitz, R.J. and Wechsler, W. Vascularization of human cerebral gliomas: a lectin-cytochemical and morphometric study. In: *Biology of Brain Tumors*, edited by M. D. Walker and D. G. T. Thomas, Martinus Nijhoff, Boston-Dordrecht-Lancaster, 1986, pp. 132–137.

188. Shapiro, J.R. and Shapiro, W. R. Clonal tumor cell heterogeneity. In: *Brain Tumor Biology*, edited by M. L. Rosemblum and C. B. Wilson, Progr. Exp. Tumor Res., Basel, Karger, V 27, 1984, pp. 49–66.

189. Shapiro, J.R., Young, W.A., and Shapiro, W.R. Isolation, karyotype and clonal growth of heterogeneous subpopulations of human malignant gliomas. Cancer Res., *41:*2349–2359, 1981.

190. Shaw, C.M., Sumi, M.S., Alvord, E.C., *et al.* Fast-neutron irradiation of glioblastoma multiforme. Neuropathological analysis. J. Neurosurg., *49:*1–12, 1978.

191. Shuangshoti, S. and Netsky, M.G. Neoplasm of mixed mesenchymal and neuroepithelial origin: relation to "monstrocellular sarcoma" or "giant-celled glioblastoma." J. Neuropath. Exp. Neur., *30:*290–309, 1971.

192. Slowik, F., Jellinger, K., Gaszò, *et al.* Gliosarcomas: histological, immunohistochemical, ultrastructural and tissue culture studies. Acta Neuropathol. (Berl.), *67:*201–210, 1985.

193. Spence, A.M. and Geraci, J.P. Combined cyclotron fast-neutron and BCNU therapy in a rat brain tumor model. J. Neurosurg., *54:*461–467, 1981.

194. Steinvåg, S.K. and Laerum, O.D. Transmission electron microscopy of cocultures between normal rat brain tissue and rat glioma cells. Anticancer Res., *5:*137–146, 1985.

195. Steinvåg, S.K., Laerum, O.D., and Bjerkvig, R. Interaction between rat glioma cells and normal rat brain tissue in organ culture. Natl. Cancer Inst., *74:*1095–1104, 1985.

196. Storring, F.K. and Duguid J.B. The vascular formations in glioblastoma. J. Pathol. Bacteriol., *68:*231–242, 1954.

197. Sturrok, R.R. Cell division in the normal central nervous system. In: *Advances in cellular neurobiology*, edited by S. Fedoroff and L. Hertz, New York, Academic Press, V. 4, 1982, p. 3.

198. Sturrok, R.R. Light microscopic identification of immature glial cells in semithin sections of the developing mouse corpus callosum. J. Anat., *122:*521–537, 1976.

199. Swenberg, J.A., Clendenon, N., Denlinger, R., *et al.* Sequential development of ethylnitrosourea-induced neurinomas: morphology, biochemistry, and transplantability. J. Natl. Cancer Inst., *55:*147–152, 1975.

200. Swenberg, J.A., Wechsler, W., and Koestner, A. The sequential development of transplacentally induced neuroectodermal tumors. J. Neuropath. Exp. Neur., *30:*202–203, 1971.

201. Szikla, G., Plond, S. Daumas-Duport, C., *et al.* Stereotaxis in management of brain tumors: three-dimensional angiography, sampling biopsies and focal irradiation using the Talairach stereotactic system. Ital. J. Neurol. Sci., *2:*83–96, 1983.

202. Tannock, I.F. Population kinetics of carcinoma cells, capillary endothelial cells and fibroblasts in a transplanted mouse mammary tumor. Cancer Res., *30:*2470–2476, 1970.

203. Todaro, G. In: *Theories of Carcinogenesis*, edited by O. H. Iversen, Washington, D.C., Hemisphere, 1988, pp. 61–80.

204. Van der Meulen, J.D.M., Houthoff, H.J., and Ebels, E.J. Glial fibrillary acidic protein in human gliomas. Neuropath. Appl. Neurobiol., *4:*177–190, 1978.

205. Velasco, M.E., Dahl, D., Roessman, U., *et al.* Immunohistochemical localization of glial fibrillary acidic protein in human glial neoplasms. Cancer, *45:*484–494, 1980.

206. Vick, N.A., Khandekar, J.D., and Bigner, D.D. Chemotherapy of brain tumors. The "blood-brain barrier" is not a factor. Arch. Neurol., *34:*523–526, 1977.

207. Vinores, S.A. and Koestner, A. Reduction of ethylnitrosourea-induced neoplastic proliferation in rat trigeminal nerves by nerve growth factors. Cancer Res., *42:*1038–1040, 1982.

208. Waggener, J.D. and Beggs, J.L. Vasculature of neural neoplasms. In: *Neoplasia in the central nervous system.*, edited by R. A. Thompson and J. R. Green, Advances in Neurobiology, New York, Raven Press, V 15, 1976, pp. 27–42.

209. Warnke, P.C., Blasberg, R.G., and Groothuis, D.R. The effect of hyperosmotic blood-brain barrier disruption on blood-to-tissue transport in ENU-induced gliomas. Ann. Neurol., *22*:300–305, 1987.

210. Waterfield, M.D., Scrace, G.T., Whittle, N., *et al.* Platelet-derived growth factor is structurally related to the putative transforming protein p28 sis of simian sarcoma virus. Nature (Lond.), *304*:35–39, 1983.

211. Wechsler, W., Kleihues, P., Matsumoto, S., *et al.* Pathology of experimental neurogenic tumors chemically induced during prenatal and postnatal life. Ann. NY Acad. Sci., *159:* 360, 408, 1969.

212. Wechsler, W. and Koestner, A. The sequential development of transplacentally induced neuroectodermal tumors. J. Neuropath. Exp. Neur., *31*:202–203, 1972.

213. Weller, R.O., Foy, M., and Cox, S. The development and ultrastructure of the microvasculature in malignant gliomas. Neuropath. Appl. Neurobiol., *3*:307–322, 1977.

214. Weller, R.O. and Griffin, R.L. Transmission and scanning electron microscopy of the microcirculation of gliomas. In: *Pathology of Cerebrospinal Microcirculation*, edited by J. Cervòs-Navarro, E. Betz, G. Ebhardt, *et al.*, Advances in Neurology, New York, Raven Press, V 20, 1978, pp. 569–575.

215. Westermark, B., Heldin, C-H., Johusson, A., *et al.* In: *Growth and Maturation Factors*, edited by G. J. Guroff, New York, Wiley, 1983, pp. 73–115.

216. Willson, N. and Duffy, P.E. Morphologic changes associated with combined BCNU and radiation therapy in glioblastoma multiforme. Neurology, *24*:465–471, 1974.

217. Yamada, K., Hayakawa, T., Ushio, Y., *et al.* Regional blood flow and capillary permeability in the ethylnitrosourea-induced rat glioma. J. Neurosurg., *55*:922–928, 1981.

218. Zanker, K.S., Stavrou, D., Osterkamp, U., *et al.* Fibrinolysis induced by rat glioma cells. J. Neurol. Sci., *38*:67–75, 1978.

219. Zimmerman, H.M. Experimental brain tumors. In: *The Biology and Treatment of Intracranial Tumors*, edited by W. S. Fields and P. C. Sharkey, Springfield, Thomas, 1962, pp. 49–62.

220. Zũlch, K.J. Biologie und Pathologie der Hirngeschwũlste. In: *Pathologische Anatomie der raumbeengenden intrakraniellen Prozesse*, edited by K. J. Zũlch and E. Christensen, Springer, Berlin, 1956.

221. Zũlch, K.J. and Mennel, H.D. Die Morphologie der durch alkylierende Substanzen erzeugten Tumoren des Nervensystems. Zbl. Neurochir., *32*:225–243, 1971.

222. Zũlch, K.J. and Wechsler, W. Pathology and classification of gliomas. In: *Progress in Neurological Surgery*, edited by H. Krayenbũhl, P. E. Maspes, and W. H. Sweet, Basel, New York, Karger, V 2, 1968, pp. 1–84.

CHAPTER 8

Differentiation and Phenotypic Expression in Human Gliomas

PAUL L. KORNBLITH, M.D., and MARSHA J. MERRILL, Ph.D.

INTRODUCTION

In the clinical management of patients with gliomas the influence of the degree of cellular differentiation on outcome is apparent (32). The difference between the relatively long range prognosis for a child with a well-differentiated astrocytoma of the cerebellum and the dismal outlook for an adult with an intrinsic cerebral glioblastoma multiforme is indeed dramatic. This contrast in clinical outcome must have a biological basis. The question that this observation raises is whether there are ways of understanding the process of glial cell differentiation which can lead to some form of therapeutic intervention to achieve partial reversal of the tumorigenic phenotype and thus improve the clinical prognosis.

The idea that cancer is a disease of developmental biology has been with us since the first descriptions of neoplasia. Within recent years evidence has accumulated that, at least in some instances, cancer cells are differentiation deficient (27, 34). That is to say that the processes of growth and maturation which occur during normal stem cell differentiation are uncoupled in the malignant cell, with cells retaining the ability to divide but losing the ability to become terminally differentiated adult cells. Some cancer cells may still retain the capacity to function as normal cells but do not because they are lacking in either the ability to produce certain regulatory factors or the ability to respond to such factors.

If this is the case then the tumorigenic phenotype may be reversible upon restoration of normal differentiation control mechanisms. Ten years ago, the experiments of Illmensee and Mintz provided tantalizing evidence that frankly malignant cells could express a normal phenotype if placed in the appropriate environment (18). These investigators injected teratocarcinoma cells into blastocytes and found that these cancer cells gave rise to normal cells in the adult animal. More recently Sachs and coworkers have demonstrated that some leukemia cells have the ability to differentiate into nonmalignant cells when supplied with the appropriate differentiation factor (25, 26). Other model systems also exist in which tumor-derived cells can be induced to express differentiated functions in the presence of various chemicals (7, 9, 21, 29, 31). Thus, at least some cancer cells do retain the ability to express a more normal phenotype and may not be irreversibly malignant.

Investigations into the differentiation of glioma cells are in their infancy in comparison to those on leukemia cells. The process of development of normal glia is not well understood and a glial stem cell population is not fully identified. However, normal glia do retain the ability to divide in a controlled manner particularly in response to injury (28), and both a glial growth factor (22, 23) and a glial maturation factor (24) have been isolated from normal brain. Inappropriate production of, or response to, these factors may be involved in the development of gliomas.

As yet the clinical efficacy of differentiating agents is untested in glioma patients and the material presented here deals with experimental studies. There have been some preliminary trials against colon cancer and brain metastases which have not as yet been completed. In this chapter, this new and potentially useful approach will be discussed with respect to the basic data obtained to this point. It should be noted that in addition to the direct effects of these differentiating agents, in some instances there appear to be synergistic effects with radiation therapy and certain cytotoxic chemotherapy agents (see below).

In a discussion of biological growth modifying agents, two groups are generally considered: those agents which alter the growth of tumor cells and those agents which effect a change in the immune response thus indirectly affecting tumor growth. This discussion will focus only on those agents which alter the tumor cell itself. The data presented in this chapter by no means constitute a comprehensive study of the problem. They merely serve to indicate the potential of the system.

METHODS FOR STUDY OF DIFFERENTIATION IN CULTURED HUMAN GLIOMA CELLS

The basic technique of our laboratory involves the use of cells derived from human glial tumors in a monolayer culture system (3). The cells are grown in Ham's F-10 nutrient medium (Gibco-Grand Island, NY) with 10% fetal calf serum (Gibco). The lines are regularly tested for mycoplasma by Dr. Del Guidice of the Frederick Cancer Center. The lines used are all derived from patients with astrocytic tumors (Grades II, III, and IV). The chemicals used as differentiation agents are N^6, O^6-dibutyryl cyclic adenosine 3′,5′-monophosphate (DBcAMP), N,N-dimethylformamide (DMF), and sodium butyrate. Cultured cells from each of the cell lines are distributed into Falcon 25-sq cm flasks. Phase contrast micrographs are used to monitor morphological changes, and daily flask counts provide data for growth curves. For immunological studies, autologous sera from the patients are used to determine autologous humoral cytotoxicity (20) and immune adherence (6).

Counting of plates is facilitated by use of the Bausch and Lomb image analysis system. The cytotoxic index is derived by the following formula:

$$CI = 1 - \frac{\text{Average no. of cells in test wells}}{\text{Average no. of cells in control wells}}$$

The data is then subjected to the student's *t* test. The analysis of plasminogen activator (PA) levels is carried out by Drs. Daniel Dexter and Janet Gross at the Glenolden Laboratories of the Dupont Corporation.

REGULATION OF THE DIFFERENTIATED PHENOTYPE IN CULTURED HUMAN GLIOMA CELLS

The study of differentiation and malignancy in normal glia and glioma derived cells is made difficult due to the extensive heterogeneity among cell lines and among cell populations within a single cell line (2, 5, 35, 39). Nevertheless, certain features are thought to be reflective of normal astroglial differentiation; these include morphology, karyotype, surface proteins, glial fibrillary acidic protein (GFAP), S-100, high affinity glutamine and gamma aminobutyric acid (GABA) uptake, and glutamine synthetase (13). Malignancy in glioblastoma-derived cells is usually characterized by the degree of expression of certain general tumor-associated parameters, including rapid growth rate, plasminogen activator, tumor angiogenesis factor, anchorage independence and loss of contact inhibition (13). Thus differentiation of glioma cells in culture is characterized by a shift away from tumor-associated behavior and/or a shift toward increased expression of one or more of the functions associated with normal glial cells.

We have examined the effects of three differentiating agents, DBcAMP, DMF, and sodium butyrate, on four parameters of glioma cell differentiation, namely, morphology, growth rate, plasminogen activator levels, and immunological responsiveness. The biological differences between high and low grade malignancies are reflected not only in the clinical prognosis but also in the behavior and morphology of the cells cultured from these tumors. In cells derived from low grade malignancies the growth rate is slower, the saturation density is lower, and the morphology is more characteristically astrocytic then in cells derived from high grade malignancies (Fig. 8.1). With DBcAMP, morphological changes were observed in 16 of 26 cultures. These changes consisted primarily of increased process formation (Fig. 8.2*B*). DMF produced morphological changes in 17 of 26 cell cultures. With DMF the changes were mainly cellular elongation, and a marked decrease in saturation density (Fig. 8.2*C*). There were 11 cultures which responded to both agents. In studies of growth inhibition, DBcAMP produced inhibition in 21 of 26 cultures and DMF in 23 of 26 cultures tested. This inhibition ranged from 39 to 96% in the DBcAMP-treated cultures and from 59 to 96% in DMF-treated cultures, but never appeared to result in terminal differentiation as cells would resume growing at their pretreatment rates 72 hours after removal from contact with the agents. In a study of 3 cul-

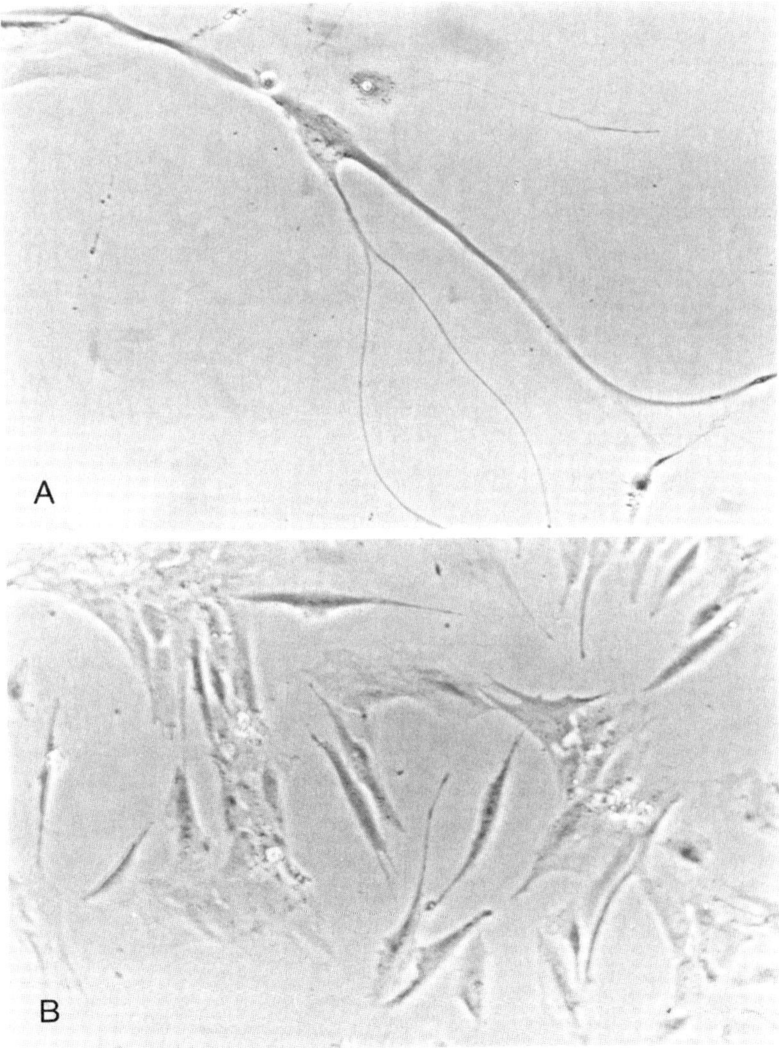

Figure 8.1. Morphology of cells cultured from low- and high-grade malignancies. Light micrographs of primary explant culture derived *A*) from a low-grade astrocytoma of a 7-month-old child and *B*) from a recurrent glioblastoma multiforme of a 50-year-old man are shown. ×100.

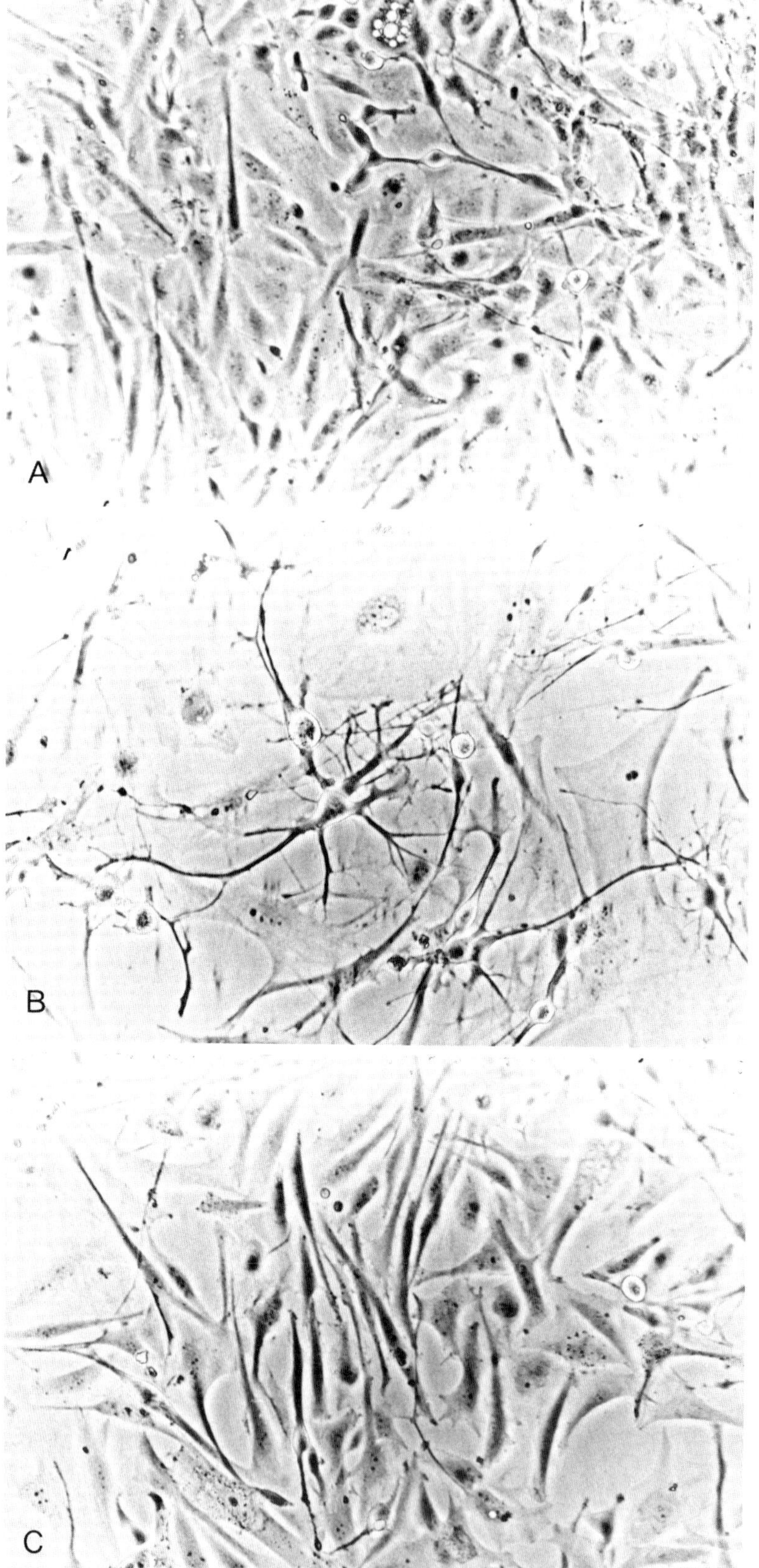
A
B
C

tures, PA levels were lowered significantly in all 3 with use of sodium butyrate. The most striking response was a decline from levels of 2.4 ± 0.5 to 0.75 ± 0.1 (PSA in mV/mg) at a sodium butyrate dose of 1 mm. In 7 cultures studied for immunological responsiveness before and after treatment with DBcAMP and DMF, two of the lines initially negative with the cytotoxic assay became positive after treatment. In general, immune adherence was not altered by treatment (Table 8.1).

Other investigators have observed that the differentiated phenotype of glial and glioma-derived cells is responsive to regulation by additional agents. Glial maturation factor (GMF) induces a morphologic change to a more differentiated appearance in normal astrocytes and in schwannoma cells but failed to induce such a change in at least some glioblastoma derived cell lines (19). Glucocorticoids have a variety of effects on cultured glioma cells (12, 14, 15). Dexamethasone induces glutamine synthetase and β-adrenergic receptors and reduces the saturation density of glioma cells. Dexamethasone, cAMP, and GMF increase high-affinity GABA uptake. Dexamethasone alters the molecular weight profile of glioma cell surface proteins to more closely resemble the profile of normal cells and also markedly reduces the level of plasminogen activator.

TABLE 8.1
Cytotoxic Index and Immune Adherence[a]

		Control		DBcAMP		DMF	
Line	Grade	CI	IA	CI	IA	CI	IA
GB	IV	0.03		0.05		0.30[b]	1:4
MC	IV	−0.05		−0.08		−0.08	
RF	IV	0.73[b]	1:8	0.88[b]	1:4	1.00[b]	1:8
FG	II	−0.25		0.15		−0.32	
LM[c]	IV	0.02		−0.02		0.15	
XN	III	0.28[b]	1:4	0.86[b]	1:2	0.31	1:1
MR	IV	−0.19		0.42[b]		0.85[b]	

[a] Taken from Gumerlock, M.K., Smith, B.H., Pollock, L.A., *et al.* Chemical differentiation of cultured human glioma cells: morphologic and immunologic effects. Surg. Forum, *32*:475–477, 1981.
[b] Positive cytotoxic index, significant to $P < 0.05$.
[c] Allogeneic serums tested; used MR serum.

CONCLUSIONS AND FUTURE DIRECTIONS

In spite of the complexities of this system, it is now clear that malignant glioma cells are responsive to differentiating agents. Many of the nonspecific differentiating agents effective in other systems are also effective in glioma cells. Sodium butyrate, an inhibitor of histone deacetylation (4, 37), reduces plasminogen activator and clonogenicity in soft agar (16). DMSO, which increases cell membrane permeability, reduces cell growth and glycosaminoglycan production (8). Both DBcAMP and dimethylformamide alter cell morphology and immunogenicity. Furthermore the distinct morphological and kinetic changes induced by these agents make the system easy to monitor. The finding that plasminogen activator, a biochemical parameter of malignancy and tumor invasiveness, is drastically altered by sodium butyrate treatment allows us to have an index of a biochemical nature with which to follow the process.

The changes in immunological status are of particular interest. Inasmuch as immune responses are so frequently detected in low grade tumors and so infrequently found in patients with the most malignant lesions, it is of importance that by using differentiation agents one can shift cultures from nonresponsive to responsive. This suggests that the use of differentiation agents as probes may provide an insight into the immunological recognition process.

The use of differentiating agents in conjunction with cytotoxic forms of therapy has not yet been examined in glioma cells. Early results from other systems appear encouraging. Sodium butyrate, presumably by alterations in chromatin structure, has been shown to enhance the cytotoxicity of nitrosoureas, nitrogen mustards, daunorubicin, UV irradiation, and x-rays in various types of cultured cells (30, 33, 38). Similarly DMSO has been shown to enhance the cytotoxicity of BCNU, *cis*-platinum, and melphalan in cultured hepatocarci-

Figure 8.2. Morphologic effects of DBcAMP and DMF on cultured glioma cells. Light micrographs of glioma cells cultured under three conditions are shown: *A*) Control, *B*) Treatment with 10^{-3}M DBcAMP for 72 hours and *C*) Treatment with 0.6% DMF for 72 hours. ×100.

noma cells (36). The polar solvents DMSO, DMF, and N-methylformamide have been shown to enhance the radiosensitivity of certain tumor cells (10, 11), although the mechanism of this enhancement is not well understood.

Although the field of differentiation of gliomas is a new one, early results suggest that gliomas are responsive to differentiating agents thus giving encouragement to the eventual possibility of modulating the tumorigenic phenotype of human glioblastomas in the clinical setting.

REFERENCES

1. Balana, A., Wiels, J., Tetaud, C., *et al.* Induction of cell differentiation in Burkitt lymphoma lines. BLA: a glycolipid marker of B-cell differentiation. Int. J. Cancer, *36:*453–460, 1985.
2. Bigner, D.D., Bigner, S.H., Pont'en, J.,*et al.* Heterogeneity of genotypic and phenotypic characteristics of fifteen permanent cell lines derived from human gliomas. J. Neuropathol. Exp. Neurol., *40:*201–229, 1981.
3. Black, P.M., Kornblith, P.L., Davison, P.F., *et al.* Immunological, biochemical, ultrastructural, and electrophysiological characteristics of a human glioblastoma-derived cell culture line. J. Neurosurg., *56:*62–72, 1982.
4. Boffa, L.C., Vidali, G., Mann, R.S., *et al.* Suppression of histone deacetylation in vivo and in vitro by sodium butyrate. J. Biol. Chem., *253:*3364–3366, 1978.
5. Cairncross, J.G., Mattes, M.J., Beresford, H.R., *et al.* Cell surface antigens of human astrocytoma defined by mouse monoclonal antibodies: identification of astrocytoma subsets. Proc. Natl. Acad. Sci., *79:*5641–5645, 1982.
6. Coakham, H.B., Kornblith, P.L., Quindlen, E.A., *et al.* Autologous humoral response to human gliomas and analysis of certain cell surface antigens: in vitro study with the use of microcytotoxicity and immune adherence assays. J. Natl. Cancer Inst., *64:*223–233, 1980.
7. Collins, J.C., Ruscetti, F.W., and Gallagher, R.E., *et al.* Terminal differentiation of human promyelocytic leukemia cells induced by dimethyl sulfoxide and other polar compounds. Proc. Natl. Acad. Sci., *75:*2458–2462, 1979.
8. Constantopoulos, G., Hawkins, C.S., and Kornblith, P.L. Dimethylsulfoxide inhibits glycosaminoglycan synthesis and cell growth in human gliomas in vitro. Trans. Am. Soc. Neurochem., *17:*223, 1986.
9. Dexter, D.L. and Hager, J.C. Maturation-induction of tumor cells using a human colon carcinoma model. Cancer, *45:*1178–1184, 1980.
10. Dexter, D.L., Lee, E.S., Bliven, S.F., *et al.* Enhancement by N-methylformamide of the effect of ionizing radiation on a human colon tumor xenografted in nude mice. Cancer Res., *44:*4942–4946, 1984.
11. Einspenner, M., Boulton, J.E., and Borsa, J. Variation of radiation sensitivity of Friend erythroleukemia cells cultured in the presence of the differentiation inducer DMSO. Radiat. Res., *97:*55-63, 1984.
12. Foster, S.J. and Harden, T.K. Dexamethasone increases beta-adrenoceptor density in human astrocytoma cella. Biochem. Pharmacol., *29:* 2151–2153, 1980.
13. Frame, M.C., Freshney, R.I., Vaughan, P.F.T., *et al.* Interrelationship between differentiation and malignancy-associated properties in glioma. Br. J. Cancer, *49:*269–280, 1984.
14. Freshney, R.I. Effects of glucocorticoids on glioma cells in culture. Exp. Cell. Biol., *52:*286–292, 1984.
15. Freshney, R.I., Sherry, A., Hassanzadah, M., *et al.* Control of cell proliferation in human glioma by glucocorticoids. Br. J. Cancer, *41:*857–866, 1980.
16. Gross, J.L., Behrens, D.L., Kornblith, P.L., *et al.* Plasminogen activator and inhibitor activity in human glioma cells: modulation by differentiating agents. Submitted for publication, 1986.
17. Gumerlock, M.K., Smith, B.H., Pollock, L.A., *et al.* Chemical differentiation of cultured human glioma cells: morphologic and immunologic effects. Surg. Forum, *32:*475–477, 1981.
18. Illmensee, K. and Mintz, B. Totipotency and normal differentiation of single teratocarcinoma cells cloned by injection into blastocyst. Proc. Natl. Acad. Sci., *73:*549–533, 1976.
19. Kato, T., Ito, J., Ishikawa, K., *et al.* The absence of differentiation-promoting response of astroglioma cells to glia maturation factor. Brain Res., *301:*83–93, 1984.
20. Kornblith, P.L., Coakham, H.B., Pollock, L.A., *et al.* Autologous serologic responses in glioma patients; correlation with tumor grade and survival. Cancer, *52:*2230–2235, 1983.
21. Leder, A. and Leder, P. Butyric acid, a potent inducer of erthyroid differentiation in cultured erythroleukemic cells. Cell, *5:*319–322, 1975.
22. Lemke, G.E. and Brockes, J.P. Glial growth factor: a mitogenic polypeptide of the brain and pituitary. Fed. Proc., *42:*2627–2629, 1983.
23. Lemke, G.E. and Brockes, J.P. Identification and purification of glial growth factor. J. Neurosci., *4:*75–83, 1984.
24. Lim, R. Glia maturation factor and other factors acting on glia. In *Growth and Maturation Factors, Vol. 3* edited by G. Guroff, pp. 119–147, John Wiley and Sons, Inc., 1985.
25. Lotem, J., Berrebi, A., and Sachs, L. Screening for induction of differentiation and toxicity to blast cells by chemotherapeutic compounds in human myeloid leukemia. Leukemia Res., *9:*249–258, 1985.
26. Lotem, J. and Sachs, L. Control of in vivo differentiation of myeloid leukemic cells. IV. Inhibition of leukemia development by myeloid

differentiation-inducing protein. Int. J. Cancer, *33:*147–154, 1984.
27. Lotem, J. and Sachs, L. Coupling of growth and differentiation in normal myeloid precursors and the breakdown of this coupling in leukemia. Int. J. Cancer, *32:*127–134, 1983.
28. Nieto-Sampedro, M., Saneto, R.P., deVellis, J., *et al.* The control of glial populations in brain: changes in astrocyte mitogenic and morphogenic factors in response to injury. Brain Res., *343:*320–328, 1985.
29. Novogrodsky, A., Rubin, A.L., and Stenzel, K.H. A new class of inhibitors of lymphocyte mitogenesis: agents that induce erythroid differentiation in Friend leukemia cells. J. Immunol., *124:*1892–1897, 1980.
30. Pani, B., Babudri, N., Giancotti, V., *et al.* Sodium butyrate affects the cytotoxic and mutagenic response of V79 chinese hamster cells to the genotoxic agents, daunorubicin and UV radiation. Mutation Res., *140:*175–179, 1984.
31. Reem, G.H. and Friend, C. Purine metabolism in murine virus-induced erythroleukemic cells during differentiation in vitro. Proc. Natl. Acad. Sci., *72:*1630–1634, 1975.
32. Salcman, M. The morbidity and mortality of brain tumors. Neurol. Clin., *3:*229–257, 1985.
33. Sankaranarayanan, K., Natarajan, A.T., Mullenders, L.H.F., *et al.* Effects of pre-treatment with sodium butyrate on the frequencies of x-ray-induced chromosomal aberrations in human peripheral blood lymphocytes. Mutation Res., *151:*269–274, 1985.
34. Scott, R.E. and Maercklein, P.B. An initiator of carcinogenesis selectively and stably inhibits stem cell differentiation: a concept that initiation of carcinogenesis involves multiple phases. Proc. Natl. Acad. Sci., *82:*2995–2999, 1985.
35. Studer, A., de Tribolet, N., Diserens, A.C., *et al.* Characterization of four human malignant glioma cell lines. Acta. Neuropathol. (Berl), *66:*208–217, 1985.
36. Tofilon, P.J., Vines, C.M., and Milas, L. Enhancement of in vitro chemotherapeutic activity by dimethylsulfoxide. Clin. Exp. Metastasis., *3:*141–150, 1985.
37. Vidali, G., Goffa, L.C., Mann, R.S., *et al.*. Reversible effects of Na-butyrate on histone acetylation. Biochem. Biophys. Res. Commun., *82:*223–227, 1978.
38. Vu, V.T., Moy, B.C., Schein, P.S., *et al.* Enhanced nitrosourea cytotoxicity in cell culture by sodium butyrate. Oncology, *42:*317–321, 1985.
39. Yung, W.K., Shapiro, J.R., and Shapiro, W.R. Heterogeneous chemosensitivities of subpopulations of human glioma cells in culture. Cancer Res., *42:*992–998, 1982.

CHAPTER 9

Cell Kinetics of Brain Tumors

TAKAO HOSHINO, M.D., D.M.Sc.

INTRODUCTION

From the clinical standpoint, brain tumors include all tumors arising in the intracranial cavity. These lesions therefore comprise a diversity of neoplastic types, each with its own growth pattern and cellular and histological characteristics. Intracranial tumors may be grouped broadly according to their origin: from nervous (neuroectodermal) tissue and blood vessels of the brain, from the coverings of the brain (mesodermal tissue), from the intracranial portions of the cranial nerves, from embryological defects, from the pituitary and pineal glands, from the cranium, and from primary malignant extracranial tumors that metastasize to the cranium. Many classification systems, based mostly on cellular origin and histological pattern, have been proposed by pathologists. The complexity and magnitude of uncertainty of these systems vary, giving rise to frequent disputes without providing an unequivocal histological diagnosis for many brain tumors. The purpose of this chapter, however, is neither to review the pathology of brain tumors nor to argue the issues underlying their classification in relation to their proliferative potential or cell kinetics. Instead, it will present a thorough discussion of the cell kinetics of human brain tumors and indicate the direction of future studies in this field.

Central nervous system tumors are unique from several points of view. They grow where the proliferative capacity is minimal and rarely metastasize outside the cerebrospinal cavity. Most patients with brain tumors die from cerebellar or cerebral herniation caused by increased intracranial pressure. Because of limited surgical accessibility, even histopathologically benign tumors may carry a clinically malignant prognosis as long as they continue to grow within the cranial cavity. Thus, the prognosis for the patient with a brain tumor depends largely on the rate of tumor growth.

The histopathological diagnosis and grading of gliomas and other brain tumors are at times ambiguous because biological malignancy has been judged largely by morphology. The number of mitoses observed in gliomas does not necessarily correlate with the rapidity of growth, for example, a glioblastoma multiforme may fail to show mitoses, whereas an oligodendroglioma, a slow-growing tumor, may show frequent mitoses. More quantitative measurements of the proliferative activity and phenotypic variability of each type of brain tumor in various states of differentiation are needed to predict survival in individual patients and to design more effective treatments for their tumors.

BASIC CONCEPTS OF CELL KINETICS

The neoplastic process can be defined as a progressive and unrestricted increase of cell population through cell reproduction in a host. Two classes of cell reproduction are recognized: cell renewal systems and expanding cell populations. Cell renewal systems, in which the total population of cells remains constant because the rate of cell death equals the rate of cell birth, are seen in many adult tissues (e.g., bone marrow, small intestinal epithelium, and skin). Expanding cell populations, in which cell birth exceeds cell death, are of two types:

normal controlled-growth systems (e.g., in embryonal tissues, fibroblastic response to injury, and regeneration of the liver after partial hepatectomy), and uncontrolled systems, characterized by neoplastic growth. The growth of both normal and tumor tissues is determined by four basic factors: the cell cycle time (T_c), the growth fraction (GF), the population doubling time (T_d), and the cell loss factor (CLF). Familiarity with these parameters is prerequisite to understanding tumor cell population kinetics.

Cell Cycle Time

The cell cycle time (T_c) is the time required for a proliferating cell to progress from one mitotic division to the next. Not all cells within a tumor have the same cycle time; rather, a range of variability exists (4). T_c as currently determined expresses the average cycle time in a specified tumor.

The cell cycle can be divided into four stages based on the nuclear DNA content. The stage most readily identified (by light microscopy) is the mitotic (M) phase, during which the previously duplicated chromosomes are shared between two daughter cells. The new daughter cells then enter the postmitotic gap (G_1), or pre-DNA synthetic phase, during which they synthesize RNA, enzymes, and proteins in preparation for the beginning of DNA synthesis. From the G_1 phase, cells enter the DNA synthesis (S) phase, in which they replicate DNA; chromosomal duplication is normally completed by the end of this phase. The end of DNA synthesis marks the beginning of another gap, the postsynthetic, or premitotic, phase (G_2), in which RNA and proteins are synthesized in preparation for the M phase of the next cycle. The proportion of cells in S phase can be identified by pulse- or flash-labeling the tissue *in vitro* or *in vivo* by briefly exposing it to a labeled DNA precursor, radioactive thymidine (i.e., [^{3}H]- or [^{14}C]-thymidine). By determining the percentage of labeled mitoses (PLM) in repeated samples, a curve can be constructed, from which the T_c and the duration of each phase can be calculated (41).

The proportion of S-phase cells labeled by a flash of [^{3}H]-thymidine, called the labeling index (LI), gives a rough approximation of the proliferative activity of the tissue being studied. However, although a high LI reflects an actively proliferating tissue, equal LIs for two tissues do not necessarily imply equal proliferative activity. The actual proliferative activity of a tumor depends not only on the proportion of cells in S phase, but also on T_c, GF, and the rate of cell loss from the tumor cell population.

Growth Fraction

The GF is an index of the proportion of proliferating cells in relation to the total tumor cell population. Few solid tumors consist entirely of proliferating cells; it is thc presence of nonproliferating cells that accounts in part for the discrepancy between estimated tumor growth calculated from the T_c and actual growth observed in experimental tumor systems. The concept of a pool of nonproliferating cells in the tumor cell population was first suggested by Baserga *et al.* (5) in 1960. Soon thereafter, Mendelsohn (52) defined this factor mathematically as the number of proliferating cells divided by the total cell population and introduced its use for the study of cell population kinetics.

Population Doubling Time

The population doubling time (T_d), usually called "doubling time," signifies the time required for the tumor cell population to double in number. The T_d of a tumor should not be confused with its T_c; they are the same only when all cells are proliferating (GF = 1.0) and there is no cell loss. The GF is less than 1.0 in many tissues and tumors. In solid tumors, T_d invariably exceeds T_c. Cells in the proliferating pool must divide more than once to double the total population because nonproliferating cells contribute nothing and cell death acts to reduce the population (69).

Cell Loss

Cell loss in a tumor is characterized by the presence of individual dead cells, massive or focal necrosis, or exfoliation of cells from the tumor mass. Quantitative estimation of the rate of such loss is, however, difficult. To express the magnitude of cell loss, Steel (69) defined the cell loss factor (CLF) as $1 - (T_p/T_d)$, where T_p is the potential, or theoretical, doubling time in the absence of cell loss. The CLF represents the rate of cell loss as a fraction of the rate at which cells are added to the total population by mitosis.

Although T_p and CLF are calculated rather than measured values, they allow the importance of cell loss as a determinant of growth rate to be compared in different tumor types. Generally, both variables are dependent on the size and nature of the tumor; as a rule, an increase in tumor size is accompanied by greater cell loss, a lower GF, and a longer T_d.

LABELING INDEX OF HUMAN BRAIN TUMORS

Autoradiographic Study by [^{3}H]Thymidine

In the past decade, the LI obtained by autoradiographic analysis of tissue exposed to a pulse of [^{3}H]-thymidine has been used to estimate the proliferative potential of human brain tumors in situ. The cell synthesizes DNA throughout the S phase, and DNA synthesis requires, among nucleotides, thymidine. Exogenous thymidine presented to a cell in the S phase will be incorporated into nuclear DNA. If the thymidine contains [^{3}H] or [^{14}C], nuclei that incorporate it can be identified by autoradiography. Thus, the LI provides a rough estimate of the proliferative activity of the tissue, as the proportion of labeled cells indicates the proportion of cells actually in proliferation cycles.

The first in vivo autoradiographic study of a human glioblastoma was performed by Johnson *et al.* (44), who injected multiple doses of [^{3}H]-thymidine intravenously into a terminally ill patient and calculated an LI of 0.6%. Chigasaki (9) studied the in vitro uptake of [^{3}H]-thymidine in biopsy specimens of a glioblastoma, an astrocytoma, and an oligodendroglioma, which were found to have LIs of 0.94%, 0.44%, and 0.33% respectively. He estimated the generation time of glioblastoma to be 45 to 60 days. A few years later, Kury and Carter (48) determined the LIs of several gliomas in vitro using a method almost identical to Chigasaki's. The LIs were 3.6% and 6.0% in two glioblastomas and 2% to 7% in five astrocytomas (grade 2 or 3), all considerably higher than those reported by Johnson *et al.* and Chigasaki. Assuming an S phase of 6 hours, Kury and Carter estimated that the generation times (approximating T_p in our terms) of glioblastomas and malignant astrocytomas were 3 to 5 days and 2 to 10 days, respectively. Fukuma *et al.* (18) injected [^{3}H]-thymidine into glioma tissue at the time of craniotomy and obtained LIs similar to those reported by Kury and Carter.

Tym (72) introduced the stathmokinetic method, adding to the flash-labeling technique the use of vinblastine sulfate, which, like colchicine, facilitates kinetic analysis by arresting and holding cells in the metaphase. Studying a single glioblastoma, Tym obtained an LI of 1.6% and calculated a G_2 phase of 5 hours, an S phase of 8 hours, and a T_c of 125 to 242 hours (5.4 to 10 days).

Hoshino and Wilson (40) administered [^{3}H]-thymidine, either with or without mitostatic agents, to 24 patients harboring various gliomas. The LI was 5 to 15% in viable areas of glioblastomas, 1% or less in well-differentiated gliomas, and intermediate in anaplastic astrocytomas, reflecting the extent of anaplasia. The LIs averaged 9.3% for glioblastomas, 4.0% for anaplastic astrocytomas, and 1% for differentiated gliomas (Table 9.1). This variable proved to have a strong correlation with the length of survival. Eight of 14 patients with a tumor LI over 5% died within 1 year after the onset of symptoms. However, all 14 died within 6 months of operation, the point at which the LI was established. In contrast, patients having tumors with an LI less than 1% had a far better prognosis, as did those with tumors having an LI of 1 to 4%, usually anaplastic astrocytomas. With few exceptions, these patients survived more than 1 year, and many lived for 5 years. This difference was statistically significant ($p = 0.001$) according to the Gehan test (19), and the median survival times for patients with a tumor LI greater than 5% and those with an LI less than 5% were 3 and 13 months, respectively (28, 40).

The tumor LI does not always correlate with the length of survival. Hoshino *et al.*

TABLE 9.1
Average Labeling Index and Median Survival Time in 28 Patients With Gliomas

Tumor Type	No. of Cases	Labeling Index[a]	Median Survival Time (mos.)[b]
Medulloblastoma	4	12.0 ± 1.3% (7.0–14.4%)	72
Glioblastoma	13	9.3 ± 1.0% (4.5–15.9%)	8
Anaplastic astrocytoma	7	4.0 ± 0.8% (2.2–8.3%)	60
Fibrillary astrocytoma	3	0.8% (0.3–0.9%)	99
Ependymoma	1	1.9%	156

[a] Values are mean ± SE; ranges are given in parentheses.
[b] From time of onset.

(30) reported that the average LI for medulloblastomas was 12.0 ± 1.3% (SE). The mean survival for patients with these tumors is approximately 6 years. The longer survival of these patients is not the result of slower tumor growth but is primarily due to improved radiotherapy techniques and to the greater radiosensitivity of medulloblastomas (6, 7, 10, 13, 26, 60, 71) compared with malignant gliomas (75). Left untreated or treated with surgery alone, both tumors grow rapidly and cause death within weeks to months, but their sensitivities to radiation are markedly divergent.

Although the results of autoradiographic studies have helped us understand the malignancy and the proliferative potential of individual tumors, these techniques have been limited mainly to patients with malignant disease and have not been used in many other brain tumors. Because the half-life of tritium exceeds 12 years, autoradiographic techniques pose a potential radiation hazard, both to normal tissues that incorporate [^{3}H]-thymidine into their DNA and to the environment, as degraded tritium is excreted from the patient continuously, even though the amount of radioactivity is negligible. In addition, the results are not available soon enough to predict the rate of tumor growth or to be considered in the design of treatment regimens in individual patients.

In the past decade, two alternatives to autoradiographic studies have been developed: DNA analysis by flow cytometry and immunohistochemical techniques using a monoclonal antibody against bromodeoxyuridine.

Flow Cytometry

In nondividing cells, the amount of nuclear DNA usually remains constant throughout the life of the cell. In most dividing cells, the DNA content immediately after division represents the diploid chromosomal complement (2C); this complement increases during DNA synthesis (4C) and then returns to the diploid state after mitosis. Using microcytophotometry, one can measure the amount of DNA in the nucleus of each cell type in a particular tissue (49, 50), but the method is time-consuming and the results are somewhat unsatisfactory in terms of resolution and statistical validity.

A more efficient and accurate way of analyzing the DNA content in individual cells is by flow cytometry (73, 74). This technique measures the amount of DNA per cell by quantitating the intensity of the fluorescence emitted by a DNA-bound dye as up to 5000 nuclei per second flow past a high-intensity laser beam. From these data, a histogram plotting the number of cells against the intensity of fluorescence can be constructed to show the frequency with which these DNA contents appear in the cell population. When the entire population consists of diploid cells, there is a single peak in the histogram; when cells with tetraploid (4C) and octaploid (8C) DNA contents are both present, multiple peaks occur at positions relative to the intensity of their fluorescence. If there are also cells synthesizing DNA before cell division, their fluorescence values fall between the 2C and 4C peaks (Fig. 9.1).

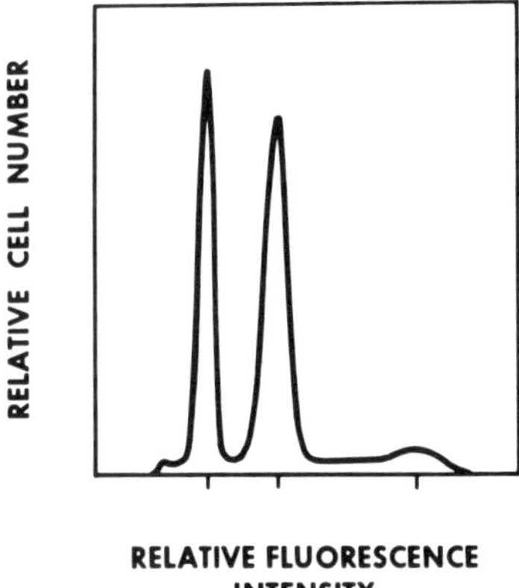

Figure 9.1. DNA histogram of human glioblastoma multiforme obtained by FCM analysis (stained with chromomycin A_3). Relative fluorescence intensity indicates the amount of DNA in each cell. Multiple DNA peaks represent multiple subpopulations (i.e., diploid, tetraploid cells, etc.).

A nuclear isolation technique for the use of flow cytometry in the study of human brain tumors has been developed by Hoshino *et al.* (35). Observations made with this technique showed that benign brain tumors, such as meningiomas, pituitary adenomas, and well-differentiated gliomas—all of which grow slowly—had a number of characteristics in common. There were very few cells in DNA synthesis; a majority of the tumor was composed of a single karyotype, using the term "karyotype" to denote cells with identical amounts of DNA in their nuclei, rather than cells with the same number of chromosomes; and there was little variability within a single tumor. The characteristics of malignant gliomas, including glioblastoma multiforme, were quite different. There was a substantial population of cells in DNA synthesis. The distribution of the nuclear DNA complement ranged from 2C to 8C, assuming that the initial peak represented diploid nuclei, and the predominant ploidy varied greatly from one area to another within the same tumor, with the nuclear population seeming to be primarily diploid in some areas and mainly tetraploid (4C) in others. Therefore, malignant gliomas are heterogeneous with respect to ploidy and to the characteristics of the populations within different areas of the same tumor. These findings have been confirmed by Frederiksen *et al.* (16), Kawamoto *et al.* (45), and Mørk *et al.* (54).

Theoretically, flow cytometry made it possible to obtain a measurement similar to the autoradiographic LI by quantitating the intensity of DNA fluorescence in individual tumor cells. Unfortunately, the difficulty of obtaining clean single-cell suspensions and the lack of sophisticated computer programs to analyze the DNA histograms have prohibited routine use of flow cytometry to measure the proliferative capacity of most human tumors. Most computer programs cannot reliably analyze DNA histograms consisting of an aneuploid population with a large coefficient of variation in each peak population and a relatively small S-phase fraction (14).

Immunocytochemistry Using Antibromodeoxyuridine Monoclonal Antibody

In 1982, Gratzner (25) developed a monoclonal antibody (MAb) that can identify nuclei containing bromodeoxyuridine (BrdU). Anti-BrdU MAb can be detected by direct conjugation of FITC (fluorescein isothiocyanate) to the antibody, by indirect conjugation of FITC using a FITC-tagged secondary antibody (15, 25, 56), or by immunoperoxidase methods (55). The immunocytochemical method requires only 2 to 3 hours to complete, and the results are available 1 to 2 days after biopsy. This is a breakthrough for studies of cell kinetics. BrdU, like [^{3}H]-thymidine, is incorporated into nuclear DNA during DNA synthesis (24, 70), but is neither radioactive nor myelotoxic at the doses used for in vivo labeling studies (32, 33, 55). Therefore, a wider variety of human tumors can be investigated.

BrdU is one of the halopyrimidines and, like thymidine, is incorporated into cellular nuclei at the time of DNA synthesis for mitosis (24, 70). Although cytocidal or teratogenic effects occur with prolonged administration of high doses (24), BrdU has been used without serious side effects as a radiosensitizing agent for brain tumors and for cancers of the head and neck (3, 38, 66). Daily infusions of BrdU (600–700 mg/m^2

IV) for several weeks can be tolerated without severe myelosuppression (3, 46, 65). The dose required to permit identification of BrdU-labeled nuclei is far below the doses used therapeutically.

Hoshino *et al.* (32) administered BrdU (150–200 mg/m^2 IV) to 18 patients with various brain tumors at the time of surgery and examined tumor tissues in three ways to determine the S-phase fraction: single-cell suspensions prepared from biopsied material were analyzed by flow cytometry (FCM) to detect 1) FITC-conjugated anti-BrdU MAb bound cells and 2) to determine the distribution of DNA and 3) tissue sections were stained using an indirect immunoperoxidase method to detect nuclei tagged with anti-BrdU MAb (Fig. 9.2). The fraction of S-phase cells in the tissue sections in this series was similar to both the percentage of BrdU-labeled nuclei and the S-phase fraction determined by FCM analysis. A similar analysis of neuroectodermal tumors (33) demonstrated that the average S-phase fraction was 10.0 ± 0.8% (SE) for glioblastoma multiforme, 8.9 ± 2.4% for highly anaplastic astrocytomas, less than 1% for moderately anaplastic (or low-grade) astrocytomas, and 13.0 ± 3.0% for medulloblastomas. These values were close to those estimated by autoradiography of tumor tissue exposed to a pulse of [^{3}H]-thymidine. Since BrdU can be used with fewer restrictions than [^{3}H]-thymidine, it can be used in cell kinetics studies of benign tumors such as pituitary adenomas, neurinomas, and meningiomas.

A bivalent fluorescence analysis of BrdU-treated cells stained with anti-BrdU antibody and with propidium iodide to demonstrate the DNA content is feasible and can be displayed as a three-dimensional histogram (Fig. 9.3). With this technique, aneuploidy and proliferative potentials for individual DNA populations can be analyzed.

Nagashima *et al.* (57) studied 21 pituitary adenomas in situ with BrdU and reported that a majority of them had a BrdU LI of less than 0.5%. Except in two cases of Nelson's syndrome, in which it was greater than 1%, the LI did not correlate with any variable, such as hormonal activity, patient age, tumor size, or the duration of signs and symptoms (Fig. 9.4). These results differ from those of Anniko *et al.* (1, 2), who analyzed DNA histograms from 47 pituitary tumors by microcytophotometry and estimated the percentage of S-phase cells to be 3.1% to 19.5%. S-phase fractions greater than 10% appear to be similar to the [^{3}H]-thymidine LI of a glioblastoma multiforme. Because pituitary adenomas grow much more slowly than other kinds of brain tumors, the results of Anniko *et al.* are difficult to accept, unless pituitary adenomas proliferate under unusual kinetic conditions, for example, extremely high cell loss or long S phase.

Hoshino *et al.* have also used BrdU label-

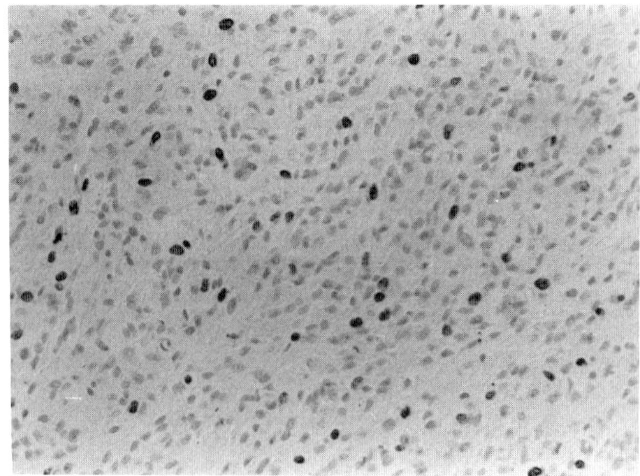

Figure 9.2. Photomicrograph showing a glioblastoma multiforme reacted with anti-BrdU monoclonal antibody, stained by the immunoperoxidase method, and counterstained with hematoxylin, ×100. Labeled cells have nuclei stained dark (with reaction products).

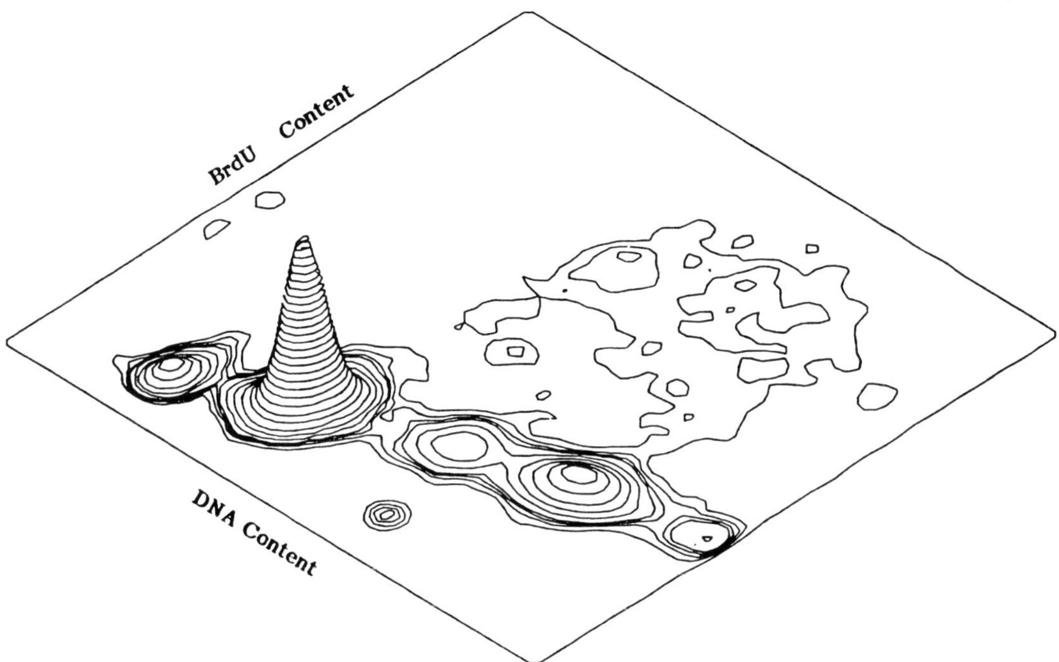

Figure 9.3. The relative DNA and BrdU content can be measured concomitantly by flow cytometry and displayed three-dimensionally; height represents the relative cell numbers. In this example, a glioblastoma multiforme, the first DNA population from the left does not show any BrdU positive cells, suggesting that this non-proliferating population probably consisted of normal cells such as lymphocytes and macrophages. The second peak represents the proliferating cell population, as BrdU-positive cells exist in the S phase DNA region. (By courtesy of Dr. Joe W. Gray, Lawrence Livermore Laboratory.)

ing techniques to study 20 meningiomas, including seven malignant meningiomas (34). The nonmalignant meningiomas showed an average LI of less than 1%, but all of the malignant meningiomas had an average LI greater than 3%. Although malignant meningiomas are not well-defined histologically, their proliferative potential can be demonstrated quite easily with BrdU labeling techniques (Fig. 9.5). Similar results were reported by Fukui *et al.* (17), Iwaki *et al.* (43), Inoue *et al.* (42), and Cho *et al.* (12). Thus, malignant evolution of meningiomas can be demonstrated reasonably well with BrdU LI. The tumor doubling time was estimated from serial computed tomographic scans of eight patients with recurrent meningiomas (11). According to their results, a semilogarithmic linear regression analysis revealed a correlation coefficient of 0.99 and T_d may be calculated with the formula $T_d = 500 \times \exp(-0.73 \times \text{LI})$. This allows a physician to determine an appropriate time of follow-up and to estimate the rate of regrowth for the remaining tumor when total removal of the tumor is not possible.

S-phase fractions of various types of neuroectodermal tumors from 327 patients are given in Table 9.2. These data and those previously reported (31, 36), demonstrate that the biological malignancy of the tumors is fairly well reflected in the S-phase fractions or LI. However, even histopathologically similar tumors showed a wide range of LIs. For example, although most moderately anaplastic astrocytomas had S-phase fractions less than 1%, some appeared to have the same proliferative potential as highly anaplastic astrocytomas.

It is important to recognize that histologically similar tumors may have different proliferative potentials. Hoshino *et al.* reported prognostic significances of the proliferative potential measured by BrdU LIs in 47 patients with low-grade astrocy-

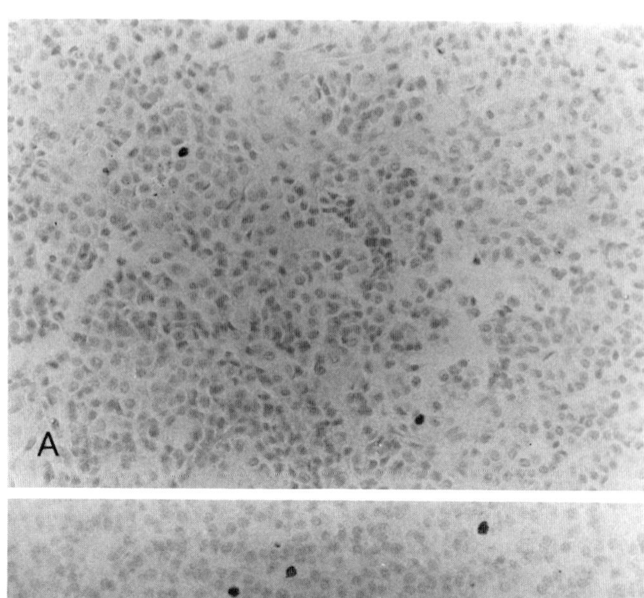

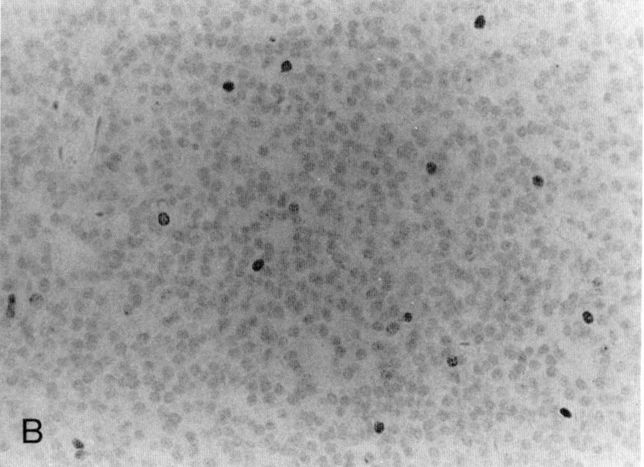

Figure 9.4. Tissue sections from *A*) a pituitary adenoma and from *B*) an adenoma in a patient with Nelson's syndrome. Both sections were stained immunohistochemically with anti-BrdU monoclonal antibody and counterstained with hematoxylin ×100. More nuclei were BrdU positive in the tissue section from the patient with Nelson's syndrome.

tomas (37). In 29 patients (60%), the tumors had LIs of less than 1%, indicating a slow growth rate; only three (10%) of these patients died of recurrent tumor during a follow-up period of up to 3 1/2 years. In contrast, of the 18 patients (40%) whose tumors had BrdU LIs of 1% or more, 12 (67%) had a recurrence and nine died during the same follow-up period.

The results of this study, although preliminary, have important implications for the treatment of these patients. Low-grade astrocytomas are not biologically uniform tumors: some follow a benign course, while others behave like malignant astrocytomas. The latter tumors should be treated as aggressively as malignant astrocytomas or glioblastomas, while low-grade gliomas with low LIs may not respond to adjuvant therapies but nevertheless have a far better prognosis as reflected by longer survival times. This issue should be evaluated as quickly as possible because aggressive radiotherapy or chemotherapy may be an inefficient treatment for tumors with low LIs, and a conservative approach (observation) may deny potentially beneficial adjuvant treatment for patients whose tumors have high LIs.

These observations are still preliminary, and correlations between histopathology, actual rate of tumor growth, response to various treatment modalities, and S-phase fraction should be studied in the future. However, cell kinetic studies using BrdU may benefit the patient by predicting pro-

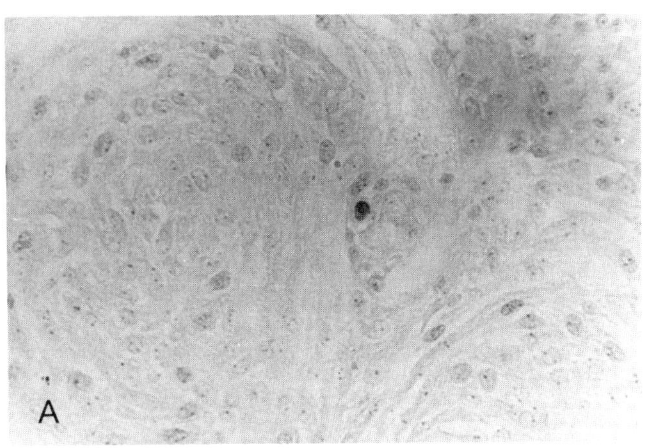

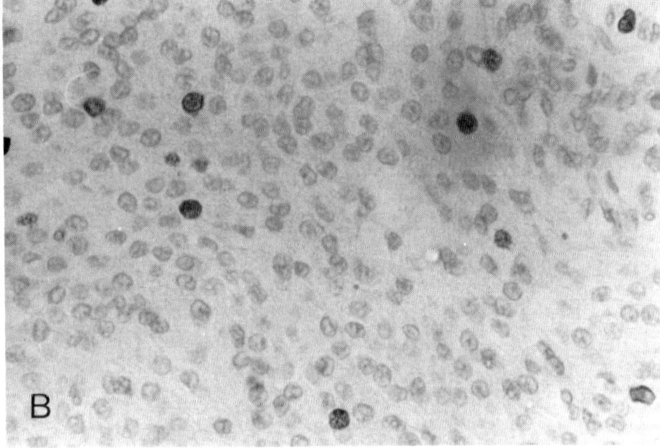

Figure 9.5. BrdU stains of *A*) a meningotheliomatous meningioma and *B*) a malignant meningioma. There are markedly more BrdU-positive nuclei in the malignant meningioma. Counterstained with hematoxylin ×400.

TABLE 9.2
BrdU Labeling Indices of 327 Neuroectodermal Tumors

Tumor Type	Labeling Index (%)			No. of Cases of LI		
	No. of Cases	Median	Range	<1%	1–5%	> 5%
Medulloblastoma	18	9.5	3.9–38.2	0	1	17
Glioblastoma multiforme	110	7.3	1.3–30.5	0	28	82
Highly anaplastic astrocytoma	63	2.7	<1.0–38.1	9	35	19
Moderately anaplastic astrocytoma	66	<1.0	<1.0–9.3	40	23	3
Ependymoma	28	<1.0	<1.0–18.9	18	8	2
Juvenile pilocytic astrocytoma	17	1.0	<1.0–4.3	8	9	0
Mixed glioma	17	2.1	<1.0–8.0	6	9	2
Ganglioglioma	8	1.0	<1.0—2.8	4	4	0
Total	327			85	117	125

liferation potential or biological malignancy and thereby supplementing the histopathological diagnosis.

DURATION OF THE S PHASE IN GLIOMAS

In contrast to the variability of the LI in different astrocytic tumors, the duration of the S phase measured by double autoradiography (29) remained within a range of 7 to 13 hours. Several factors may influence the duration of the S phase in vivo, but the uniformity of this variable in astrocytomas of widely differing behavior indicates that degree of differentiation (or dedifferentiation) is not one of them. The duration of the S phase (T_s) and the LI can be used to calculate the turnover time. This basic parameter of cell kinetics is defined as the time required for a given number of cells to replace their population, assuming a constant rate of cell production, and is expressed as $(T_S/LI) \times 100$. Although it usually concerns normal and cell renewal systems and is ordinarily not applied to an expanding system such as tumor, the turnover time can help us to understand the proliferative potential of a tumor.

The turnover time for malignant gliomas is on the order of a few days to a week, and in astrocytomas it approaches 2 months. In tumors with an expected potential doubling time (T_p) of over 100 hours, multiplying the turnover time by a conversion factor of 0.7 yields the T_p (69). According to these calculations, malignant gliomas, including glioblastomas double the size of their viable area in less than 5 days in the absence of cell loss. However, at a symptom-producing size of 50 to 100 g, glioblastomas seem unlikely to double their volume every week or so. To explain this discrepancy, we must assume extensive cell loss within the tumor. A tentative calculation, assuming a potential doubling time of 1 week and a clinically reasonable ("actual") doubling time of 5 to 6 weeks, yields a cell loss factor between 0.80 and 0.85 (80 to 85%) (29). This, surprisingly, is not high when compared to the cell loss estimated in other tumors, e.g., 95% for head and neck tumors (63) and 70% for melanomas (68).

GROWTH FRACTION AND CELL CYCLE TIME

Hoshino and Wilson (40) proposed to estimate growth fraction (GF) and T_c by applying the method of Mendelsohn (52) in combination with the stathmokinetic method developed by Puck and Steffen. The results are shown in Table 9.3. The GFs of malignant gliomas varied from 0.14 to 0.44, with a mean of 0.31 ± 0.10 (SD). Only areas of tumor exhibiting no microscopic necrosis and fairly homogenous labeling were scored. Consequently, the GF would be smaller if one considered the entire tumor, including its large nonviable portion. If one half of the tumor is necrobiotic (a reasonable estimate in glioblastomas), the GF would be reduced by half, in this case making the GF of glioblastomas closer to 15% than to the calculated 30%. Yoshii *et al.* (76) measured GFs of various brain tumors by intravenous infusion of

TABLE 9.3
Labeling Index, Growth Fraction, and Cell Cycle Time in Seven Glioblastomas and Two Anaplastic Astrocytomas

Cases	Labeling Index (%) (Mean ± SD)	Growth Fraction (Mean ± SD)	Cell Cycle Time (hr) (Mean ± SD)
Glioblastoma			
1	15.9 ± 3.4	0.44 ± 0.13	145.0 ± 63.4
2	11.0 ± 1.4	0.40 ± 0.14	151.7 ± 33.8
3	8.6 ± 3.1	0.39 ± 0.10	64.1 ± 12.9
4	15.5 ± 4.6	0.35 ± 0.11	55.8 ± 11.6
5	9.8 ± 2.6	0.32 ± 0.10	55.4 ± 11.5
6	13.0 ± 3.2	0.29 ± 0.07	
7	5.1 ± 1.2	0.21 ± 0.06	36.4 ± 16.6
Anaplastic astrocytoma			
1	2.3 ± 3.7	0.25 ± 0.03	43.9 ± 7.1
2	3.4 ± 1.0	0.14 ± 0.06	52.3 ± 26.5

BrdU every 8 hours for 3 days, thus labeling all the cells in the cycling pool with BrdU. The GFs ranged from 9.1 to 46.5% in malignant gliomas, 2.0 to 6.7% in low-grade gliomas, and 11.2 to 43.2% in metastatic brain tumors. These figures appear to coincide with the results of Hoshino and Wilson (40), although the methods of measurement were different.

Recently, a monoclonal antibody produced against a nuclear antigen from a cell line derived from a Hodgkin's lymphoma was reported to recognize a nuclear antigen found in proliferating cells (23). In vitro, this antibody (Ki-67) reacted with G_1, S, and G_2, M phase cells but not with nonproliferating G_0 cells (20–22, 62), thus identifying GF. Kleiheus *et al.* (47), Burger *et al.* (8), Ostertag *et al.* (59), Roggendorf *et al.* (64), and Zuber *et al.* (77) measured the LIs of brain tumors with Ki-67 and all reported LIs similar to those obtained with BrdU in the same kinds of tumors. Previous studies have shown that GF of brain tumors is much larger than the S-phase fraction (40, 76) and therefore larger than the Ki LIs reported by those authors, even taking into consideration a recent report that some noncycling cells that entered the G_1 phase did not react with Ki-67 (22). Although Nishizaki *et al.* (58) demonstrated some positive correlation of Ki-67 with BrdU LIs, the real usefulness of this antibody awaits the further characterization of the antigen and clarification of what it detects; among the possibilities are by-products of cycling cells, enzymes, or substrates required for cellular proliferation. Moreover, it is not clear how or by what intracellular or extracellular processes the antigen is synthesized or metabolized.

Even though considerable variability exists in the T_cs calculated from different samples of each tumor, Hoshino and Wilson (40) demonstrated that the average values for the tumors were similar, excepting the two glioblastomas. When combined, the values yielded a mean T_c of 3 days, or 75.6 ± 45.7 hours (SD). From these results, the low LIs observed in slow-growing brain tumors were assumed to result from a low GF rather than from a prolonged T_c.

CHARACTERISTIC PROLIFERATION PATTERNS IN GLIOBLASTOMAS AND ANAPLASTIC AND LOW-GRADE GLIOMAS

All intracranial gliomas are clinically malignant, regardless of the degree of histological differentiation or anaplasia, because without appropriate treatment they are fatal to the host. Neoplasms originating in other tissues of the body, for example, polyps in the digestive system, are not always life-threatening and are clearly different from invasive fast-growing tumors such as adenocarcinoma and scirrhous carcinoma, which are fatal without early appropriate treatment. The histological malignancy of such tumors correlates fairly well with the prognosis.

Most gliomas are classified as glioblastoma multiforme, as anaplastic astrocytomas of varying degree, or as well-differentiated tumors such as fibrillary astrocytoma, oligodendroglioma, or ependymoma. Tumors in this latter group are separated by vague diagnostic borderlines. Some clinicians assume that well-differentiated, or "low-grade" gliomas, are "benign" because they usually grow very slowly and patients who have them survive longer than those with anaplastic gliomas or glioblastoma multiforme. Even low-grade gliomas, however, have some malignant characteristics, such as the lack of a clear border between the tumor and surrounding brain and the tumor's invasiveness in normal tissue.

In performing cell kinetic studies of various human gliomas, Hoshino *et al.* (39) made several interesting observations. Autoradiographic analysis of tissue samples obtained at biopsy and subsequently at autopsy showed that some of the glioblastomas diluted out the labeled cells in the 2- to 4-month interval between labeling and autopsy, whereas the other glioblastomas and the anaplastic astrocytomas retained labeled neoplastic cells in parts of the tumors at autopsy after intervals of 3 weeks to 5 months after labeling. Most patients whose tumors contained foci of labeled cells at autopsy survived longer. Hoshino *et al.* concluded that certain neoplastic cells in anaplastic astrocytomas and some glioblastomas appear either to limit cell division or to differentiate even in an environment favorable to cell proliferation. Glioblastomas belonging to the latter category could be regarded as an extreme variety of anaplastic astrocytoma, originating as astrocytoma and then undergoing malignant transformation to the histological characteristics of glioblastoma multiforme, probably meeting Scherer's criteria for a "secondary glioblastoma" (67). In contrast, the glioblastomas in the former category are malignant from the beginning, like scirrhous carcinomas.

Hoshino postulated two mechanisms that might be responsible for the inherent slowness of growth in low-grade gliomas (27). The first concerns the mode of proliferation. Evidence from kinetic studies suggests that well-differentiated or low-grade gliomas proliferate conservatively: only one of two daughter cells retains mitotic activity, and the other stops dividing. The second mechanism concerns the possible lack of traffic between the noncycling and the cycling pool. If the cycling population does not increase and only sterile noncycling cells are added as a tumor grows, the GF decreases steadily. Thus, partial resection of these tumors effectively reduces the number of cells in the proliferating pool, resulting in further retarded growth. In contrast, glioblastomas have a higher GF and frequent movement between noncycling and cycling populations. Because their growth seems to be depressed by crowding, partial resection might stimulate cells in the nonproliferating pool to move into the proliferating pool, causing more rapid growth and only a temporary reduction in the proliferating population.

Malignant astrocytomas or anaplastic astrocytomas consist basically of astrocytes with various anaplastic foci. They appear to carry both types of proliferation patterns intermingled in the tissue. The rapidity of tumor growth depends also on the timing of anaplastic changes in preexisting, well-differentiated astrocytomas and the extent of anaplastic foci in the tumor. The correlation between LI at biopsy and the postoperative survival time shows that once anaplastic transformation begins, the growth rate of the tumor simulates that of glioblastoma, and the anaplastic foci overwhelm the growth of the tumor as a whole.

Although it cannot be substantiated for lack of a suitable experimental model, this hypothesis may afford a working model of the biological behavior of tumors whose proliferative activities are morphologically similar but whose response to a particular treatment may vary enormously (51). Thus, further verification of the cell kinetics of these tumors is extremely important. Sophisticated use of BrdU labeling techniques, combined with autoradiographic and flow cytometric analysis, may help to elucidate these issues.

ACKNOWLEDGMENT

This work was supported in part by grant PDT-159 from the American Cancer Society and by grants CA-13525 and CA-50210 from the National Cancer Institute.

REFERENCES

1. Anniko, M., Holm, L.E., and Wersall, J. Aggressive pituitary tumor growth. Arch. Otorhinolaryngol., *283:*53–62, 1983.
2. Anniko, M., Tribukait, B., and Wersall, J. Significance of high percentage of S phase cells in human pituitary tumors. O.R.L. J. Otorhinolaryngol. Related Spec., *45:*177–186, 1983.
3. Bagshaw, M.A., Doggett, R.L.S., Smith, K.C., *et al.* Intra-arterial 5-bromodeoxyuridine and x-ray therapy. Am. J. Roentgenol., *99:*886–894, 1967.
4. Barrett, J.C. A mathematical model of the mitotic cycle and its application to the interpretation of percentage labeled mitosis data. J. Natl. Cancer Inst., *37:*443–450, 1966.
5. Baserga, R., Kisieleski, W.E., and Halvorsen, K. *et al.* A study on the establishment and growth of tumor metastases with tritiated thymidine. Cancer Res., *20:*910–917, 1960.
6. Bloom, H.J.G., Wallace, E.N.K., and Henk, J.M. The treatment and prognosis of medulloblastoma in children. Am. J. Roentgenol., *105:*43–62, 1969.
7. Bongartz, E.B., Bamberg, M., Nau, H.E., *et al.* Optimal therapy in medulloblastoma. Acta. Neurochir., *50:*117–125, 1979.
8. Burger, P.C., Shibata, T., and Kleiheus, P. The use of the monoclonal antibody Ki-67 in the identification of proliferating cells: application to surgical neuropathology. Am. J. Surg. Pathol., *10:*611–617, 1986.
9. Chigasaki, H. Studies on the DNA synthesis function of glial cells by means of [^{3}H]-thymi-

dine microradioautography (Japanese). Brain Nerve (Tokyo), *15:*767–781, 1963.

10. Chin, H.W. and Maruyama, Y. Early response and long-term results in the radiotherapy of childhood medulloblastoma. J. Neurooncol., *1:*53–59, 1983.
11. Cho, K.G., Hoshino, T., Nagashima, T., *et al.* Prediction of tumor doubling time in recurrent meningiomas. J. Neurosurg., *65:*790–794, 1986.
12. Cho, K.G., Hoshino, T., Nagashima, T., *et al.* Proliferative potential of malignant and nonmalignant meningiomas. In: *Brain Oncology,* edited by M. Chatel, F. Darcel, and J. Pecker, pp. 79–81. Dordrecht, The Netherlands, Martinus Hijhoff, 1987.
13. Cumberlin, R., Luk, K.H., Wara, W.M., *et al.* Medulloblastoma. Treatment results and effect on normal tissues. Cancer, *43:*1014–1020, 1979.
14. Dean, N.P. Methods of data analysis in flow cytometry. In: *Techniques in Cell Cycle Analysis,* edited by J.W. Gray and Z. Darzynkiewicz, pp. 207–250, Clifton, N.J., Humana Press, 1987.
15. Dolbeare, F., Gratzner, H., Pallavicini, M.G., *et al.* Flow cytometric measurement of total DNA content and incorporated bromodeoxyuridine. Proc. Natl. Acad. Sci. *80:*5573– 5577, 1983.
16. Frederiksen, P., Reske-Nielsen, E., and Bichel, P. Flow cytometry in tumors of the brain. Acta. Neuropathol. (Berl.), *41:*179–183, 1978.
17. Fukui, M., Iwaki, T., Sawa, H., *et al.* Proliferative activity of meningiomas as evaluated by bromodeoxyuridine uptake examination. Acta. Neurochir. (Wien.), *81:*135–141, 1986.
18. Fukuma, S., Taketomo, S., Ueda, S., *et al.* Autoradiographic studies on human brain tumors using local labeling with [^{3}H]-thymidine in vivo (Japanese). Brain Nerve (Tokyo), *21:*1029–1035, 1969.
19. Gehan, E.A. A generalized Wilcoxon test for comparing arbitrarily singly-censored samples. Biometrika, *52:*203–223, 1965.
20. Gerdes, J. An immunohistological method for estimating cell growth fractions in rapid histopathological diagnosis during surgery. Int. J. Cancer, *35:*169–171, 1985.
21. Gerdes, J., Dallenbach, F., and Lennert, K. Growth fractions in malignant non-Hodgkins's lymphomas (NHL) as determined in situ with the monoclonal antibody Ki-67. Hematol. Oncol., *2:*365–371, 1984.
22. Gerdes, J., Lamke, H., Baisch, H., *et al.* Cell cycle analysis of a cell proliferation-associated human nuclear antigen defined by the monoclonal antibody Ki-67. J. Immunol., *133:* 1710–1715, 1984.
23. Gerdes, J., Schwab, U., Lemke, H., *et al.* Production of a mouse monoclonal antibody reactive with a human nuclear antigen associated with cell proliferation. Int. J. Cancer, *31:*13–20, 1983.
24. Goz, B. The effects of incorporation of 5-halogenated deoxyuridines into the DNA of eukaryotic cells. Pharmacol. Rev., *29:*249–272, 1978.
25. Gratzner, H.G. Monoclonal antibody to 5-bromo- and 5-iododeoxyuridine: a new reagent for detection of DNA replication. Science, *218:*474–476, 1982.
26. Hirsh, J.F., Renier, O., Czerniehow, P., *et al.* Medulloblastoma in childhood. Survival and functional results. Acta. Neurochir., *48:*1–15, 1979.
27. Hoshino, T. A commentary on the biology and growth kinetics of low-grade and high-grade gliomas. J. Neurosurg., *61:*895–900, 1984.
28. Hoshino, T. The cell kinetics of gliomas: its prognostic value and therapeutic implications. In: *Multidisciplinary Aspects of Brain Tumor Therapy,* edited by P. Paoletti, M.D. Walker, G. Butti, and R. Knerich, pp. 105–112. Amsterdam, Elsevier/North Holland, 1979.
29. Hoshino, T., Barker, M., Wilson, C.B., *et al.* Cell kinetics of human gliomas. J. Neurosurg., *37:*15–26, 1972.
30. Hoshino, T., Kobayashi, S., Townsend, J.J., *et al.* A cell kinetic study on medulloblastomas. Cancer, *55:*1711–1713, 1985.
31. Hoshino, T., Nagashima, T., Cho, K.G., *et al.* S-phase fraction of human brain tumors in situ measured by uptake of bromodeoxyuridine. Int. J. Cancer, *38:*369–374, 1986.
32. Hoshino, T., Nagashima, T., Murovic, J., *et al.* Cell kinetic studies of *in situ* brain tumors with bromodeoxyuridine. Cytometry, *6:*627–632, 1985.
33. Hoshino, T., Nagashima, T., Murovic, J.A., *et al.* *In situ* cell kinetic studies on human neuroectodermal tumors using bromodeoxyuridine. J. Neurosurg., *64:*453–459, 1986.
34. Hoshino, T., Nagashima, T., Murovic, J.A., *et al.* Proliferative potential of human meningiomas of brain. A cell kinetic study with bromodeoxyuridine. Cancer, *58:*1466–1472, 1986.
35. Hoshino, T., Nomura, K., Wilson, C.B., *et al.* The distribution of molecular DNA from human brain tumor cells. Flow cytometric studies. J. Neurosurg., *49:*13–21, 1978.
36. Hoshino, T., Prados, M., Wilson, C.B., *et al.* Prognostic implications of bromodeoxyuridine labeling index (BUdR LI) in human gliomas. J. Neurosurg., *69:*839–842, 1988.
37. Hoshino, T., Rodriguez, L.A., Cho, K.G., *et al.* Prognostic implications of the proliferative potential of low-grade astrocytomas. J. Neurosurg., *69:*839–842, 1988.
38. Hoshino, T. and Sano, K. Radiosensitization of malignant brain tumors with bromouridine (thymidine analogue). Acta. Radiol. Ther. Phys. Biol., *8:*15–21, 1969.
39. Hoshino, T., Townsend, J.J., Muraoka, I., *et al.* An autoradiographic study of human gliomas: growth kinetics of anaplastic astrocytoma and glioblastoma multiforme. Brain, *103:*967–984, 1980.

40. Hoshino, T. and Wilson, C.B. Cell kinetic analysis of human malignant brain tumors (gliomas). Cancer, *44*:956–962, 1979.
41. Howard, A. and Pelc, S.R. Synthesis of deoxyribonucleic acid in normal and irradiated cells and its relation to chromosome breakage. Heredity (Suppl.), *6*:261–273, 1953.
42. Inoue, H., Tamura, M., Koizumi, H., *et al.* Clinical pathology of malignant meningiomas. Acta. Neurochir., *73*:179–191, 1984.
43. Iwaki, T., Takeshita, I., Fukui, M., *et al.* Cell kinetics of the malignant evolution of meningothelial meningioma. Acta. Neuropathol. (Berl.), *74*:243–247, 1987.
44. Johnson, H.A., Haymaker, W.E., Rubini, J.R., *et al.* A radioautographic study of a human brain and glioblastoma multiforme after the in vivo uptake of tritiated thymidine. Cancer, *13*:636–642, 1960.
45. Kawamoto, K., Herz, F., Wolley, R.C., *et al.* Flow cytometric analysis of the DNA distribution in human brain tumors. Acta. Neuropathol. (Berl.), *46*:39–44, 1979.
46. Kinsella, T.J., Russo, A., Mitchell, J.B., *et al.* A phase I study of intermittent intravenous bromodeoxyuridine (BUdR) with conventional fractionated irradiation. Int. J. Radiat. Oncol. Biol. Phys., *10*:69–76, 1984.
47. Kleihues, P., Shibata, T., Landolt, A.M., *et al.* Assessment of the growth fraction in human brain tumors as defined by the monoclonal antibody Ki-67. J. Neurooncol., in press, 1990.
48. Kury, G. and Carter, H.D. Autoradiographic study of human nervous system tumors. Arch. Pathol., *80*:38–42, 1965.
49. Leuchtenberger, C. Quantitative determination of DNA in cells by Feulgen microspectrophotometry. In: *General Cytochemical Methods, Vol. 1*, edited by J.F. Danielli, pp. 219–278. New York, Academic Press, 1958.
50. Leuchtenberger, C., Leuchtenberg, R., and Davis, A.M. A microspectrophotometric study of the deoxyribose nucleic acid (DNA) content in cells of normal and malignant human tissues. Am. J. Pathol., *30*:65–85, 1954.
51. Levin, V.A., Wilson, C.B., Davis, R.L., *et al.* A phase III comparison of BCNU, hydroxyurea, and radiation therapy to BCNU and radiation therapy for treatment of primary malignant gliomas. J. Neurosurg., *51*:526–532, 1979.
52. Mendelsohn, M.L. Autoradiographic analysis of cell proliferation in spontaneous breast cancer of C3H mouse. III. The growth fraction. J. Natl. Cancer. Inst., *28*:1015–1029, 1962.
53. Mitchell, J.B., Kinsella, T.J., Russo, A., *et al.* Radiosensitization of hematopoietic precursor cells (CFUc) in glioblastoma patients receiving intermittent intravenous infusions of bromodeoxyuridine (BUdR). Int. J. Radiat. Oncol. Biol. Phys., *9*:457–463, 1983.
54. Mørk, S.J. and Laerum, O.D. Modal DNA content of human intracranial neoplasms studied by flow cytometry. J. Neurosurg., *53*:198–204, 1980.
55. Nagashima, T., De Armond, S.J., Murovic, J., *et al.* Immunocytochemical demonstration of S phase cells by anti-bromodeoxyuridine monoclonal antibody in human brain tumor tissues. Acta. Neuropathol. (Berl.), *67*:155–159, 1985.
56. Nagashima, T. and Hoshino, T. Rapid detection of S phase cells by antibromodeoxyuridine monoclonal antibody in 9L brain tumor cells in vitro and in situ. Acta. Neuropathol. (Berl.), *66*:12–17, 1985.
57. Nagashima, T., Murovic, J.A., Hoshino, T., *et al.* The proliferative potential of human pituitary tumors *in situ*. J. Neurosurg., *64*:588–593, 1986.
58. Nishizaki, T., Orita, T., Furutani, Y., *et al.* Flow-cytometric DNA analysis and immunohistochemical measurement of Ki-67 and BUdR labeling indices in human brain tumors. J. Neurosurg., *70*:379–384, 1989.
59. Ostertag, C.B., Volk, B., Shibata, T., *et al.* The monoclonal antibody Ki-67 as a marker for proliferating cells in stereotactic biopsies of brain tumors. Acta. Neurochir., *89*:117–121, 1987.
60. Park, T.S., Hoffman, H.J., Hendrick, E.B., *et al.* Medulloblastoma: Clinical presentation and management. J. Neurosurg., *58*:543–552, 1983.
61. Puck, T.T. and Steffen, J. Life cycle analysis of mammalian cells. I. A method of localizing metabolic events within the life cycle, and its application to the action of colcemide and sublethal doses of X-irradiation. Biophys. J., *3*:379–397, 1963.
62. Ralfkiaer, E., Stein, H., Bosq, J., *et al.* Expression of a cell-cycle associated nuclear antigen (Ki-67) in cutaneous lymphoid infiltrates. Am. J. Dermatopathol., *8*:37–43, 1986.
63. Refsum, S.B. and Berdal, P. Cell loss in malignant tumors in man. Eur. J. Cancer., *3*:235–236, 1967.
64. Roggendorf, W., Schuster, T., and Peiffer, J. Proliferative potential of meningiomas determined with the monoclonal antibody Ki-67. Acta. Neuropathol., *73*:361–364, 1987.
65. Russo, A., Gianni, L., Kinsella, T.J., *et al.* Pharmacological evaluation of intravenous delivery of 5-bromodeoxyuridine to patients with brain tumors. Cancer Res., *44*:1702–1705, 1984.
66. Sano, K., Hoshino, T., and Nagai, M. Radiosensitization of brain tumor cells with a thymidine analogue (bromouridine). J. Neurosurg., *28*:530–538, 1968.
67. Scherer, H.J. The pathology of cerebral gliomas. J. Neurol. Psychiatry., *3*:147–177, 1940.
68. Shirakawa, S., Luca, J.K., Tannock, I., *et al.* Cell proliferation in human melanoma. J. Clin. Invest., *49*:1188–1199, 1970.
69. Steel, G.G. Cell loss from experimental tumors. Cell Tissue Kinet., *1*:193–207, 1968.
70. Szybalski, W. X-ray sensitization by halopyrimi-

dines. Cancer Chemother. Rep., *58:*539–557, 1974.

71. Tokars, R.P., Stutton, H.G., and Griem, M.L. Cerebellar medulloblastoma: results of a new method of radiation treatment. Cancer, *43:* 129–136, 1979.
72. Tym, R. Distribution of cell doubling times in in vivo human cerebral tumors. Surg. Forum., *20:*445–447, 1969.
73. Van Dilla, M.A., Steinmetz, L.L., David, D.T., *et al.* High-speed cell analysis and sorting with flow systems: Biological applications and new approaches. Nucl. Sci., *21:*714–720, 1974.
74. Van Dilla, M.A., Trujillo, T.T., Mullaney, P.F., *et al.* Cell microfluorometry: A method for rapid fluorescence measurement. Science, *163:* 1213–1214, 1969.
75. Walker, M.D., Strike, T.A., and Sheline, G.E. An analysis of dose-effect relationship in the radiotherapy of malignant gliomas. J. Radiat. Oncol. Biol. Phys., *5:*1725–1731, 1979.
76. Yoshii, Y., Maki, Y., Tsuboi, K., *et al.* Estimation of growth fraction with bromodeoxyuridine in human central nervous system tumors. J. Neurosurg., *65:*659–663, 1986.
77. Zuber, P., Hamou, M.F., and Tribolet, N. Identification of proliferating cells in human gliomas using the monoclonal antibody Ki-67. Neurosurgery, *22:*364–368, 1988.

SUGGESTED READINGS

Baserga, R. (ed.): *The Cell Cycle and Cancer.* New York, Dekker, 1971.

Cleaver, J.E. *Thymidine Metabolism and Cell Kinetics.* Amsterdam, Elsevier/North Holland, 1967.

Hoshino, T. Cellular aspects of human brain tumors (gliomas). In: *Advances in Cellular Neurobiology, vol 2,* edited by S. Fedoroff and L. Hertz. New York, Academic Press, 1981.

Steel, G.G. *Growth Kinetics of Tumors.* Oxford, Oxford University Press, 1977.

PART III

The Cell Biology of Brain Tumors

Chapter 10

In Vitro Growth of Brain Tumors

YISHENG LEE, M.D., Ph.D., CAROL J. WIKSTRAND, Ph.D., PETER A. HUMPHREY, M.D., Ph.D., SANDRA H. BIGNER, M.D., HENRY S. FRIEDMAN, M.D., FOTIOS D. VRIONIS, M.D., M.P.H., and DARELL D. BIGNER, M.D., Ph.D.

INTRODUCTION

The lack of progress in the treatment of human gliomas (66) and medulloblastomas (51) has prompted the investigation of many of the inherent biological characteristics of brain tumors such as cellular heterogeneity, low vascular permeability to drugs, low immunogenicity, small growth fraction, and other factors that may be responsible for resistance to therapy. Advances in understanding in all these areas will be necessary to design new approaches to diagnosis and therapy (11, 51). Our ability to define these phenomena and their molecular mechanisms at the cellular level would not be possible without the in vitro establishment of brain tumor cell lines.

A comprehensive review of cultured human glial and glioma cells has been recently published (35); notable in this overview was the conclusion that, of all human tumors, gliomas as a family have been the "easiest" tissues from which to establish permanent cell lines. Dating from the first report of the successful cultivation of malignant glioma cells by Fischer in 1925 (46), several groups have reported the establishment of cell lines from tumors of the central nervous system (CNS) (10, 52, 53, 100, 105, 120, 175). In comparison to the overall success rate of 6% for cell line establishment from all types of human tumor biopsy material reported by Giard *et al.* (63), the approximately 12% success rate which these authors obtained with gliomas was encouraging. As methods of tumor explantation continued to improve during the 1970s, more cell lines derived from "astrocytomas" and "glioblastomas" were reported; by 1977 Fogh *et al.* (48) listed 11 such lines demonstrably free of HeLa cell contamination. Of these lines, five were established to be tumorigenic in athymic mice (47). By the early 1980s, over 70 established lines derived from human gliomas had been reported. An excellent summary of these lines and annotated references to their characterization, including chromosome analysis, marker protein measurements, tumorigenicity, viral expression, and antigenicity are provided by Collins (35).

In contrast to the experience with gliomas, continuous medulloblastoma cell lines have been notoriously difficult to establish. The most extensively studied medulloblastoma cell line (TE-671) was established by McAllister *et al.* (106) after 21 attempts. However, recent cytogenetic analysis, DNA fingerprinting, and the expression of muscle-type nicotinic acetylcholine receptors and intermediate filament protein desmin established that TE-671 is a subline of the human rhabdomyosarcoma cell line RD, previously established in McAllister's Laboratory (159). No cell line survived beyond 15 passages in our initial trials of medulloblastoma cell line explantation over a period of 2 years (52). The characteristic in vivo cellular behavior of medulloblastoma cells, such as leptomeningeal infiltration and cerebrospinal pathway metastasis (134), led to the use of suspension culture techniques (119) and injections of freshly resected tumors into the "immunologically privileged" intracranial site with further animal immunosuppression (52). The establishment of D283 Med and D341 Med in our laboratory (52, 53) reflected the success of such an approach. To date, except for cell line Daoy (79), our laboratory has established the largest collection of human medulloblastoma cell lines including D283 Med (52), D341 Med (53), D384 Med, and D425 Med (116).

As human brain tumor lines are too numerous for detailed description, in the first half of this chapter we intend to provide an overview of the methods of explantation; the isolation of purified CNS cell populations, which has a bearing on the characterization of cultured brain tumor cell populations; the markers of cell types in the CNS; and the use of karyotyping for the "fingerprinting" of individual cell lines. We will then discuss the experimental use of these cell lines in various analyses of brain tumor studies. Lastly, animal brain tumor models will be examined, as a very limited number of experimental animal models have been used in brain tumor research, but those established have provided us with a wealth of knowledge in brain tumor biology.

METHODS OF EXPLANTATION AND INITIAL CULTURE

General Techniques

The most frequently used techniques for human brain tumor explantation to in vitro culture are certainly not unique to this type of tumor. The origin of the basic explant and trypsinization techniques discussed below are thoroughly discussed by Gilden *et al.* (64) and Wroblewska *et al.* (180) in their two-part study of the "long-term" culture of cells from normal brain tissue.

The desired goal of a crude suspension of tumor material relatively free of contaminating erythrocytes and stromal elements can be achieved by either mechanical or enzymatic disruption, followed by appropriate filtration, centrifugation, and hypotonic treatment. If the best characterized and most widely used glioma and medulloblastoma lines are listed by method of explantation, it is apparent that the majority of these lines were obtained following mechanical disaggregation of tumor biopsy material. Several investigators [Pontén and Mcintyre (120): U-105 MG, U-118 MG, U-138 MG, U-251 MG; Giard *et al.* (63): A-172; Westermark (175): U-343 MG, U-373 MG, U-410 MG; Shapiro *et al.* (148): eight cell lines and clones, successfully grown for short term studies; Friedman *et al.* (52): D283 Med; Friedman *et al.* (53): D341 Med; and Oakes *et al.* (116): D384 Med and D425 Med] have reported the successful establishment of astrocytoma-, glioblastoma-, and medulloblastoma-derived cell lines by this simplest of methodologies. With minor variations on the theme, the method used by all of these investigators was basically as follows. Freshly resected tumor tissue, placed in sterile phosphate-buffered saline or tissue culture medium (to be discussed in the section below on early culture), with or without fetal calf serum, is dissected free of macroscopically observable normal brain, hemorrhagic, and necrotic areas and is rinsed in sterile medium. Following mincing with blades or iris scissors into fragments approximately 1-3 mm^3, one of two routes can be followed. For standard explant culture, the fragments can be placed directly in tissue culture flasks or petri dishes containing very small amounts of complete tissue culture medium to allow for adherence, followed by complete submersion in medium after the fragments have become attached to the culture vessel. Alternatively, the fragments may be further dissociated by mincing followed by aspiration through a large (19- to 22-gauge) needle. This procedure usually yields small clusters of cells as well as individual cells and filamentous and lipid fragments (148). Such crude suspensions can be plated directly following dilution in complete medium, or separated further by passage through stainless steel or nylon meshes with pore sizes ranging from 50 to 1000 μm (68) and/or fractionation on sucrose or Ficoll density gradients (68). Elimination of erythrocyte contamination is readily performed by hypotonic lysis in cold 0.83% NH_4Cl supplemented with $KHPO_4$ for human cells. In general, however, a higher proportion of success has been achieved with preparations plated at the crude suspension level. Also as described earlier, direct injection of cell homogenate prepared from newly biopsied tumors to the "immunologically privileged" intracranial site in immunosuppressed animals apparently increased the success rate of medulloblastoma cell line production, possibly as this approach provides an intermediate in vivo environment before in vitro growth. Some tumor lines, such as the human giant cell glioblastoma line D-212 MG (15), can only be carried in athymic nude mice and in a special organ culture (matrix) system (78) but not in monolayer or spheroid systems.

Success has also been achieved by the use of enzymatic digestion of tumor tissue dissected free of normal or necrotic tissue and then minced, as described above. Most of the long-term cell lines obtained by this method were dissociated by trypsin (0.125% in 0.8% NaCl, 0.02% KCl, 0.02% $KH_2HPO_4.7H_2O$, without Ca^{2+} and Mg^{2+}) as reported by Bigner *et al.* (10) for cell lines D-32 MG, D-37 MG, D-54 MG, and D-65 MG and lines (13) D-245 MG, D-247, D-259 MG, and D-263 MG by Friedman *et al.* (52) for D283 Med; and by Maunoury (105). Other investigators have reported the alternative use of collagenase (161) or an enzyme cocktail composed of collagenase, hyaluronidase, pronase, and DNAase in serum-free medium (13, 176). In general, enzymatic digestion of the tissue minces is allowed to proceed at room temperature in a trypsinization flask with constant agitation for 5 to 60 minutes. Aliquots of generated crude cell suspension can be removed and plated at various intervals following centrifugation to remove enzyme followed by resuspension in complete medium. Mesh filtration and erythrocyte lysis are performed if necessary. Pontén (119) has reported the derivation of a subclone of U-251 MG, U-251 MGsp, by differential trypsinization of an early passage of the parent line but this method has not been reported elsewhere.

Recently, the induction of multicellular spheroid formation by cells isolated from human tumor material described by Wibe *et al.* (176) has been successfully applied to human glioma cell lines (33, 38) and human brain tumor biopsy material (37, 38). Briefly, this technique involves the generation of a crude cell suspension by enzymatic disruption followed by plating in tissue culture vessels base-coated with agar which prevents cell adhesion. Within days, floating multicellular spheroids can be seen. The initial use for such cultures is not for cell line establishment but for chemosensitivity assays. Anecdotally, the new medulloblastoma lines D283 Med, D341 Med, D384 Med, and D425 Med recently reported by Friedman *et al.* (52, 53) and Oakes *et al.* (116) all spontaneously grew as multicellular spheroids and are totally anchorage independent.

Despite the fact that the spheroid culture system provides a three-dimensional pattern of histological organization and a better expressed and organized extracellular matrix (65, 111) similar to that observed in vivo, and can be reproducibly used for chemosensitivity analysis, it fails to preserve structural and functional integrity and probably also the tumor heterogeneity of human gliomas (38). Organ culture, on the other hand, retains the original cellular interrelationships and has been used as an analog of the in vivo state of human and experimental gliomas (131, 132, 152). In organ culture, tissue fragments of 1 to 3 mm^3 in size are cultured and supported on a platform (coverslips) or a porous matrix (sponge foam) which is exposed to a moist gas or air phase on the surface of a relatively large volume of stationary nutrient medium (72, 74, 131). This culture technique has been especially helpful in enhancing morphological and biochemical differentiation in a variety of human and experimental gliomas and medulloblastomas (72, 78, 131, 152), probably through conditions favoring the development of cells in G_0 state by increased cell-to-cell contacts and the nutritional, metabolic, pH, and oxygen tension gradients generated in the explants (74). The organ culture system also has been used in combination with multicellular spheroids in a confrontation culture system to study tumor invasion in both human and experimental brain tumors (21, 85, 86, 126, 157). However, only minimal cell growth is maintained in vitro (38) and there are no qualitative measurements to distinguish tumor cell response from that of normal cells in the explants in a chemosensitivity assay (76). This limits the applicability of organ culture systems.

Initial Culture of Newly Explanted Lines

The relative ease with which brain tumor cell lines are established is complemented by the basically uncomplicated demands of outgrowing glioma lines. A subsequent section will deal with growth factors, growth factor receptors, and their function and action in the growth control of brain tumor cell lines. This brief section simply reviews the basic culture conditions well tolerated by brain tumor cell lines.

A variety of basic tissue culture media, all essentially variants of Eagle's Minimal Essential Medium (MEM) have been reported: MEM (97, 180), Waymouth (148), McCoy's 5A (62), Hams F10 (37), RPMI 1640 (105), and Richter's ZO-MEM (10). With the exception of Shapiro *et al.* (148), who report the use of 20% fetal calf serum (FCS), almost all investigators routinely supplement the medium with approximately 5 to 10% serum and exogenous glutamine. Some cell lines which initially appear to grow best in 20% serum medium readily adapt to 10% FCS medium (10). Cell cultures are uniformly incubated at 37°C in a 5% CO_2 humid atmosphere and fed when the pH of the culture medium drops. Subculture of these predominantly anchorage-dependent lines is usually performed by incubation in 0.125 to 0.25% trypsin, 0.02% EDTA, or a combination of the two (10, 97, 119, 148). The required split ratio varies widely from cell line to cell line, from 1:2 (D-18 MG) to 1:5 (D-54 MG) (10).

Lindgren and Westermark (97) have observed that, like explanted normal glial cells, glioma cells will respond to increased density by becoming blocked at G_1, but that this block becomes operative at a much higher density for glioma cells. This, coupled with the much reduced serum concentration required for the initiation of DNA synthesis, results in the comparatively high rate of proliferation by cultured glioma cells. Additionally, unlike normal glia, glioma cells grow in agarose gels (32) and have been reported to migrate through them to adhere to plastic (37). The relative insensitivity of cultured glioma cells to heat, survival being significantly compromised only at temperatures >43°C or following decreases in pH, further attests to the hardiness of these cells in culture (62).

ISOLATION OF PURIFIED POPULATIONS

In an effort to conduct studies of growth, differentiation, and metabolism of cells of the CNS without the undefined and complicating influences of serum, several groups have developed serum-free defined media, or "chemically defined" (CD) media for the in vitro culture of cells (24, 25, 43, 83, 107, 109, 110, 117). In general, the transition from FCS-supplemented medium to basal media requires supplementation with a surface precoating treatment and various hormones, depending upon the cell types being selected.

Extensive work in the area of substratum requirements and defined media for many CNS-derived cell types has been performed (22–25, 107, 135). Perhaps the best review of the contribution of the extracellular matrix (ECM) to the successful culture of these cells is provided in Bottenstein (24). The complex functions of the naturally elaborated ECM have been successfully substituted for various cell types by pretreatment of vessel surfaces with collagen, polylysine, fibronectin (24), or various synthetic polymeric amines (133). Cell types differ in their substratum requirements. Whereas established cell lines of glial origin (U-251 MG sp) or neural origin (B104 rat neuroblastoma) adhere well to surfaces coated with polylysine and fibronectin (24), these substances will not substitute for the ECM required by primary cultures of neurons, which adhere and extend neurites best on collagen-treated surfaces. Primary cultures of astrocytes require polylysine and fibronectin (24, 110), however, if epidermal growth factor (EGF) is provided in the culture medium, Bottenstein (24) maintains that the need for fibronectin is eliminated.

As the needs for attachment vary, so do the requirements for growth of glial cell lines versus those for neuronal cell lines. Bottenstein (24) has reported the formulation of several media: the N series and the G series. The N series, for the support of neuronal cell lines, is based on a 1:1 ratio of Dulbecco's modified Eagles (DME) and Ham's F12 and contains insulin, transferrin, progesterone, and putrescine. The G series, for glial lines, is based on DME alone and must therefore contain biotin, but omits the putrescine and progesterone, replacing the latter with hydrocortisone. Whereas the glial fibrillary acidic protein (GFAP)-positive glioblastoma line U-251 MGsp can be grown in a basic G medium without insulin, the culture of primary astrocytes requires the addition of EGF and insulin (24), and the growth of glial tumor cells is significantly enhanced by EGF, but not other nervous system tumors (primitive neuroectodermal tumors and various tumors of neuroepithelial/mesenchymal origin) (50). The results of Morrison and de Vellis (110) are in general agreement, although these authors included putrescine and prostaglandins in their CD astrocyte medium. Patel *et al.* (117) described the use of brief cytosine arabinoside treatment (48 hours) of EGF-stimulated astroglial cells in a CD medium to enrich neuronal populations. Purified oligodendroglia have been reported to require only polylysine for attachment, but a more complete CD medium including insulin, progesterone, hydrocortisone, transferrin, and putrescine in a DME:F12 ratio of 3:1, which is primarily a "neuronal" cocktail (83), has been shown to support an oligodendrocyte-enriched population demonstrating cell differentiation in culture that parallels in vivo development. The modification of such CD media consisting of DME:F12 ratio 1:1 supplemented with insulin, sodium selenite, putrescine, and D+ galactose allowing the long-term survival of mature oligodendrocyte pure cultures was recently described (43). Despite the intricacies of these various formulations, it is apparent that the differential use of CD media which are totally nonsupportive of some types of cell growth can be used as a selective factor in CNS cell culture.

MARKERS FOR BRAIN TUMORS

Markers for Cell Types in the Central Nervous System

As briefly reviewed by Walker *et al.* (166), the use of cell-specific markers with immunocytochemical methods has proven to be the most reliable way of distinguishing different types of nervous system-derived cells in culture. Although several monoclonal antibodies with highly unique patterns of reactivity for tumors of the CNS have been reported (for comprehensive tables see references 177 and 70), the reliable, definitive, biochemically defined markers of nervous system cell type conventionally used are listed in Table 10.1.

TABLE 10.1.
Conventionally Used Markers of Normal Nervous System Cell Types

Marker	Cellular Location	References
S-100	Glial cells, neuroendocrine cells, Schwann cells, satellite cells of sympathetic ganglia, oligodendroglia	164 41 177
GFAP	Astrocytes, ependymal cells, Bergmann glia	183 118 42
Tetanus toxin	Neurons, type 2 astrocytes	108 133
Neuron specific enolase (NSE)	Neurons, neuroendocrine system (APUD cells)	130 164
Myelin basic protein	Schwann cells, oligodendroglia	121 83
Galactocerebroside	Oligodendrocytes	112 121
2′,3′-Cyclic nucleotide 3′-phosphodiesterase	Oligodendrocytes	83

These markers can be used to distinguish between the major lineages potentially represented in cultures of normal CNS material. Among these, GFAP is the best known and most widely used. With GFAP-specific monoclonal antibodies, both normal and neoplastic astroglial cells can be identified. It must be remembered, however, as discussed extensively by Collins (35), that endothelial, epithelial, and contaminating lymphocyte populations derived from explanted CNS tissue can also contribute to outgrowing populations. Moreover, extreme caution in the interpretation of either the cell lineage or differentiation status of neoplastic cells on the basis of individual "marker" expression must be exercised. Many cell lines in culture that are derived from neoplastic brain tumors have major ploidy and structural chromosome changes and, through gene amplification and rearrangement, may cease to express normal CNS-associated markers.

Morphology and Cytogenetics

As with cultured cell lines of any origin, a perpetual problem with brain tumor cell lines is to assure that they are individually distinct and derived from the tumor and patient of origin. Glioma cell lines generally can be grouped into four morphologic patterns termed fibroblastic, epithelioid, fascicular, and glial (Fig. 10.1). Within these groups, however, individual lines may closely resemble one another. Furthermore, glioma lines may be impossible to distinguish from lines derived from other tumor types by morphology alone. Glioma lines exhibiting a fibroblastic growth pattern, for example, may resemble normal fibroblasts or cultured sarcomas.

The most reliable means for establishing the individuality of cultured cell lines is cytogenetics. Karyotypic analysis of primary malignant human gliomas revealed predominantly normal or near-diploid stemlines with statistically significant numerical deviations such as gains of chromosome 7, loss of chromosome 10, structural abnormalities of 9p and 19q, and occurrence of double minutes (17). Most gliomas with double minutes have been shown to contain amplification of the c-*erb* B gene, which encodes for the epidermal growth factor receptor (EGFR); a few cases revealed c-*myc*, n-*myc* or *gli* amplification (17, 20, 82, 163, 178). Karyotypes of established glioma lines most commonly contain stemlines or modal numbers in the near-triploid region (14, 101–103). Less commonly, near-tetraploid and near-pentaploid populations dominate. A small proportion (5 to 10%) maintain near-diploid karyotypes. Regardless of the chromosome counts, all established glioma lines studied to date have shown complex patterns with gains and losses of whole chromosomes as well as structurally abnormal chromosomes (marker chromosomes) formed by translocation and deletions. Although identical marker chromosomes have occasionally been described in a small number of glioma lines, most lines contain numerous markers as well as many numerical deviations. Thus, the karyotypic profile for each line, consisting of its modal chromosome number, numerical deviations, and specific marker chromosomes, is distinctive and this "fingerprint" can be used to distinguish each glioma line from all others. Karyotype of seven medulloblastoma biopsies in direct preparation and/or short-term cultures derived therefrom reveal structural abnormalities quite different from gliomas. Medulloblastomas contain mainly deletions and unbalanced translocations of chromosomes 1, 3, 17, and 20 resulting in partial trisomy (18). The most common structural abnormality is i [17q], which may be associated with tumor progression (18, 31).

A few established glioma lines have been followed karyotypically over spans of at least one hundred in vitro passages (104, 123, 124). Some changes inevitably occur such as gains or losses of entire copies of normal or abnormal chromosomes, the emergence of new chromosomal markers, or occasional doubling of the whole chromosome complement. Due to the multiple parameters which comprise each glioma line's karyotypic profile, however, it is still possible to confirm the identity of an individual line. The D-54 MG glioma line has been studied karyotypically after intracerebral transplantation in immunosuppressed

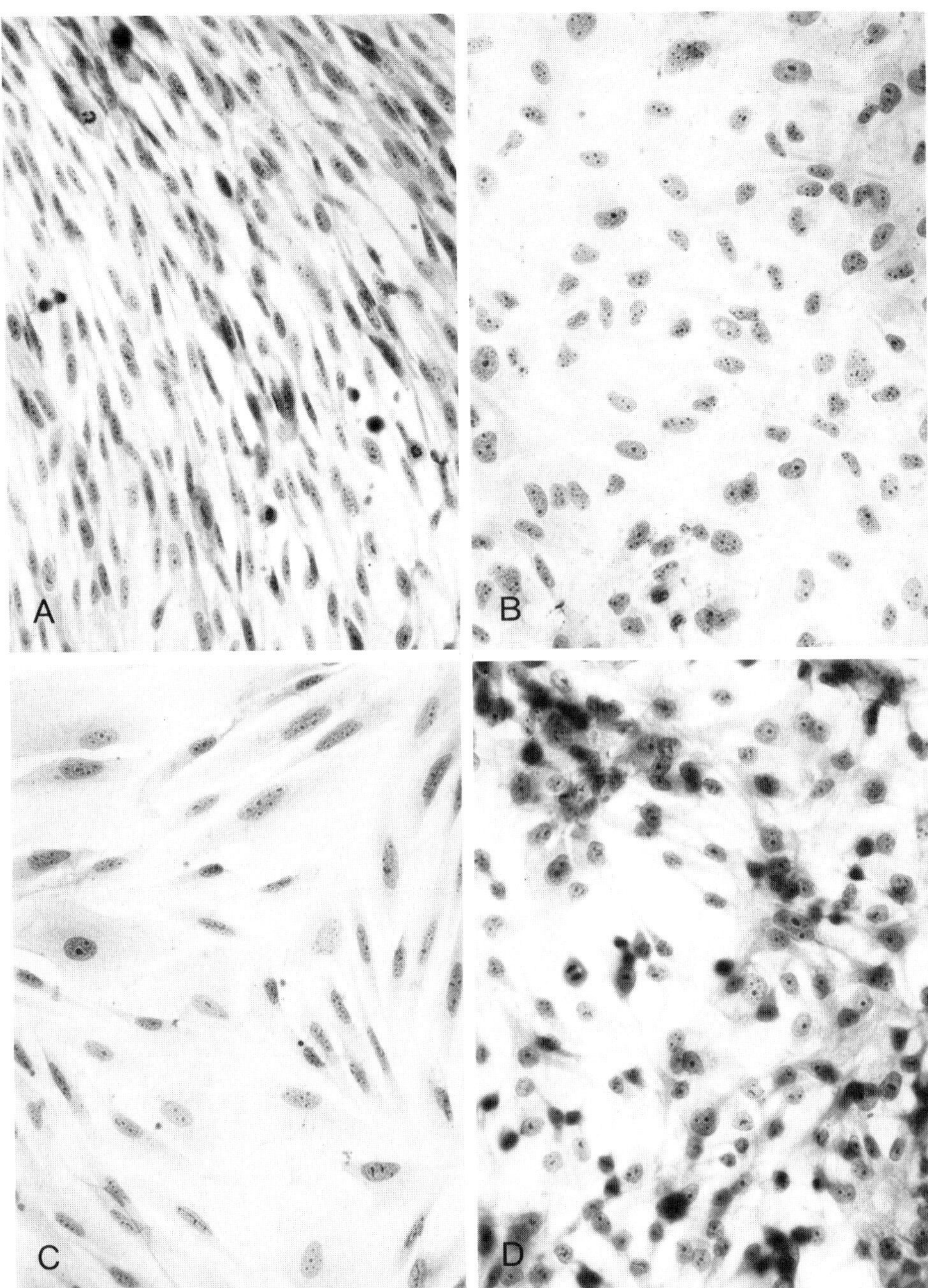

Figure 10.1. The four most common morphologic patterns of permanent human glioma-derived cell lines. *A*) Fibroblastic U-410 MG. *B*) Epithelioid D-32 MG. *C*) Fascicular U-343 MG. *D*) Glial D-54 MG. Papanicolaou stain ×250.

rats (1, 136), and D283 Med medulloblastomas have been karyotyped following subcutaneous and intracerebral transplantation into athymic mice (52). In all instances the karyotypes remained virtually unchanged, allowing unequivocal identification of the xenografts. Recent chromosomal analysis also demonstrated that most subcutaneous xenografts derived from seven human glioblastomas retained karyotypes (double minutes, marker chromosomes, and structural abnormalities) similar to those seen in original tumors (19).

A more difficult problem when dealing with putative human glioma-derived cell lines is to substantiate that they truly originated in a glioma, since most of these lines do not express GFAP, the only currently reliable marker of glial derivation. Similarly, the origin of putative medulloblastoma-derived cell lines may be difficult to confirm. In several instances, biopsies of malignant gliomas and medulloblastomas have been karyotyped and the chromosomal evolution of the tumors followed after the cell lines were established in culture (16, 52, 53). Although some of these lines doubled their chromosome number and acquired new markers, the structural abnormalities and the general chromosomal distribution seen originally were generally retained allowing confirmation of the identity of the cultured cells with the tumor from which they were derived (Fig. 10.2).

EXPERIMENTAL APPLICATIONS OF BRAIN TUMOR CELL LINES

The addition of chemotherapy to the current treatment regimen of surgical resection and radiation for both glioma and medulloblastoma has failed to provide clear survival benefit. Even though the failure may be multifactorial in nature involving factors such as cell hypoxia, the distribution of cells in the cell cycle, cellular and genetic heterogeneity, drug resistance, and drug delivery, the lack of a relevant and reliable drug evaluation system for choosing chemotherapeutic agents individually tailored for each brain tumor patient may have been the most responsible factor. Several in vitro and in vivo chemosensitivity models using both human medulloblastoma and glioma cell lines have been established for such a purpose (37, 38, 51, 142).

In vitro analyses can be performed either with "short-term" assays such as vital dye exclusion, inhibition of radiolabeled nucleic acid and amino acid incorporation (76, 160), a growth inhibition assay, or with "long-term" systems such as the double layer clonogenic assay in soft agar and the multicellular spheroid inhibition assay (38). The advantages and disadvantages of each assay technique have been reviewed (75, 80). Since much evidence has demonstrated how tissue culture conditions can influence in vitro results, not only between different laboratories but also between experiments (128, 150), it is extremely important to establish the reliability of each assay system with rigorous controls (84). Using a microtitration assay with 35 *S*-methionine incorporation inhibition as the end point, Thomas *et al.* (162) have demonstrated a correlation between the in vitro procarbazine and CCNU sensitivity of biopsied human glioma tissue and the clinical relapse free interval of patients from whom the tumors were derived.

Similar chemosensitivity results can be achieved with long-term clonogenic assay and multicellular spheroid assays established for brain tumors. The response parameters of the clonogenic assays are derived by linear regression analysis of the relationship between percentage of colony formation and log drug concentration. Such an assay helped to demonstrate the chemosensitivity of human medulloblastoma cell lines D283 Med and Daoy to melphalan and phenyl ketocyclophosphamide (54). The determination of drug sensitivity in spheroid assays is made by studying spheroid size increase delay and the clonogenicity of the treated spheroid cells. This assay system is especially ideal for the investigation of the structural features of solid tumors which may influence cell cycle characteristics, cell differentiation, drug penetration and delivery, and effect of hypoxia on radiosensitivity. Darling *et al.* (37) reported that 83.4% of biopsy samples (n = 46) yielded spheroids. Of these, 34.8% generated sufficient numbers for a chemosensitivity assay. Moreover, all the human es-

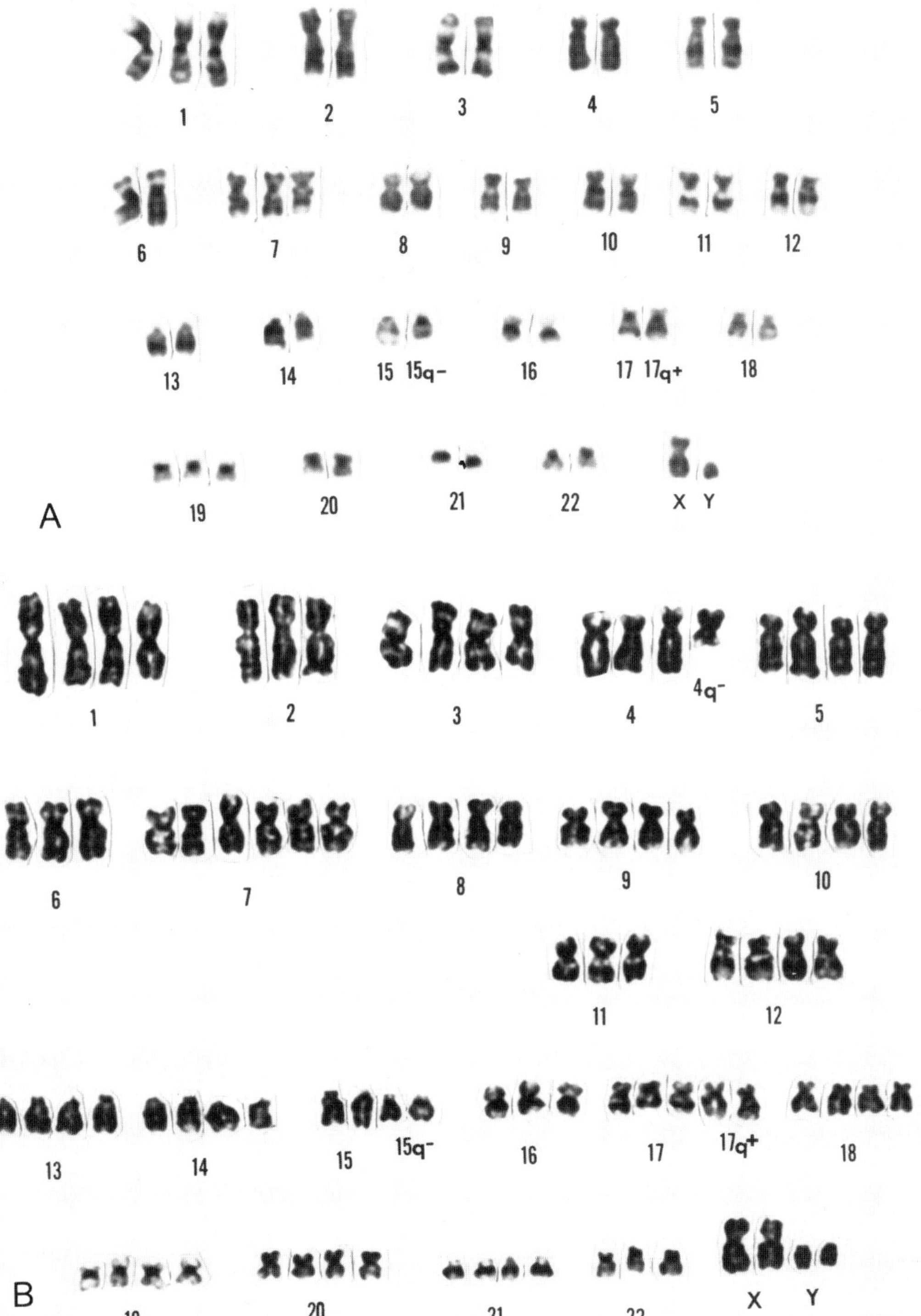

Figure 10.2. *A*) The stemline karyotype of the original biopsy of D-245 MG shows a reciprocal translocation between chromosomes 15 and 17 and extra copies of chromosomes 1, 7, and 19. Giemsa-trypsin banding ×1200. *B*) In passage 86, D-245 MG has doubled its chromosome number but retains 2 copies of the 15q− and 17q+ chromosomes seen in the original biopsy. Giemsa-trypsin banding ×1200.

tablished cell lines tested to date produce spheroids under appropriate conditions (38). Such findings can then be applied to in vivo systems for further analysis.

The in vivo study of human brain tumors can be performed in athymic mice or rats bearing either subcutaneous or intracranial xenografts exposed to potentially tumoricidal drugs or vehicles by various routes (i.e., intraperitoneal, intravenous, intracarotid, and intrathecal administration) usually at the 10% lethal dose (30, 56, 59). The response of subcutaneous tumors is assessed by tumor growth delay and that of intracranial tumors by median survival prolongation. Earlier studies also indicated that, for drugs with assumed or measured plasma concentration equal to or lower than ID75 (the in vitro dose at which there is a 75% reduction in the number of colonies formed), there is a good correlation between in vitro and subcutaneous tumor chemosensitivity for the TE-671 cell line (56). Chemotherapeutic agents effective in experimental gliomas include carmustine, procarbazine, diaziquone, PCNU, melphalan, cyclophosphamide, and fludarabine (140–142), whereas melphalan, cyclophosphamide, iphosphamide, and thiotepa are active in human medulloblastoma cell lines and transplantable xenografts (54, 57). These experimental data established the basis for Phase II clinical trials of gliomas with cyclophosphamide (142) and medulloblastomas with melphalan (58). Recent reports of increased melphalan activity in intracranial medulloblastomas and glioma xenografts following glutathione depletion by buthionine sulfoximine have provided an additional strategy in brain tumor therapy (55, 153, 154). The therapeutic efficacy of radioiodinated antitenascin monoclonal antibody in subcutaneous and intracranial glioma xenografts (89, 90) has led to further studies in human patients (184). Moreover, the findings of differential drug sensitivity between subcutaneous and intracranial tumors (51) and the benefit of intracarotid agent administration (29, 88) further highlights one of the unique problems of human brain tumors: the existence of the blood-brain barrier. For a rational therapeutic design, the use of cell lines in in vitro and in vivo models is both necessary and complementary.

Brain tumor cell lines have also been utilized in the investigations of the role of growth factors in human glioma growth (146, 174). The two most extensively characterized glial-binding growth factors are epidermal growth factor and platelet-derived growth factor (PDGF). Both growth factors are related to oncogenes. The PDGF β-chain gene is the cellular homologue and proto-oncogene of the viral oncogene v-*sis* and the EGF receptor gene is the cellular homologue and proto-oncogene of the viral *erb*-B oncogene. Less well characterized is the role of the transforming growth factors in glioma growth.

PDGF purified to homogeneity is a basic protein with a molecular size of approximately 30,000 daltons and consists of two peptide chains denoted A and B of roughly 16,000 and 14,000 daltons, respectively (129, 158). It is a potent growth factor for cultured glial cells (172). Evidence for PDGF synthesis by glioma cells has been obtained at the mRNA and protein levels (9, 44, 113–115). Transcripts of c-*sis* mRNA were detected by nick-translated simian sarcoma virus *sis* DNA in three of five glioblastomas (44). A PDGF-like protein, which resembled PDGF structurally, immunologically, and functionally, was demonstrated to be expressed by the human glioma cell line U-343 MGa cl 2 (113, 115). Moreover, glioma PDGF production correlated with both an immature phenotype and glioma cell growth rate (114). The endothelial hyperplasia characteristic of glioblastoma may be due to the strong coexpression of PDGF B chain/c-*sis* and PDGF receptor mRNA in endothelial cells present in glioblastoma (73). Finally, glioblastoma cells themselves have been shown to coexpress PDGF A chain, PDGF B chain, and PDGF-β subunit receptor mRNA (73). These findings implicate PDGF in glioma growth control, and it has been hypothesized that autocrine and paracrine activation of the PDGF receptor may be operational in the growth of the vasculature in gliomas and of the glioma cells themselves (73, 114).

EGF, a 6045-dalton protein, has been

demonstrated to stimulate the growth of mouse astrocytes, neonatal rat glial cells, and normal human glial cells in culture (27, 151, 168, 171). Neoplastic glial cells are also responsive to EGF. For example, EGF induces cell migration of glioma cells in culture (173) and also enhances the invasiveness of glioma cells into brain spheroids in culture (98). EGF has also been demonstrated to significantly enhance the growth of glioma tumor cells in both serum-free short-term cultures (50) and in established cell lines requiring serum for growth (170).

The main investigational focus of the role of EGF in neoplastic glial growth has centered on the EGFR. The EGFR gene, the c-*erb* B proto-oncogene, is often amplified and highly expressed in malignant human gliomas. In biopsy tissue, 40% of gliomas showed EGFR gene amplification (95, 96, 178), and this amplification was invariably associated with high expression of the receptor (178). The amplified receptor genes appear to be located in extrachromosomal rings known as double minute chromosomes (20). EGFR gene rearrangement is associated with gene amplification and the expression of low molecular weight, truncated EGFR proteins (77, 99, 181). Recently, it has been demonstrated that the basis for the expression of the low molecular weight EGFR protein forms can be traced to deletion mutations of the gene itself (179). These deletions are always located in the extracellular domain and seem to segregate according to the size and location of the deletion. One deletion has resulted in a c-*erb* B-like protein, with deletion of most of the extracellular domain (77, 179). This EGFR may function similarly in conferring a growth advantage; that is, deletion of the EGF-binding domain in these proteins may result in a constitutively activated state which allows for uncontrolled growth and proliferation. Double minute formation and EGFR gene amplification, rearrangement, and mutations are all maintained when human gliomas are grown in xenograft form (77), but are apparently lost under culture conditions; in culture only 1 of 22 astrocytoma cell lines showed EGFR gene amplification (45). It has been hypothesized that the loss of gene amplification in culture may reflect the constancy of in vitro selective pressures compared to the inconstancy of in vivo selective pressures (165). A wide range of EGFR expression from 10^4 to 10^6 EGFR molecules per cell has been observed (4, 45, 155, 182) and, in culture, most EGFRs seem to possess functionally intact EGF-binding and kinase domains. Truncated EGFRs have not been found in glioma cell cultures but an EGFR with an inactive kinase (169) and a high molecular weight form of the EGFR have been found (156). Both the normal-sized, overexpressed EGFR and variant EGFR molecules may be of critical importance in glioma cell propagation.

Only a few studies on transforming growth factors and gliomas have been performed. Transforming growth factor-β (TGF-β), a potent growth inhibitor of many tumor cell lines, also inhibited the growth of glioblastoma cell line in soft agar but did not affect monolayer growth (71). Transforming growth factor-α (TGF-α), which exhibits structural homology with EGF and binds to the EGFR with high affinity, is synthesized mainly by transformed cells. Several studies have demonstrated increased TGF-α immunoreactivity in both cultured glioma cells and in glioma biopsies compared to non-neoplastic glial cells (61, 137). Thus, similar to glioma cells' coexpression of PDGF ligand and receptor, they may also express (or overexpress) both TGF-α and its receptor, the EGFR, resulting in autocrine and/or paracrine growth stimulation of glioma cells.

Another application of brain tumor cell lines, very likely as significant as their use in the study of the known growth factors (EGF, PDGF), lies in the identification of unknown transforming sequences present in brain tumor cell DNA. The presence of a transforming gene termed "*neu*" (138) was identified by NIH 3T3 cell transfection assay with DNA extracted from the ethylnitrosourea-induced rat neuroblastoma cell line B104 (149). The *neu* gene encodes a 185-kilodalton plasma membrane phosphoprotein (p-185) which can be precipitated by polyclonal antibodies against the EGFR (138). Sequence analysis of the *neu* oncogene predicts an overall structure of its product similar to that of the EGFR, reflected in 82% homology of the putative intracytoplasmic tyrosine kinase domain of the *neu* gene product (7). However, *neu* oncogene is distinct from the EGFR gene in that its human counterpart (c-*erb* B-2) is mapped to chromosome 17, whereas the EGFR (c-*erb* B-1) gene is on chromosome 7 (60). This suggests that p-185 is a growth factor receptor for a still unidentified ligand (7). In vitro studies showed that monoclonal antibody 7.16.4, which reacts with p-185, inhibits the anchorage independent growth of *neu* transformed cells in soft agar, and this inhibition correlates well with the down modulation of p-185 expression caused by the same antibody (39). Moreover, treatment with 7.16.4 inhibits the tumorigenic growth of *neu*-transformed NIH 3T3 cells and the growth of the rat neuroblastoma cell line (B104) from which *neu* was initially identified in nude mice and in syngeneic rats (40). Although the normal function of the *neu* gene product presently remains obscure, its significance in transformation seems to be more well defined. Recently, a mechanism of *neu* activation valid in the rat model was documented. It was found that there were two versions of the *neu* oncogene, a normal and a transforming allele that differ from each other in a single amino acid in the transmembrane domain of the *neu*-encoded protein. All rat tumor cell lines (B103, B104, B50 and B82) containing activated *neu* oncogenes possess the same mutation, suggesting a mechanism identical to that postulated for the rat oncogene (8). However, other mechanisms of *neu* gene activation may apply in other systems. The human counterpart of the rat *neu* oncogene (termed c-*erb* B-2) (40) has been demonstrated to be amplified in one salivary adenocarcinoma (144), one mammary carcinoma (81), and one MKN-7 gastric cancer cell line (60). The aforementioned account of the biological significance of the *neu* oncogene places new emphasis upon the importance of chemically induced neuroectodermal tumors and cell lines derived thereof in gene transfer experiments and in the identification of novel tumor specific antigens.

ANIMAL BRAIN TUMOR MODELS

Much research concerning brain tumors has involved animal cell lines (see works discussed above). However, the incidence of spontaneous animal CNS tumors in certain strains of dogs, rats, and the inbred VM/Dk strain mouse (12), although generally equal to the human incidence (1.2%), is too low to allow consistent and reproducible models. The most commonly used animal brain tumor cell lines in experimental neuro-oncology have thus involved chemically and virally induced gliomas in mice and rats, where up to 100% tumor incidence has been observed. The inducing agents most frequently employed are polycyclic aromatic hydrocarbons (methylcholanthrene, benzypyrene, and dibenzanthracene), *N*-nitroso compounds (*N*-methylnitrosourea, MNU; and *N*-ethylnitrosourea, ENU), RNA tumor viruses (Rous sarcoma virus, murine sarcoma virus, and simian sarcoma virus), and DNA tumor viruses (human adenovirus 12 and simian vacuolating virus, SV-40) (12). In vitro culture and characterization have been attempted in both spontaneous and induced glioma models, with variable success. The explantation and cell line establishment methodologies are similar to those of human brain tumor cell line production. This has lead to the production of many animal glioma cell lines (Table 10.2).

The most commonly used models with in vivo and in vitro components include murine ependymoblastoma lines GL261, Ep, EpA, and GL26 and the rat glioma lines C-6, 9L, and RG-2 (139). Animal models are generally divided into transplantable tumor models and cell lines. In the syngeneic models, the gliomas can be maintained either as cell lines or as continuously transplantable tumors. Otherwise, the in vitro cell lines usually can only be introduced in immunosuppressed animals or into an immunologically privileged site. Except for C-6, which is used mainly for in vitro studies as it is derived from outbred

TABLE 10.2.
Animal Brain Tumor Cells

Tumors	Inducing Agents	Animal Species/Strain	Tumor Type	GFAP[a]	References
P497					
P540	Spontaneous	Mouse VM/Dk	Astrocytoma	–	145
P560					
GL261	Methylcholanthrene	Mouse C3H	Ependymoblastoma	nd	143
Ep					
EpA	Methylcholanthrene	Mouse C57BL/6	Ependymoblastoma	nd	2
GL26					139
C-6	N-Methylnitrosourea	Random-bred Wistar	Glioma	+[b]	5
		Furth rat			139
9L	N-Methylnitrosourea	Inbred CD Fischer 344	Gliosarcoma	–	6
					3
RG-2	N-Ethylnitrosourea	Inbred CD Fischer 344	Glioma	–	28
S69-c15	Avian sarcoma virus	Inbred CD Fischer 344	Anaplastic astrocytoma	–	34
S70-cli	(B-77)				36
S635c15	Avian sarcoma virus	Inbred CD Fischer 344	Anaplastic astrocytoma	++	87
	(Schmidt-Ruppin)				

[a] –, negative expression; +, positive expression; nd, no data.
[b] Induction by dbcAMP, dexamethasone, norepinephrine, or organ culture.

animals, all other cell lines are transplantable in their respective syngeneic hosts which provide the opportunity to study the correlation and difference between in vitro and in vivo cell behaviors. EpA and GL26 have been used in the NCl drug screening program in which nitrosoureas and procarbazine, effective chemotherapeutic agents against human brain tumors, were shown to prolong survival in mice bearing transplanted tumors; mithramycin, vincristine, and methotrexate were not effective in either the models or clinical trials (67, 147). C-6, a rat glial stem cell line, has been used for the study of astrocytic differentiation, as its GFAP expression can be increased by dibutyryl cyclic AMP (122), norepinephrine (26), high cell density (49), and organ culture (94). 9L, on the other hand, is used mostly for cell kinetic and drug and radiation sensitivity studies (92, 127, 167); both in vitro and in vivo models are available for 9L and RG-2 cell lines and are ideal for drug delivery and therapy design studies. For immunological analysis, S69-cl5, an avian sarcoma virus-induced rat astrocytoma cell line, has been shown to express a common (69) as well as a glioma-associated antigen (91).

Even though the cell lines discussed previously were all derived from morphologically identified astroglial tumors, few retained differentiation markers in prolonged in vitro passages. The analysis of 104 experimental gliomas induced by transplacental application of ENU in CDF rats showed GFAP immunoreactivity only in a low fraction of tumor astrocytes and the commonly used RG-2 cell line exhibited no GFAP in culture but some GFAP-positive tumor cells were noted in intracerebral xenografts (125). These could well be reactive astrocytes of the host. The recently described cell line S635cl5 (87), derived from an anaplastic astrocytoma induced by the avian sarcoma retrovirus in the F-344 rat, expressed the astrocytic differentiation marker GFAP both in transplanted tumors and in cultured cells after over 100 passages in vitro. The cellular morphology and architecture of the transplanted intracranial tumors were highly similar to those of the original tumor. In vitro growth was characterized by a short population doubling time (18.82 hours) and a high colony formation efficiency (90.8%). Intracranial transplantation produced consistent survival curves and the blood flow and blood-to-tissue transport constants were very homogeneous, similar to those observed with RG-2. Further studies in tumor sensitivity to chemotherapeutic agents and radiation in both cultured cells and tumors will be most useful.

CONCLUSION

Although research using both human and animal cell lines has provided a tremendous amount of information in brain tumor biology and therapeutic design, the inherent differences between in vitro and in vivo conditions such as culture artifacts and in vivo metabolism, and between animal and human systems such as spontaneous incidence, tumor growth rate, immunogenicity, vasculature, and drug metabolism, all warrant a careful approach in applying data derived from in vitro systems and animal model experiments to the human condition. For example, the karyotypes of most glioma-derived cell lines are near tetraploid or near-triploid, but most biopsied gliomas are near-diploid, and most of the animal cell lines were derived from chemically or virally induced tumors which may not be immunogenically equivalent to spontaneous tumors. Morphologically, endothelial proliferation can usually be identified in transplanted brain tumors; however, the glomeruloid formation characteristic in human glioblastoma multiforme has not been seen in either animal or human glioma cell line-induced xenografts. In terms of drug sensitivity, procarbazine, which is effective in both human patients and the mouse ependymoblastoma model, was not demonstrably beneficial in rat models. The serum half-life of BCNU, which is a useful parameter in both humans and animals, was much shorter in humans (93). These differences, which may be species specific, should be carefully considered in the interpretation of results derived from cell line and animal model studies.

ACKNOWLEDGMENT:

This work is supported by NINCDS Grants KO7 NSOO958-02, P50 NS20023-04 and NCI Grants CA 11898, CA 43722, and CA 44640. We thank Ms. Bonnie Lynch for her secretarial assistance and Ms. Ann Tamariz for editorial assistance.

REFERENCES

1. Adams, C., Bullard, D. E., Bigner, S.H., *et al.* Intracerebral transplantation of D-54 human glioma line in immunosuppressed rats. In: *Biology of Brain Tumor,* edited by M.D. Walker and D.G.T. Thomas, pp. 97–195. Boston, Martinus Nijhoff, 1986.
2. Ausman, J.I., Shapiro, W.R., and Rall, D.P. Studies on the chemotherapy of experimental brain tumors: development of an experimental model. Cancer Res., *30:*2394–2400, 1970.
3. Barker, M., Hoshino, T., Gurcay, O., *et al.* Development of an animal brain tumor model and its response to therapy with 1,3-bis(2-chloroethyl)-1-nitrosourea. Cancer Res., *33:*976–986, 1973.
4. Bell, D., Harsh, G. IV, Rosenblum, M., *et al.* Numeric structural alterations of chromosome 7 in human brain tumor: correlation with expression of epidermal growth receptors (EGFR) (abstr.) AACR Proc. *27:*37, 1986.
5. Benda, P., Lightbody, J., Sato, G., *et al.* Differentiated rat glial cell strain in tissue culture. Science, *161:*370–371, 1968.
6. Benda, P., Someda, K., Messer, J., *et al.* Morphological and immunochemical studies of rat glial tumors and clonal strains propagated in culture. J. Neurosurg., *34:*310–323, 1971.
7. Bergmann, C.I., Hung, M.C., and Weinberg, R.A. The neu oncogene encodes an epidermal growth factor receptor-related protein. Nature (Lond.), *319:*226–230, 1986.
8. Bergmann, C.I., Hung, M.C., and Weinberg, R.A. Multiple independent activations of the neu oncogene by a point mutation altering the transmembrane domain of p-185. Cell, *45:*649–657, 1986.
9. Betsholtz, C., Heldin, C.H., Nister, M., *et al.* Synthesis of a PDGF-like growth factor in human glioma and sarcoma cells suggests the expression of the cellular homologue to the transforming protein for simian sarcoma virus. Biochem. Biophys. Res. Commun., *117:*176–182, 1983.
10. Bigner, D.D., Bigner, S.H., Pontén, J., *et al.* Heterogeneity of genotypic and phenotypic characteristics of fifteen permanent cell lines derived from human gliomas. J. Neuropathol. Exp. Neurol., *40:*201–229, 1981.
11. Bigner, D.D., Pedersen, H.B., Bigner, S.H., *et al.* A proposed basis for the therapeutic resistance of gliomas. Semin. Neurol., *1:*169–179, 1981.
12. Bigner, D.D. and Swenberg, J.A. (eds.) *Janisch and Schreiber's Experimental Tumors of the Central Nervous System.* Kalamazoo, MI, Upjohn Press, 1977.
13. Bigner, S.H., Friedman, H.S., Biegel, J.A., *et al.* Specific chromosomal abnormalities characterize four established cell lines derived from malignant human gliomas. Acta Neuropathol. (Berl.), *72:*86–97, 1986.
14. Bigner, S.H., Mark, J., and Bigner, D.D. Chromosomal composition of four permanent culture cell lines derived from human gliomas. Cancer Genet. Cytogenet., *10:*335–349, 1983.

15. Bigner, S.H., Mark, J., Schold, S.C., Jr., *et al.* A serially transplanted human giant cell glioblastoma that maintains a near-haploid stem line. Cancer Genet. Cytogenet., *18:*141–154, 1985.
16. Bigner, S.H., Mark, J., and Bigner, D.D. Chromosomal progression of malignant human gliomas from biopsy to establishment as permanent lines in vitro. Cancer Genet. Cytogenet., *24:*163–176, 1987.
17. Bigner, S.H., Mark, J., Burger, P.C., *et al.* Specific chromosomal abnormalities in malignant human gliomas. Cancer Res., 88:405–411, 1988.
18. Bigner, S.H., Mark, J., Friedman, H.S., *et al.* Structural chromosomal abnormalities in human medulloblastoma. Cancer Genet. Cytogenet., *30:*91–101, 1988.
19. Bigner, S.H., Schold, S.C., Jr., Friedman, H.S., *et al.* Chromosomal composition of malignant human gliomas through serial subcutaneous transplantation in athymic mice. Cancer Genet. Cytogenet., *40:*111–120, 1989.
20. Bigner, S.H., Wong, A.J., Mark, J., *et al.* Relationship between gene amplification and chromosomal deviations in malignant human gliomas. Cancer Genet. Cytogenet., *29:*165–170, 1987.
21. Bjerknes, R., Bjerkvig, R., and Laerum, O. Phagocytic capacity of normal and malignant rat glial cells in culture. J. Natl. Cancer Inst., *78:*279–288, 1987.
22. Bottenstein, J.E. Differentiated properties of neuronal cell lines. In: *Functionally Differentiated Cell Lines,* edited by G.H. Sato, pp. 155–184. New York, Alan R. Liss, 1981.
23. Bottenstein, J.E. Culture methods for growth of neuronal cell lines in defined media. In: *Cell Culture Methods for Molecular and Cell Biology, Vol. 4,* edited by D. Barnes, D. Sirbasku, and G. Sato. pp. 3–13. New York, Alan R. Liss, 1984.
24. Bottenstein, J.E. Growth and differentiation of neural cells in defined media. In: *Cell Culture in the Neurosciences,* edited by J.E. Bottenstein and G.H. Sato. pp. 3–43. New York, Plenum Press, 1985.
25. Bottenstein, J.E. and Sato, G. H. Growth of a rat neuroblastoma cell line in serum-free supplemented medium. Proc. Natl. Acad. Sci. USA, *76:*514–517, 1979.
26. Browning, E. T. and Ruina, M. Glial fibrillary acidic protein: norepinephrine stimulated phosphorylation in intact C-6 glioma cells. J. Neurochem., *42:*718–726, 1984.
27. Brunk, U., Schellens, J., and Westermark, B. Influence of epidermal growth factor (EGF) on ruffling activity, pinocytosis and proliferation of cultured human glial cells. Exp. Cell Res., *103:*295–302, 1976.
28. Bullard, D.E. and Bigner, D.D. Animal models and virus induction of tumors. In: *Brain Tumors: Scientific Basis, Clinical Investigation, and Current Therapy,* edited by D.G.T. Thomas and D.I. Graham. pp. 51–84. London, Boston, Butterworths, 1980.
29. Bullard, D.E., Bigner, S.H., and Bigner, D.D. Comparison of intravenous versus intracarotid therapy with 1,3-Bis(2-chloroethyl)-1-nitrosourea in a rat brain tumor model. Cancer Res., *45:*5240–5245, 1985.
30. Bullard, D.E., Schold, S.C., Jr., Bigner, S.H., *et al.* Growth and chemotherapeutic response in athymic mice of tumors arising from human glioma-derived cell lines. J. Neuropathol. Exp. Neurol., *40:*410–427, 1981.
31. Callen, D.F., Cirocco, L., and Moore, L.A. der(11)t(8;11) in two medulloblastomas. A possible non-random cytogenetic abnormality. Cancer Genet. Cytogenet., *38:*255–260, 1989.
32. Carlsson, J., Collins, P., and Brunk, U. Plasma membrane motility and proliferation of human glioma cells in agarose and monolayer cultures. Acta Pathol. Microbiol. Immunol. Scand. [A], *86:*45–55, 1978.
33. Carlsson, J., Nilsson, K., Westermark, B., *et al.* Formation and growth of multicellular spheroids of human origin. Int. J. Cancer, *31:*523–533, 1983.
34. Cloyd, M.W. and Bigner, D.D. Surface morphology of normal and neoplastic rat cells. Am J. Pathol., *88:*29–52, 1977.
35. Collins, V.P. Cultured human glial and glioma cells. Int. Rev. Exp. Pathol., *24:*135–202, 1983.
36. Copeland, D.D., Cloyd, M.W., Weschsler, W., *et al.* Surface morphology of avian sarcoma virus and ethyl-nitrosourea transformed rat neuroectodermal cells and human glioblastoma cells in organ and monolayer culture. In: *Scanning Electron Microscopy, Part V,* edited by O. Johari and R.P. Becker, pp. 93–100. The Ninth Scanning Electron Microscopy Symposium, Toronto, 1976.
37. Darling, J.L., Oktar, N., and Thomas, D.G.T. Multicellular tumour spheroids derived from human brain tumors. Cell Biol. Int. Rep., *7:*23–30, 1983.
38. Darling, J.L., Oktar, N., and Thomas, D.G.T. In vitro chemosensitivity testing of human brain tumours using multicellular spheroids. Adv. Biosci., *58:*121–134, 1986.
39. Drebin, J.A., Link, V.C., Stern, D.F., *et al.* Down-modulation of an oncogene protein product and reversion of the transformed phenotype by monoclonal antibodies. Cell, *41:*695–706, 1985.
40. Drebin, J.A., Link, V.C., Weinberg, *et al.* Inhibition of tumor growth by a monoclonal antibody reactive with an oncogene-encoded tumor antigen. Proc. Natl. Acad. Sci. USA, *83:*9129–9133, 1986.
41. Eng, L.F. and Bigbee, J.W. Immunocytochemistry of nervous system specific antigens. In: Adv. Neurochem., *3:*43–98, 1978.
42. Eng., L.F. and DeArmond, S.J. Immunochemistry of the glial fibrillary acidic protein.

Prog. Neuropathol., *5:*19–39, 1983.

43. Espinosa de los Monteros, A., Roussel, G., Neskovic, N.M., *et al.* A chemically defined medium for the culture of mature oligodendrocytes. J. Neurosci. Res., *19:*202–211, 1988.

44. Eva, A., Robbins, K.C., Andersen, P.R., *et al.* Cellular genes analogous to retroviral oncogenes are transcribed in human tumour cells. Nature (Lond.), *295:*116–119, 1982.

45. Filmus, J., Pollak, M.N., Cairncross, J.G., *et al.* Amplified, overexpressed and rearranged epidermal growth factor receptor gene in a human astrocytoma cell line. Biochem. Biophys. Res. Commun., *131:*207–215, 1985.

46. Fischer, A. Observations on the division of sarcoma cells in vitro. J. Cancer. Res., *9:*71–84, 1925.

47. Fogh, J., Fogh, J.M., and Orfeo, T. One hundred and twenty-seven cultured human tumor cell lines producing tumors in nude mice. J. Natl. Cancer Inst., *59:*221–225, 1977.

48. Fogh, J., Wright, W.C., and Loveless, J.D. Absence of HeLa cell contamination in 169 cell lines derived from human tumors. J. Natl. Cancer Inst., *58:*209–214, 1977.

49. Frame, M.C., Freshney, R.I., and Vaughan, P.F.T. Interrelationship between differentiation and malignancy-associated properties in glioma. Br. J. Cancer, *49:*269–280, 1984.

50. Frappaz, D., Singletary, S.E., Spitzer, G., *et al.* Enhancement of growth of primary metastatic fresh human tumors of the nervous system by epidermal growth factor in serum-free short term culture. Neurosurgery, *23:*355–359, 1988.

51. Friedman, H.S., Bigner, S.H., Schold, S.C. Jr., *et al.* The use of experimental models of human medulloblastoma in the design of rational therapy. In: *Biology of Brain Tumor,* edited by M.D. Walker and D.G.T. Thomas, pp. 405–409. Boston, Martinus Nijhoff, 1986.

52. Friedman, H.S., Burger, P.C., Bigner, S.H., *et al.* Establishment and characterization of the human medulloblastoma cell line and transplantable xenograft D283 Med. J. Neuropathol. Exp. Neurol., *44:*592–605, 1985.

53. Friedman, H.S., Burger, P.C., Bigner, S.H., *et al.* Phenotypic and genotypic analysis of a human medulloblastoma cell line and transplantable xenograft (D341 Med) demonstrating amplification of c-myc. Am. J. Pathol., *130:*472–484, 1988.

54. Friedman, H.S., Colvin, O.M., Skapek, S.X., *et al.* Experimental chemotherapy of human medulloblastoma cell lines and transplantable xenografts with bifunctional alkylating agents. Cancer Res., *48:*4189–4195, 1988.

55. Friedman, H.S., Colvin, O.M., Griffith, O.W., *et al.* Increased melphalan activity in intracranial human medulloblastoma and glioma xenografts following buthionine sulfoximine-mediated glutathione depletion. J. Natl. Cancer Inst., *81:*524–527, 1989.

56. Friedman, H.S., Schold, S.C., Jr., Muhlbaier, L.H., *et al.* In vitro versus in vivo correlations of chemosensitivity of human medulloblastoma. Cancer Res., *44:*5145–5149, 1984.

57. Friedman, H.S., Schold, S.C. Jr., and Bigner, D.D. Chemotherapy of subcutaneous and intracranial human medulloblastoma xenografts in athymic mice. Cancer Res., *46:*224–228, 1986.

58. Friedman, H.S., Schold, S.C., Jr., Mahaley, M.S., *et al.* Phase II treatment of medulloblastoma and pineoblastoma with melphalan: clinical therapy based on experimental model of human medulloblastoma. J. Clin. Oncol., *7:*904–911, 1989.

59. Fuchs, H.E., Archer, G.A., Colvin, O.M., *et al.* Activity of intrathecal 4-hydroperoxycyclophosphamide in a nude rat model of human neoplastic meningitis. Cancer Res., *50:*1954–1959, 1990.

60. Fukushige, S.-I., Matsubara, K.-I., Yoshida, M., *et al.* Localization of a novel v-erb B-related gene, c-erb-B-2, on human chromosome 17 and its amplification in a gastric cancer cell line. Mol. Cell Biol., *6:*955–958, 1986.

61. Gerosa, M.A., Talarico, D., Fognani, C., *et al.* Overexpression of N-ras oncogene and epidermal growth factor receptor gene in human glioblastomas. J. Natl. Cancer Inst., *81:*63–67, 1989.

62. Gerweck, L.E., and Richards, B. Influence of pH on the thermal sensitivity of cultured human glioblastoma cells. Cancer Res., *41:*845–849, 1981.

63. Giard, D.J., Aaronson, S.A., Todaro, G.J., *et al.* In vitro cultivation of human tumors: establishment of cell lines derived from a series of solid tumors. J. Natl. Cancer Inst., *51:*1417–1423, 1973.

64. Gilden, D.H., Devlin, M., Wroblewska, Z., *et al.* Human brain in tissue culture. I. Acquisition, initial processing, and establishment of brain cell cultures. J. Comp. Neurol., *161:*295–306, 1975.

65. Glimelius, B., Norling, B., Nederman, T., *et al.* Extracellular matrices in multicellular spheroids of human glioma origin: Increased incorporation of proteoglycans and fibronectin as compared to monolayer cultures. Acta Pathol. Microbiol. Immunol. Scand., *96:*433–444, 1988.

66. Green, S.B., Byar, D.P., Walker, M.D., *et al.* Comparisons of carmustine, procarbazine, and high-dose methylprednisolone as additions to surgery and radiotherapy for the treatment of malignant gliomas. Cancer Treat. Rep., *67:*121–132, 1983.

67. Hagesawa, H., Shapiro, W.R., Posner, J.B., *et al.* Effect of 1-(4-amino-2-methyl-5-pyrimidinyl)methyl-3-(2-chloroethyl)-3-nitrosourea hydrochloride on experimental brain tumors. Cancer Res., *39:*2687-2690, 1979.

68. Haglid, K.G., Hamberger, A., Carlsson, C.-A., *et al.* Glial cell characteristics in bulk-prepared cell fractions from human brain tumours. Acta Neuropathol. (Berl.), *40:*243–247, 1977.

69. Harwood, S.E., Bigner, D.D., Wechsler, W., *et al.* Antigens shared by rat schwannomas, neuroblastomas and a testicular interstitial cell carcinoma. Cancer Res., *37:*3379–3384, 1977.
70. He, X., Skapek, S.X., Wikstrand, C.J., *et al.* Phenotypic analysis of four human medulloblastoma cell lines and transplantable xenografts. J. Neuropathol. Exp. Neurol., *48:*48–68, 1989.
71. Helseth, E., Unsgaard, G., Dalen, A., *et al.* The effects of type beta transforming growth factor in proliferation and epidermal growth factor receptor expression in a human glioblastoma cell line. J. Neurooncol., *6:*269–276, 1988.
72. Herman, M.M. and Rubinstein, L.J. Divergent glial and neuronal differentiation in a cerebellar medulloblastoma in an organ culture system: in vitro occurrence of synaptic ribbons. Acta Neuropathol. (Berl.), *65:*10–24, 1984.
73. Hermansson, M., Nister, M., Betsholtz, C., *et al.* Endothelial cell hyperplasia in human glioblastoma: coexpression of mRNA for platelet-derived growth factor (PDGF) B chain and PDGF receptor suggests autocrine growth stimulation. Proc. Natl. Acad. Sci. USA, *85:*7748–7752, 1988.
74. Hess, J.R., Michaud, J., Sobel, R.A., *et al.*The kinetics of human glioblastomas maintained in an organ culture system. An in vitro autoradiography study. Acta Neuropathol. (Berl.), *61:*1–9, 1983.
75. Hill, B.T. An overview of correlations between laboratory tests and clinical responses. In: *Human Tumour Drug Sensitivity Testing In Vitro,* edited by P.P. Dendy and B.T. Hill, pp. 235–249. London, Academic Press, 1983.
76. Hill, B.T. Methodologies for in vitro growth of human 'solid' tumours and their applications. In: *Advances in Biosciences. Brain Tumors: Biopathology and Therapy,* edited by M.A. Gerosa, M.L. Rosenblum, and G. Tridente, pp. 3–13. Oxford, Pergamon Press, 1986.
77. Humphrey, P.A., Wong, A.J., Friedman, H.S., *et al.* Amplification and expression of the epidermal growth factor receptor (EGFR) gene in human glioma (HGL) xenografts. Cancer Res., *48:*2231–2238, 1988.
78. Ibayashi, N., Herman, M.M., Boyd, J.C., *et al.* Kinetics and glial fibrillary acidic (GFA) protein production in a transplantable human giant cell glioblastoma (D-212 MG) of near haploid karyotype maintained in an organ culture system. An immunohistochemistry study. Neuropathol. Appl. Neurobiol., *16:* 27–37, 1990.
79. Jacobsen, P.F., Jenkyn, D.J., and Papatimitriou, J.M. Establishment of a human medulloblastoma cell line and heterotransplantation into nude mice. J. Neuropathol. Exp. Neurol., *44:*472–485, 1985.
80. Kimmel, D.W., Shapiro, J.R., and Shapiro, W.R. In vitro drug sensitivity testing in human gliomas. J. Neurosurg., *66:*161–171, 1987.
81. King, C.R., Kraus, M.H., and Aaronson, S.A. Amplification of a novel v-erb B-related gene in a human mammary carcinoma. Science, *229:*974–976, 1985.
82. Kinzler, K.W., Bigner, S.H., Bigner, D.D., *et al.* Identification of an amplified highly expressed gene in a human glioma. Science, *236:*70–73, 1987.
83. Koper, J.W., Lopes-Cardozo, M., Romijn, H.J., *et al.* Culture of rat cerebral oligodendrocytes in a serum-free, chemically defined medium. J. Neurosci. Methods., *10:*157–169, 1984.
84. Kovach, J.S. In vitro models as guides to clinical chemotherapy. Adv. Biosci., *58:*49–57, Oxford, Pergamon Press, 1986.
85. Laerum, O.D., Bjerkvig, R., Steinsvag, S.K., *et al.* Invasiveness of primary brain tumors. Cancer Metastasis Rev., *3:*223–263, 1984.
86. Laerum, O.D., Steinvag, S., and Bjerkvig, R. Cell and tissue culture of the central nervous system: recent developments and current applications. Acta Neurol. Scand., *72:*529–549, 1985.
87. Lee, Y.S., Bigner, S.H., Eng, L.F., *et al.* A glial fibrillary acidic protein expressing and tumorigenic cell line derived from an avian sarcoma virus induced rat astrocytoma. J. Neuropathol. Exp. Neurol., *45:*704–720, 1986.
88. Lee, Y.S., Bullard, D.E., Wikstrand, C.J., *et al.* Comparison of monoclonal antibody delivery to intracranial glioma xenografts by intravenous (IV) and intracarotid (IC) administration. Cancer Res., *47:*1941–1946, 1987.
89. Lee, Y.S., Bullard, D.E., Humphrey, P.A., *et al.* Treatment of intracranial human glioma xenografts with ^{131}I-labeled anti-tenascin monoclonal antibody 81C6. Cancer Res., *48:*2904–2910, 1988.
90. Lee, Y.S., Bullard, D.E., Zalutsky, M.R., *et al.* Therapeutic efficacy of antiglioma mesenchymal extracellular matrix ^{131}I-radiolabeled murine monoclonal antibody in a human glioma xenograft model. Cancer Res., *48:*559–566, 1988.
91. Lee, Y.S., Wikstrand, C.J., and Bigner, D.D. Glioma-associated antigen defined by monoclonal antibodies against an avian sarcoma virus-induced rat astrocytoma. J. Neuroimmunol., *13:*183–202, 1986.
92. Leith, J.T., Schilling, W.A., and Wheeler, K.T. Cellular radiosensitivity of a rat brain tumor. Cancer, *35:*1545–1550, 1975.
93. Levin, V.A., Hoffman, W., and Weinkam, R.J. Pharmacokinetics of BCNU in man: a preliminary study of 20 patients. Cancer Treat. Rep., *62:*1305–1312, 1978.
94. Liao, C.L., Eng, L.F., Herman, M.M., *et al.* Glial fibrillary acidic protein-solubility characteristics, relation to cell growth phases and cellular localization in rat C-6 glioma cells: an immunoradiometric and immunohistologic study. J. Neurochem., *30:*1181–1186, 1978.
95. Libermann, T.A., Nusbaum, H.R., Razon, N.,

et al. Amplification, enhanced expression and possible rearrangement of EGF receptor gene in primary human brain tumors of glial origin. Nature (Lond.), *313:*144–147, 1985.

96. Libermann, T.A., Razon, N., Bartal, A.D., *et al.* Expression of epidermal growth factor receptors in human brain tumors. Cancer Res., *44:*753–760, 1984.

97. Lindgren, A. and Westermark, B. Serum requirement and density dependent inhibition of human malignant glioma cells in culture. Exp. Cell Res., *104:*293–299, 1977.

98. Lund-Johansen, M., Bjerkvig, R., Engebräten, O., *et al.* Interactions between human glioma spheroids from permanent cell lines and rat brain cell aggregates. 1. Studies in a chemically defined medium. 2. Possible role of the EGF-receptor during expansive tumor growth and invasion (abstr.). J. Neurooncol., *7:*318, 1989.

99. Malden, L.T., Novak, U., Kaye, A.M., *et al.* Selective amplification of the cytoplasmic domain of the epidermal growth factor receptor gene in glioblastoma multiforme. Cancer Res., *48:*2711–2714, 1988.

100. Manuelidis, L. and Manuelidis, E.E. Surface growth characteristics of defined normal and neoplastic neuroectodermal cells in vitro. Prog. Neuropathol., *4:*235–266, 1979.

101. Mark, J., Pontén, J., and Westermark, B. G-band analysis of an established cell line of a human malignant glioma. Humangenetik, *22:*323–326, 1974.

102. Mark, J., Pontén, J., and Westermark, B. Cytogenetical studies with G-band techniques of established cell lines of human malignant gliomas. Hereditas, *78:*304–308, 1974.

103. Mark, J., Pontén, J., and Westermark, B. Origin of the marker chromosomes in an established hypotriploid glioma cell line studied with G-band technique. Acta Neuropathol. (Berl.), *29:*223–228, 1974.

104. Mark, J., Westermark, B., and Pontén, J. Banding patterns in human glioma cell lines. Hereditas, *87:*243–260, 1977.

105. Maunoury, R. Establishment and characterization of 5 human cell lines derived from a series of 50 primary intracranial tumors. Acta Neuropathol. (Berl.) *39:*33–41, 1977.

106. McAllister, R.M., Isaacs, H., Rongey, R., *et al.* Establishment of a human medulloblastoma cell line. Int. J. Cancer, *20:*206–212, 1977.

107. Michler-Stuke, A., and Bottenstein, J.E. Proliferation of glial-derived cells in defined media. J. Neurosci. Res., *7:*215–228, 1982.

108. Mirsky, R., Wendon, L.M.B., Black, P., *et al.* Tetanus toxin: a cell surface marker for neurons in culture. Brain Res., *148:*251–259, 1978.

109. Morrison, R.S. and Vellis, J. de. Growth of purified astrocytes in a chemically defined medium. Proc. Natl. Acad. Sci. USA, *78:*7205–7209, 1981.

110. Morrison, R.S. and Vellis, J. de. Preparation of a chemically defined medium for purified astrocytes. In: *Cell Culture Methods for Molecular and Cell Biopsy, Vol. 4,* edited by D. Barnes, D. Sirbasku, and G. Sato, pp. 15–22. New York, Alan R. Liss, Inc., 1984.

111. Nederman, T., Norling, B., Glimelius, B., *et al.* Demonstration of an extracellular matrix in multicellular tumor spheroids. Cancer Res., *44:*3090–3097, 1984.

112. Neskovic, N.M., Rebel, B., Harth, S., *et al.* Biosynthesis of galactocerebrosides and glucocerebrosides in glial cell lines. J. Neurochem., *37:*1363–1370, 1981.

113. Nister, M., Heldin, C.-H., Wateston, A., *et al.* A glioma-derived analog to platelet-derived growth factor: demonstration of receptor competing activity and immunological crossreactivity. Proc. Natl. Acad. Sci. USA, *81:*926–930, 1984.

114. Nister, M., Heldin, C.-H., and Westermark, B. Clonal variation in the production of a platelet-derived growth factor-like protein and expression of corresponding receptors in a human malignant glioma. Cancer Res., *46:*332–340, 1986.

115. Nister, M., Wedell, B., Betsholtz, C., *et al.* Evidence for progressional changes in the human malignant glioma line U-343 MGa: Analysis of karyotype and expression of genes encoding the subunit chains of platelet-derived growth factor. Cancer Res., *47:*4953–4960, 1987.

116. Oakes, W.J., Friedman, H.S., Bigner, S.H., *et al.* Successful laboratory growth and analysis of CUSA-obtained medulloblastoma samples. Technical report. J. Neurosurg., *72:*821–823, 1990.

117. Patel, A.J., Seaton, P., and Hunt, A. A novel way of removing quiescent astrocytes in a culture of subcortical neurons grown in a chemically defined medium. Brain Res., *470:*283–288, 1988.

118. Pegram, C.N., Eng, L.F., Wikstrand, C.J., *et al.* Monoclonal antibodies reactive with epitopes restricted to glial fibrillary acidic proteins of several species. Neurochem. Pathol., *3:*119–138, 1985.

119. Pontén, J. Neoplastic human glial cells in culture. In: *Human Tumors Cells In Vitro,* edited by J. Fogh, pp. 175–206. New York, Plenum Press, 1975.

120. Pontén, J. and Macintyre, E.H. Long term culture of normal and neoplastic human glia. Acta Pathol. Microbiol. Immunol. Scand. [A], *74:*465-486, 1968.

121. Raff, M.C., Mirsky, R., Fields, K.L., *et al.* Galactocerebroside is a specific cell-surface antigenic marker for oligodendrocytes in culture. Nature, *274:*813–816, 1978.

122. Raju, T.R., Bignami, A., and Dahl, D. Glial fibrillary acidic protein in monolayer cultures of C-6 glioma cells: effect of aging and dibutyryl cyclic AMP. Brain Res., *200:*225–230, 1980.

123. Ray, J.A., Bello, M.J., Ramos, C., *et al.* Serial cytogenetic study of a human glioma cell

line. Cancer Genet. Cytogenet., *8:*287–295, 1983.

124. Ray, J.A., Bello, M.J., Campos, J.M. de, *et al.* Cytogenetic follow-up from direct preparation to advanced in vitro passages of a human malignant glioma. Cancer Genet. Cytogenet., *41:*175–183, 1989.

125. Reifenberger, G., Bilzer, T., Seitz, R.J., *et al.* Expression of vimentin and glial fibrillary acidic protein in ethylnitrosourea-induced rat gliomas and glioma cell lines. Acta Neuropathol. (Berl.), *78:*270–282, 1989.

126. Ridder, L.I. de, Laerum, O.D., Mork, S.J., *et al.* Invasiveness of human glioma cell lines in vitro: relation to tumorigenicity in athymic mice. Acta Neuropathol. (Berl.), *72:*207–213, 1987.

127. Rodriguez, A. and Alpen, E.L. Feeder cells and cell survivals in spheroids and monolayers. Int. J. Radiat. Biol., *41:*111-117, 1982.

128. Rosenblum, M.L., Emma, D.A., Kleppe-Hoifodt, H., *et al.* Brain tumor stem cells: influence of different culture conditions. Adv. Biosci., *58:*83–86, 1986.

129. Ross, R. Platelet-derived growth factor. Lancet, *1:*1179–1182, 1989.

130. Royds, J.A., Taylor, C.B., and Timperley, W.R. Enolase isoenzymes as diagnostic markers. Neuropathol. Appl. Neurobiol. *11:*1–16, 1985.

131. Rubinstein, L.J., Herman, M.M., and Foley, V.L. In vitro characteristics of human glioblastomas maintained in organ culture systems. Light microscopy observations. Am. J. Pathol., *71:*61-80, 1973.

132. Rubinstein, L.J. and Herman, M.M. Studies on the differentiation of human and experimental gliomas in organ culture systems. Recent Results Cancer Res., *51:*35–51, 1975.

133. Ruegg, U.T. and Hefti, F. Growth of dissociated neurons in culture dishes coated with synthetic polymeric amines. Neurosci. Lett., *49:*319–324, 1984.

134. Russell, D.S. and Rubinstein, L.J. *Pathology of Tumours of the Nervous System,* ed. 4 Baltimore, Williams & Wilkins, 1977.

135. Rutka, J.T. The K.G. McKenzie Award Lecture, 1986. Effects of extracellular matrix proteins on the growth and differentiation of an anaplastic glioma cell line. Can. J. Neurol. Sci., *13:*301–306, 1986.

136. Saris, S.C., Bigner, S.H., and Bigner, D.D. Transplantation of human glioma-derived tumors into the brains of immuno-suppressed rats. J. Neurosurg., *60:*582–588, 1984.

137. Samuels, V., Barrett, J.M., Bockman, S., *et al.* Immunocytochemical study of transforming growth factor expression in benign and malignant gliomas. Am. J. Pathol., *134:*895–902, 1989.

138. Schechter, A.L., Stern, D.F., Vaidyanathan, L., *et al.* The neu oncogene: an erb-B-related gene encoding a 185,000-Mr tumour antigen. Nature (Lond.), *312:*513–516, 1984.

139. Schold, S.C., Jr., and Bigner, D.D. A review of animal brain tumor models which have been used for therapeutic studies. In: *Oncology of The Nervous System,* edited by M. Walker, pp. 31–63. Boston, Martinus-Nijhoff, 1982.

140. Schold, S.C., Jr. and Bigner, D.D. Treatment of five subcutaneous human glioma tumor lines in athymic mice with carmustine, procarbazine and mithramycin. Cancer Treat. Rep., *67:*811–819, 1983.

141. Schold, S.C., Jr., Friedman, H.S., Bjornsson, T., *et al.* Treatment of human glioma and medulloblastoma tumor lines in athymic mice with diaziquone and diaziquone-based drug combinations. Cancer Res., *44:*2352–2357, 1984.

142. Schold, S.C. Jr., Friedman, H.S., and Bigner, D.D. Therapeutic profile of the human glioma line D-54 MG in athymic mice. Cancer Treat. Rep., *71:*849–850, 1987.

143. Seligman, A.M. and Shear, M.J. Studies in carcinogenesis. VIII. Experimental production of brain tumors in mice with methylcholanthrene. Am J. Cancer, *37:*364–399, 1939.

144. Semba, K., Kamata, N., Toyoshima, K., *et al.* A v-erb B-related protooncogene, c-erb B-2, is distinct from the c-erb-1/epidermal growth factor-receptor gene and is amplified in a human salivary gland adenocarcinoma. Proc. Natl. Acad. Sci. USA, *82:*6497–6501, 1985.

145. Serano, R.D., Pegram, C.N., and Bigner, D.D. Tumorigenic cell culture lines from a spontaneous VM/Dk murine astrocytoma (SMA). Acta Neuropathol. (Berl.), *51:*53–64, 1980.

146. Shapiro, J.R. Biology of gliomas: heterogeneity, oncogenes and growth factors. Semin. Oncol., *13:*4–15, 1986.

147. Shapiro, W.R., Ausman, J.I., and Rall, D.P. Studies of the chemotherapy of experimental brain tumors: evaluation of 1,3-bis(2-chloroethyl)-1-nitrosourea, cyclophosphamide, mithramycin, and methotrexate. Cancer Res., *30:*2401–2413, 1970.

148. Shapiro, J.R., Yung, W.K.A., and Shapiro, W.R. Isolation, karyotype, and clonal growth of heterogeneous subpopulations of human malignant gliomas. Cancer Res., *41:*2349–2359, 1981.

149. Shih, C., Padhy, L., Murray, M., *et al.* Transforming gene of carcinomas and neuroblastomas introduced into mouse fibroblasts. Nature, *290:*261–264, 1981.

150. Shoemaker, R.H., Wolpert-DeFilippes, M.K., Kern, D.H., *et al.* Application of a human tumor colony-forming assay to new drug screening. Cancer Res., *45:*2145–2153, 1985.

151. Simpson, D.L., Morrison, R., Vellis, J. de, *et al.* Epidermal growth factor binding and mitogenic activity on purified populations of cells from the central nervous system. J. Neurosci. Res., *8:*453–462, 1982.

152. Sipe, J.C., Rubinstein, L.J., Herman, M.M., *et al.* Ethylnitrosourea-induced astrocytomas: morphologic observations on rat tumors maintained in tissue and organ culture sys-

tems. Lab. Invest., *31*:571–579, 1974.

153. Skapek, S.X., Colvin, O.M., Griffith, O.W., *et al.* Enhanced melphalan cytotoxicity following buthionine sulfoximine-mediated glutathione depletion in a human medulloblastoma xenograft in athymic mice. Cancer Res., *48*:2764–2767, 1988.
154. Skapek, S.X., Colvin, O.M., Griffith, O.W., *et al.* Buthionine sulfoximine-mediated depletion of glutathione in intracranial human glioma-derived xenografts. Biochem. Pharmacol., *37*:4313–4317, 1988.
155. Steck, P.A., Gallick, G.E., Maxwell, S.A., *et al.* Expression of the epidermal growth factor receptor and associated glycoprotein on cultured human brain tumor cells. J. Cell Biochem., *32*:1–10, 1986.
156. Steck, P.A., Lee, P., Hung, M.-C., *et al.* Expression of an altered epidermal growth factor receptor by human glioblastoma cells. Cancer Res., *48*:5433–5439, 1988.
157. Steinsvag, S.K., Laerum, O.R., and Bjerkvig, R. Interaction between rat glioma and normal rat brain tissue in organ culture. J. Natl. Cancer Inst., *74*:1095–1104, 1985.
158. Stiles, C.D. The molecular biology of platelet-derived growth factor. Cell, *33*:653–655, 1983.
159. Stratton, M.R., Darling, J., Pilkington, G.J., *et al.* Characterization of the human cell line TE671. Carcinogenesis, *10*:899–905, 1989.
160. Thomas, D.G.T. and Darling, J.L. In vitro chemosensitivity of human brain tumour tissue cultures and its relationship with relapse free interval. In: Adv. Biosci., *58*:135–143, 1986.
161. Thomas, D.G.T., Darling, J.L., Freshney, R.I., *et al.* In vitro chemosensitivity assay of human glioma by scintillation autofluorography. In: *Multidisciplinary Aspects of Brain Tumor Therapy,* edited by P. Pooletti, M.D. Walker, G. Butti, and R. Knerich. pp. 19–35. Amsterdam, Elsevier Biomedical Press, 1979.
162. Thomas, D.G.T., Darling, J.L., Paul, E.A., *et al.* Assay of anti-cancer drugs in tissue culture: relationship of relapse free interval (RFI) and in vitro chemosensitivity in patients with malignant cerebral glioma. Br. J. Cancer, *51*:525–532, 1985.
163. Trent, J., Meltzer, P., Rosenblum, M., *et al.* Evidence for rearrangement, amplification, and expression of c-myc in a human glioblastoma. Proc. Natl. Acad. Sci. USA, *83*:470–473, 1986.
164. Trojanowski, J.Q. and Lee, V.M.Y. Monoclonal and polyclonal antibodies against neural antigens: diagnostic applications for studies of central and peripheral nervous system tumors. Hum. Pathol., *14*:281–285, 1983.
165. Wahl, G.M. The importance of circular DNA in mammalian gene amplification. Cancer Res., *49*:1333–1340, 1989.
166. Walker, A.G., Chapman, J., Bruce, C.B., *et al.* Immunocytochemical characterization of cell cultures grown from dissociated 1-2 day post-natal rat cerebral tissue. J. Neuroimmunol., *7*:1–20, 1985.
167. Wallen, C.A., Michaelson, S.M., and Wheeler, K.T. Evidence for an unconventional radiosensitivity of rat 9L subcutaneous tumor. Radiat. Res., *84*:529–541, 1980.
168. Wang, S.L., Shiverick, K.T., Ogilvie, S., *et al.* Characterization of epidermal growth factor receptors in astrocytic glial and neuronal cells in primary culture. Endocrinology, *124*:240–247, 1989.
169. Wells, A., Bishop, J.M., and Helmeste, D. Amplified gene for the epidermal growth factor receptor in a human glioblastoma cell line encodes an enzymatically inactive protein. Mol. Cell. Biol., *8*:4561–4565, 1988.
170. Werner, M.H., Humphrey, P.A., Bigner, D.D., *et al.* Growth effect of epidermal growth factor (EGF) and a monoclonal antibody against the EGF receptor in five glioma cell lines. Acta Neuropathol. (Berl.), *77*:196–201, 1988.
171. Westermark, B. Density dependent proliferation of human glia cells stimulated by epidermal growth factor. Biochem. Biophys. Res. Commun., *69*:304–310, 1976.
172. Westermark, B., Heldin, C.-H., Elk, B., *et al.* Biochemistry and biology of platelet-derived growth factor. In: *Growth Factors and Maturation Factors, Vol. 1,* edited by G. Guroff. pp. 73–115. New York, Wiley, 1983.
173. Westermark, B., Magnusson, A., and Heldin, C.-H. Effect of epidermal growth factor on membrane motility and cell locomotion in cultures of clonal glioma cells. J. Neurosci. Res., *8*:491–507, 1982.
174. Westermark, B., Nister, M., and Heldin, C.-H. Growth factors and oncogenes in human malignant glioma. Neurol. Clin., *3*:785–799, 1985.
175. Westermark, B., Pontén, J., and Hugosson, R. Determinants for the establishment of permanent tissue culture lines from human gliomas. Acta Pathol. Microbiol. Immunol. Scand. [A], *81*:791–805, 1973.
176. Wibe, E., Berg, J.P., Tveit, K.M., *et al.* Multicellular spheroids grown directly from human tumour material. Int. J. Cancer, *34*:21–26, 1984.
177. Wikstrand, C.J. and Bigner, D.D. Use of monoclonal antibodies in neurobiology and neuro-oncology. In: *Monoclonal Antibodies in Cancer,* edited by S. Sell and R. Reisfeld, pp. 365–397. Clifton, N.J., The Humana Press, 1985.
178. Wong, A.J., Bigner, S.H., Bigner, D.D., *et al.* Increased expression of the EGF receptor gene in malignant gliomas is invariably associated with gene amplification. Proc. Natl. Acad. Sci. USA, *84*:6899–6903, 1987.
179. Wong, A.J., Ruppert, J.M., Bigner, S.H., *et al.* Structural alterations of the epidermal growth factor receptor gene in human gliomas. Nature, Submitted, 1990.
180. Wroblewska, Z., Devlin, M., Gilden, D.H., *et*

al. Human brain in tissue culture II. Studies of long-term cultures. J. Comp. Neurol., *161*:307–316, 1975.

181. Yamazaki, H., Fukui, Y., Ueyama, Y., *et al.* Amplification of the structurally and functionally altered epidermal growth factor receptor gene (c-erb B) in human brain tumors. Mol. Cell. Biol., *8*:1816–1820, 1988.

182. Yung, W.K.A., Gallick, G.E., Waterfield, M.D., *et al.* Expression of epidermal growth factor in culture human brain tumor cells (abstr.). J. Neurooncol., *4*:98, 1985.

183. Yung, W.K.A., Luna, M., and Borit, A. Vimentin and glial fibrillary acidic protein in human brain tumors. J. Neurooncol., *3*:35–38, 1985.

184. Zalutsky, M.R., Moseley, R.P., Coakham, H.B., *et al.* Pharmacokinetics and tumor localization of ^{131}I-labeled anti-tenascin monoclonal antibody 81C6 in patients with gliomas and other intracranial malignancies. Cancer Res., *49*:2807–2813, 1989.

CHAPTER 11

Biological Markers of Glial and Primitive Tumors

WILLEMINA M. MOLENAAR, M.D., Ph.D., and JOHN Q. TROJANOWSKI M.D., Ph.D.

INTRODUCTION

For many years the classification of brain tumors has been largely based on a morphological comparison of tumor cells with cells in the mature nervous system (171). In the absence of acceptable nonneoplastic, mature counterparts, tumors have been named after putative progenitor cells, e.g., medulloblastomas were named after the hypothetical medulloblast. However, solid evidence for the presumed origin of a neoplasm from a normal precursor cell is often lacking. The plethora of names applied to some neoplasms attests to the lack of objective scientific data on the nature of some of these tumors. In addition, morphological appearances may be deceiving; dissimilar appearing neoplasms may in fact be of the same type and similar appearing neoplasms may be totally unrelated to each other. The differential diagnosis of small cell neoplasms exemplifies this problem. Recent advances in immunology, cell biology and neurobiology have added a new dimension to tumor classification by providing a molecular basis for the comparison of neoplastic and nonneoplastic cells. The recognition of specific markers for the different cell types which comprise the central (CNS) and the peripheral nervous system (PNS) has improved our understanding of basic aspects of normal nervous system ontogeny and function and of neoplastic events (8, 57, 70, 182, 224). With continued improvements in such technologies as monoclonal antibody (MA) production, DNA cloning, immuno(histo)chemistry and in situ hybridization, the pace of acquisition of new knowledge in these areas will certainly quicken.

An ideal tumor marker from the point of view of diagnosis would be one which is expressed only by neoplastic cells of a given type. Ideally it should be possible to exploit such molecules for therapeutic purposes as well as early diagnosis. Despite the efforts of a large number of outstanding investigators, the identification of tumor specific markers has remained an elusive goal. In the absence of such markers, oncofetal antigens, i.e. antigens expressed only in ontogeny and by malignant cells, represent a reasonable compromise. Another reasonable alternative is the use of cell type specific markers, i.e. antigens restricted to only one class of cells, whether immature, mature or transformed.

This chapter discusses some of the innovations which are already changing the way clinicians evaluate and treat glial and primitive tumors of the CNS. These innovations are a direct result of the recognition of a vast array of antigens which are expressed by restricted populations of nervous system cells. With a combination of biochemical, immunochemical and immunohistochemical methods an increasing number of such molecular markers are being identified and characterized (8, 18, 23, 57, 70, 98, 150, 159, 161, 182, 208, 224, 227, 228). The markers discussed here are a small subset of nervous system specific molecules which have already been studied in normal brain or appear to be promising markers of glial and primitive brain tumors. Although they may be useful in a variety of different studies of tumor biology, this chapter emphasizes their potential for improving the diagnosis and classification of this group of tumors. It is anticipated that some of the more recently discovered CNS antigens not included in the present discussion will be exploited in future studies of brain tumors. Similarly, the rapidly evolving body of data on the expression of oncogenes in human malignancies will unmistakably lead to new approaches to the diagnosis and therapy of cancer (16). Consideration of these data is beyond the scope of the present review. It is also impossible to devote adequate attention to the technical aspects of these innovative methods. However, it cannot be emphasized enough that these important facets of modern immunology and cell biology should not be regarded as minor technical procedures. The essential probes in studies of antigens have been either monoclonal antibodies (MAs), or conventional antisera (AS) and it is absolutely essential that the interpretation of diagnostic tests which employ MAs or AS and modern immunological techniques be based on a solid understanding of the principles underlying these methods. Several detailed reviews considering such subjects as antibody production and characterization, the nature of an antigenic determinant or epitope, immunochemical methods and immunohistochemical procedures have appeared (8, 10, 53, 154, 190). Some general interpretive problems will be discussed and attention will be given to pitfalls in the use of certain markers in the discussion of glial and primitive brain tumors. However, since many of these problems are due to limitations in the immunochemical and immunohistochemical methods used to detect these markers, reference to more detailed reviews is necessary.

THE INTERPRETATION OF MARKER STUDIES

The results obtained with MAs or AS as to cell type specific antigens in brain tumors have to be interpreted cautiously and false negative or false positive findings should be avoided. In previous studies we have addressed the issue of false negative and false positive results in normal tissue, using MAs antibodies to neurofilament (NF) or glial filament (GF) proteins (83, 110, 112, 201, 211). It is apparent from these studies that no detail of tissue preparation and immunohistochemical processing is too trivial to merit attention and serious evaluation. Prospective studies of tumors processed by a variety of different methods are required if a better understanding of this potential problem is to be developed. The integration of immunohistochemistry into the diagnostic pathology laboratory will require new attitudes and approaches to the handling of biological materials by pathologists, if reliable immunohistochemical results are to be obtained using human tissues. MAs certainly help to standardize the immunochemical reagents used in diagnostic pathology, but they must still be used under appropriate conditions. For example, highly concentrated MAs with well-defined specificities may immunostain nonspecifically or yield false negative results if they are not used in a proper dilutional "window" (32). Further, MAs, no matter what their specificity or affinity, will not recognize a molecule if its epitopes are destroyed prior to its exposure to the MA. These issues may present a greater obstacle to the application of MAs for the detection of biological markers in brain tumors than the production and rigorous characterization of the MAs themselves.

As with the characterization of an MA, no single method will permit the confident conclusion that the protein detected in a tissue section is the same as the immunogen used to produce the MA being applied. Where possible immunochemical confirmation of the identity of an antigen recognized in tissue sections by immunochemistry is desirable. The evaluation of human brain tumors by both immunochemical and immunohistochemical methods may help to eliminate the risk of false-positive and false-negative results in immunohistochemical preparations. However, the use of the immunoblot method for this purpose is not without pitfalls as well. For example, the presence of degradation products arising from intermediate filament (IF) proteins in rapidly dividing tumors or tumors with necrosis may complicate analysis by this method. Furthermore, since some biological markers are relatively ubiquitous (for example, the neurofilament (NF) proteins in the nerves present throughout the body), it may be difficult to examine the antigens of neoplastic cells independent from normal, nonneoplastic structures presenting the same antigens.

CELL TYPE SPECIFIC BIOLOGICAL MARKERS FOR GLIAL AND PRIMITIVE BRAIN TUMORS

Cell type specific markers are not only of potential usefulness for the diagnosis of brain tumors, but they may also be exploited in the treatment of these neoplasms. For example, the de novo appearance or increased levels of such markers in the blood or cerebrospinal fluid could permit the early recognition of a brain tumor. The recognition of such markers in a brain biopsy would allow irrelevant diagnostic considerations to be eliminated from consideration. The biological markers of different CNS cell types which may be relevant in this respect are listed in Table 11.1. The function of most of these molecules is unknown. Nevertheless, many have been extensively studied and both amino acid composition data and partial gene sequences are available on some of them.

Of the markers listed in Table 11.1, the different classes of intermediate filaments (IF) appear to be among the most promising cell type specific markers under both normal and pathological conditions. Antibodies specific for each of these proteins are being used with increasing frequency in both applied and basic science studies of disease processes. Since the five classes of IF (neuro-, glial, vimentin, desmin and keratin filaments) are comprised of a family of polypeptides which are biochemically and immunochemically related, they will be discussed together as a group after the other markers are considered. Similarly, neuron specific enolase and nonneuronal enolase are discussed together as are the carbonic anhydrases and the neuroendocrine markers.

For a variety of reasons, a number of putative brain specific molecules or probes used for the identification of subsets of neurons and glia are not listed in Table 11.1, or if listed are not extensively considered here. This group includes S-100 protein, lectins, and markers of lymphoid and vascular elements. The calcium binding protein S-100, despite its initial promise as a marker of normal and neoplastic neurons and glia, has been clearly shown to be expressed by a wide variety of nonneural cells (23, 76, 141). Although S-100 surely plays an important role in calcium metabolism and possibly other cellular processes, its utility as a diagnostic marker for studies of brain tumors is questionable. The use of lectins to characterize tumors arising from different cell types or in different organs is actively under investigation. The results of such studies have recently been reviewed (33). Finally, the markers for lymphoid

TABLE 11.1.
Cell Type-Specific Markers of the Mature Central Nervous System[a]

Cell Type	Specific Marker or Antigen
Neurons	Neurofilament proteins* Neuron-specific enolase Cholera toxin "receptors" Tetanus toxin "receptors" Neurotransmitters and peptide hormones
Astrocytes	Glial and vimentin filament proteins* Nonneuronal enolase Carbonic anhydrase II
Oligodendroglia	Myelin basic protein and other myelin related proteins and glycolipids Carbonic anhydrase II
Epithelial cells	Keratin filament proteins* Epithelial membrane antigen
Lymphoid cells	Vimentin filament protein* B and T cell markers
Vascular cells	Desmin and vimentin filament proteins* Factor VIII

[a]This table lists the better characterized antigens or markers putatively specific for different cell types of the mature mammalian CNS. Although the distribution of these antigens has been relatively well-characterized in the normal, mature CNS of mammals, information concerning the distribution of these molecules in CNS cells affected by neoplastic and non-neoplastic disease states is incomplete. Furthermore, evidence from studies of the developing CNS suggests that some of these antigens may be expressed in immature but not in mature forms of these cells. For example, developing, but not mature oligodendroglia, have been found to express both GFAP and MBP. The *asterisks* identify the family of related polypeptides which comprise intermediate filaments, the cell type specific cytoskeletal elements present in most mammalian cells. Markers for epithelial cells (as seen in the pituitary gland), lymphoid and vascular cells are not discussed in detail since neoplastic cells derived from such elements are uncommonly found in glial and primitive brain tumors.

cells and vascular cells are listed for completeness in the table, but are not discussed here since lymphoid and vascular elements are, in general, incidental findings in glial and primitive brain tumors. The use of these markers as diagnostic probes has been reviewed elsewhere (18, 22, 23, 70, 73, 87, 94, 123, 124, 198).

Neuron-Specific and Nonneuronal Enolase

The enolase isoenzymes are a group of five dimeric proteins comprised of combinations of three different 40- to 50-kilodalton subunits: gamma, alpha and beta (120). They are enzymes of the glycolytic pathway that catalyze the interconversion of 2-phospho-D-glycerate and phosphoenolpyruvate. Neuron-specific enolase (NSE), originally termed 14-3-2 protein, is a homodimer composed of two gamma subunits. In the normal nervous system, NSE is restricted in its distribution to neurons of the CNS and PNS. Nonneuronal enolase (NNE), also termed liver enolase, is a homodimer of two alpha subunits and is the most widely distributed enolase isoenzyme. In the CNS it is found in glial cells but not in neurons or nonglial cell types. The third homodimer is formed from two beta subunits and is termed muscle enolase because it is restricted to muscle cells. Heterodimers comprised of an alpha and a beta, or an alpha and a gamma subunit exist, but their tissue distribution is not well described. However, cells of the diffuse neuroendocrine system (DNS), also called dispersed neuroendocrine cells (DNCs) or APUD (*A*mine *P*recursor *U*ptake and *D*ecarboxylation) cells, contain both immunoreactive alpha and gamma subunits under normal circumstances (120).

Because NSE is largely restricted to CNS and PNS neurons under normal circumstances, it was speculated that antibodies to NSE could be used for the identification of tumors of neuronal origin (23, 120, 213). Since the expression of NSE is developmentally regulated, it was possible that NSE might be used for the prognostic assessment of neoplasms in the expectation that more antigen would be expressed by better differentiated tumors and less by poorly differentiated neoplasms. Initial reports using antibodies to NSE as diagnostic reagents were encouraging (23, 57, 70, 76, 120, 213, 221).

However, two obstacles arose which seemed to preclude the use of this antigen as a neuronal marker under pathological conditions. First, it was appreciated that a group of MAs raised against NSE also recognized NNE, indicating that similar or identical epitopes were shared by both alpha and beta enolase subunits (74). This problem could be surmounted by the production of a larger library of MAs some of which should be specific for one or the other of the two subunits (177, 200). A more challenging problem was the observation that NSE is present in normal nonneuronal cells (78) and inducible under a large variety of pathological conditions (23, 221). NSE has now been detected in glial neoplasms, reactive astrocytes and in nonneuroepithelial tumors such as carcinomas and lymphomas (23, 221).

At present therefore, NSE appears to be a molecule which is an important marker for normal CNS and PNS neurons and the expression of the gamma enolase subunit can distinguish cells of the DNS from other nonneuronal cell types (23, 120). NSE also appears promising as a probe for the classification of tumors arising in the DNS (23, 120). However, antibodies against NSE are of limited use as reagents for the selective detection of tumors of neuronal origin or for the recognition of neuronal differentiation in a tumor.

Cholera Toxin "Receptors"

Cholera toxin (CT) is the exotoxin of *Vibrio cholerae*, the organism responsible for cholera, an intestinal infection leading to watery diarrhea, dehydration and metabolic acidosis (85). CT is an 84-kilodalton polypeptide comprised of 5 binding or B subunits (each with a mol wt of 11.5-kilodalton) and an active or A subunit of mol wt 28-kilodalton which is the toxic fragment. The A and B subunits are linked by noncovalent interactions. The A subunit contains an A-1 (mol wt 21kD) and an A-2 (mol wt 7kD) subunit linked by disulfide bonds. CT, through the B subunit, binds to monosialoganglioside (GM1), the membrane "receptor" for CT, and is internalized. This leads to diarrhea via an A-1 subunit mediated activation of cyclic AMP. The B subunit is nontoxic. Although "receptors" for CT are present on mucosal cells of the intestine, and other cells, neurons are particularly rich in GM1. CT has thus been used as a marker for neurons in culture. For example, a recent report utilized CT and anti-CT MAs to identify neurons in culture (145). These included primary cultures of normal CNS and PNS neurons and a rat pheochromocytoma cell line which expresses the phenotypic features of neurons after exposure to nerve growth factor. Cultured Schwann cells, fibroblasts and glial cells were negative. Since GM1 is expressed by CNS glial cells, although to a lesser extent than by neurons, caution should be exercised in the interpretation of results obtained using CT as a recognition molecule for cell types within or outside the CNS. Nevertheless, studies such as the one just described suggest that CT or the B subunit of CT may be of potential use in diagnostic studies of human brain tumors.

Tetanus Toxin "Receptors"

Tetanus toxin (TT) is a potent neurotoxin produced by the gram positive bacillus *Clostridium tetani* (19). Like CT, TT is comprised of a binding subunit and a toxic subunit and is internalized after binding to its "receptors", i.e. di- and trisialogangliosides. In its extracellular form, TT has a mol wt of 150 kilodalton and is comprised of two polypeptide chains of mol wt 100-kilodalton and 50-kilodalton linked by disulfide bonds. Although the mode of action of TT is unknown, it has been demonstrated that the heavy subunit is nontoxic and mediates the binding of TT to the cell surface; the light subunit mediates the toxic effects of TT.

A number of studies have employed TT, like CT, as a probe for identifying neurons in culture (19, 57, 99). Because of the toxicity of TT, nontoxic fragments have been developed for investigative use. For example, Koulakoff *et al.* (99) have recently described the use of a 46-kilodalton nontoxic fragment of TT, designated the IIc fragment, for studies of neuronal differentiation in the developing mouse nervous system. The IIc fragment, produced by papain digestion of native TT, was incubated with cells and localized on the cell surface of neurons using an anti-TT AS and a rhodamine labeled anti-immunoglobulin antibody. To what extent it would be feasible to apply this approach to studies of human brain tumors remains to be determined. In addition, the distribution of other potential TT binding sites needs to be assessed. For example, gangliosides on the plasma membrane of thyroid cells, which are part of the receptor for thyrotropin, also bind iodinated TT (19). Nevertheless, the initial studies on the use of TT and its nontoxic derivatives for the detection of neurons are encouraging. Further studies must evaluate the usefulness of these probes in neurooncology.

Myelin Basic Protein and Other Myelin Proteins and Glycolipids

CNS myelin is comprised of a number of different proteins and glycolipids, some of which are also present in PNS myelin. The major CNS myelin proteins are myelin basic protein (MBP), myelin associated glycoprotein (MAG), P2 protein, proteolipid and Wolfgram proteins (79, 227). MAG, P0, P1 and P2 are some of the major proteins of PNS myelin. Galactocerebroside (GalC) is a major glycolipid present in both CNS and PNS myelin which is expressed on the cell surface of oligodendrocytes and Schwann cells.

MBP comprises about 30% of myelin proteins and is one of the best studied of the myelin proteins. It has a mol wt of 18 kilodaltons and is thought to be identical to or nearly identical to P1 protein in PNS myelin. MBP contains an encephalitogenic portion which is responsible for the induction of experimental allergic encephalomyelitis but its function under normal circumstances is not understood. In embryogenesis, MBP can be detected in the cytoplasm of oligodendroglial cells by immunohistochemistry, but in the mature CNS it is localized in myelin sheaths, specifically, the major dense line of myelin lamellae, and not in the cell bodies of oligodendrocytes (83, 88, 146, 191). Recent studies with antibodies to MBP and glial fibrillary acidic protein (GFAP) indicate that immature human glial cells transiently express both GFAP and MBP (30). In the adult nervous system this does not appear to be the case although tumors diagnosed by conventional criteria as pure oligodendrogliomas have been observed to contain a variable number of GFAP positive cells. In primary cultures of rat optic nerve cells, the culture medium can be manipulated such that cells express both GFAP and GalC (157). Thus it appears that a common glial progenitor cell, under the influence of environmental cues, is programmed to become a mature astrocyte (GFAP positive, GalC negative), or a mature oligodendrocyte (GalC positive, GFAP negative), and express the phenotypic features of either of these terminally differentiated glial cell types. These important observations, as discussed later, have implications for the use of cell type specific molecules as potential histogenetic markers.

Using immunofluorescence and either antiserum or MAs specific for GalC, this antigen has been shown to be a reliable marker for myelin forming cells, especially in primary cultures of CNS or PNS cells (157, 158, 167). However, its usefulness as a biological marker for neoplastic human oligodendroglial cells has not been explored as yet. Although antibodies specific for P2 and P0 have been used for the study of extra-CNS tumors (139), antibodies to CNS myelin proteins have not been successfully used to study CNS tumors. One report has demonstrated MBP in the neural foci commonly seen in human teratomas; however, the immunoreactivity was confined to myelin sheaths and was not seen in the cytoplasm of the myelin forming cells of teratomas (206). Nevertheless, the presence of MBP appeared to correlate with the presence of mature elements and the absence of immature elements in these tumors and therefore appears to be promising for the prognostic evaluation of human teratomas.

Carbonic Anhydrase Isoenzymes

Carbonic anhydrase (CA) isoenzymes are a multigene family of zinc metalloenzymes which catalyze the reversible hydration of carbon dioxide and other compounds (197). The mammalian CA isoenzymes are proteins composed of about 260 amino acid residues for which a considerable amount of structural and gene sequence data exist. A low activity (CAI) and high activity (CAII) isoenzyme have been described. A recently identified third isoenzyme is designated CAIII. It appears to be less active enzymatically than CAI and CAII. The structures of all three isoenzymes are similar, and human CAI and CAII are 60% homologous with respect to their amino acid composition, although a large number of CAI and CAII variants, due to amino acid substitutions, have been recognized in humans.

CA isoenzymes are widely distributed in plants and animals and in different mammalian tissues, as might be expected considering their important function (197). CA activity can be demonstrated in tissue histochemically using Hansson's cobalt-phosphate method, but this technique does not discriminate between the different CA isoenzymes in situ. Using AS for the different CA isoenzymes, the distribution of CAI, CAII and CAIII can be independently mapped with immunohistochemical methods. With this approach, CAIII has been found principally in muscle and a few other tissues. In thus appears to have a more limited distribution than CAI and CAII. Although CAII is the most widely distributed isoenzyme, in brain it appears to be found predominantly in oligodendroglia and to a lesser extent in astrocytes and choroid plexus epithelium. CAII does not appear to be expressed by neurons, but this is controversial (197). A recent study in human tissues documented the presence of immunoreactive CAII in oligodendrocytes, but not in astrocytes and neurons of the cerebrum and cerebellum (103). Two oligodendrogliomas which were examined by the same methods were negative for immunoreactive CAII. This may reflect altered genetic expression, metabolism, etc. of CAII in these neoplasms. Issues such as these will require further investigation. CAII may prove to be a useful biological marker for glial neoplasms, but this remains to be determined by future investigations.

Neuroendocrine Markers

The recognition of a system of dispersed neuroendocrine cells (DNCs) has provided a conceptual link between the nervous system and the endocrine system. The DNCs share with neurons the ability for uptake and decarboxylation of amine precursors (i.e. APUD cells; for review: ref. 5). However, they deliver these transmitters not by way of synapses, as neurons do, but by way of the bloodstream, as endocrine organs, or by local diffusion (101). The close relations between neuroendocrine cells and neurons are presumably best exemplified by, and most extensively studied in, the adrenal medulla, where both chromaffin cells and neurons express neurofilaments (6, 136, 209). Morcover, the development of a chromaffin or neuronal phenotype in medullary cells appears to be influenced by local factors (4, 115, 144, 214). Neuroendocrine tumors may share neurofilament positivity with neural tumors and keratin positivity with epithelial tumors. On this basis, it has been suggested that "neural" and "epithelial" neuroendocrine tumors should be distinguished (65, 66).

The following reviews some of the markers which may be used to further explore the relations between neuroectodermal and neuroendocrine tumors.

Synaptophysin

Synaptophysin is an integral membrane glycoprotein originally isolated and characterized by Wiedenmann *et al.* (225) from presynaptic vesicles in bovine brain neurons. Recent studies suggest that its function is in the Ca^{++} dependent release of neurotransmitters (162, 199). Since the development of MAs to synaptophysin (225, 226) the glycoprotein has been probed for in many normal tissues and neoplasms, but it has been reported that its immunoreactivity is dependent on tissue fixation (86). Synaptophysin has been demonstrated in many central and peripheral neurons, in adult adrenal medulla and in many neuroendocrine cells (65, 86, 225, 226). In developing rat cerebellar cortex synaptophysin expression was found to increase with maturation, but it was present already before synapses were established (106). In human fetal adrenal medulla synaptophysin expression was demonstrable as early as the 9th gestational week (136).

To date, synaptophysin has been used as a marker for neuroendocrine differentiation in many neoplasms (64–66, 75, 131, 132, 134, 183, 225, 226) and it has been demonstrated in both peripheral (66, 75, 131, 132, 226) and central neuroectodermal tumors (64–66, 134, 183). In our study (132) synaptophysin expression was more prominent in ganglion cells of ganglioneuroblastomas and ganglioneuromas than in the primitive cells of neuroblastomas, a phenomenon which may be related to an increase of synaptophysin expression during maturation (106). Moreover, in the CNS, synaptophysin was expressed in primitive neuroectodermal tumors (PNETs), but not in other tumor types and may thus serve as an aid in the histopathological diagnosis (64, 134). The demonstration of synaptophysin in neuroectodermal tumors lends support to the suggestion that these tumors may be considered as the "neural" branch of the family of neuroendocrine tumors.

Chromogranin A

Chromogranin A is the major constituent of the proteins isolated from vesicles in adrenal chromaffin cells (187) and has a mol wt of 70- to 80-kilodaltons. With the aid of MAs chromogranin A has been demonstrated in a wide variety of neuroendocrine cells and their tumors (42, 77, 116–118, 142). The protein has also been demonstrated in neurons of the peripheral and central nervous system, at least in nonhuman mammals, where it was localized either in the perikarya or in the region of the axon terminals (42, 187). Although chromogranin A has been demonstrated in peripheral neuroblastomas, ganglioneuroblastomas and ganglioneuromas (75, 132), we are not aware of reports of its presence in tumors of the CNS.

Moc-antibodies

Moc-antibodies represent a panel of MAs raised against small cell lung carcinoma (44–48, 156), an example of an "epithelial" member of the neuroendocrine family. These MAs have been tested on a wide range of normal fetal and adult human tissues and neoplasms, but the molecular structure of the antigens which they recognize is not fully known. On the basis of their immunoreactivity with normal and tumor tissues, three different subsets may be defined, i.e., (*a*) a neural/neuroendocrine subset, reacting with most neuroendocrine and neural structures and tumors, (*b*) an epithelial subset, reacting with neuroendocrine and epithelial structures and their tumors and (*c*) a neural subset, reacting with neuroendocrine tumors and, in normal tissues, primarily with neural structures. MAs of the neural/neuroendocrine subset appeared to be highly reactive with both peripheral and central neuroectodermal tumors (133). In contrast to the findings with synaptophysin, reactivity with these Moc-antibodies was observed in PNETs as well as in astrocytomas and ependymomas. MAs of the neural subset were reactive with ganglioneuroblastomas and ganglioneuromas but only to a limited extent with neuroblastomas and hardly at all with central tumors. Obviously, these MAs need further evaluation. However, the available data suggest that they may evolve to be markers for the level of differentiation in neuroectodermal tissues rather than markers for cell lineage. The epithelial subset, which was basically unreactive with all tested neuroectodermal tumors, may serve to distinguish the "neural" from the "epithelial" members of the neuroendocrine family.

Neuropeptides

Perhaps the most direct link between cells of the neuroendocrine system and those of the nervous system is their sharing of polypeptides, which may serve as hormones or neurotransmitters. Although the function of polypeptides in the neuroendocrine system has long been established, their significance for the normal human brain has only recently gained acceptance (84, 101). Surprisingly, a recent study (186) showed that neonatal rat astrocytes also produce neuropeptides. In line with the identification of polypeptides in normal neurons, several neuropeptides have now been demonstrated in neuroectodermal tumors of both the PNS (117, 127) and the CNS (64, 194). These data indicate that the similarities between the neuroendocrine system and the nervous system may remain in the neoplastic state.

Intermediate Filament Proteins

The polypeptides which comprise intermediate filaments (IFs) are a family of different classes of developmentally regulated proteins which are biochemically quite similar (89, 105). IFs are filamentous structures, 10 nm, in diameter, so named because they are intermediate in diameter between actin filaments (4–6 nm) and microtubules (22–24 nm). By conventional transmission electron microscopy the different classes are indistinguishable except for NFs which have distinctive sidearm projections (89, 170, 223). IFs form part of the cytoskeleton of nearly all mammalian cells, but their precise function is unknown (104, 170, 223). Each class of IFs, with the exception of vimentin filaments, is restricted to limited cell types, at least in mature cells (68, 216).

At least five types of IFs can be distinguished (Table 11.2) according to their cell type specific expression patterns in mature cells and the intron and exon structure of their genes (149, 150, 189, 223). Types I-IV are cytoplasmic filaments, while the type V IFs, comprised of lamins (125, 189), are present within the nucleus. Type I and type II keratins are expressed primarily in epithelial cells, at least in mammals (137, 161, 216), but a wider distribution of keratins in other, non-epithelial, cell types now seems likely based on recent studies of submammalian species (59, 97, 169). Type III IFs exhibit a heterogeneous pattern of cellular expression and this class of IFs includes desmin, vimentin and glial filaments. These IFs are expressed primarily in muscle, mesenchymal and glial cells, respectively. A fourth type III IF, known as peripherin or the neuron-specific type III IF, has been described recently and added to the family of IFs (2, 153, 155). Peripherin is found in a subset of CNS and PNS neurons. The type IV IFs are neurofilaments (NFs) which are much more widely expressed in

TABLE 11.2.
Intermediate Filament Proteins[a]

IF Class	Type	Polypeptide Composition	Normal Distribution
Keratin filaments	I and II	A family of 20 different polypeptides ranging from 40 to 68 kilodaltons	Keratinizing and nonkeratinizing epithelial cells
Glial filaments	III	51-kilodalton protein	Astroglia, rarely ependymal cells
Vimentin filaments	III	57-kilodalton protein	Mesenchymal cells, coexpressed with other IF classes
Desmin filaments	III	53-kilodalton protein	Smooth, striated and cardiac muscle
Peripherin	III	57-kilodalton protein	A subset of CNS and PNS neurons
Neurofilaments	IV	68-, 150-, and 200-kilodalton protein subunits	CNS and PNS neurons, axons and dendrites
Lamin	V	60–70 kilodaltons	Cell nuclei

[a] This table lists the major classes of IF proteins, their type as defined by their expression pattern in mature cells and the intron/exon structure of their genes, the polypeptides which comprise them and the cells in which they are found under normal circumstances.

CNS and PNS neurons than peripherin. They differ considerably from the other cytoplasmic IFs because of their unique intron/extron structure, heteropolymeric composition of three different subunits, large subunit size and extensive phosphorylation of the two large neurofilament (NF) subunits (see below).

Antibodies to IF proteins were first introduced into pathology for the diagnostic evaluation of human tumors by Duffy *et al.* (51) and Deck *et al.* (40) in 1977 and 1978. These investigators used antibodies against GFAP, produced by Eng and co-workers to identify neoplastic astrocytes in a group of human brain tumors. They concluded that tumors with cells that expressed GFAP were astrocytomas, i.e., they were derived from astrocytes. The early studies of GFAP expression subsequently led to the development of three important hypotheses concerning the expression of IF proteins in normal and neoplastic cells:

a) IFs are composed of immunochemically distinct proteins

b) IF proteins are relatively cell type specific

c) Neoplastic cells express the same IF proteins as their presumed progenitor cells. These hypotheses are the essential assumptions on which the use of these markers in diagnostic pathology is based; they continue to be the subject of intensive research. Thus far, with few qualifications, these hypotheses appear to be substantiated.

The introduction of anti-GFAP antibodies in neuropathology soon led to the use of antibodies to vimentin, keratin and desmin for diagnostic studies of extra-CNS tumors in general pathology (3, 67, 69, 100, 130, 150, 159, 161, 222). More recently, anti-NF antibodies have been used for the diagnosis of CNS (95, 96, 201–203, 208, 210) and extra-CNS (7, 28, 31, 112, 138, 140, 147, 163, 166, 172, 185, 206) tumors with similar effectiveness. In addition, it is becoming clear that IF proteins are implicated in a wide variety of nonneoplastic conditions such as alcoholic liver disease and senile dementia of the Alzheimer type (26, 49, 170, 178–181, 229). Thus, antibodies specific for different IF polypeptides are being used with increasing frequency not only for the assessment of neoplastic lesions but also in basic and applied studies of a large variety of nonneoplastic lesions.

It has become clear since the original observations by Deck *et al.* and Duffy *et al.*, that the interpretation of immunohistochemical studies which employ anti-IF specific antibodies is not as straight forward as might have appeared several years ago. For instance, the lack of objective criteria which permit the discrimination of reactive from neoplastic cells is a limitation in the use of cell type specific markers. This may be exemplified by the use of anti-NF and anti-GFAP MAs to detect neurons and astrocytes in gangliogliomas. Since NF and GFAP are cell type specific markers for neurons and astrocytes, respectively, it is clear that the cells in the tumor which express NF proteins are neurons or neuron-like cells, and those which express GFAP in the tumor are astrocytes. However, since the antibodies do not discriminate between normal and neoplastic cells, subjective cytological criteria must be applied in order to determine if these cells are indeed neoplastic. Thus, of the three labeled neurons in Figure 11.1G, only the two binucleated cells are definitely neoplastic. It is possible that the abnormal appcarance or composition of the IF of neoplastic cells may aid in the differentiation of reactive from neoplastic cells. For example, aggregates of immunoreactive NF proteins have thus far only been seen in diseased and not in normal neurons (109, 111).

Three classes of IF predominate in the CNS and its tumors, i.e., NFs, GFAP and vimentin and each of them will be discussed in more detail.

Neurofilaments

NFs are type IV IFs and are composed of heteropolymers of three different subunits. The three subunits have molecular weights of 68, 150, and 200 kilodaltons and are referred to as low (L), medium (M) and high (H) molecular weight subunits (107, 108, 114, 143, 175, 176, 212). All three subunits are widely expressed in neurons of the CNS and PNS. With the exception of a report that NF-L is present in chicken erythrocytes (71), NF proteins have not been detected in normal cells other than neurons and adrenal chromaffin cells (136, 209). NFs have been demonstrated in neoplasms of presumed neuronal (Table 11.3), as well as in some tumors of presumed nonneuronal (Table 11.4) origin (e.g. Merkel cell tumors).

A wide variety of MAs to different NF subunits is now available and several of them also recognize the phosphorylation state of NF-M and NF-H (107, 178, 208, 212). However, it is important to emphasize that tissue preparative methods significantly affect the immunoreactivity of these antigens. For example, extensive evaluation of the fixation dependent alterations in NF subunit immunoreactivity in neuronal cell bodies, axons and dendrites revealed dramatic differences in the apparent distribution of NF subunit antigens as a result of the use of different fixatives (83, 212). This is an important point to keep in mind in the study of brain and other tumors.

Glial Filaments

The first polypeptide to be identified as the major component of an IF class was a glial protein, a 50- to 52-kilodalton protein which Eng and co-workers initially isolated over 15 years ago from multiple sclerosis plaques and termed glial fibrillary acidic protein or GFAP (15, 54–56). In the CNS GFAP is expressed by fibrous astrocytes (but only by reactive and not normal protoplasmic astrocytes), rare ependymal cells, cerebellar radial glia and Mueller cells of the retina. Mature oligodendrocytes do not express GFAP, but, in the developing nervous system of the rat, cells which transiently express both GFAP and MBP have been detected (30). This finding is of interest in view of a recent study (17) which suggests that coexpression of GFAP and oligodendroglial markers may also occur in human astrocytomas. MAs have been reported which recognize GFAP, but a num-

Figure 11.1. Immunoperoxidase studies of cerebellar PNETs (A-E) and other pediatric brain tumors. *A*) Neuropil staining for tau protein (paraffin section); *B*) perikaryal staining for NF-M- (frozen section); *C*) H&E demonstrating follicular pattern (paraffin section); *D*) follicular, neuropil staining for MAP-2 in the same case as in *C*) (frozen section); *E*) predominantly follicular staining for GFAP in the same case as *C*) and *D*) (frozen section); *F*) cytoplasmic staining for EMA in an atypical teratoid tumor (paraffin section) and *G*) staining for NF-M/H+ of binucleated neurons in a ganglioglioma (*arrows*, paraffin section). f, follicle, N, neuropil. Bar corresponds to 25 μm in *G*), to 50 μ in A), B) and F) and to 100μ in C) and D). (Reprinted with permission from Molenaar, W.M., Jansson, D., Gould, V.E., *et al.* Molecular markers of primitive neuroectodermal tumors (PNETs) and other pediatric central nervous system tumors. Monoclonal antibodies to neuronal and glial antigens distinguish subsets of PNETs. Lab. Invest., *61*:635–643, 1989.)

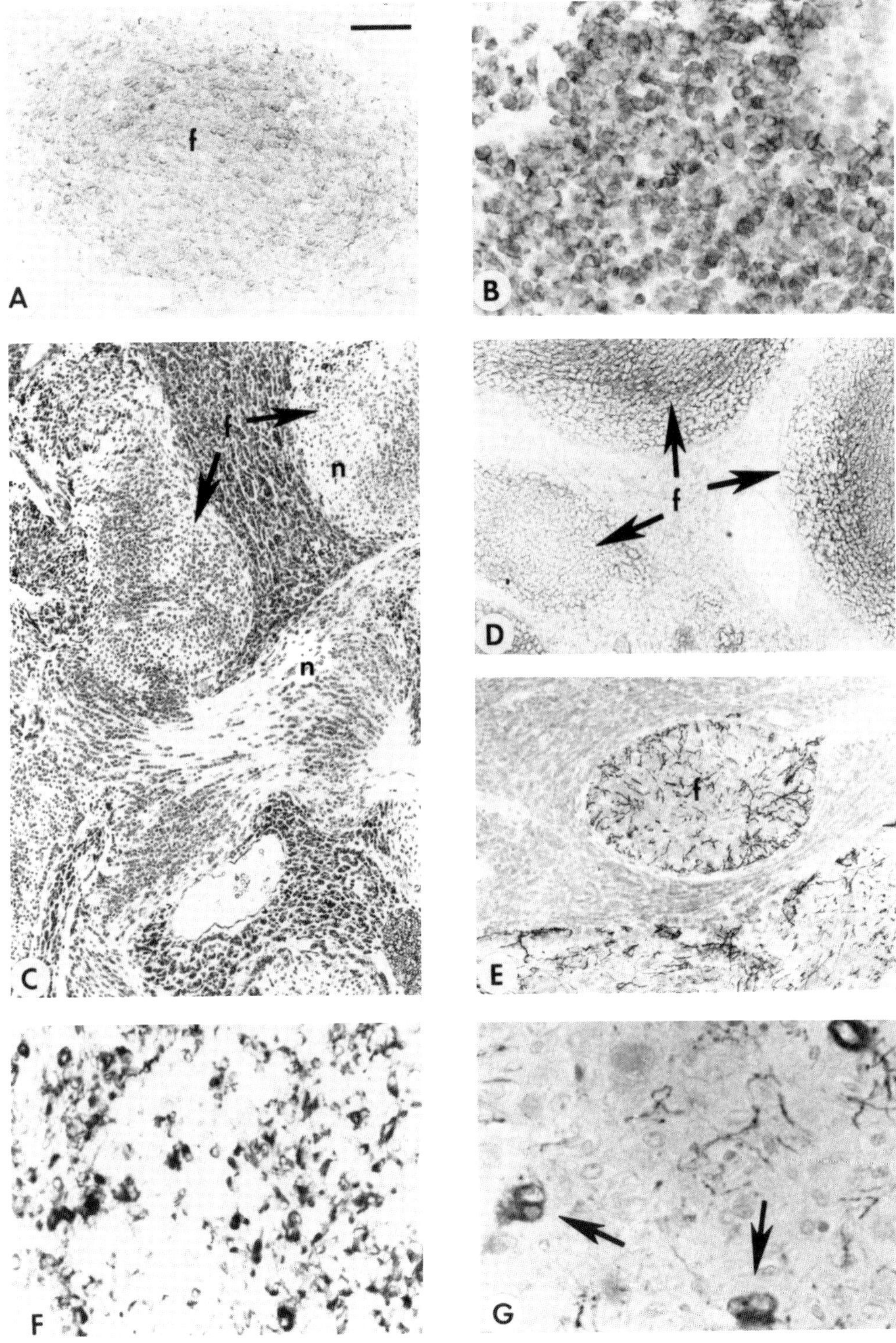
A
f
B
C
f
n
n
D
f
E
f
F
G

TABLE 11.3.
CNS Tumors with NF- or GFAP-Positive Cells[a]

Tumor	NF	GFAP
Astroblastoma	−	+
Astrocytoma	−	+
Cerebral neuroblastoma	+	+
Choroid plexus papilloma	−	+
Ependymoma	−	+
Ganglioglioma	+	+
Gemistocytic astrocytoma	−	+
Hemangioblastoma	−	+
Medulloblastoma*	+	+
Mixed glioma	−	+
Oligodendroglioma	−	−
Pineoblastoma*	+	+
Pineocytoma	−	+
Pituitary adenoma	−	+
Pleomorphic xanthoastrocytoma	NT	+
Retinoblastoma*	−	+
Subependymal giant cell astrocytoma	−	+
Subependymoma	−	+

[a]Common CNS tumors found to express either or both NF and GFAP are listed here. These data are summarized, among others, from the following references: 23, 24, 40, 41, 50–52, 55, 72, 128, 135, 147, 161, 196, 202, 203, 222. NT, not tested. Tumors indicated with an * are included in the group of tumors designated primitive neuroectodermal tumors (9, 165, 166).

TABLE 11.4.
Extracranial Tumors with NF or GFAP-Positive Cells[a]

Tumor	NF	GFAP
Carcinoid	+	−
Esthesioneuroblastoma	+	−
Ewing's sarcoma	+	−
Ganglioneuroblastoma	+	+
Ganglioneuroma	+	+
"Merkel cell tumor" of the skin	+	−
Neuroblastoma	+	+
Oat cell carcinoma	+	−
Paraganglioma	+	−
Pheochromocytoma	+	−
Pleomorphic adenoma	−	+
Teratoma	+	+

[a]Extracranial neoplasms which express NF and/or GFAP are listed here. This table summarizes data obtained, among others, from the following references: 55, 112, 132, 147, 161, 216, 222. The expression of NFs in a Ewing's sarcoma is a personal observation, which is in keeping with findings in cell lines (29).

ber of them recognize epitopes present on GFAP and other IF proteins such as NF subunits and vimentin (39, 67, 110) as well. Thus it is likely that MAs to GFAP contain species of antibodies which recognize epitopes common to more than one class of IF proteins. This may explain some of the controversy surrounding the localization of GFAP in the PNS and in cells outside the CNS and PNS (20, 38, 55, 80, 91–93, 230).

In addition to the sites mentioned above, immunoreactive GFAP has been reported in Schwann cells, enteric glia, cells in all portions of the pituitary gland, Kupfer cells of the liver, the iris, lens epithelium, and in some tumors not generally considered to be of glial origin, such as pleomorphic adenomas (1, 20, 24, 38, 55, 80, 126, 188, 205, 220). To what extent the localization of GFAP in cells outside the CNS might represent cross-reaction of anti-GFAP antisera with vimentin protein or other proteins remains to be shown. Eng and co-workers have convincingly demonstrated that lens epithelial cells contain a protein which is immunochemically identical to GFAP in CNS glia (80). Similar combined immunohistochemical and immunochemical studies will help to resolve this issue in other organs.

Vimentin

The major polypeptide of the IF of mesenchymal cells is vimentin, a 57-kilodalton protein (104, 148, 189, 222). Vimentin has a wide distribution and is seen in such mature cells as fibroblasts, chondrocytes, lymphoid cells, and endothelial cells. Vimentin may also coexist in some mature cells with any of the other classes of IF. In the immature mammal, vimentin may be expressed in a cell before it becomes differentiated only to be replaced later by another class of IF appropriate for the differentiated cell type (11, 105, 148, 195, 217). In addition, vimentin is expressed in neoplasms or in vitro even by cells that do not express it in vivo (63, 109, 111, 160). The mechanisms regulating the induction of vimentin in vitro are unclear, but increased levels of vimentin, as well as NF, can be induced in a rat pheochromocytoma cell line by nerve growth factor (109, 111). Thus of all classes of IF vimentin is the least cell type specific. However, since vimentin is expressed in embryogenesis prior to GFAP or NF in astrocytes and neurons, respectively, its presence or absence may be of prognostic significance. This notion remains to be tested, since there is little information available on the usefulness of antivimentin antibodies for the diagnostic evaluation of human brain tumors.

MAs specific for vimentin have been produced. Some recognize only the 57 kilodalton protein known to comprise this class of IFs, while others recognize epitopes present on other IF proteins as well (39, 69, 110).

Studies of Human Glial and Primitive Brain Tumors with Antibodies to Intermediate Filaments

To date, several studies have been published applying MAs to IF proteins to astrocytic tumors of the adult and pediatric CNS. As expected, these demonstrate that astrocytomas express GFAP as well as vimentin (29, 40, 50, 51, 82, 130, 134, 135, 173, 219). Somewhat unexpectedly, it has been reported that some tumor cells are also immunoreactive for keratin proteins (34). However, such "aberrant" keratin expression has now been described for several nonepithelial tumors and even normal cells, including amphibian optic nerve astrocytes (97, 169).

Not only astrocytomas, but also gangliogliomas, ependymomas and rhabdoid (14, 90) and malignant teratoid tumors (113) were found to express GFAP (37, 128, 129, 135). As mentioned above, gangliogliomas combine GFAP expression (Fig. 11.1G) with expression of NF proteins, whereas the other three tumor types combine GFAP expression with expression of vimentin and an epithelial marker, i.e. keratin and/or epithelial membrane antigen (Fig. 11.1F; refs. 36, 37, 128, 129, 135).

Among the tumors of the CNS the group of primitive neuroectodermal tumors (PNETs) takes a special position. As the name implies, such tumors are composed of primitive cells of presumed neuroectodermal origin (9, 64, 65). They almost exclusively occur in children and are most frequently located in the cerebellum, where they are called medulloblastomas (168, 171, 215). However, they may occur in adults and at other sites and other names have been given to histologically similar tumors according to their site (168, 171, 215). Several studies of such tumors using MAs and AS to GFAP (25, 95, 96, 102, 119, 121, 152, 201), to vimentin (201) and to NFs (25, 35, 95, 96, 201, 218) have been reported. These studies indicate that GFAP is the most frequently expressed IF, followed by vimentin, whereas NFs are expressed only in a limited number of cases. However, most of these studies were performed on formalin-fixed material. In a recent prospective study (135) we examined a large group of pediatric CNS tumors, either fixed in Bouin's fixative or fresh frozen, for immunologic evidence of neuronal or glial differentiation by probing them with a panel of well-defined and extensively characterized MAs. Since it has become increasingly clear that the recognition of NFs by different MAs may depend on the phosphorylation state of the NF proteins (21, 107, 178, 202, 203, 208, 212), MAs and AS that recognize phosphorylated, non-phosphorylated or phosphorylation independent NF subunit epitopes were used. With these antibodies NF expression was demonstrated in 20 out of 37 PNETs of the CNS (Fig. 11.1*B*). Neuronal differentiation was further substantiated by immunoreactivity for the neuronal microtubule-associated protein MAP2 (Fig. 11.1*D*) in six and for tau-protein (Fig. 11.1A) in 13 of these cases. The staining pattern for NF as well as for MAP2 and tau protein was either perikaryal or diffuse in fine fibrillary extensions of the tumor cells (neoplastic neuropil). In contrast to older studies (25, 219) NF proteins were demonstrated in cells that were morphologically primitive and indistinguishable from their nonreactive neighbors. Another interesting finding that emerged is the pattern of expression of NF subunits and phosphoisoforms (Table 11.5). Thus, it was found that the nonphosphorylated phosphoisoform of NF-M was most frequently expressed, usually with NF-L. Phosphorylated NF-M and especially NF-H were expressed only in cases that also expressed nonphosphorylated NF-M with or without NF-L. Moreover, only poorly phosphorylated NF-H was expressed and not intermediate or heavily phosphorylated NF-H. These findings are reminiscent of the changes that occur during normal mammalian development, i.e. NF-M and NF-L

TABLE 11.5.
Neural Markers in PNETS

PNET	NF-L	NF-M^{ind}	NF-M/H^{-}	NF-M^{+}	NF-H/M^{+}	NF-H^{+}	Tau	MAP2	GFAP
1	+++	+++	+++	+++	++	++	−	−	R
2	+++	+++	+++	+++	++	++	−	−	++
3	+	+++	+++/P	+++	−	+	+/P	−	+
4	+++	+++	++	++	+++	−	−	−	+
5	+++	+++	+++	++	++	−	+/P	−	+
6	+	++	+/P	++	−	+	−	−	+
7	P	++	−	+	+/P	−	−	−	+
8	+	−	++/P	−	−	−	+/P	P	++
9	++	++	+	+	−	−	−	−	+
10	−	+	+/P	−	−	−	++/P	P	E
11	−	+	+	−	−	−	P	−	−
12	−	−	+/P	−	−	−	−	P	−
13	−	−	+/P	−	−	−	P	−	+
14	−	P	P	P	P	P	P	P	+++
15	−	P	P	P	−	−	P	P	+
16	−	P	P	−	−	−	P	−	R
17	−	−	P	−	−	−	P	−	+
18	−	−	P	−	−	−	P	P	R
19	−	−	P	−	−	−	P	−	R
20	−	−	P	−	−	−	P	−	−
21	−	−	−	−	−	−	−	−	+++
22	−	−	−	−	−	−	−	−	+++
23	−	−	−	−	−	−	−	−	++
24	−	−	−	−	−	−	−	−	++
25	−	−	−	−	−	−	−	−	+
26	−	−	−	−	−	−	−	−	+
27	−	−	−	−	−	−	−	−	E
28	−	−	−	−	−	−	−	−	E
29	−	−	−	−	−	−	−	−	E
30	−	−	−	−	−	−	−	−	E
31	−	−	−	−	−	−	−	−	E
32	−	−	−	−	−	−	−	−	E
33	−	−	−	−	−	−	−	−	R
34	−	−	−	−	−	−	−	−	R
35	−	−	−	−	−	−	−	−	−
36	−	−	−	−	−	−	−	−	−
37	−	−	−	−	−	−	−	−	−

[a] Summary of the results obtained with Mabs to NF-protein isoforms, MAPs and GFAP. The numbers in the first column refer to case numbers. Results of Mabs with similar recognition patterns are combined and Mabs that gave no positive results in any case are omitted. M/H$^{ind,\ -,\ +}$: Mabs that recognize NF-isoforms independent of phosphorylation, only in nonphosphorylated state or only in phosphorylated state, respectively. For further details on antibodies see refs. 27, 78, 107, and 110. −, no staining; +, scattered positive tumor cells; ++, groups of positive tumor cells; +++, confluent fields of positive tumor cells; P, neuropil staining; R, positive cells identified as reactive astrocytes; E, positive cells equivocal, i.e., reactive astrocytes or tumor cells.

appear before NF-H and NF-M, and NF-M and NF-H are first synthesized and then phosphorylated (11, 12, 27, 58, 151, 184, 193). It thus appears that the least neuronally differentiated PNETs have a NF complement comparable to very early neuronal development, but that even the most neuronally differentiated PNETs have not reached a fully mature state as far as NFs are concerned. The findings in PNETs contrast with those in neuroectodermal tumors of the peripheral nervous system, where all of 12 studied neuroblastomas expressed NF, including NF-H in nine of them (132). They also differ from gangliogliomas in the CNS and ganglioneuroblastomas and ganglioneuromas in the PNS, which express all NF subunits, including heavily phosphorylated NF-H (132, 135).

The expression of GFAP in nonastrocytomas of the CNS has been a matter of debate. It has been discussed by many authors (25, 95, 96, 119, 171, 174) that it is difficult to distinguish GFAP positive tumor cells from incarcerated nonneoplastic astrocytes. However, the reports of GFAP positive cells with astrocytic morphology in the subarachnoid space in infiltrating medulloblastoma (171) and in bone marrow (171) and lymph node (62) metastases of cerebellar medulloblastomas certainly suggest that differentiated astrocytes may form an integral part of these tumors. In six of our cases GFAP immunoreactive cells with ample cytoplasm and widely branching extensions were observed and these cells were interpreted as reactive astrocytes. However, in 18 cases unequivocal staining of tumor cells was observed, which was particularly prominent in frozen sections (Figs. 11.1E, 11.2). In several of these cases confluent areas of GFAP-positive cells with "primitive" morphologic features were observed, which undoubtedly

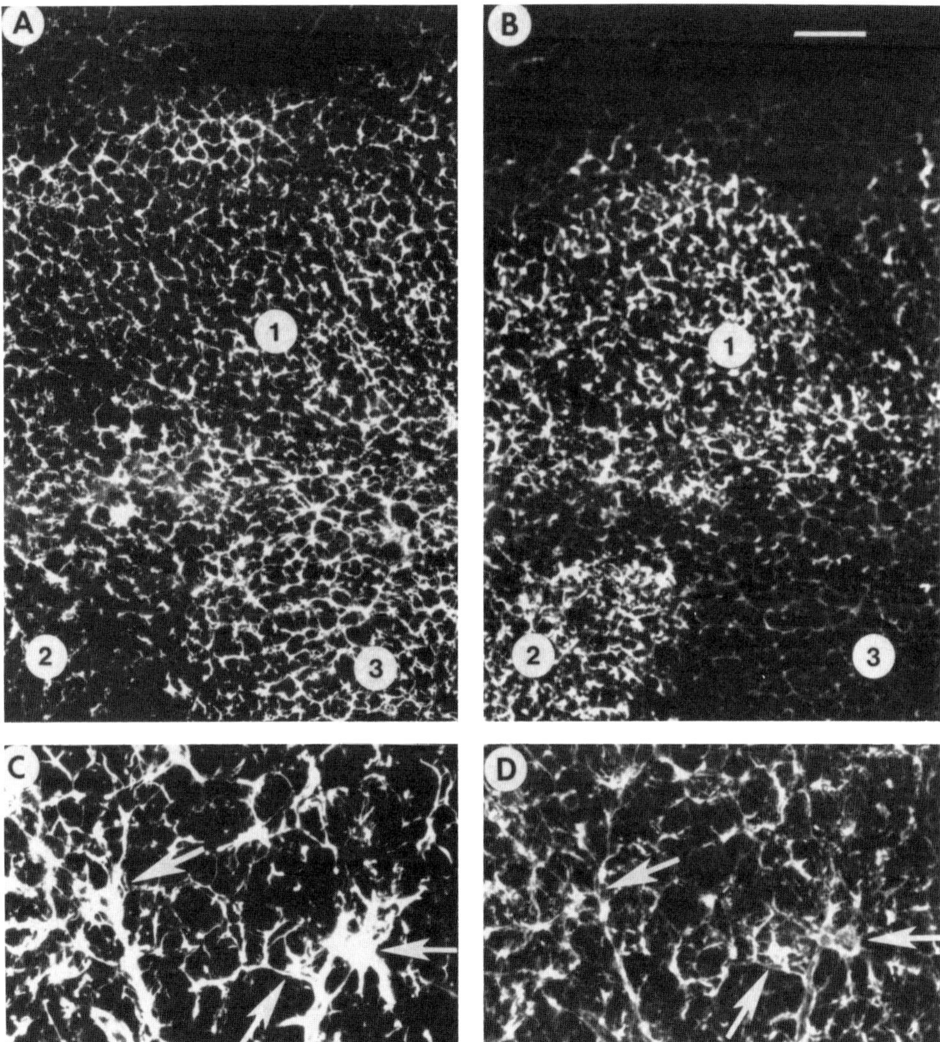

Figure 11.2. Double-fluorescence in a cerebellar PNET. *A*) and *C*) staining for GFAP (fluoresceinated isothiocyanate) and *B*) and *D*) staining for NF-M/H$^-$ (rhodamine) in the same areas as in *A*) and *C*), respectively. *1*) area positive for both GFAP and NF-M/H$^-$, *2*) area positive for NF-M/H$^-$ only and *3*) area positive for GFAP only. Arrows indicate the same cells in *C*) and *D*) positive for both GFAP and NF-M/H$^-$. Bar corresponds to 50μm in *A*) and *B*) and to 25μm in *C*) and *D*). (Reprinted with permission from Molenaar, W.M., Jansson, D., Gould, V.E., *et al.* Molecular markers of primitive neuroectodermal tumors (PNETs) and other pediatric central nervous system tumors. Monoclonal antibodies to neuronal and glial antigens distinguish subsets of PNETs. Lab. Invest., *61*:635–643, 1989.)

represent tumor cells with glial differentiation. In double-labeling immunofluorescence studies some of these primitive cells appeared to be positive for both NF proteins and GFAP, suggesting a bipotential differentiation. In the same way as for neuronal differentiation the acquisition of immunologically detectable astrocytic proteins apparently precedes the emergence of morphologically recognizable astrocytic features. In cases with well-defined follicles a GFAP-positive network was often observed, especially at the margins of the follicles, a pattern also described by Katsetos *et al.* (96). The topographical relation between the NF-protein positive neoplastic neuropil in the follicles and this GFAP-positive network strongly suggests a highly organized differentiation along both neuronal and glial lines and raises the question of mutual differentiation induction. It thus seems that GFAP expression in tumor cells may cover the full range of differentiation, i.e., from very primitive cells, which may be bipotential, on the one end to highly, presumably terminally differentiated cells, on the other. Here again a comparison with peripheral neuroectodermal tumors is of interest. In our cases GFAP expression was not observed in primitive cells, but it was described in such cells by Carlei *et al.* (28). In our cases it was present in ganglioneuroblastomas and ganglioneuromas in cells that presumably represent terminally differentiated nonmyelinating Schwann cells (92, 93). In these tumors but not in PNETs of the CNS myelin basic protein was also expressed, most likely representing myelinating Schwann cells (92, 93). Although central and peripheral neuroectodermal tumors, which have been grouped together (9, 43), definitely have similarities, the above findings on NF expression suggest that, overall, the peripheral tumors have a higher level of differentiation than their central counterparts.

In addition to NF and GFAP, all of 22 PNETs studied in frozen material appeared to express vimentin (64). Somewhat unexpectedly, isolated cells in three PNETs were immunoreactive for cytokeratins, again reflecting the "promiscuity" of keratin IFs, also observed in astrocytomas. In four PNETs immunoreactivity for desmin was demonstrated, an observation in line with earlier morphologic observations of smooth or skeletal muscle differentiation in cerebellar medulloblastomas (164, 165, 175).

Studies of Cell Lines of Primitive Brain Tumors with Antibodies to Intermediate Filaments

Three cell lines derived from human medulloblastomas have been described, i.e., D283 MED (61), DAOY (89) and D341 MED (60). A fourth cell line, TE671, initially described as a medulloblastoma cell line (122) was recently found to be a rhabdomyosarcoma cell line (192). Based on its karyotype and the presence of a number of polypeptides that are specific to, or preferentially expressed by neurons, D283 MED was considered to be comprised largely of tumor cells with a neuron-like phenotype (81, 204). Both this cell line and the later established D341 MED were found to express NF proteins, but not GFAP. However, the NF expression in both cell lines differed from the adult in vivo situation. Thus, NF-M and NF-H were expressed in a much larger percentage of D283 MED cells than NF-L, whereas in D341 MED NF-L was not expressed at all and NF-M and NF-H only by a minority of cells (5–25%). Nevertheless, these cell lines provided the first evidence that medulloblastomas contain a population of neoplastic cells that is capable of cell division and the expression of NF proteins, i.e., the IF proteins of committed embryonic and mature, nondividing cells. In a recent study (207) the expression of NF subunits and phosphoisoforms was further studied during the cell cycle in D283 MED cells. These studies were prompted by previous work which demonstrated that NF-L and NF-M are expressed prior to NF-H in postmitotic neurons and that NF-M attains its mature state of phosphorylation more rapidly than NF-H (11, 27, 58). Using two parameter flow cytometry with propidium iodide as the first marker and MAs to NF subunits as the second, it was found that all three NF subunits are expressed throughout the cell cycle. This may indicate that the regulation of NF expression in D283 MED cells is different from normal mature neurons, where the induction of NF expression is a postmitotic event. It remains to be seen whether this difference relates to the neoplastic state of these cells or to their in vivo conditions.

The third medulloblastoma cell line that was established, DAOY, differs from the other two in that it expresses neither NF proteins nor GFAP. However, several other neuroectodermal and glioma associated antigens were demonstrated, suggesting that this cell line is of a glial lineage. This finding is in keeping with the notion derived from immunohistochemical studies on tumor tissue that PNETs, or medulloblastomas, may reveal neuronal and/or glial differentiation.

CONCLUSIONS

In the absence of tumor specific markers, antigens or molecules restricted to different CNS cell types can be exploited in order to more objectively evaluate human brain tumors. Delineation of the lines of differentiation permissible within a given tumor using such probes may assist in the rational classification of primary brain neoplasms. In addition, the presence of certain markers may reflect the differentiation level of a certain tumor, which in turn may be of prognostic significance. Thus, the information gleaned from studies of human neoplasms with cell type specific markers may lead to improvements not only in the diagnosis, but also in the management of CNS tumors.

More fundamentally, a better understanding of the state of differentiation of the types of cells from which a tumor arises may permit the events leading to the neoplastic transformation to be probed in a more meaningful manner. For example, cells which have attained a specific level of differentiation may be especially vulnerable to undergo neoplastic transformation. However, in order to use cell type specific molecules as histogenetic markers, more basic information on the expression of such molecules in embryogenesis is needed.

Numerous cell type specific markers have been defined, largely as a result of the introduction of monoclonal antibody technology. However, only a few appear to be of potential use for the diagnostic assessment of tumors of the CNS. Among those discussed in this review, the intermediate filament proteins, and especially NF proteins and GFAP appear most promising in this regard. A number of advances in the diagnostic evaluation of human glial and primitive brain tumors brought about by studies of these neoplasms with antibodies specific for NF proteins and GFAP are discussed here. In the group of primitive brain tumors this led to the recognition of four subgroups: (*a*) those expressing both NF proteins and GFAP, (*b*) those expressing NF proteins, (*c*) those expressing GFAP, and (*d*) those expressing neither NF proteins nor GFAP. The pattern of expression of NF subunits and phospho-isoforms appeared to be reminiscent of the events during normal mammalian development. The findings in cell lines of primitive tumors corroborate those observed in tissue sections. In addition, they demonstrate some basic differences between normal and neoplastic cells, such as the expression of NF proteins in dividing tumor cells, but only in postmitotic normal neurons.

ACKNOWLEDGMENTS

Appreciation is expressed to Dr. N.K. Gonatas for support and to Drs. V.M.-Y. Lee, W.W. Schlaepfer, and L.B. Rorke for advice and helpful collaboration throughout many phases of the studies discussed here. Ms. M.A. Obrocka, Ms. T. Schuck, Mr. P. Newman, and Ms. A. O'Brien contributed invaluable technical assistance to many aspects of this work. Drs. J. Chatten, R.J. Packer, and L.B. Rorke kindly contributed tissue from the Children's Hospital of Philadelphia. Dr. W.M. Molenaar spent a sabbatical year at the University of Pennsylvania Medical School as a Fulbright Scholar, during the time she participated in several of the studies reviewed here.

REFERENCES

1. Achstaetter, T., Moll, R., Anderson, A., *et al.* Expression of glial filament protein (GFP) in nerve sheaths and non-neural cells re-examined using monoclonal antibodies, with special emphasis on the co-expression of GFP and cytokeratins in epithelial cells of human salivary glands and pleomorphic adenomas. Differentiation, *31*:206–227, 1986.
2. Aletta, J.M., Angeletti, R., Liem, R.K.H., *et al.* Relationship between the nerve growth fac-

tor-regulated clone 73 gene product and the 58-kilodalton neuronal intermediate filament protein (peripherin). J. Neurochem., *51:*1317–1320, 1988.
3. Altmannsberger, M., Osborn, M., Schauer, A., *et al.* Antibodies to different intermediate filament proteins. Cell type specific markers on paraffin-embedded human tissues. Lab. Invest., *45:*427–434, 1981.
4. Anderson, D.J. and Axel, R. A bipotential neuroendocrine precursor whose choice of cell fate is determined by NGF and glucocorticoids. Cell, *47:*1079–1090, 1986.
5. Andrew, A. The APUD concept: where has it led us? Br. Med. Bull., *38:*221–225, 1982.
6. Bader, M.F., Georges, E., Mushynski, W.E., *et al.* Neurofilament proteins in cultured adrenal chromaffin cells. J. Neurochem. *43:* 1180–1193, 1984.
7. Bannasch, P., Zerban, H., and Mayer, D. The cytoskeleton in tumor cells. Pathol. Res. Pract., *175:*196–211, 1982.
8. Barnstable, C.J., Akagawa, K., Hofstein, R., *et al.* Monoclonal antibodies that label discrete cell types in the mammalian nervous system. Cold Spring Harbor Symp. Quant. Biol. *48:*863–876, 1983.
9. Becker, L.E. and Hinton, D. Primitive neuroectodermal tumors of the central nervous system. Hum. Pathol. *14:*538–550, 1983.
10. Benjamin, D.C., Berzofsky, J.A., East, I.J., *et al.* The antigenic structure of proteins: A reappraisal. Annu. Rev. Immunol. *2:*67–101, 1984.
11. Bennett, G.S. Changes in intermediate filament composition during neurogenesis. Curr. Top. Dev. Biol., *21:*151, 1987.
12. Bennett, G.S. and DiLullo, C. Expression of neurofilament protein by the precursors of a subpopulation of ventral spinal cord neurons. Dev. Biol., *107:*94, 1985.
13. Bigbee, J.W., Bigner, D.D., Pegram, C. *et al.* Study of glial fibrillary acidic protein in a human glioma cell line grown in culture and as a solid tumor. J. Neurochem., *40:*460–467, 1983.
14. Biggs, P.J., Garen, P.D., Powers, J.M., *et al.* Malignant rhabdoid tumor of the central nervous system. Hum. Pathol., *18:*332–337, 1987.
15. Bignami, A., Eng, L.F., Dahl, D., *et al.* Localization of the glial fibrillary acidic protein in astrocytes by immunofluorescence. Brain Res., *43:*429–435, 1972.
16. Bishop, M.J. Cellular oncogenes and retroviruses. Annu. Rev. Biochem., *52:*301–354, 1983.
17. Bishop, M. and DelaMonte, S.M. Dual lineage of astrocytomas. Am. J. Pathol., *135:*517–527, 1989.
18. Birkmayer, G.D. Tumor markers of the central nervous system: biological basis and clinical relevance. Cancer Detect. Prevent., *6:*317–324, 1983.
19. Bizzini, B. Tetanus toxin. Microbiol. Rev., *43:*224–240, 1979.
20. Bjorklund, H., Dahl, D., Olson, L., *et al.* Glial fibrillary acidic protein-like reactivity in the iris: development, distribution and reactive changes following transplantation. J. Neurosci., *4:*978–988, 1984.
21. Black, M.M. and Lee, V.M.-Y. Phosphorylation of neurofilament proteins in intact neurons: demonstration of phosphorylation in cell bodies and axons. J. Neurosci., *8:*3296–3305, 1988.
22. Bohling, T., Paetau, A., Ekblom, P., *et al.* Distribution of endothelial and basement membrane markers in angiogenic tumors of the nervous system. Acta Neuropathol., *62:*67–72, 1983.
23. Bonnin, J.M. and Rubinstein, L.J. Immunohistochemistry of central nervous system tumors. Its contribution to neurosurgical diagnosis. J. Neurosurg. *60:*1121–1133, 1984.
24. Bonnin, J.M., Rubinstein, L.J., Papasozomenos, S.C., *et al.* Subependymal giant cell astrocytoma. Significance and possible cytogenetic implications of an immunohistochemical study. Acta Neuropathol. *62:*185–193, 1984.
25. Burger, P.C., Grahmann, F.C., Bliestle, A., *et al.* Differentiation in the medulloblastoma. A histological and immunohistochemical study. Acta Neuropathol., *73:*115–123, 1987.
26. Carden, M.J., Lee, V.M.-Y., and Schlaepfer, W.W. 2,5-Hexadione neuropathy is associated with the covalent crosslinking of neurofilament proteins. Neurochem. Pathol., *5:*25–35, 1986.
27. Carden, M.J., Trojanowski, J.Q., Schlaepfer, W.W., *et al.* Two-stage expression of neurofilament polypeptides during rat neurogenesis with early establishment of adult phosphorylation patterns. J. Neurosci., *7:* 3489–3504, 1987.
28. Carlei, F., Polak, J.M., Ceccamea, A., *et al.* Neuronal and glial markers in tumours of neuroblastic origin. Virchows. Arch. (A), *404:*313–324, 1984.
29. Cavazzana, A.O., Miser, J.S., Jefferson, J., *et al.* Experimental evidence for a neural origin of Ewing's sarcoma. Am. J. Pathol., *127:*507–518, 1987.
30. Choi, B.H. and Kim, R.C. Expression of glial fibrillary acidic protein in immature oligodendroglia. Science, *223:*407–409, 1984.
31. Christen, B., Trojanowski, J.Q., and Pietra, G.G. Immunohistochemical demonstration of phosphorylated and nonphosphorylated forms of human neurofilament subunits in human pulmonary carcinoids. Hum. Pathol. *18:*997–1001, 1987.
32. Ciocca, D.R., Adams, D.J., Bjercke, R.J., *et al.* Monoclonal antibody storage conditions, and concentration effects on immunohistochemical specificity. J. Histochem. Cytochem., *31:*691–696, 1983.

33. Coggi, G., Dell'Orto, P., Bonoldi, E., *et al.* Lectins in diagnostic pathology. *Lectins, Vol. III*, edited by T.C. Bag-Hansen and G.A. Spengler, pp. 87–103. Berlin, Walter de Gruyter & Co., 1983.
34. Cosgrove, M., Fitzgibbons, P.L., Sherrod, A., *et al.* Intermediate filament expression in astrocytic neoplasms. Am. J. Surg. Pathol. *13:*141–145, 1989.
35. Cruz-Sanchez, F.F., Rossi, M.L., Hughes, J.T., *et al.* Medulloblastoma. An immunohistochemical study of 50 cases. Acta Neuropathol., *79:*205–210, 1989.
36. Cruz-Sanchez, F.F., Rossi, M.L., Esiri, M.M., *et al.* Epithelial membrane antigen expression in ependymomas. Neuropathol. Appl. Neurobiol., *14:*197–205, 1988.
37. Cruz-Sanchez, F.F., Rossi, M.L., Hughes, J.T., *et al.* An immunohistological study of 66 ependymomas. Histopathology, *13:*443–454, 1988.
38. Dahl, D., Chi, N.H., Miles, L.E., *et al.* Glial fibrillary acidic (GFA) protein in Schwann cells: fact or artifact. J. Histochem. Cytochem., *30:*912–918, 1982.
39. Debus, E., Weber, K. and Osborn, M. Monoclonal antibodies specific for glial fibrillary acidic (GFA) protein and for each of the neurofilament triplet polypeptides. Differentiation, *25:*193–203, 1983.
40. Deck, J.H.N., Eng., L.F., Bigbee, J., *et al.* The role of glial fibrillary acidic protein in the diagnosis of central nervous system tumors. Acta Neuropathol., *42:*183–190, 1978.
41. Deck, J.H.N. and Rubinstein, L.J. Glial fibrillary acidic protein in stromal cells of some capillary hemangioblastomas: significance and possible implications of an immunoperoxidase study. Acta Neuropathol., *54:* 173–181, 1981.
42. Deftos, L.J., Linnoila, R.I., Carney, D.N., *et al.* Demonstration of chromogranin A in human neuroendocrine cell lines by immunohistology and immunoassay. Cancer *62:*92–97, 1988.
43. Dehner, L.P. Peripheral and central primitive neuroectodermal tumors. A nosologic concept seeking a consensus. Arch. Pathol. Lab. Med., *110:*997–1005, 1986.
44. DeLey, L., Berendsen, H., Spakman, H., *et al.* Neuroendocrine and epithelial antigens in SCLC. Lung Cancer, *4:*42–44, 1988.
45. DeLey, L., Broers, J., Ramaekers, F., *et al.* Monoclonal antibodies in clinical and experimental pathology of lung cancer. In: *Application of monoclonal antibodies in tumor pathology*, edited by D.J. Ruiter, G.J. Fleuren, and S. O. Warnaar, pp. 191–210. Amsterdam, Martinus Nijhoff Publ. Amsterdam, 1986.
46. DeLey, L., Poppema, S., Nuland, J.K., *et al.* Neuroendocrine differentiation antigen on human lung carcinoma and Kulchitski cells. Cancer Res., *45:*2192–2200, 1985.
47. DeLey, L., Postmus, P.E., Poppema, S., *et al.* The use of monoclonal antibodies for the pathological diagnosis of lung cancer. In: *Lung Cancer: Basic and Clinical Aspects*, edited by A.H. Hansen, pp. 31–48. Boston, Martinus Nijhoff publishers, 1986.
48. DeLey, L., TerHaar, J.G., Schwander, E., *et al.* Small cell lung cancer and embryonic lung epithelium share monoclonal antibody defined neuro-endocrine related antigens. Chest 91(Suppl), 1987.
49. Denk, H. and Krepler, R. The cytoskeleton in pathologic conditions. Pathol. Res. Pract., *175:*180–195, 1982.
50. Duffy, P.E., Graff, L., Huang, Y.Y., *et al.* Glial fibrillary acidic protein in ependymomas and other brain tumors. Distribution, diagnostic criteria, and relation to formation of processes. J. Neurol. Sci., *40:*133–146, 1979.
51. Duffy, P.E., Graf, L., and Rapport, M.M. Identification of glial fibrillary acidic protein by the immunoperoxidase method in human brain tumors. J. Neuropathol. Exp. Neurol., *36:*645–652, 1977.
52. Duffy, P.E., Huang, Y.Y., and Rapport, M.M. Glial fibrillary acidic protein in giant cell tumors of brain and other gliomas. A possible relationship to malignancy, differentiation and pleomorphism of glia. Acta Neuropathol., *52:*51–57, 1980.
53. Edwards, P.A.W. Some properties and applications of monoclonal antibodies. Biochem. J., *200:*1–10, 1981.
54. Eng, L.F. Glial fibrillary acidic protein (GFAP): the major protein of glial intermediate filaments in differentiated astrocytes. J. Neuroimmunol., *8:*203–214, 1985.
55. Eng, L.F. and DeArmond, S.J. Immunocytochemical studies of astrocytes in normal development and disease. Adv. Cell. Neurobiol., *3:*145–171, 1982.
56. Eng, L.F., Vanderhaeghen, J.J., Bignami, A., *et al.* An acidic protein isolated from fibrous astrocytes. Brain Res., *28:*351–354, 1971.
57. Esiri, M.M. Immunohistological techniques in neuropathology. In: *Recent Advances in Neuropathology*, edited by W.T. Smith and J.B. Cavanaugh, pp. 1–28. New York, Churchill Livingstone, 1982.
58. Foster, G.A., Dahl, D., and Lee, V.M.-Y. Temporal and topographic relationships between the phosphorylated and non-phosphorylated epitopes of the 200kDa neurofilament protein during development in vitro. J. Neurosci., *7:*2651–2663, 1987.
59. Franke, W.W., Jahn, L., and Knapp, A.C. Cytokeratins and desmosomal proteins in certain epithelioid and nonepithelial cells. In: *Cytoskeletal proteins in tumor diagnosis: current communications in molecular biology*, edited by M. Osborn and K. Weber, p. 151. Cold Spring Harbor Laboratory, Cold Spring Harbor, NY, 1989.
60. Friedman, H.S., Burger, P.C., Bigner, S.H., *et al.*

Phenotypic and genotypic analysis of human medulloblastoma cell line and transplantable xenograft (D341 MED) demonstrating amplification of c-myc. Am. J. Pathol., *130:*472–484, 1988.
61. Friedman, H.S., Burger, P.C., Bigner, S.H., *et al.* Establishment and characterization of the human medulloblastoma cell line and transplantable xenograft D283 MED. J. Neuropathol. Exp. Neurol., *44:*592–605, 1985.
62. Ghobrial, M., Velasco, M., Ross, E., *et al.* Astrocytic differentiation in metastatic medulloblastoma (abstr.). Lab. Invest., *60:*33A, 1989.
63. Gould, V.E. The co-expression of distinct classes of intermediate filaments in human neoplasms. Arch. Pathol. Lab. Med. *109:* 984–985, 1985.
64. Gould, V.E., Jansson, D.S., Molenaar, W.M., *et al.* Primitive neuroectodermal tumors of the central nervous system. Patterns of expression of neuroendocrine markers and all classes of intermediate filaments. Lab. Invest., in press, 1990.
65. Gould, V.E., Lee, I., Wiedenmann, B., *et al.* Synaptophysin: a novel marker for neurons, certain neuroendocrine cells and their neoplasms. Hum. Pathol. *17:*979–983, 1986.
66. Gould, V.E., Wiedenmann, B., Lee, I., *et al.* Synaptophysin expression in neuroendocrine neoplasms as determined by immunocytochemistry. Am. J. Pathol., *126:*243–257, 1987.
67. Gown, A.M. and Vogel, A.M. Monoclonal antibodies to intermediate filament proteins of human cells: unique and cross-reacting antibodies. J. Cell Biol., *95:*414–424, 1982.
68. Gown, A.M. and Vogel, A.M. Monoclonal antibodies to human intermediate filament proteins. II. Distribution of filament proteins in normal human tissues. Am. J. Pathol., *114:* 309–321, 1984.
69. Gown, A.M. and Vogel, A.M. Anti-intermediate filament monoclonal antibodies: tissue specific tools in tumor diagnosis. Surv. Synth. Pathol. Res., *3:*369–385, 1984.
70. Grahm, D.R., Thomas, D.G.T., and Brown, I. Nervous system antigens. Histopathology *7:*1–21, 1983.
71. Granger, B.L. and Lazarides, E. Expression of the major neurofilament subunit in chicken erythrocytes. Science, *221:*553–556, 1983.
72. Grant, J.W. and Gallagher, P.J. Pleomorphic xanthoastrocytoma: immunohistochemical methods for differentiation from fibrous histiocytomas with similar morphology. Am. J. Surg. Pathol., *10:*336–342, 1986.
73. Guarda, L.A., Ordonez, N.G., Smith, J.L., *et al.* Immunoperoxidase localization of Factor VIII in angiosarcomas. Arch. Pathol. Lab. Med., *106:*515–516, 1982.
74. Haan, E.A., Boss, B.D., and Cowan, W.M. Production and characterization of monoclonal antibodies against the "brain-specific" proteins 14-3-2 and S-100. Proc. Natl. Acad. Sci. USA, *79:*7585–7589, 1982.
75. Hachitanda, Y., Tsuneyoshi, M., and Enjoji, M. Expression of pan-neuroendocrine proteins in 53 neuroblastic tumors. An immunohistochemical study with neuron-specific enolase, chromogranin and synaptophysin. Arch. Pathol. Lab. Med., *113:*381–384, 1989.
76. Haglid, K., Carlsson, C.A., and Starvou, D. An immunological study of human brain tumors concerning the brain specific proteins S-100 and 14.3.2 Acta Neuropathol. *24:*187–196, 1973.
77. Hagn, C., Schmid, K.W., Fischer-Colbrie, R., *et al.* Chromogranin A, B and C in human adrenal medulla and endocrine tissues. Lab. Invest., *55:*405–411, 1986.
78. Haimoto, H., Takahashi, Y., Koshikawa, T., *et al.* Immunohistochemical localization of gamma-enolase in normal human tissues other than nervous and neuroendocrine tissues. Lab. Invest., *52:*257–263, 1985.
79. Hashim, G.A. (ed). *Myelin Chemistry and Biology: Progress in Clinical and Biological Research, Vol.*49. New York, Alan R. Liss, 1980.
80. Hatfield, J.S., Skoff, R.P., Maisel, H., *et al.* Glial fibrillary acidic protein is localized to the lens epithelium. J. Cell Biol., *98:*1895–1898, 1984.
81. He, X., Skapek, S.X., Wikstrand, C.J., *et al.* Phenotypic analysis of four human medulloblastoma cell lines and transplantable xenografts. J. Neuropathol. Exp. Neurol., *48:*48–68, 1989.
82. Herpers, M.J.H.M., Ramaekers, F.C.S., Aldeweireldt, J., *et al.* Co-expression of glial fibrillary acidic protein- and vimentin-type intermediate filaments in human astrocytomas. Acta Neuropathol., *70:*333–339, 1986.
83. Hickey, W.F., Lee, V.M.-Y., Trojanowski, J.Q., *et al.* Immunohistochemical application of monoclonal antibodies against myelin basic protein and neurofilament triplet protein subunits: Advantages over antisera and technical limitations. J. Histochem. Cytochem., *31:*1126–1135, 1983.
84. Hoekfelt, T., Millhorn, D., Seroogy, K., *et al.* Coexistence of peptides with classical neurotransmitters. In: *Regulatory peptides*, edited by J. Polak, pp. 154–191. Birkhaeuser Verlag, Basel, 1989.
85. Holmgren, J. and Svennerholm, A.M. Cholera and the immune response. Prog. Allergy, *33:*106–109, 1983.
86. Hoog, A., Gould, V.E., Grimelius, L., *et al.* Tissue fixation methods alter the immunohistochemical demonstrability of synaptophysin. Ultrastruct. Pathol., *12:*673–678, 1988.
87. Houthoff, H.J., Poppema, S., Ebels, E.J., *et al.* Intracranial malignant lymphomas. A morphologic and immunocytologic study of twenty cases. Acta Neuropathol., *44:*203–210, 1978.

88. Itoyama, Y., Sternberger, N.H., Kies, M.W., *et al.* Immunocytochemical method to identify myelin basic protein in oligodendroglia and myelin sheaths of the human nervous system. Ann. Neurol., *7:*157–166, 1980.
89. Jacobsen, P.F., Jenkyn, D., and Papadimitriou, J.M. Establishment of a human medulloblastoma cell line and its heterotransplantation into nude mice. J. Neuropathol. Exp. Neurol., *44:*472–485, 1985.
90. Jakate, S.M., Marsden, H.B., and Ingram, L. Primary rhabdoid tumor of the brain. Virchows Arch.(A), *412:*393–397, 1988.
91. Jessen, K.R. and Mirsky, R. Glial cells in the enteric nervous system contain glial fibrillary acidic protein. Nature, *286:*736–737, 1980.
92. Jessen, K.R., Mirsky, R. Nonmyelin-forming schwann cells coexpress surface proteins and intermediate filaments not found in myelin-forming cells: a study of Ran-2, A5E3 antigen and glial fibrillary acidic protein. J. Neurocytol., *13:*923–934, 1984.
93. Jessen, K.R. and Mirsky, R. Glial fibrillary acidic polypeptides in peripheral glia. Molecular weight, heterogeneity and distribution. J. Neuroimmunol., *8:*377–393, 1985.
94. Jurco, S. III, Nadji, M., Harvey, D.G., *et al.* Hemangioblastomas: histogenesis of the stromal cell studied by immunocytochemistry. Hum. Pathol., *13:*13–18, 1982.
95. Katsetos, C.D., Herman, M.M., Frankfurter, A., *et al.* Cerebellar desmoplastic medulloblastomas: a further immunohistochemical characterization of the reticulin-free pale islands. Arch. Pathol. Lab. Med., *113:*1019–1029, 1989.
96. Katsetos, C.D., Liu, H.M., and Zacks, S.I. Immunohistochemical and ultrastructural observations on Homer Wright (neuroblastic) rosettes and the "Pale islands" of human cerebellar medulloblastomas. Hum. Pathol., *19:* 1219–1227, 1988.
97. Knapp, A.C. and Franke, W.W. Spontaneous losses of control of cytokeratin gene expression in transformed nonepithelial human cells occurring at different levels of regulation. Cell, *59:*67–79, 1989.
98. Kohler, G. and Milstein, C. Continuous cultures of fused cells secreting antibody of predefined specificity. Nature, *256:*495–497, 1975.
99. Koulakoff, A., Bizzini, B., and Berwald-Netter, Y. A correlation between the appearance and the evolution of tetanus toxin binding cells and neurogenesis. Devel. Brain Res., *5:*139–147, 1982.
100. Krepler, H., Denk, D., Hartlieb, U., *et al.* Antibodies to intermediate filament proteins as molecular markers in clinical tumor pathology. Pathol. Res. Pract., *175:*212–226, 1982.
101. Krieger, D.T. Brain peptides: what, where and why?, Science, *222:*975–985, 1983.
102. Kumanishi, T., Wahiyama, K., Watabe, K., *et al.* Glial fibrillary acidic protein in medulloblastomas. Acta Neuropathol., *67:*1–5, 1985.
103. Kumpulainen, T. Immunohistochemical localization of human carbonic anhydrase isoenzymes. Ann. N.Y. Acad. Sci., *429:*359–368, 1984.
104. Lazarides, E. Intermediate filaments as mechanical integrators of cellular space. Nature, *283:*249–253, 1980.
105. Lazarides, E. Intermediate filaments: a chemically heterogeneous, developmentally regulated class of proteins. Annu. Rev. Biochem., *51:*219–250, 1982.
106. Leclerc, N., Beesley, P.W., Brown, I., *et al.* Synaptophysin expression during synaptogenesis in the rat cerebellar cortex. J. Comp. Neurol., *280:*197–212, 1989.
107. Lee, V.M.-Y., Carden, M.J., Schlaepfer, W.W., *et al.* Monoclonal antibodies distinguish several differentially phosphorylated states of the two largest rat neurofilament subunits (NF-H and NF-M) and demonstrate their existence in the normal nervous system of adult rats. J. Neurosci., *7:*3474–3488, 1987.
108. Lee, V.M.-Y., Otvos, L., Carden, M.J., *et al.* Identification of the major multiphosphorylation site in mammalian neurofilaments. Proc. Natl. Acad. Sci. U.S.A., *85:*1–5, 1988.
109. Lee, V.M.-Y. and Page, C. Dynamics of nerve growth factor-induced neurofilament and vimentin filament expression and organization in PC12 cells. J. Neurosci., *4:*1705–1714, 1984.
110. Lee, V.M.-Y., Page, C., Wu, H.L., *et al.* Monoclonal antibodies against gel excised glial filament proteins and their reactivity with other intermediate filament proteins. J. Neurochem., *42:*25–32, 1984.
111. Lee, V.M.-Y., Trojanowski, J.Q., and Schlaepfer, W.W. Induction of neurofilament triplet proteins in PC12 cells by nerve growth factor. Brain Res., *238:*169–180, 1982.
112. Leff, Y.L., Brooks, J.S.J., and Trojanowski, J.Q. Expression of neurofilament and neuron-specific enolase in small cell tumors of skin using immunocytochemistry. Cancer, *56:* 625–631, 1985.
113. Lefkowitz, I.B., Rorke, L.B., Packer, R.J., *et al.* Atypical teratoid tumor of infancy: definition of an entity (abstr.). Ann. Neurol., *28:* 448, 1987.
114. Liem, R.K.H., Yen, S.-H., Salomon, G.B., *et al.* Intermediate filaments in nervous tissue. J. Cell Biol., *79:*637–645, 1979.
115. Livett, B.G. The secretory process in adrenal medullary cells. In: *Cell Biology of the Secretory Process*, edited by M. Cantin. pp. 309–358. Basel, S. Karger, 1984.
116. Lloyd, R.V., Cano, M., Rosa, P., *et al.* Distribution of chromogranin A and secretogranin I (chromogranin B) in neuroendocrine cells and tumors. Am. J. Pathol., *130:*296–304, 1988.

117. Lloyd, R.V., Sisson, J.C., Shapiro, B., *et al.* Immunohistochemical localization of epinephrine, norepinephrine, catecholamine-synthesizing enzymes, and chromogranin in neuroendocrine cells and tumors. Am. J. Pathol., *125:*45–54, 1986.
118. Lloyd, R.V. and Wilson, B.S. Specific endocrine tissue marker defined by a monoclonal antibody. Science, *222:*628–630, 1983.
119. Mannoji, H., Takeshita, I., Fukui, M., *et al.* Glial fibrillary acidic protein in medulloblastoma. Acta Neuropathol., *55:*63–69, 1981.
120. Marangos, P.J., Polak, J.M., and Pearse, A.G.E. Neuron-specific enolase: A probe for neurons and neuroendocrine cells. TINS *5:*193–196, 1982.
121. Marsden, H.B., Kumar, S., Kahn, J., *et al.* A study of glial fibrillary acidic protein (GFAP) in childhood brain tumours. Int. J. Cancer, *31:*439–445, 1983.
122. McAllister, R.M., Isaacs, H., Rongey, R., *et al.* Establishment of a human medulloblastoma cell line. Int. J. Cancer, *20:*206–212, 1977.
123. McComb, R.D., Jones, T.R., Pizzo, S.V., *et al.* Localization of Factor VIII/von Willebrand factor and glial fibrillary acid protein in the hemangioblastoma: implications for stromal cell histogenesis. Acta Neuropathol. *56:*207–213, 1982.
124. McComb, R.D., Jones, T.R., Pizzo, S.V., *et al.* Specificity and sensitivity of immunohistochemical detection of Factor VIII/von Willebrand factor antigen in formalin-fixed paraffin-embedded tissue. J. Histochem. Cytochem. *30:*371–372, 1982.
125. McKeon, F.D., Kirshner, M.W., and Caput, D. Homologies in both primary and secondary structure between nuclear envelope and intermediate filament proteins. Nature, *319:*463–468, 1986.
126. Memoli, V.A., Brown, E.F., and Gould, V.E. Glial fibrillary acidic protein (GFAP) immunoreactivity in peripheral nerve sheath tumors. Ultrastruct. Pathol. *7:*269–275, 1984.
127. Mendelsohn, G., Eggleston, J.C., Olson, J.L., *et al.* Vasoactive intestinal polypeptide and its relationship to ganglion cell differentiation in neuroblastic tumors. Lab. Invest. *41:*144–149, 1979.
128. Miettinen, M., Clark, R., and Virtanen, I. Intermediate filament proteins in choroid plexus and ependyma and their tumors. Am. J. Pathol. *123:*231–240, 1986.
129. Miettinen, M., Lehto, V.P., Dahl, D., *et al.* Differential diagnosis of chordoma, chondroid and ependymal tumors as aided by anti-intermediate filament antibodies. Am. J. Pathol., *112:*160–169, 1983.
130. Miettinen, M., Lehto, V.P., and Virtanen, I. Antibodies to intermediate filament proteins in the diagnosis and classification of human tumors. Ultrastruct. Pathol., *7:*83–107, 1984.
131. Miettinen, M., and Rapola, J. Synaptophysin—an immunohistochemical marker for childhood neuroblastoma. Acta Pathol. Microbiol. Immunol. Scand. Sect. A. *95:* 167–170, 1987.
132. Molenaar, W.M., Baker, D.L., Pleasure, D., *et al.* The neuroendocrine and neural profiles of neuroblastomas, ganglioneuroblastomas and ganglioneuromas. Am. J. Pathol., *136:* 375–382, 1990.
133. Molenaar, W.M., DeLey, L., and Trojanowski, J.Q. Neuroectodermal tumors of the peripheral and the central nervous system share neuroendocrine antigens with small cell lung carcinomas. submitted.
134. Molenaar, W.M., Jansson, D., Gould, V.E., *et al.* The immunophenotype of central primitive neuroectodermal tumors (PNETs) (abstr.). J. Neuropathol. Exp. Neurol. *48:*359, 1989.
135. Molenaar, W.M., Jansson, D., Gould, V.E., *et al.* Molecular markers of primitive neuroectodermal tumors (PNETs) and other pediatric central nervous system tumors. Monoclonal antibodies to neuronal and glial antigens distinguish subsets of PNETs. Lab. Invest. *61:*635–643, 1989.
136. Molenaar, W.M., Lee, V.M.-Y., and Trojanowski, J.Q. Early fetal acquisition of the chromaffin and neuronal immunophenotype by human adrenal medullary cells. An immunohistological study using monoclonal antibodies to chromogranin A, tyrosine hydroxylase and neuronal cytoskeletal proteins. Exp. Neurol., *108:*1–9, 1990.
137. Moll, R., Franke, W.W., Schiller, D.L., *et al.* The catalogue of human cytokeratins: patterns of expression in normal epithelia, tumors and cultured cells. Cell *31:*11–24, 1982.
138. Moll, R., Osborn, M., Hartschuh, W., *et al.* Variability of expression and arrangement of cytokeratin and neurofilaments in cutaneous neuroendocrine carcinomas (Merkel cell tumors): immunocytochemical and biochemical analysis of twelve cases. Ultrastruct. Pathol., *10:*473–495, 1986.
139. Mukai, M. Immunohistochemical localization of S-100 protein and peripheral nerve myelin proteins (P2 protein, PC protein) in granular cell tumors. Am. J. Pathol. *112:*139–146, 1983.
140. Mukai, M., Torikata, C., Iri, H., *et al.* Expression of neurofilament triplet proteins in human neural tumors. An immunohistochemical study of paraganglioma, ganglioneuroma, ganglioneuroblastoma and neuroblastoma. Am. J. Pathol., *122:*28–35, 1986.
141. Nakamura, Y., Becker, L.E., and Marks, A. Distribution of immunoreactive S-100 protein in pediatric brain tumors. J. Neuropathol. Exp. Neurol. *43:*136–145, 1983.
142. Nolan, J., Trojanowski, J.Q., and Hogue-Angeletti, R.A. Neurons and neuroendocrine cells contain chromogranin: detection of the molecule in normal bovine tissues by immunochemical and immunohistochemical

methods. J. Histochem. Cytochem. *33*:791–798, 1985.

143. Norton, W. and Goldman, J.E. Neurofilaments. In: Bradshaw, R.A. Schneider, D.M. (eds): *Proteins of the Nervous System*, ed 2, pp. 301–329. New York, Raven Press, 1980.

144. Ogawa, M., Ishikawa, T., and Ohta, H. Transdifferentiation of endocrine chromaffin cells into neuronal cells. Curr. Top. Dev. Biol., *20*:99–110, 1986.

145. Okada, E., Maeda, T., and Watanabe, T. Immunocytochemical study of cholera toxin binding sites by monoclonal anti-cholera toxin antibody in neuronal tissue culture. Brain Res. *242*:233–241, 1982.

146. Omlin, F.X., Webster, deF.H., Palkovits, C.G., *et al.* Immunocytochemical localization of basic protein in major dense line regions of central and peripheral myelin. J. Cell Biol., *95*:242–248, 1982.

147. Osborn, M., Dirk, T., Käser, H., *et al.* Immunohistochemical localization of neurofilaments and neuron-specific enolase in 29 cases of neuroblastoma. Am. J. Pathol., *122*:433–442, 1986.

148. Osborn, M. and Weber, K. Tumor diagnosis by intermediate filament typing: a novel tool of surgical pathology. Lab. Invest. *48*:372–394, 1983.

149. Osborn, M. and Weber, K. Intermediate filament proteins: a multigene family distinguishing major cell lineages, TIBS, *11*:469–472, 1986.

150. Osborn, M., Weber, K. (eds.), *Cytoskeletal Proteins in Tumor Diagnosis: Current Communications in Molecular Biology.* Cold Spring Harbor, NY, Cold Spring Harbor Laboratory, 1989.

151. Pachter, J.S. and Liem, R.K.H. The differential appearance of neurofilament triplet polypeptides in the developing rat optic nerve. Dev. Biol., *193*:200–210, 1984.

152. Palmer, J.O., Kasselberg, A.G., and Netsky, M.G. Differentiation of medulloblastoma. Studies including immunohistochemical localization of glial fibrillary acidic protein. J. Neurosurg., *55*:161–169, 1981.

153. Parysek, L.M. and Goldman, R.D. Distribution of a novel 57kDa intermediate filament (IF) protein in the nervous system. J. Neurosci. *8*:555–563, 1988.

154. Polak, J.M., Van Noorden B. (eds.) *Immunocytochemistry: Practical Applications in Pathology and Biology.* Bristol, John Wright & Sons, 1983.

155. Portier, M.M., DeNechaud, B., and Gros, F. Peripherin, a new member of the intermediate filament protein family. Dev. Neurosci. *6*:335–344, 1983/1984.

156. Postmus, P.E., Hirschler-Schulte, T.J.W., DeLey, L., *et al.* Diagnostic application of a monoclonal antibody against small cell lung cancer. Cancer, *57*:60–63, 1986.

157. Raff, M.C., Miller, R.H., and Noole, M. A glial progenitor cell that develops in vitro into an astrocyte or an oligodendrocyte depending on culture medium. Nature, *303*:390–396, 1983.

158. Raff, M.C., Mirsky, R., Fields, K.F., *et al.* Galactocerebroside: a specific cell surface antigenic marker for oligodendrocytes in culture. Nature, *274*:813–816, 1978.

159. Ramaekers, F., Puts, J., Kant, A. *et al.* Differential diagnosis of human carcinomas, sarcomas and their metastases using antibodies to intermediate filaments. Eur. J. Cancer Clin. Oncol., *18*:1251–1257, 1982.

160. Ramaekers, F.C.S., Haag, D., Kant, A., *et al.* Co-expression of keratin and vimentin type intermediate filaments in human metastatic carcinoma cells. Proc. Natl. Acad. Sci. U.S.A., *80*:2618–2622, 1983.

161. Ramaekers, F.C.S., Puts, J.J.G., Moesker, O., *et al.* Antibodies to intermediate filament proteins in the immunohistochemical identification of human tumours: an overview. Histochem. J. *15*:691–713, 1983.

162. Rehm, H., Wiedenmann, B., and Betz, H. Molecular characterization of synaptophysin, a major calcium-binding protein of the synaptic vesicle membrane. EMBO J., *5*:535–541, 1986.

163. Roessmann, U., Velasco, M.E., Gambetti, P. *et al.* Neuronal and astrocytic differentiation in human neuroepithelial neoplasms: an immunohistochemical study. J. Neuropathol. Exp. Neurol., *42*:113–121, 1983.

164. Rorke, L.B. The cerebellar medulloblastoma and its relationship to primitive neuroectodermal tumors. J. Neuropathol. Exp. Neurol. *42*:1–15, 1983.

165. Rorke, L.B., Gilles, F.H., David, R.L., *et al.* Revision of the World Health Organization classification of brain tumors for childhood brain tumors. Cancer, *56*:1869–1886, 1985.

166. Ross, R.A., Ciccarone, V., Meyers, M.B., *et al.* Differential expression of intermediate filaments and fibronectin in human neuroblastoma cells. In: *Advances in Neuroblastoma Research*, edited by A.E. Evans. New York, Alan R. Liss Inc., 1987.

167. Rostami, A., Eccelston, P.A., Lisak, R.P., *et al.* Generation and biological properties of a monoclonal antibody to galactocerebroside. Brain Res., *298*:203–208, 1984.

168. Rubinstein, L.J. Embryonal central neuroepithelial tumors and their differentiating potential. A cytogenetic view of a complex neuro-oncological problem. J. Neurosurg. *62*:795–805, 1985.

169. Rungger-Braendle, E., Achstaetter, T., and Franke, W.W. An epithelium-type cytoskeleton in glial cells: astrocytes of amphibian optic nerves contain cytokeratin filaments and are connected by desmosomes. J. Cell Biol. *9*:705–716, 1989.

170. Rungger-Braendle, E. and Gabbiani, G. The role of cytoskeletal and cytocontractile elements in pathologic processes. Am. J. Pathol. *110*:359–393, 1983.

171. Russell, D. and Rubinstein, L.J. *Pathology of Tumors of the Nervous System*, ed. 5. Baltimore, William & Wilkins, 1989.
172. Sasaki, A., Ogawa, A., Nakazato, Y., *et al.* Distribution of neurofilament protein and neuron-specific enolase in peripheral neuronal tumours. Virchows Arch. (A), *407:*33–41, 1985.
173. Schiffer, D., Giordana, M.T., Mauro, A., *et al.* Immunohistochemical demonstration of vimentin in human cerebral tumors. Acta Neuropathol. *70:*209–219, 1986.
174. Schindler, E. and Gulotta, F. Glial fibrillary acidic protein in medulloblastomas and other embryonic CNS tumors of children. Virch. Arch., *398:*263–275, 1983.
175. Schlaepfer, W.W. Neurofilaments of mammalian peripheral nerve. In: *Neurofilaments*, edited by G.A. Marotta, pp. 57–85. Minneapolis, University of Minneapolis Press, 1983.
176. Schlaepfer, W.W. and Freeman, L.A. Neurofilament proteins of rat peripheral nerve and spinal cord. J. Cell Biol., *78:*653–662, 1978.
177. Schmechel, D.E. Gamma-subunit of the glycolytic enzyme enolase: non-specific or neuron specific? Lab. Invest., *52:*239–242, 1985.
178. Schmidt, M.L., Carden, M.J., Lee, V.M.-Y., *et al.* Phosphate dependent and independent neurofilament epitopes in the axonal swellings of patients with motor neuron disease and controls. Lab. Invest. *56:*282–294, 1987.
179. Schmidt, M.L., Gur, R.E., Gur, R.C., *et al.* Intraneuronal and extracellular neurofibrillary tangles exhibit mutually exclusive cytoskeletal antigens. Ann. Neurol. *23:*184–189, 1988.
180. Schmidt, M.L., Lee, V.M.-Y., Hurtig, H., *et al.* Properties of antigenic determinants that distinguish neurofibrillary tangles in progressive supranuclear palsy and Alzheimer's disease. Lab. Invest. *59:*460–466, 1988.
181. Schmidt, M.L., Lee, V.M.-Y., and Trojanowski, J.Q. Analysis of epitopes shared by Hirano bodies and neurofilament proteins in normal and Alzheimer's disease hippocampus. Lab. Invest., *60:*513–522, 1989.
182. Schnitzer, J., Sommer, I., Lagenaur, C., *et al.* Immunological characterization of cell types in the cerebellum. In: *Clinical and Biological Aspects of Peripheral Nerve Diseases*, edited by L. Battistin, G.A. Hasnim, and A. Lajtha, pp. 301–319. New York, A.R. Liss, 1983.
183. Schwechheimer, K., Wiedenmann, B., and Franke, W.W. Synaptophysin: a reliable marker for medulloblastomas. Virchows Arch. (A), *411:*53–59, 1987.
184. Shaw, G. and Weber, K. Differential expression of neurofilament triplet proteins in brain development. Nature, *298:*277–292, 1982.
185. Shea, T.B., Sihag, R.K., and Nixon, R.A. Neurofilament triplet proteins of NB2a/d1 neuroblastoma: posttranslational modification and incorporation into the cytoskeleton during differentiation. Dev. Brain Res. *43:* 97–109, 1988.
186. Shinoda, H., Marini, A.M., Cosi, C., *et al.* Brain region and gene specificity of neuropeptide gene expression in cultured astrocytes. Science, *245:*415–417, 1989.
187. Somogyi, P., Hodgson, A.J., DePotter, R.W., *et al.* Chromogranin immunoreactivity in the central nervous system. Immunochemical characterization, distribution and relationship to catecholamine and enkephalin pathways. Brain Res. Rev. *8:*193–230, 1984.
188. Stead, R.H., Qizilbash, A.H., Kontozoglou, T., *et al.* An immunohistochemical study of pleomorphic adenomas of the salivary gland: glial fibrillary acidic protein-like immunoreactivity identifies a major myoepithelial component. Hum. Pathol. *19:*32–40, 1988.
189. Steiner, P.M. and Roop, D.R. Molecular and cellular biology of intermediate filaments. Ann. Rev. Biochem. *57:*593–625, 1988.
190. Sternberger, L.A. *Immunocytochemistry*, ed. 2. New York, Wiley, 1979.
191. Sternberger, N.H., Itoyama, Y., Kies, M.W., *et al.* Myelin basic protein demonstrated immunocytochemically in oligodendroglia prior to myelin sheath formation. Proc. Natl. Acad. Sci. USA, *75:*2521–2524, 1978.
192. Stratton, M.R., Darling, J., Pilkington, G.J., *et al.* Characterization of the human cell line TE671, Carcinogenesis *10:*899–905, 1989.
193. Szaro, B.G., Lee, V.M.-Y., Gainer, H. Spatial and temporal expression of phosphorylated and nonphosphorylated forms of neurofilament proteins in the developing nervous system of *Xenopus laevis*. Dev. Brain Res., *48:*87–103, 1989.
194. Takahashi, H., Wakabayashi, K., Kawai, K., *et al.* Neuroendocrine markers in the central nervous system neuronal tumors (gangliocytoma and ganglioglioma). Acta Neuropathol., *77:*237–243, 1989.
195. Tapscott, S.J., Bennett, G.S., Toyama, Y., *et al.* Intermediate filament proteins in the developing chick spinal cord. Dev. Biol. *86:*40–54, 1981.
196. Tascos, N.A., Parr, J., and Gonatas, N.K. Immunocytochemical study of the glial fibrillary acidic protein in human neoplasms of the nervous system. Hum. Pathol., *5:*454–458, 1982.
197. Tashian, R.E., Hewett-Emmett, D. (eds). *Biology and Chemistry of the Carbonic Anhydrases, Vol.* 429. Ann N.Y. Acad. Sci., 1984.
198. Taylor, C.R., Russell, R., Lukes, R.J., *et al.* An immunohistochemical study of immunoglobulin content of primary central nervous system lymphomas. Cancer, *41:*2197–2205, 1978.
199. Thomas, L., Hartung, K., Langosch, D., *et al.* Identification of synaptophysin as a hexameric channel protein of the synaptic vesicle membrane. Science, *242:*1050–1053, 1988.

200. Thomas, P., Battifora, H., Manderino, G.L., *et al.* A monoclonal antibody against neuron-specific enolase. Am. J. Clin. Pathol., *88:* 145–152, 1987.

201. Tremblay, G.F., Lee, V.M.-Y., Trojanowski, J.Q. Expression of vimentin, glial filament and neurofilament proteins in primitive childhood brain tumors. A comparative immunoblot and immunoperoxidase study. Acta Neuropathol., *68:*239–244, 1985.

202. Trojanowski, J.Q. Neurofilament proteins and human nervous system tumors. J. Histochem. Cytochem., *35:*999–1003, 1987.

203. Trojanowski, J.Q. Cytoskeletal proteins and neuronal tumors. In: Diagnostic Immunopathology, edited by R.B. Colvin, A.K. Bhan, and R.T. McCluskey, pp. 225–243. New York, Raven Press, 1988.

204. Trojanowski, J.Q., Friedman, H.S., Burger, P.C., *et al.* A rapidly dividing human medulloblastoma cell line (D283 MED) expresses all three neurofilament subunits. Am. J. Pathol., *126:*358–363, 1987.

205. Trojanowski, J.Q., Gordon, D., Obrocka, M.A., *et al.* Developmental expression of neurofilament and glial filament proteins in the developing human pituitary gland. Dev. Brain Res., *13:*229–239, 1984.

206. Trojanowski, J.Q. and Hickey, W.F. Human teratomas express differentiated neural antigens: an immunohistochemical study with monoclonal antibodies against neurofilaments, glial filaments and myelin basic protein. Am. J. Pathol., *115:*383–389, 1984.

207. Trojanowski, J.Q., Kelsten, M.L., and Lee, V.M.-Y. Phosphate dependent and independent neurofilament protein epitopes are expressed throughout the cell cycle in human medulloblastoma (D283) cells. Am. J. Pathol. *135:*74–758, 1989.

208. Trojanowski, J.Q. and Lee, V.M.-Y. Anti-neurofilament monoclonal antibodies: Reagents for the evaluation of human neoplasms. Acta Neuropathol., *59:*155–158, 1983.

209. Trojanowski, J.Q. and Lee, V.M.-Y. Expression of neurofilament antigens by normal and neoplastic human adrenal chromaffin cells. N. Engl. J. Med. *313:*101–104, 1985.

210. Trojanowski, J.Q., Lee, V.M.-Y., Pillsbury, N., *et al.* Neuronal origin of human esthesioneuroblastoma demonstrated with anti-neurofilament monoclonal antibodies. N. Engl. J. Med., *307:*159–161, 1982.

211. Trojanowski, J.Q., Lee, V.M.-Y., and Schlaepfer, W.W. Neurofilament breakdown products in degenerating rat and human peripheral nerves. Ann. Neurol. *16:*349–355, 1984.

212. Trojanowski, J.Q., Obrocka, M.A., and Lee, V.M.-Y. Distribution of neurofilament subunits in neurons and neuronal processes: immunohistochemical studies of bovine cerebellum with subunit-specific monoclonal antibodies. J. Histochem. Cytochem. *33:* 557–563, 1985.

213. Tsokos, M., Chandra, R.S., and Triche, T.J. Neuron-specific enolase in the diagnosis of neuroblastoma and other small round cell tumors in children. Hum. Pathol., *15:*575–584, 1984.

214. Unsicker, K. Differentiation and phenotypical conversion of adrenal medullary cells: the effects of neuronotrophic, neurite-promoting, hormonal and neuronal signals. In: *Neurohistochemistry: Modern Methods and Applications*, edited by P. Panula, H. Päiväriuta, and S. Soinila. pp. 183–206. New York, Alan R. Liss, 1986.

215. Vandenberg, S.R., Herman, M.M., and Rubinstein, L.J. Embryonal central neuroepithelial tumors: current concepts and future challenges. Cancer Metast. Rev., *5:*343–364, 1987.

216. VanMuyen, G.N.P., Ruiter, D.J., and Warnaar, S.O. Intermediate filaments in Merkel cell tumors. Hum. Pathol., *16:*590–595, 1985.

217. VanMuyen, G.N.P., Ruiter, D.J., and Warnaar, S.O. Coexpression of intermediate filament polypeptides in human fetal and adult tissues. Lab. Invest., *57:*359–369, 1987.

218. Valasco, M.E., Dahl, D., Roessmann, U., *et al.* Immunohistochemical localization of glial fibrillary acidic protein in human glial neoplasms. Cancer, *45:*484–494, 1980.

219. Velasco, M.E., Ghobrial, M.W., Ross, E.R. Neuron-specific enolase and neurofilament protein as markers of differentiation in medulloblastoma. Surg., Neurol., *23:*177–182, 1985.

220. Velasco, M.E., Roesmann, U., and Gambetti, P. The presence of glial fibrillary acidic protein in the human pituitary gland. J. Neuropathol. Exp. Neurol., *41:*150–163, 1982.

221. Vinores, S.A., Bonnin, J.M., Rubinstein, L.J., *et al.* Immunohistochemical demonstration of neuron-specific enolase in neoplasms of the CNS and other tissues. Arch. Pathol. Lab. Med., *108:*536–540, 1984.

222. Virtanen, I., Miettinen, M., Lehto, V.P., *et al.* Diagnostic application of monoclonal antibodies to intermediate filaments. Ann. N.Y. Acad. Sci., *455:*635–648, 1984.

223. Weber, K. and Osborn M. Cytoskeleton: definition, structure and gene regulation. Pathol. Res. Pract., *175:*128–145, 1982.

224. Weiner, H.L. and Hauser, S.L. Neuroimmunology. II. Antigenic specificity of the nervous system. Ann. Neurol., *12:*499–509, 1982.

225. Wiedenmann, B. and Franke, W.W. Identification and localization of synaptophysin, integral membrane glycoprotein of Mr 38,000 characteristic of presynaptic vesicles. Cell, *41:*1017–1028, 1985.

226. Wiedenmann, B., Franke, W.W., Kuhn, C., *et al.* Synaptophysin: a marker protein for neuroendocrine cells and neoplasms. Proc. Natl.

Acad. Sci. USA, *83*:3500–3504, 1986.

227. Whitaker, J.N. The protein antigens of peripheral nerve myelin. Ann. Neurol., *9* (Suppl): 56–64, 1981.

228. Wikstrand, C.J., Bourdon, M.A., Pegram, C.N., *et al.* Human fetal brain antigen expression common to tumors of neuroectodermal tissue origin. Gliomas, neuroblastomas, and melanomas. J. Neuroimmunol., *3*:43–62, 1982.

229. Yachnis, A.T., Trojanowski, J.Q., Memmo, M., *et al.* Expression of neurofilament proteins in the hypertrophic granule cells of Lhermitte-Duclos disease: an explanation for the mass effect and the myelination of parallel fibers in the disease state. J. Neuropathol. Exp. Neurol., *47*:206–216, 1988.

230. Yen, S.H. and Fields, K.L. Antibodies to neurofilament, glial filament and fibroblastic intermediate filament proteins bind to different cell types in the nervous system. J. Cell Biol., *88*:115–126, 1981.

CHAPTER 12

Immunocompetence of Patients with Malignant Glioma

HAROLD F. YOUNG, M.D., RANDALL E. MERCHANT, Ph.D.
and MICHAEL L. J. APUZZO, M.D.

INTRODUCTION

Patients with the diagnosis of malignant glioma face a dismal prognosis. The survival curve of these patients is fixed and prolongation of life, much less quality life, has been only increased in miniscule fashion by modern techniques of surgery, irradiation and/or chemotherapy. In fact, some therapists, neurosurgeons as well as oncologists, take a nihilistic approach to glioma therapy or use palliative steroids only. All of the present therapeutic approaches are self-limited and therefore it behooves investigators to carefully examine the status of these patients with malignant gliomas in order to design more effective modes of therapy. It is our intention in this chapter to examine the immunocompetence of patients with gliomas. We will examine *(a)* the general immunocompetence of patients with gliomas, the evidence for glioma-specific antigens (Ags), *(b)* the concept of immunological privilege of the brain, and *(c)* the previous and current applications of immunotherapy for malignant gliomas.

GENERAL IMMUNOCOMPETENCE OF PATIENTS WITH MALIGNANT GLIOMA

The relationship of host immunocompetence to neoplasia is well-documented in the literature. Altered states of immunity, especially cell-mediated immunity, are associated with neoplastic growth (4). It is held that immunosuppression is related to the onset of neoplastic disease, but it is still argued whether the onset of neoplastic disease is the result of or the cause of neoplasia. In humans, there are some statistical claims that under certain circumstances immunological reactions have some association with malignant disease. Immunosuppressive therapy or immunodeficiency diseases are also associated with an increased incidence of malignancy. In a review of 4000 cases of renal transplants, Doll and Kinlen reported there were 42 cases of malignant disease (26). In another series of 200 cases of ataxia-telangiectasia, 14 patients developed malignant tumors, mainly lymphomas and among 90 cases of Wiskott-Aldrich syndrome, 11 patients developed primary malignant lymphoma (78, 89). Both conditions are T-cell deficiency states with thymus aplasia. Immunosuppression thus appears to play an important role in tumor development.

The concept of immunological surveillance was first proposed in 1958 by Erlich and Thomas and later elaborated on by Burnet who attempted to explain how the immune system defends against malignancy (19). Theoretically, neoplastic cell transformation is a continuum that is consistently recognized and destroyed by the cellular immune system acting as a surveillance system. Experimental support for the surveillance theory is found in manipulations known to inhibit the immune response, such as total body radiation, neonatal thymectomy, or treatment with antilymphocyte serum. Whether or not the theory of immune surveillance is too simplistic, it is an attractive hypothesis which should be kept in mind when considering the general immune status of patients with gliomas since glioblastoma is a malignancy and, like systemic cancer, has a profound influence on the immune system.

Patients harboring gliomas have a marked, generalized depression of immune competence affecting both cellular and humoral immune mechanisms. Immune deficiencies are present in the preoperative period, prior to radiotherapy, chemotherapy or steroid administration. Brooks *et al.* and Mahaley *et al.* have defined a significant degree of anergy in patients with malignant gliomas (15, 17, 59). Cell-mediated immune mechanisms have received the most attention because of their role in delayed hypersensitivity reactions (DHRs), allograft rejection, reactions against virus-infected target cells, and tumor cell lysis. Cell-mediated immunity is depressed as evidenced by impaired DHRs to common skin test Ags such as *Candida,* mumps, PPD, and streptokinase, the inability to become sensitized to dinitrochlorobenzene, and diminished blastogenic responses of peripheral blood lymphocytes (PBL) to mitogens and alloantigens in vitro. Mahaley *et al.* studied DHRs and lymphocyte counts in 42 patients with glioblastoma multiforme and 17 others with anaplastic gliomas (59). At the time of surgery, DHRs and the percentage of the patients responding to two or more skin-test Ags were subnormal and the magnitude of the cellular anergy was proportional to the presence and extent of anaplasia. The degree of cellular anergy also paralleled the progression of the tumor and sequential evaluation showed that a continuing reduction in certain immune parameters could signify tumor recurrence. Specific studies on circulating T-lymphocytes have demonstrated a general depression of T cell number and function in patients with malignant gliomas (16, 85, 116). We examined the in vitro blastogenic response of glioma patients' PBL to T cell mitogens and saw that 50% of patients with glioblastoma multiforme demonstrated a depressed mitogenic response while lymphocytes from patients with low-grade astrocytomas did not (116). Depressed PBL proliferation may also result from insufficient interleukin-2 (IL-2) production and/or expression of IL-2 receptors by stimulated lymphocytes (28, 113). Elliott suggested that T cells of glioma patients have an "intrinsic" defect in their ability to synthesize IL-2 and its receptors (28).

We reported several years ago that plasma from patients with glioblastoma inhibits the blastogenic response of PBL from normal blood donors, while plasma from patients with low grade astrocytomas has no effect (116). This implied the presence of an inhibitory factor within the sera of patients with high-grade glioma, a finding which has been subsequently supported by others. This blocking activity, though not specifically identified, appeared to be at least partially responsible for the impairment of cell-mediated immune responses in patients with glioblastoma multiforme. It remains unclear, however, whether the appearance of the blocking factor is important in the progression of a benign astrocytoma into a highly malignant glioblastoma. The blocking factor may alter the host-tumor relationship, and block the host's immunosurveillance mechanisms needed to suppress the benign astrocytoma over long periods of time.

Suppressor factors have been described that specifically block cytotoxicity of glioma cells in culture by peripheral blood leukocytes from glioma patients (51, 53). The identity of this humoral suppressor factor was unknown, although the suppressor activity was reported to migrate in the IgG fraction of serum. Recently, immunosuppressive factors have been described in brain tumor cyst fluid as well which suppressed mitogen-induced activation of lymphocytes from normal individuals (48). Serum and cerebrospinal fluid (CSF) from the same patients had little suppressive effect. This immunosuppressive factor, therefore, appeared to be mainly secreted by the tumor. Recently, the mediator, transforming growth factor-beta$_2$ (TGF-β_2), a 12.5-kilodalton peptide, has been found to be secreted by a variety of tumor cells in vitro including those obtained from glioblastomas (24, 30, 83, 112). Fontana and co-workers reported that TGF-β_2 inhibited T cell proliferation and generation of immune responses in vitro by interfering with IL-2 dependent pathways (24, 30, 112).

Mononuclear cell populations in peripheral blood of glioma patients have been studied extensively. Although there is a depletion of T-lymphocytes in these patients, the effects of altered immunoregulatory function remain controversial. Leukocytes from glioma patients demonstrate enhanced suppressive immunoregulatory cell functions due to a subclass of suppressor cells as well as other cells of monocytic origin (13). Actually, there may be a shift in T lymphocyte subpopulations toward a relative excess of T-suppressor lymphocytes, and a relative elevation of suppressor cells in patients prior to surgery. It is not yet known why this disturbance in T-cell subpopulations or immunoregulation occurs in patients with malignant glial tumors.

The assays designed to demonstrate the cytotoxic capabilities of lymphocytes in patients with gliomas have yielded conflicting results. Hitchcock *et al.* studied Ag preparations used for in vivo testing by polyacrylamide gel electrophoresis (42). They showed that the "glioma-specific" antigenically active fractions in tests of cutaneous delayed hypersensitivity contained antigenic components shared with normal white matter, contradicting a premise of a specific response. Levy in well-controlled studies investigated the specificity of lymphocyte-mediated in vitro cytotoxic reactions in a series of patients with primary brain tumors (54). Specific tumor-directed lymphocyte cytotoxicity was found in 35/41 patients. Lymphocytes of each patient and controls were tested for tumor specificity against 9 to 12 different cell lines. The targets were from early-passage cultures and included both neoplastic and normal cells from a given patient as well as allogenic tumor cells of types both related and unrelated to the patient's tumor. Cytotoxic responses were abolished by prior absorption of the lymphocytes on appropriate cell monolayers affirming some specificity. In the patients with gliomas, direct assays showed that cytotoxicity was directed against two different antigenic determinants. One was found on cells from all glial tumors, regardless of the degree of anaplasia: a common glioma Ag. The other was expressed on anaplastic gliomas, melanomas, and fetal cells, but not on well-differentiated gliomas, normal adult glial cells, fetal fibroblasts, or other tumors. The presence of this second Ag was believed to be due to the common origin of melanocytes and glial cells from the ectodermal cells of the neural tube. However, more recent studies of cytotoxicity have only occasionally demonstrated apparent tumor-specific cytotoxicity in vitro. For example, Woosley *et al.* found significant cytotoxicity in only 7/36 patients with anaplastic gliomas (111). The cumulative data suggest that cell-mediated cytotoxicity, if it does occur in vivo, is probably inadequate to halt a growing glioma.

Studies of humoral immune responses have been meager when compared to the effort to define the cell-mediated status of patients with malignant brain tumors. Immunoglobulin levels are essentially normal, with the exception of elevated serum IgM (61). Following immunization with tetanus and influenza vaccines, patients with malignant gliomas show an initial, but unsustained, rise in antibody (Ab) titers. The ability to mount an effective humoral response to a novel Ag is also significantly impaired. It is as yet unknown whether this impairment in Ab response is due to a B-cell defect or a basic defect in processing and recognition of any new Ag.

The presence of a specific humoral antiglioma response is unsettled although immunoglobulins have been detected bound to CNS tumors (109). Since the target Ags are unknown, this does not guarantee a specific tumor response since IgG binds to myelin, neurons, and glia (1). Patients studied by Kornblith *et al.* showed significant autologous serologic responses in 15/20 patients with Grades I, II, and III astrocytomas, but only 5/22 patients with Grade IV glioblastoma had cytotoxic sera (50). The authors' observation that the presence of cytotoxic Ab correlated with a better prognosis can be challenged on the basis that the Ab was found most frequently in the sera of patients with lower grade malignancies. As shown by Woosley *et al.*, postoperative sera from only 20% of the patients were specifically cytotoxic in vitro and sera from normal controls were often cytotoxic for glioma cells used as targets (111). Yet, some well-controlled studies have reported glioma-specific activity remaining in an occasional patient following extensive absorption to remove contaminating Abs (79).

Even in those patients where Ab or cell-mediated cytotoxicity can be demonstrated against tumor cells in vitro, the rejection of neoplasms usually does not occur in vivo. The broad, nonspecific immunosuppression previously discussed may be paramount, but other specific tumor escape mechanisms may be operative. The Hellstroms first proposed the concept of specific humoral blocking factors that may act by coating the antigenic sites of the tumor, thus preventing recognition by cytotoxic lymphocytes (39). This factor was thought to be an Ag-Ab complex that masked a specific Ag (93). Ag-Ab complexes can induce suppressor T cells and the latter probably causes enhanced tumor growth (32). It is now apparent that blocking factors may activate suppressor T-cell subsets to elaborate glycoproteins which are the active agents that interfere with effector cell subsets. At the same time, suppressor macrophages also elaborate mediators, such as prostaglandins, which impair the development of effector cells too, principally by inhibiting the proliferation of T-cell precursors. Another possible mechanism of blockade is one in which a soluble Ag may block cytotoxic T lymphocytes (CTLs) via interaction with specific receptors. This type of specific alteration may affect either the expression of already sensitized T cells or may prevent precursors of Ag-sensitive cells from turning into functional CTLs. Thus, tolerance is produced in the host to the Ag. Also, the Ag released by the tumor could combine with lymphocyte receptors and inactivate them which could explain the described nonimmunoglobulin suppressor factor found in tumor cyst fluid (48). Thus, blocking may be very important in patients with gliomas and may play a role in immunosuppression via various mechanisms.

Whether surgery can restore immunocompetence is questionable since there is invariably tumor left behind and all adjunctive therapies following surgery are usually also immunosuppressive and limited in their application. However, newer techniques of radiotherapy such as brachytherapy and the development of new chemotherapeutic agents and combinations of agents can be expected to reduce tumor cell numbers to such an extent as to significantly reduce their immunosuppressive influence.

IMMUNOLOGIC PRIVILEGE OF THE BRAIN

When a foreign skin graft is transplanted from one individual to another, rejection occurs unless the donor and recipient are identical twins. Medawar, however, observed that if foreign skin was implanted into the brain of a rabbit it was not rejected (65). He concluded that the brain was "an immunologically privileged site," meaning that Ags within the brain did not evoke an afferent response because the brain lacked a lymphatic system and because immunocytes in the circulation were prevented entry into the CNS by the blood-brain barrier (BBB). Previously, Murphy and Sturm found that tumors which were rejected when transplanted subcutaneously would often grow when transplanted into the brain (72).

This concept of the brain's immune privilege, however, has not stood the test of time. Scheinberg *et al.* showed that chemically induced ependymomas from inbred mice could be successfully transplanted 100% of the time into the brains of other animals of the same strain but only 10–35% of the time into allogeneic mice (87, 88). If the ependymomas were cured by irradiation, rejection of subsequent tumor implants occurred whether in the skin or in the brain. Also, irradiation of subcutaneous (SC) tumor implants resulted in a significant number of animals refractory to subsequent intracerebral or SC implants. If mice were previously immunized with tumor cells in complete Freund's adjuvant, there was inhibition of growth in 85% of subsequent implants. Reconfirmation of these findings has been interpreted to demonstrate incomplete immunological privilege. Not only is there evidence for intracerebral graft rejection and a systemic immune response secondary to intracerebral implants, but in patients with brain tumors there is the entry of effector cells from the systemic circulation into the brain tumor. Ridley and Cavanaugh made the initial observation that more than 50% of malignant gliomas show characteristic infiltration of lymphocytes and monocytes in perivascular and diffuse sections of the tumor (82). This infiltration is similar to the histological picture of successful host vs. graft rejection specimens and has been confirmed by many other authors (14, 70, 76, 97). Though there is not universal agreement on these observations in terms of correlation with survival, nevertheless it is this evidence that has encouraged investigators to pursue and test a variety of immunotherapeutic approaches for the treatment of patients with gliomas. It may be that this recruitment of lymphocytes represents a too feeble and ineffective immune response that constitutes a major reason for the failure of the immune system to prevent tumor growth. The nature and function of intratumoral lymphoid populations are also disputed. The infiltrates are believed to be predominantly composed of T cells and macrophages (70, 94). Von Hanwehr *et al.* characterized the blood mononuclear cells infiltrating CNS tumors using monoclonal antibodies (mAbs) and found a predominance of T cells with the suppressor/cytotoxic phenotype (103).

The original concept that the brain is an immunologically privileged site, therefore, can no longer be supported. Rather a much stronger argument can be made for "partial" privilege on the basis of *(a)* intracerebral graft rejections, *(b)* induction of a systemic immune response secondary to intracerebral implants, and *(c)* entry of leukocytic effectors of hematologic origin into areas of pathological alteration of the BBB as occurs in neoplasia, trauma, or inflammatory processes.

GLIOMA-SPECIFIC ANTIGENS

For over 30 years, it has been known that neoplastic cells express Ags some of which are shared by normal cells as well as other antigens which are unique. Unfortunately, in regard to the CNS, special problems arise when considering the above statement. There are now large numbers of CNS Ags which have been characterized and it is clear that many are evident throughout the vertebrate fila (107). Some of the best studied Ags are intracellular in location, including S-100 protein, 14-3-2 protein, glial fibrillary acidic protein, alpha-2 glycoprotein, and myelin basic protein. Also, a large number of reported interspecies brain-associated Ags are also co-expressed on human lymphoid cells and fetal brain cells (33).

In 1936, Siris using rabbit antiserum demonstrated similar reactivity profiles in complement fixation assays against aqueous extracts of normal brain or glioblastoma tissue (92). Since then, numerous investigators have shown that glial tumors share certain antigenic determinants with normal brain. It has been observed that the expression of normal brain Ags decreases with increasing malignancy, suggesting that these Ags are expressed by less anaplastic cells and are absent from anaplastic cells. To date, however, no one has defined the existence of any additional or unique glioma-specific antigens (GSAs).

Several authors have extensively studied the sera of patients with gliomas. Trouillas used sera from patients immunized with extracts of their own tumors to demonstrate a common Ag shared by glioblastomas, astrocytomas, and fetal brain (98). Coakham *et al.* studied the sera from 25 patients with malignant gliomas (22). They used microcytotoxicity and immune adherence assays to describe reactivity and defined several categories of glioma surface Ags: *(a)* common to glioma cells, but not shared with other tissues; *(b)* shared by astroctyoma, neuroblastoma, meningioma, ependymoma, and melanoma tissue; *(c)* shared with fetal tissue; and *(d)* widely distributed on many diverse cell types.

The alternative approach to the problem of GSAs is the study of glioma Ags through the utilization of heteroantisera. Difficulties are encountered here because interspecies preparation of antisera may lack specificity of response. Identification of GSAs is also complicated by the polyclonal nature of the Ab preparations and the large number of contaminating reactivities that need be removed by extensive adsorption studies. Nevertheless, much important work has been done in this area since the initial work of Siris in 1936, when he concluded that glioma Ags did not differ from those of normal brain (92). Coakham used rabbit antisera adsorbed by normal brain to demonstrate cytotoxicity against cultured astrocytoma cells that could not be adsorbed by fetal brain, meningioma, or other tumors (21). Wahlstrom *et al.*, using normal brain-adsorbed rabbit antisera, demonstrated immunofluorescence in 15/15 glioblastoma cell lines and no reactivity against nonglial cell lines (104). Preadsorption with glioblastoma Ags abolished all reactivity. Wikstrand and co-workers performed very carefully controlled studies using heteroantisera (107, 108). They extensively adsorbed primate antisera raised against glioblastoma tissue and cell lines. These reacted against all gliomas tested but not against unrelated tumors as evidenced by complement-mediated lysis and indirect immunofluorescence assays. Adsorption with normal adult or fetal brain, however, abolished reactivity against many of the target glioma cell lines.

Hybridoma technology is now revolutionizing our approaches to the serological definition of cell surface molecules. Monoclonal Abs are produced by the hybrid progeny that result from the fusion of a myeloma cell with a normal immunoglobulin-secreting B cell. The probability that the resulting hybrid will secrete an Ab specific for GSAs is improved if the B cell parent can be derived from the spleen of hyperimmunized animals or even from B cells taken from glioma biopsy tissue. Monoclonal Abs have resulted in the description of various categories of Ags: some restricted to gliomas, those expressed by most glioma cells thus far tested, some shared by gliomas and fetal brain, and some widely distributed on tissue of neuroectodermal origin (18, 90, 108, 110). Even among cells of experimental cell lines there is remarkable heterogeneity in regard to expression of Ags (8).

It is anticipated that mAbs will solve many of the adsorption problems in the use of heteroantisera (49). The most serious problem which will then remain will be to overcome the histological and biochemical heterogenicity of cells which exist within each class of glioma and from different populations of cells within a given tumor. Indeed, recent studies indicate that there are Ags apparently restricted to glioma cells, as well as Ags shared with a variety of neoplastic and nonneoplastic cell types in the brain (18, 110). Specific mAbs have been produced which recognize some of these epitopes and some have been used in glioma imaging studies as well as in phase I immunotherapeutic investigations (see next section).

IMMUNOTHERAPY FOR GLIOMA

Even though patients with a malignant glioma typically have impaired cell-mediated immune functions, the observation that tumors often show lymphocytic infiltration and that this might positively correlate with survival (14, 25, 70, 76, 82) has spawned experimentation with immunotherapy as a fourth treatment modality. Much of the experimental work has centered on the use of adoptively transferred lymphoid cells, cytokines, mAbs, and nonspecific immunostimulants in an attempt to restore and/or enhance reactivity of the patient's immune system for their tumor. Even though these early attempts to manipulate a patient's immune system and the use of immunotherapy have yielded rather poor responses in terms of tumor rejection, many of the early immunotherapy trials were performed with limited knowledge of the immune system, much less the immune system as it relates to the CNS. Also, many of these studies were uncontrolled, nonrandomized studies on patients with recurrent tumors who had failed conventional therapies and who in most cases had a poor clinical status and required high dosages of corticosteroids to control peritumoral edema. Nevertheless, we will briefly review some of the early trials for their historical merit so one can appreciate how they laid the foundation for immunotherapies currently under investigation.

Active Specific Immunotherapy

Historically, whenever one considers immunotherapy, either in the treatment or prevention of diseases, it has been specific immunization that has led to the greatest success. As a cancer therapy, active specific immunization should sensitize patients to Ags present on their tumors. Immunogens thus far employed include autologous tumor cells, antigenically related cultured tumor cell lines, tumor extracts that retain tumor-specific antigenicity, or cross-reacting Ags of viral or bacterial nature. Inoculation with live cells is considered to be more effective than inoculation with killed cells or cell extracts. With this form of immunotherapy for glioma, there is theoretically some risk of induction of allergic (autoimmune) encephalitis since patients receive material derived from the CNS. The risk of such a cross-reactive immune response to Ags shared by brain and autologous tumor tissue is probably increased when adjuvants are included.

It is not surprising that active specific immunotherapy was the first form of immunotherapy applied to patients with gliomas. In 1960, Bloom made the first attempt to induce an immune response in a patient with malignant glioma by SC inoculation of viable autologous tumor cells (11). A total of 15 ml of glioma cell suspension was injected into 12 sites distributed over both thighs. The tumor grew locally at 10/12 injection sites and the patient's clinical status continued to worsen. At autopsy, there was no evidence of rejection of the tumor in the brain and tumor cells were found in regional lymph nodes of the thigh.

A year later, Grace *et al.* reported on their attempts at immunization with autologous tumor cells in six patients with glioblastoma multiforme (34). Tumors grew at the site of SC injection in two patients but two others strongly rejected the tumor inoculation and had positive DHRs when tested intradermally with saline extracts of both normal brain and tumor, suggesting a degree of nonspecific immunoreaction. In the two patients whose inocula grew, there was no positive skin test reaction with the same Ags. Although survival was not improved in the patients with delayed hypersensitivity to glioma Ags, there must have been an immune response determining the success or failure of the inoculations.

Almost a decade later, Trouillas and Lapras reported on their studies of 20 glioma patients who were treated postoperatively with viable autologous cells with and without Freund's adjuvant, injected in 4–10 inoculations (100). In all their patients, the implanted glioma cells did not grow and they all developed DHRs to glioma extracts. About the same time, Febvre *et al.* reported the development of DHRs to lyophilized glioma cells following immunization with autologous glioma cells (29).

In 1973, Trouillas reported on a randomized trial in 65 patients utilizing active immunotherapy with saline extracts of autologous tumor and Freund's adjuvant (99). Patients were randomized into four treatment groups postoperatively. Immunotherapy alone was given to 10 patients, 18 received immunotherapy plus irradiation, 20 had only radiotherapy, and 17 received no additional therapy. The median survival time of the patients receiving immunotherapy alone was 7.4 months; equivalent to the survival time of patients treated with radiotherapy alone. Combined immunotherapy and irradiation increased median survival time to over 10 months. Of the 28 patients receiving immunotherapy, 24 developed DHRs to autologous tumor cells during therapy and cytotoxic, complement-binding Abs for cultured glioma cells. Histopathological studies performed on six members of the immunotherapy group demonstrated lymphocytic and plasmacytic infiltration in four cases. The other two samples were examined more than seven months after immunotherapy, suggesting the effect is short-lived.

About the same time, Bloom *et al.* reported the results of a randomized prospective clinical trial using lethally irradiated autologous tumor cells in glioma patients following radical surgery and whole-brain radiation (10). Of the 62 patients entered in this trial, 27 received the cellular therapy and 10 of these received multiple SC inoculations. Unfortunately, insufficient necrotic tissue limited most patients to one inoculation and no attempt was made to select immunocompetent patients for this study. In only six patients did a local reaction occur at the site of injection and intradermal skin tests with small aliquots of irradiated cells were negative in all patients. Patients who received active immunotherapy did not survive longer than the control groups of patients.

Ommaya in 1976 and Albright in 1977 reported on their attempts to induce intracerebral DHRs in 10 patients with malignant astrocytomas following surgery and radiotherapy (3, 75). Five patients received CCNU chemotherapy alone; two received immunotherapy alone; and three received combined therapy. Immunotherapy was a monthly intradermal inoculation with BCG and semi-monthly inoculations with neuraminidase-treated autologous tumor cells. Injections of PPD were done directly into the tumor site. For 4/5 patients receiving immunotherapy, histopathological comparisons of tumor before and after treatment revealed a slight-to-moderate increase in the inflammatory response after immunotherapy. This response, however, did not extend to the periphery of the tumor. All 10 patients had their tumors recur within 12 months of therapy.

In 1983, Mahaley *et al.* reported on 20 glioma patients treated by active immunization within 4 weeks of craniotomy (58). To be eligible for treatment, each patient had to have a Karnofsky functional rating of 70 or higher, an absolute PBL count of more than 1000 cells/mm^3, skin test responses to at least one of four recall Ags, peripheral blood T-cell numbers equal to or greater than half that of normals, and no steroid therapy at the time of entry into the study. Patients were immunized with irradiated cells from one of two cultured human glioma cell lines and BCG was included as an adjuvant with the first inoculation. Inoculations were repeated monthly and levamisole was given concurrently, while whole-brain radiation therapy and BCNU chemotherapy were started one month after the first inoculation. As the disease progressed serial immunological testing confirmed gradual decline in DHRs, lymphocyte counts, and T cells. Only three patients developed cutaneous hypersensitivity to the tumor cell Ag, and all but one patient produced serum Ab against the immunizing glioma cell line. The Ab response was directed mainly against the fetal bovine serum proteins incorporated into the cultured glioma cells and against the foreign Major Histocompatibility Complex (MHC) Ags on cells. It appeared that active immunization resulted in the production of specific antiglioma activity. There was also a pronounced difference in the 12- and 18-month survival between the two groups receiving the two different cell lines.

Active Nonspecific Immunotherapy

Nonspecific immune stimulation uses adjuvants or substances that are not antigenically similar to the tumor in order to enhance the general immunocompetence of the host. Adjuvants may be administered systemically or directly into the lesion. In animal experiments of nonintracranial neoplasms, intralesional injection results occasionally in tumor regression, while systemic therapy is ineffective in animals with established tumors (6).

Nonspecific immunotherapy for malignant glioma has been used in a small number of uncontrolled studies to date. In 1978, Selker reported on six patients treated with the microbial agent, *Corynebacterium parvum,* a bacterium which stimulates cellular immunity and should prevent the formation of blocking Ab (91). No conclusions could be drawn regarding survival, but increased intracranial pressure was noted in all patients with mass lesions, a possible pitfall with this form of therapy. In 1976, Miki *et al.* used intradermal inoculations of BCG to stimulate immune responses in 45 patients who initially had a negative PPD reaction (69). Approximately 65% of the glioma patients converted to PPD positive and of those, more than 50% survived more than 3 years after surgery. Patients injected with BCG whose PPD remained negative had a survival rate at 3 years comparable to that of the uninoculated controls, i.e. approximately 12%.

In 1981, Mahaley reported on a randomized, controlled trial of levamisole treatment in patients who had had surgery, radiotherapy, and BCNU chemotherapy previously (62). The levamisole-treated group did not demonstrate any alteration of serial immune responses in cellular or humoral immunity nor was there any evidence of Ab-mediated cellular cytotoxicity against autologous glioma targets in vitro. During therapy, no changes were noted in measurements made of nonspecific immune competence, including DHRs, peripheral blood counts, and serum IgM levels. There was also no difference in survival in the treated group versus the control group, agreeing with a concurrent glioma model in rats where levamisole also failed to prolong survival.

It appears that using nonspecific immunostimulation to boost general immunocompetence in patients with gliomas may find a place in combination with other forms of cellular immunotherapy (active or adoptive) or as a form of intralesional therapy.

Adoptive Immunotherapy

This therapy attempts to confer immunocompetence to the host by transfer of cellular elements of the immune system. Autologous or allogenic lymphocytes may be administered systemically or locally into the tumor. Since most patients with cancer and as mentioned above, patients with glioblastoma, have broad immunosuppression due to their tumor burden as well as their previous chemotherapy or radiotherapy, adoptive therapy holds some theoretical advantages since it can be administered in combination with more conventional forms of cancer therapy.

In 1972, Takakura *et al.* reported on the infusion of allogenic bone marrow cells systemically into eight infants and children with a variety of malignant neoplasms (96). Up to 10 infusions of 50 ml of ABO-compatible marrow from healthy adults were administered. Although the therapy was shown to be safe, no conclusions could be reached in this study because of the small number of patients and varying histological tumor types.

In 1977, we conducted a nonrandomized trial involving 17 patients with recurrent glioblastoma multiforme (115). Autologous leukocytes (buffy coat) were obtained by leukapheresis, washed, concentrated and immediately injected directly into the intracranial tumors via an Ommaya reservoir. Survival appeared to be longer than expected in some of the patients. One patient had a remarkable clinical improvement and long survival. Extended survival was noted in those patients who had a longer interval between diagnosis and immunotherapy and probably signaled a low level of antitumor activity in those patients. Autopsies performed in six patients revealed extensive tumor necrosis, although there were no histopathologic effects which could be definitely ascribed to the immunotherapy.

From these and other early studies, conclusive judgments could not be made with regard to the efficacy of adoptive immunotherapy for glioma as none of these small, nonrandomized trials demonstrated either an immune reaction or increased survival. Over the past few years, however, dramatic inroads have been made in lymphocyte culture methodology and in our understanding of how biological response modifiers work in vitro and in vivo. The availability of purified biologics and improved culture methods have encouraged continued investigation of this immunotherapeutic modality (see below). We believe that the large trials required to judge therapeutic benefits of adoptively transferred autologous lymphocytes can now be performed.

Biologics

With the development of recombinant DNA technology and large-scale production methods, quantities of purified human cytokines, such as the interferons, interleukins, and various other growth or antitumor factors, can now be produced economically in quantities needed for clinical applications. So far, treatments involving these "manufactured" cytokines, particularly recombinant interferon-alpha (IFN-alpha) and interleukin-2 (rIL-2), have produced significant tumor regressions in a variety of cancers but have shown only limited activity in CNS malignancies.

The three classes of IFN (alpha, beta, and gamma) are now available in recombinant form and their antiglioma activities have been clinically tested in recent years. For all IFNs, the mechanism of antitumor action is believed to be by direct cytotoxicity and increased MHC expression on tumor cells (38). Indirectly, the IFNs stimulate the tumoricidal activities of natural killer cells and macrophages. In one of the first trials of systemic IFN-beta, Sano *et al.* reported that 7/42 patients with recurrent anaplastic astrocytomas had complete or partial responses lasting 4 or more weeks (86). Nagai and co-workers also found that administration of IFN-beta either locally or systemically reduced glioma mass in some patients (73). However, Duff *et al.*, in a phase II trial in which IFN-beta was injected both IV and intratumorally for glioblastoma, observed no clear improvement in mean survival (27). More recently, Yung *et al.* reported on a multicenter phase I/II trial of systemic IFN-beta in recurrent glioma patients that showed a partial or objective response in 15/65 cases and a stable disease rate of 51% (117). Mahaley's group, however, saw no evidence of response in seven patients given IV IFN-beta for up to 12 weeks (60). Three of their patients' CT scans indicated stable disease while progression was seen in the other four.

Ueda *et al.* conducted a phase II clinical trial with IFN-alpha in 15 patients with recurrent glioma and reported tumor regressions in six patients (101). In a later trial, Mahaley and co-workers treated 17 patients with recurrent gliomas with an intensive 8-week course of systemic IFN-alpha (63). CT scans indicated reduced tumor burdens in six patients. They also observed frequent but reversible neurotoxicity manifested as somnolence, disorientation and/or memory loss. Mahaley's group also recently completed testing of systemic IFN-gamma in 14 patients with recurrent glioma (57). Most patients experienced fever, chills, and nausea. Only one patient demonstrated CT evidence of tumor regression and most showed progression of their disease over the eight week course of therapy. Although these initial trials of IFNs for glioma have been disappointing, their efficacy may improve by combination with chemotherapeutic agents or other biologics. Along this line, our current rIL-2 clinical trial will determine if repeated, direct, intracavitary injections of rIL-2 in combination with systemic recombinant IFN-alpha, constitutes a safe adjunctive treatment with other, more conventional cytoreductive therapeutic modalities (67).

In response to mitogenic or antigenic stimuli, T cells divide and secrete a variety of "interleukins", proteins which serve as communication links between lymphoid cells. These cytokines orchestrate immune reactions by providing the necessary signals for amplification or suppression. Interleukin-2 was initially called T cell growth factor by Morgan *et al.* (71) who purified it in 1976. We now know that in addition to its well-defined effect on T and B lymphocyte proliferation, IL-2 amplifies the tumoricidal activity of a class of non-B, non-T lymphocytes such that they express what has become known as lymphokine-activated killer (LAK) activity (35, 36, 40, 41). These cells express non-MHC-restricted cytotoxicity for tumor cell lines in vitro and some experimental tumors in vivo. For clinical trials, lymphocytes demonstrating LAK activity are usually produced by culture of peripheral blood mononuclear cells (MNC) for 3–7 days in media containing 100-1500 U human rIL-2 (41).

Immunotherapy with systemic rIL-2 alone or combined with adoptive transfer of autologous cells having LAK activity is currently being tested in patients with a variety of malignancies. To date, systemic rIL-2 therapies have produced sustained clinical responses only in patients with metastatic melanoma or renal cell carcinoma (84) although metastatic lesions from all tumor types have failed to respond when located within the confines of the CNS.

Jacobs and colleagues were the first to show that LAK cells which were toxic for autologous tumor could be generated in vitro from PBL of glioma patients (46). We have also produced LAK activity from glioblastoma patients' blood MNC under serum-free culture conditions, although there was a wide range of tumoricidal activity which appeared to correlate inversely with steroid dependency (66, 68). In vitro production of LAK activity from PBL of steroid-dependent patients was significantly less than that generated by patients not taking the drug. This observation was consistent with that of Grimm *et al.*, who showed that hydrocortisone abrogated the generation of LAK activity at pharmacologic doses (37) and our studies which indicated that the induction of LAK cell activity was inhibited in a dose-dependent manner with continuous exposure to physiologically relevant levels of dexamethasone, hydrocortisone, prednisolone, or methylprednisolone in vitro (64).

Intralesional injection of LAK cells alone or with rIL-2, has proven to be safe for a variety of malignancies and has also avoided the toxicity seen after systemic administration (2, 68, 80). Interleukin-2 injected into tumor attracts circulating lymphocytes and activates the infiltrating lymphocytes to become more cytotoxic for tumor cells (12, 74, 102). Human rIL-2 will also attract circulating NK cells (12, 74) and we believe that this may prove relevant to in situ targeting of activated effector cell populations into sites of brain tumor as well. For these reasons, nearly all of the clinical trials involving rIL-2 for glioma have favored an intralesional approach. These trials have also usually included a concomitant local administration of autologous lymphoid cells activated with rIL-2, phytohemagglutinin, or both.

Jacobs *et al.* were the first to report on a clinical trial of autologous LAK cells and/or rIL-2 injected into the cerebral tissue surrounding the cavity remaining after resection of a recurrent glioblastoma (47). Five patients were injected with only LAK effectors, four others with rIL-2 alone, and one patient received LAK cells and rIL-2. They did not observe severe toxicity, and at 3 months following surgery and treatment, nine patients showed a stable clinical course and no CT evidence of tumor progression.

Over the past few years, we and a number of other groups have conducted additional clinical trials of human rIL-2 alone or in combination with autologous lymphocytes expressing *in vitro* LAK activity in order to define toxicity and indicate its potential efficacy in patients with high-grade glioma (5, 44, 45, 46, 55, 66, 68, 114). Since Jacobs' trial indicated that intracerebral injections of factor and cells were safe, all of these later trials have chosen a direct route: injection into the cystic cavity remaining after tumor excision, and/or neural parenchyma surrounding the site of tumor excision. In our patients, craniotomy combined with immunotherapy frequently triggered temporary headache and lethargy (66, 68). We believed these symptoms of increased intracranial pressure resulted from cerebral edema since MRI and CT scans consistently indicated greater than expected amounts of edema around the surgery site. Our preclinical animal studies had indicated that an intracerebral rIL-2 injection produced edema in normal brain and increased peritumoral edema in an animal model of glioma (105, 106). None of the patients showed any MRI or CT evidence nor did any postmortem studies provide any indication that any secondary disease process developed in the brain as a consequence of the immunotherapy. When tumors recurred or progressed, they remained histologically identical to the original lesion. Our results and those of others indicate that single or multiple injections of rIL-2 alone or in combination with autologous LAK cells represent safe, but as yet, noncurative therapies, although the fact that sustained clinical responses have been reported, suggests that such therapies may slow a recurrence of tumor at the site of treatment. Efforts to improve outcome from IL-2-based immunotherapies for malignant glioma are continuing with manipulation of rIL-2 dosing and scheduling and also with combinations of rIL-2 and other recombinant cytokines. We believe that a maintenance arm involving rIL-2 may be needed following adoptive transfer at surgery to perpetuate the antitumor effects of cellular and/or cytokine immunotherapy.

Passive Immunotherapy

Studies of passive immunotherapy have been limited until recently because of technical difficulties. While many investigators have described Abs that react with glioma cells in vitro; the use of heterologous and xenogeneic polyclonal antisera requires extensive adsorption against normal cells to remove unwanted and cross-reacting activities. In the past, humoral immunity has been considered a minor factor in tissue graft and tumor cell destruction in vivo in the unsensitized host. Serotherapy also carries the inherent risk of the formation of blocking factors in vivo, i.e., Ag-Ab complexes may form in vivo and cause tumor enhancement, and increased rate of tumor growth. Antibodies which are unable to bind complement or Fc receptors on macrophages may bind specifically to tumor associated Ags and will block the antigenic sites so they are no longer recognized by cytotoxic effectors. The tumor may also escape immune control as immune complexes interact with specific receptors on CTLs. In the early 1970s, Mahaley *et al.* administered a radioiodinated xenogeneic antiglioma Ab preparation in order to demonstrate the expression of glioma-associated Ags in vivo and found that the Abs localized in glioma tissue (56).

The availability of large quantities and varieties of mAbs has provoked new interest in serotherapy for the treatment of patients with brain tumors. A number of murine mAbs have now been developed which recognize determinants on the surface of glioma cells with a high degree of specificity and allow precise tumor imaging and selective delivery of isotopes or toxins to the site of tumor (9, 18, 52, 118, 119). One of the more extensively studied of these antiglioma mAbs has been 81C6 which reacts with an epitope on tenascin, an extracellular matrix glycoprotein found in primary brain tumors but not in normal CNS tissues. In one of the first preclinical radioimmunotherapy experiments, Blasberg and co-workers showed that [^{125}I]-labelled 81C6 crossed the vasculature of a human glioma xenograft in an athymic mouse and bound to the tumor associated Ag in detectable amounts (9). Furthermore, high levels of the mAb were retained in the xenograft for 3–5 days resulting in high isotope exposure. This study, however, also showed that the distribution of the mAb was heterogenous in glioma. Zlautsky *et al.* recently administered [^{131}I]-labelled 81C6 into the carotid artery ipsilateral to tumor in seven patients with malignant brain lesions (118). While labeled mAb accumulated in the tumor at concentrations sufficient for imaging by gamma camera, the uptake of mAb was quite variable in tumor samples from individual patients. These authors suggested that heterogeneity with regard to vascular permeability and antigenic expression accounted for these differences. Indeed, many in the field agree that the major difficulty for mAb therapies has been that uptake of mAb into solid tumor is never uniform and because of this, most of the current clinical trials now underway involve delivery of mAbs into the subarachnoid space to treat tumor that has invaded this compartment (7, 52). Lashford *et al.* intrathecally administered one of several [^{131}I]-labeled mAbs in five patients with leptomeningeal tumors (52). The mAb chosen for therapy depended on the immunophenotype of the tumor and its distribution in the CSF was monitored by radioimmunoscintigraphy. They reported clinical improvement and an objective response (i.e., clearance and/or decrease in numbers of malignant cells from the CSF) in 4/5 patients. Furthermore, these responses were sustained for 7–24 months.

Clearly, this area of investigation is constantly evolving and we have but only begun to understand the potential efficacy of antitumor therapy using specific mAbs. This therapy can be expected to become more important as new ways are defined to enhance delivery of mAbs into glioma and new mAbs to glioma Ags are produced that have better specificity.

FUTURE OF IMMUNOTHERAPY OF PATIENTS WITH BRAIN TUMORS

Even with the availability of safe imaging by CT and MRI, brain tumors are well established by the time of diagnosis. All forms of presently known therapy: surgery, irradiation and chemotherapy, though each effective in its own right, are limited when applied to the human brain. Thus, there is a need to evaluate immunotherapy, and continued research needs to be done on this important area of therapy. It is also becoming increasingly clear, however, that if immunotherapy is ever to become a viable treatment modality for patients with brain tumor, immunotherapies involving tumor cells, leukocytes, and/or biologics must work in spite of or overcome the immunosuppressive activity of corticosteroids. These drugs have pleiotropic effects on immune functions (20, 23, 95): *(a)* inhibiting lymphocyte proliferation; *(b)* decreasing expression of histocompatibility Ags on Ag-processing cells; *(c)* preventing destruction of microorganisms ingested by macrophages; *(d)* inhibiting cytokine production; *(e)* suppressing production of immunoglobulins; *(f)* partially diminishing the expression of receptors for IL-2 on lymphocytes (31, 81), and *(g)* inhibiting NK activity (43, 77). As mentioned earlier, physiologic levels of steroid significantly inhibit the generation of LAK activity. Until better drugs are developed to combat peritumoral edema, conservative use of steroids or their replacement with nonsteroidal compounds should be encouraged during immunotherapy.

CONCLUSIONS

Patients with malignant glioma present a special challenge to all who care for them. Even though almost 2 decades have passed since the development of CT scanning of the brain, these tumors are usually not diagnosed until they are large masses deep in the white matter. By this time, the patients are symptomatic and their cellular immune functions are significantly compromised. However, it has also been shown that immunological reactions do occur in the CNS and that the circulating immune system is not completely separated from the brain by the BBB, especially as it is defective in the glial tumors. Therefore, the use of immunotherapy remains a viable option worthy of further research and application along with conventional, cytoreductive therapeutic modalities.

Ways of improving the immunocompetence of glioma patients as well as the testing of recombinant cytokines and glioma-specific mAbs have been investigated for only the past few years. Immunotherapies using mixtures of cytokines alone or in combination with cellular therapies and/or chemotherapeutic agents have shown some promise in other malignancies and may also prove effective for glioma. The preliminary investigations with mAb have been encouraging especially in light of the fact that radioimmunotherapy and immunotoxin therapy do not require a fully functional immune system to be efficacious and can be useful even in glioma patients immunosuppressed by their tumor or by corticosteroids. Certainly the constantly evolving developments in hybridoma and recombinant DNA technologies are encouraging and we can reasonably expect a wide variety of immunotherapeutic options for brain tumors to develop in the future.

Patients with primary malignancies of the CNS remain among the best suited for immunotherapy trials because they usually have a single, localized lesion readily identified by CT scan and they are not debilitated by paraneoplastic factors such as malnutrition and cachexia which often appear in patients with other forms of cancer. We are hopeful that over the next decade, we will witness a pronounced increase in the number of prospective, randomized immunotherapy trials necessary to determine safe and effective new treatments for patients with malignant glioma.

REFERENCES

1. Aarli, J.A., Aparicio, S.R., Lumsden, C.E., *et al.* Binding of normal human IgG to myelin sheaths, glia and neurons. Immunology, *28:*17–85, 1975.
2. Adler, A., Stein, J.A., Kedar, E., *et al.* Intralesional injection of interleukin-2–expanded autologous lymphocytes in melanoma and breast cancer patients: A pilot study. J. Biol. Resp. Modif., *3:*491–500, 1984.
3. Albright, L., Seab J.A., and Ommaya A.K. Intracerebral delayed hypersensitivity reactions in glioblastoma multiforme patients. Cancer, *39:*1331–1336, 1977.
4. Apuzzo, M.L. and Mitchell M.S. Immunological aspects of intrinsic glial tumors. J. Neurosurg., *55:*1–18, 1981.
5. Barba, D., Saris, S.C., Holder, C., *et al.* Intratumoral LAK cell and interleukin-2 therapy of human gliomas. J. Neurosurg., *70:*175–182, 1989.
6. Bast, R.C., Zbar, B., Borsos, T., *et al.* BCG and cancer. N. Engl. J. Med., *290:*1413–1420, 1974.
7. Benjamin, J.C., Moss, T., Moseley, R.P., *et al.* Cerebral distribution of immunoconjugate after treatment for neoplastic meningitis using an intrathecal radiolabeled monoclonal antibody. Neurosurgery, *25:*253–258, 1989.
8. Bigner, D.D., Bigner, S.H., Ponten, J., *et al.*

Heterogeneity of genotypic and phenotypic characteristics of fifteen permanent cell lines derived from human gliomas. J. Neuropathol. Exp. Neurol., *40:*201–229, 1981.

9. Blasberg, R.G., Nakagawa, H., Bourdon, M.A., *et al.* Regional localization of a glioma-associated antigen defined by monoclonal antibody 81C6 *in vivo:* kinetics and implications for diagnosis and therapy. Cancer Res., *47:*4432–4443, 1987.
10. Bloom, H.J.G., Peckham, M.J., Richardson, A.E., *et al.* Glioblastoma multiforme: a controlled trial to assess the value of specific active immunotherapy in patients treated by radical surgery and irradiation. Br. J. Cancer, *27:*253–267, 1973.
11. Bloom, W.H., Carstairs, K.C., Crompton, M.R., *et al.* Autologous glioma transplantation. Lancet, *2:*77–78, 1960.
12. Bottazzi, B., Introna, M., Allavena, P., *et al. In vitro* migration of human large granular lymphocytes. J. Immunol., *134:*2316–2321, 1985.
13. Braun, D.P., Penn, R.D., Flannery, A.M., *et al.* Immunoregulatory cell function in peripheral blood leukocytes of patients with intracranial gliomas. Neurosurgery, *10:*203–209, 1982.
14. Brooks, W.H., Markesbery, W.R., Gupta, G.D., *et al.* Relationship of lymphocyte invasion and survival of brain tumor patients. Ann. Neurol., *4:*219–224, 1978.
15. Brooks, W.H., Netsky, M.G., Normansell, D.E., *et al.* Depressed cell-mediated immunity in patients with primary intracranial tumors. Characterization of a humoral immunosuppressive factor. J. Exp. Med., *136:* 1631–1647, 1972.
16. Brooks, W.H., Roszman, T.L., Mahaley, M.S. *et al.* Immunobiology of primary intracranial tumours. Analysis of lymphocyte subpopulations in patients with primary brain tumours. Clin. Exp. Immunol., *29:*61–66, 1977.
17. Brooks, W.H., Roszman, T.L., Rogers, A.S. Impairment of rosette-forming T lymphocytes in patients with primary intracranial tumors. Cancer, *37:*1869–1873, 1976.
18. Bullard, D.E., Adams, C.J., Coleman, R.E., *et al. In vivo* imaging of intracranial human glioma xenografts comparing specific with nonspecific radiolabeled monoclonal antibodies. J. Neurosurg., *64:*257–262, 1986.
19. Burnet, F.M. Immunological aspects of malignant disease. Lancet, *1:*1171–1174, 1967.
20. Claman, H.N. Anti-inflammatory effects of corticosteroids. Clin. Immunol. Allergy, *4:* 317–329, 1984.
21. Coakham, H. Surface antigen(s) common to human astrocytoma cells. Nature, *250:*328–330, 1974.
22. Coakham, H.B., Kornblith, P.L., Quindlen, E.A., *et al.* Autologous humoral response to human gliomas and analysis of certain cell surface antigens: *in vitro* study with the use of microcytotoxicity and immune adherence assays. J. Natl. Cancer Inst., *64:*223–233, 1980.
23. Cupps, T.R. and Fauci, A.S. Corticosteroid-mediated immunoregulation in man. Immunol. Rev., *65:*133–155, 1982.
24. de Martin, R., Haendler, B., Hofer-Warbinek, R., *et al.* Complementary DNA for human glioblastoma-derived T cell suppressor factor, a novel member of the transforming growth factor-beta gene family. EMBO J., *6:*3673–3677, 1987.
25. DiLorenzo, N., Palma, L., and Nicole, S. Lymphocytic infiltration in long-survival glioblastoma: possible host's resistance. Acta. Neurochir., *39:*27–33, 1977.
26. Doll, R. and Kinlen, L. Immunosurveillance and cancer: epidemiological evidence. Br. Med. J., *4:*420–422, 1970.
27. Duff, T., Borden, E., Bay, J., *et al.* Phase II trial of interferon-beta for treatment of recurrent glioblastoma multiforme. J. Neurosurg., *64:*408–413, 1986.
28. Elliott, L.H., Brooks, W.H., and Roszman, T.L. Role of interleukin-2 (IL-2) and IL-2 receptor expression in the proliferative defect observed in mitogen-stimulated lymphocytes from patients with gliomas. J. Natl. Cancer Inst., *78:*919–922, 1987.
29. Febvre, H., Maunoury, R., Constans, J.P., *et al.* Reactions d'hypersensibilitie retardee avec des lignees de cellules tumorales humaines cultivees *in vitro* chez des malades portears de tumeurs cerebrales malignes. Int. J. Cancer, *10:*221–223, 1972.
30. Fontana, A., Hengartner, H., de Tribolet, N., *et al.* Glioblastoma cells release interleukin 1 and factors inhibiting interleukin 2-mediated effects. J. Immunol., *132:*1837–1844, 1984.
31. Frey, B.M., Walker, C., Frey, F.J., *et al.* Pharmacokinetics and pharmacodynamics of three prednisolone prodrugs. Effect on circulating lymphocyte subsets and function. J. Immunol., *133:*2479–2487, 1984.
32. Gershon, R.K., Birnbaum-Mokyr, M., and Mitchell, M.S. Activation of suppressor T cells by tumor cells and specific antibody. Nature, *250:*594–596, 1974.
33. Golub, E.S. Connections between the nervous, hematopoietic and germ-cell systems. Nature, *399:*483, 1982.
34. Grace, I.T., Perese, D.M., Metzgar, R.S., *et al.* Tumor autograft responses in patients with glioblastoma multiforme. J. Neurosurg., *18:*159–167, 1961.
35. Grimm, E.A., Mazumder, A., Zhang, H.Z., *et al.* Lymphokine-activated killer cell phenomenon:lysis of natural killer-resistant fresh solid tumor cells by interleukin 2-activated autologous human peripheral blood lymphocytes. J. Exp. Med., *155:*1823–1841, 1982.
36. Grimm, E.A., Mazumder, A., and Rosenberg, S.A. *In vitro* growth of cytotoxic human lymphocytes. V. Generation of allospecific cyto-

toxic lymphocytes to nonimmunogenic antigen by supplementation of *in vitro* sensitization with partially purified T cell growth factor. Cell Immunol., *70:*248–259, 1982.

37. Grimm, E.A., Muul, L.M., and Wilson, D.J. The differential inhibitory effects exerted by cyclosporine and hydrocortisone on the activation of human cytotoxic lymphocytes by recombinant interleukin-2 versus allospecific CTL. Transplantation, *39:*537–540, 1985.
38. Gutterman, J.U., Blumenschein, G.R., Alexanian, *et al.* Leukocyte interferon-induced tumor regression in human metastatic breast cancer, multiple myeloma, and malignant lymphoma. Ann. Intern. Med., *93:*399–406, 1980.
39. Hellstrom, K.E. and Hellstrom, I. Lymphocyte-mediated cytotoxicity and blocking serum activity to tumor antigens. Adv. Immunol., *18:*209–277, 1974.
40. Henney, C., Kuribayashi, K., Kern, D., *et al.* Interleukin-2 augments natural killer cell activity. Nature, *291:*335–338, 1981.
41. Herberman, R.B., Hiserodt, J., Vujanovic, N., *et al.* Lymphokine-activated killer cell activity. Characteristics of effector cells and their progenitors in blood and spleen. Immunol. Today, *8:*178–181, 1987.
42. Hitchcock, M.H., Hollinshead, A.C., Chretien, P., *et al.* Soluble membrane antigens of brain tumors. I. Controlled testing for cell-mediated immune responses in a long surviving glioblastoma multiforme patient. Cancer, *40:*660–666, 1977.
43. Holbrook, N.J., Cox, W.J., and Horner, H.C. Direct suppression of natural killer activity in human peripheral blood leukocyte cultures by glucocorticoids and its modulation by interferon. Cancer Res., *43:*4019–4025, 1983.
44. Ingram, M., Jacques, S., Freshwater, D.B., *et al.* Salvage immunotherapy of malignant glioma. Arch. Neurol., *122:*1483–1486, 1987.
45. Ingram, M., Shelton, C.H., Jacques, S., *et al.* Preliminary clinical trial of immunotherapy for malignant glioma. J. Biol. Resp. Modif., *6:*489–498, 1987.
46. Jacobs, S.K., Wilson, D.J., Kornblith, P.L., *et al.* Killing of human glioblastoma by interleukin-2-activated autologous lymphocytes. J. Neurosurg., *64:*114–117, 1986.
47. Jacobs, S.K., Wilson, D.J., Kornblith, P.L., *et al.* Interleukin-2 or autologous lymphokine-activated killer cell treatment of malignant glioma: Phase I trial. Cancer Res., *46:*2101–2104, 1986.
48. Kikuchi, K. and Neuwelt, E.A. Presence of immunosuppressive factors in brain-tumor cyst fluid. J. Neurosurg., *59:*790–799, 1983.
49. Kohler, G. and Milstein, C. Continuous cultures of fused cells secreting antibody of predefined specificity. Nature, *256:*495–497, 1975.
50. Kornblith, P.L., Coakham, H.B., Pollack, L.A., *et al.* Autologous serologic responses in glioma patients. Correlation with tumor grade and survival. Cancer, *52:*2230–2235, 1983.
51. Kumar, S. and Taylor G. Specific immunocytotoxicity and blocking factors in the tumors of the central nervous system. Br. J. Cancer, *28:*135–141, 1973.
52. Lashford, L.S., Davies, A.G., Richardson, R.B., *et al.* A pilot study of [^{131}I] monoclonal antibodies in the therapy of leptomeningeal tumors. Cancer, *61:*857–868, 1988.
53. Levy, N.L. Cell-mediated cytotoxicity and serum-mediated blocking: evidence that their associated determinants on human tumor cells are different. J. Immunol., *121:*916–922, 1978.
54. Levy, N.L. Specificity of lymphocyte-mediated cytotoxicity in patients with primary intracranial tumors. J. Immunol., *121:*903–915, 1978.
55. Lillehei, K.O., Kruse, C.A., Mitchell, D.H., *et al.* Adoptive immunotherapy of recurrent glioma using interleukin-2 stimulated lymphocytes. Surg. Forum., in press, 1989.
56. Mahaley, M.S. Experiences with antibody production from human glioma tissue. Prog. Exp. Tumor Res. *17:*31–39, 1972.
57. Mahaley, M.S., Bertsch, L., Cush, S., *et al.* Systemic gamma-interferon therapy for recurrent gliomas. J. Neurosurg., *69:*826–829, 1988.
58. Mahaley, M.S., Bigner, D.D., Dudka, L.F., *et al.* Immunobiology of primary intracranial tumors. Part 1. Active immunization of patients with anaplastic human glioma cells. J. Neurosurg., *59:*201–207, 1983.
59. Mahaley, M.S., Brooks, W.H., Roszman, T.L., *et al.* Depressed cell-mediated immunity in patients with primary intracranial tumors. Part 1: Studies of the cellular and humoral immune competence of brain-tumor patients. J. Neurosurg., *46:*467–476, 1977.
60. Mahaley, M.S., Dropcho, E.J., Bertsch, L., *et al.* Systemic beta-interferon therapy for recurrent gliomas: a brief report. J. Neurosurg., *71:*639–641, 1989.
61. Mahaley, M.S., Gillespie, G.Y., Gillespie, R.P., *et al.* Immunobiology of primary intracranial tumors. Part 8. Serological responses to active immunization of patients with anaplastic gliomas. J. Neurosurg., *59:*208–216, 1983.
62. Mahaley, M.S., Steinbok, P., Aronin, P., *et al.* Immunobiology of primary intracranial tumors. Part 4. Levamisole as an immune stimulant in patients and in the ASV glioma model. J. Neurosurg., *54:*220–227, 1981.
63. Mahaley, M.S., Urso, M.B., Whaley, R.A., *et al.* Immunobiology of primary intracranial tumors. Part 10. Evaluation of the therapeutic efficacy of interferon in the treatment of recurrent gliomas. J. Neurosurg., *63:*719–725, 1986.
64. McVicar, D.W., Merchant, R.E., Merchant,

L.H., *et al.* Corticosteroids inhibit the generation of lymphokine-activated killer (LAK) activity. Cancer Immunol. Immunother., *29:*211–218, 1989.

65. Medawar, P.B. Immunity to homologous grafted skin. III. The fate of skin homografts transplanted to the brain, to subcutaneous tissue, and to the anterior chamber of the eye. Br. J. Exp. Pathol., *29:*58–69, 1948.
66. Merchant, R.E., Grant, A.J., Merchant, L.H., *et al.* Adoptive immunotherapy for recurrent glioblastoma multiforme using lymphokine activated killer (LAK) cells and recombinant interleukin-2. Cancer, *62:*665–671, 1988.
67. Merchant, R.E., McVIcar, D.W., Merchant, L.H., *et al.* Treatment of patients with recurrent glioblastoma by repeated intralesional injections of recombinant interleukin-2 (rIL-2) alone or in combination with systemic interferon-alpha (Abstract). J. Neuro.-Oncol., *7:*S19, 1989.
68. Merchant, R.E., Merchant, L.H., Cook, S.H.S., *et al.* Intralesional infusion of lymphokine-activated killer (LAK) cells and recombinant interleukin-2 (rIL-2) for the treatment of patients with malignant brain tumor. Neurosurgery, *23:*725–732, 1988.
69. Miki, Y., Sano, K., Takakura, K., *et al.* Adjuvant immunotherapy with BCG for malignant brain tumors. Neurol. Med. Chir., *16:*357–364, 1976.
70. Morantz, R.A., Wood, G.W., Foster, M., *et al.* Macrophages in experimental and human brain tumors. Part 2. Studies of the macrophage content of human brain tumors. J. Neurosurg., *50:*305–311, 1979.
71. Morgan, D.A., Ruscetti, F.W., and Gallo, R.C. Selective *in vitro* growth of T-lymphocytes from normal bone marrows. Science, *193:*1007–1008, 1976.
72. Murphy, J.B. and Sturm, E. Conditions determining transplantability of tissues to the brain. J. Exp. Med., *38:*183–197, 1923.
73. Nagai, M. and Arai, T. Clinical effect of interferon in malignant brain tumours. Neurosurgery Rev., *7:*55–64, 1984.
74. Natuk, R.J. and Welsh, R.M. Chemotactic effect of human recombinant interleukin 2 on mouse activated large granular lymphocytes. J. Immunol., *139:*2737–2743, 1987.
75. Ommaya, A.K. Immunotherapy of gliomas: a review. Adv. Neurol., *15:*337–359, 1970.
76. Palma, L., DiLorenzo, N., and Guidetti, B. Lymphocytic infiltrates in primary glioblastomas and recidivous gliomas. Incidence, fate, and relevance to prognosis in 228 operated cases. J. Neurosurg., *49:*854–861, 1978.
77. Pedersen, B.K. and Beyer, J.M. Characterization of the *in vitro* effects of glucocorticosteroids on NK cell activity. Allergy, *41:*220–224, 1986.
78. Penn, I. and Starzl, T.E. Malignant tumors arising *de novo* in immunosuppressed organ transplant recipients. Transplantation, *14:* 407–417, 1972.
79. Pfreundschuh, M., Shiku, H., Takahashi, T., *et al.* Serological analysis of cell surface antigens of malignant human brain tumors. Proc. Natl. Acad. Sci. USA, *75:*5122–5126, 1978.
80. Pizza, G., Severini, G., Menniti, D. *et al.* Tumor regression after intralesional injection of interleukin 2 in bladder cancer. Int. J. Cancer, *34:*359–367, 1984.
81. Reed, J.C., Abidi, A.H., Alpers, J.D., *et al.* Effect of cyclosporin A and dexamethasone on interleukin 2 receptor gene expression. J. Immunol., *137:*150–154, 1986.
82. Ridley, A. and Cavenaugh, J.B. Lymphocytic infiltration in gliomas: Evidence of possible host resistance. Brain, *94:*117–124, 1971.
83. Rook, A.H., Kehrl, J.H., Wakefield, L.M., *et al.* Effects of transforming growth factor beta on the functions of natural killer cells: depressed cytolytic activity and blunting of interferon responsiveness. J. Immunol., *136:*3916–3920, 1986.
84. Rosenberg, S.A., Lotze, M.T., Muul, L.M., *et al.* A progress report on the treatment of 157 patients with advanced cancer using lymphokine-activated killer cells and interleukin-2 or high-dose interleukin-2 alone. N. Engl. J. Med., *316:*889–897, 1987.
85. Roszman, T.L. and Brooks, W.H. Immunobiology of primary intracranial tumours. III. Demonstration of a qualitative lymphocyte abnormality in patients with primary brain tumours. Clin. Exp. Immunol., *39:*395–402, 1980.
86. Sano, K., Nagai, M., Takakura, K. *et al.* Effects of Hu IFN-beta on gliomas. 3rd Annual International Congress for Interferon Research, 1982.
87. Scheinberg, L.C., Edelman, F.L., and Levy, W.A. Is the brain "an immunologically privileged site"? I. Studies based on intracerebral tumor homotransplantation and isotransplantation to sensitized hosts. Arch. Neurol., *11:*248–264, 1964.
88. Scheinberg, L.C., Kotsilimbas, D.G., Kargf, R., *et al.* Is the brain "an immunologically privileged site"? III. Studies based on homologous skin grafts to the brain and subcutaneous tissues. Arch. Neurol., *15:*62–67, 1966.
89. Schneck, S.A. and Penn, I. *De novo* brain tumors in renal transplant recipients. Lancet, *1:*983–986, 1971.
90. Schnegg, J.F., Diserens, A.C., Carrel, S., *et al.* Human glioma-associated antigens detected by monoclonal antibodies. Cancer Res., *41:*1209–1213, 1981.
91. Selker, R.G., Wolmark, N., Fisher, B., *et al.* Preliminary observations on the use of *Corynebacterium parvum* in patients with primary intracranial tumors: effects on intracranial pressure. J. Surg. Oncol., *10:*299–303, 1978.
92. Siris, J.H. Concerning the immunological specificity of glioblastoma multiforme. Bull. Neurol. Inst. NY., *4:*597–601, 1936.
93. Sjogren, H.O., Hellstrom, I., Bansal, S.C., *et al.* Suggestive evidence that "blocking antibod-

ies" of tumor-bearing individuals may be antigen-antibody complexes. Proc. Natl. Acad. Sci. USA., *68:*1372–1375, 1971.

94. Stavrou, D., Anzil, A.P., Weidenbach, W., *et al.* Immunofluorescence study of lymphocyte infiltration in gliomas. Identification of T-lymphocytes. J. Neurol. Sci., *33:*275–282, 1977.
95. Stevenson, J.R. and Taylor, R. Effects of glucocorticoid and antiglucocorticoid hormones on leukocyte numbers and function. In. J. Immunopharmacol., *10:*1–6, 1988.
96. Takakura, K., Miki, Y., Kubo, O., *et al.* Adjuvant immunotherapy for malignant brain tumors. Jpn. J. Clin. Oncol., *2:*109–120, 1972.
97. Takeuchi, J. and Barnard, R.O. Perivascular lymphocytic cuffing in astrocytomas. Acta. Neuropathol., *35:*265–271, 1976.
98. Trouillas, P. Carcino-fetal antigen in glial tumors. Lancet, *2:*552, 1971.
99. Trouillas, P. Immunologie et immunotherapie active des tumeurs cerebrales. Etat actuel. Rev. Neurol., *128:*23–38, 1973.
100. Trouillas, P. and Lapras, C. Immunotherapie active des tumeurs cerebrales. A propos de 20 cas. Neurochirurgie, *16:*143–170, 1970.
101. Ueda, S., Hirakawa, K., Suzuki, K., *et al.* Interferon therapy for brain tumor patients. No Shinkei Geka, *10:*149–154, 1982.
102. Vaage, J. Local and systemic effects during interleukin-2 therapy of mouse mammary tumors. Cancer Res., *47:*4296–4298, 1987.
103. Von Hanwehr, R.I., Hofman, F.M., Taylor, C.R., *et al.* Mononuclear lymphoid populations infiltrating the microenvironment of primary CNS tumors. Characterization of cell subsets with monoclonal antibodies. J. Neurosurg., *60:*1138–1147, 1984.
104. Wahlstrom, T., Linder, E., Saksela, E., *et al.* Tumor specific membrane antigens in established cell lines from gliomas. Cancer, *34:*274–279, 1974.
105. Watts, R.G. and Merchant, R.E. Histopathological observations of a rat glioma following an intralesional injection of human recombinant interleukin-2 (rIL-2) (abstr.). Cytokine, 1989.
106. Watts, R.G., Wright, J.L., Atkinson, L.L., *et al.* Histopathologic and blood-brain barrier changes in rats induced by an intracerebral injection of human recombinant interleukin-2. Neurosurgery, *49:*202–208, 1989.
107. Wikstrand, C.J. and Bigner, D.D. Surface antigens of human glioma cells shared with normal adult and fetal brain. Cancer Res., *39:*3235–3243, 1979.
108. Wikstrand, C.J., Mahaley, M.S., and Bigner, D.D. Surface antigenic characteristics of human glial brain tumor cells. Cancer Res., *37:*4267–4275, 1977.
109. Wood, G.W., Morantz, R.A., Tilzer, S.A., *et al.* Immunoglobulin bound *in vivo* to Fc receptor-positive cells in human central nervous system tumors. J. Natl. Cancer. Inst., *64:*411--418, 1980.
110. Workshop on monoclonal antibodies against gliomas and other neuroectodermal-derived tumors. J. Neuroimmunol., *3:*237–243, 1982.
111. Woosley, R.E., Mahaley, M.S., Mahaley, J.L., *et al.* Immunobiology of primary intracranial tumors. Part 3. Microcytotoxicity assays of specific immune responses of brain tumor patients. J. Neurosurg., *47:*871–885, 1977.
112. Wrann, M., Bodmer, S., de Martin, R., *et al.* T cell suppressor factor from human glioblastoma cells is a 12.5-kd protein closely related to transforming growth factor-beta. EMBO, *6:*1633–1636, 1987.
113. Yosihida, S., Takai, N., and Tanaka, R. Functional analysis of interleukin-2 in immune surveillance against brain tumors. Neurosurgery, *21:*627–630, 1987.
114. Yoshida, S., Tanaka, R., Takai, N., *et al.* Local administration of autologous lymphokine-activated killer cells and recombinant interleukin-2 to patients with malignant brain tumors. Cancer Res., *48:*5011–5016, 1988.
115. Young, H., Kaplan, A., and Regelson, W. Immunotherapy with autologous white cell infusions ("lymphocytes") in the treatment of recurrent glioblastoma multiforme. Cancer, *40:*1037–1044, 1977.
116. Young, H.F., Sakalas, R., and Kaplan, A.M. Inhibition of cell-mediated immunity in patients with brain tumors. Surg. Neurol., *5:*19–23, 1976.
117. Yung, W.K.A., Prados, M., Levin, V., *et al.* Recombinant beta interferon in patients with recurrent malignant gliomas (abstr). J. Neuro-Oncol., *7:*S32, 1989.
118. Zalutsky, M.R., Moseley, R.P., Coakham, H.B., *et al.* Pharmacokinetics and tumor localization of [^{131}I]-labeled anti-tenascin monoclonal antibody 81C6 in patients with gliomas and other intracranial malignancies. Cancer Res., *49:*2807–2813, 1989.
119. Zovickian, J. and Youle, R.J. Efficacy of intrathecal immunotoxin therapy in an animal model of leptomeningeal neoplasia. J. Neurosurg., *68:*767–774, 1988.

CHAPTER 13

The Blood-Brain Barrier

MICHAEL SALCMAN, M.D., and RICHARD D. BROADWELL, Ph.D.

The nature and existence of the blood-brain barrier (BBB) have been subjects of debate and speculation for nearly 100 years (14). Prior to the turn of the century, experiments by Ehrlich (48) suggested that blood-borne intravital drugs had limited penetration within the brain. Other investigators observed that many substances introduced to the cerebrospinal fluid (CSF) entered the brain parenchyma readily, whereas the same substances administered systemically did not (39, 50, 88). The apparent absence of an extracellular space, suggested by electron microscopy in the 1950s, led investigators to question the existence of the BBB. Morphological studies employing electron dense tracers in the 1960s settled the issue with identification of the barrier at the level of the endothelial cell (18, 19, 87). From these studies, the selective permeability of the BBB in creating the internal milieu of the central nervous system (CNS) assumed increased meaning (15). More recently, the presence or absence of a functional BBB has become significant to the imaging and treatment of many neurological disorders.

THE BLOOD-BRAIN BARRIER DEFINED

The selective permeability of the BBB in regulating the passage of substances between the plasma and brain interstitial fluid is predicated upon the specialized nature of the nonfenestrated endothelial cell. In contrast to *patent* junctional complexes among endothelia in extracerebral vessels, the intercellular clefts of cerebral endothelia are closed by circumferential belts of tight junctions (Fig. 13.1). Electron dense tracers such as horseradish peroxidase (HRP) and lanthanum introduced to luminal and abluminal surfaces fail to penetrate the tight junctional complexes (Fig. 13.2). Following intravenous administration of HRP, the tracer protein is excluded from the brain parenchyma wherever interendothelial tight junctions are present but is evident within brain parenchyma adjacent to the circumventricular organs (e.g., median eminence, area postrema, etc.) which possess permeable, fenestrated endothelia (Fig. 13.3). A similar pattern of staining is observed with Evans blue dye bound to albumin and by immunohistochemical localization of endogenous albumin and IgG (33b). While the tight junctional complex precludes extracellular passage of blood-borne macromolecules between BBB endothelia, secondary lysosomes inherent to these endothelia serve to restrict or inhibit the transendothelial transfer (transcytosis) of these macromolecules (5, 22, 23, 26, 33).

Blood-borne proteins enter cerebral endothelia rapidly and appreciably by the processes of fluid or bulk phase endocytosis (Fig. 13.4), adsorptive endocytosis, and receptor-mediated endocytosis (22, 23). Secondary lysosomes within BBB endothelia are involved in the degradation of blood-borne protein entering the cell by each of the three endocytic processes (22, 23). Contrary to numerous reports within the literature, endocytic vesicles have not been demonstrated unequivocally to pass through the BBB endothelium in large numbers from the luminal to the abluminal surface to discharge their contents into the perivascular clefts (5, 6, 22, 23, 26, 33).

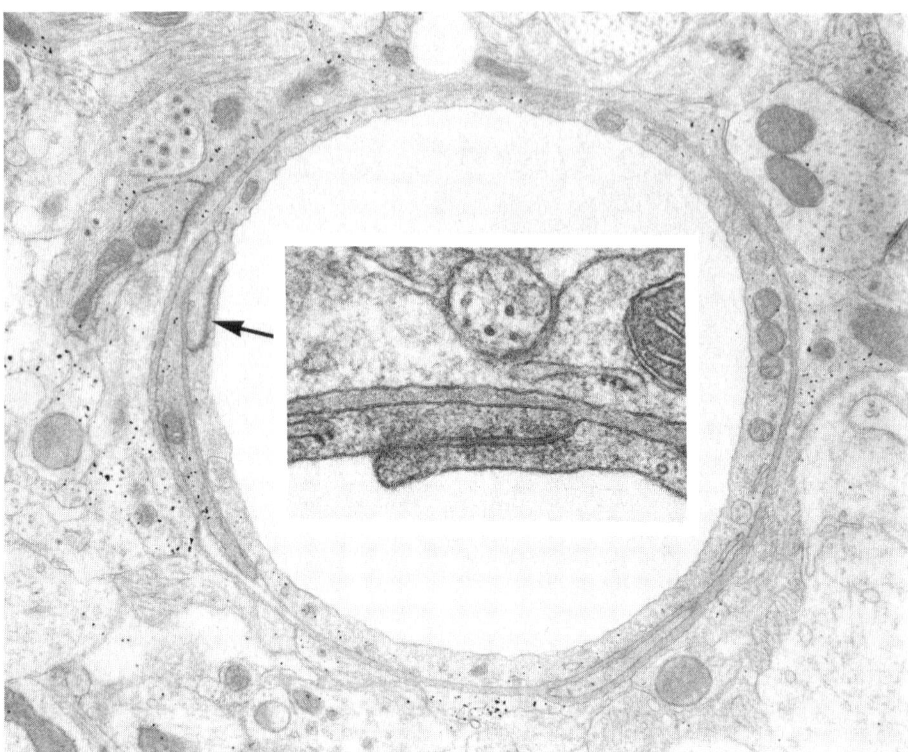

Figure 13.1. At the ultrastructural level, the mammalian blood-brain barrier from 1 day neonatal age to the adult exhibits circumferential belts of tight junctional complexes (*arrow* and *inset*) between continguous, nonfenestrated endothelial cells. The tight junctions preclude the bidirectional passage of nonlipid-soluble macromolecules between the blood and brain interstitial fluid.

Careful morphological investigations of BBB endothelia exposed to tracers disclose that suspected intraendothelial "transfer vesicles" are not what they seem. When peroxidase is administered into the lateral cerebral ventricle, the tracer moves extracellularly into the parenchyma to reach the abluminal face of the BBB and fills suspected abluminal and intraendothelial "vesicles." These "vesicular profiles" are revealed as static pits or invaginations in the abluminal plasma membrane (Fig. 13.5). That the abluminal pits are not representative of vesicles is confirmed by analysis of serial ultrathin sections (5, 23, 30) and by three-dimensional image reconstruction (35, 36). Conceivably, permeability changes in BBB endothelia to blood-borne macromolecules are related to endothelial cell damage or to compromised tight junctional complexes.

Nevertheless, a population of the abluminal surface pits in BBB endothelia *may* indeed represent intraendothelial transfer vesicles that have fused with the abluminal plasmalemma for exocytosis of their contents. A growing body of morphological (23, 26) and biochemical (45, 49, 79, 95, 101) evidence is available to support the adsorptive and receptor-mediated transcytoses of blood-borne proteins and peptides through the BBB. The adsorptive transcytosis of lectins (e.g., wheat germ agglutinin, cationized proteins) involves binding of the lectin to the luminal surface plasmalemma with the internalized membrane-associated lectin being directed eventually to the Golgi complex. Once the Golgi saccules are reached, the molecule can be packaged for intracellular transport and exocytosis at the abluminal surface (22, 23, 26). Adsorptive transcytosis through the BBB has the

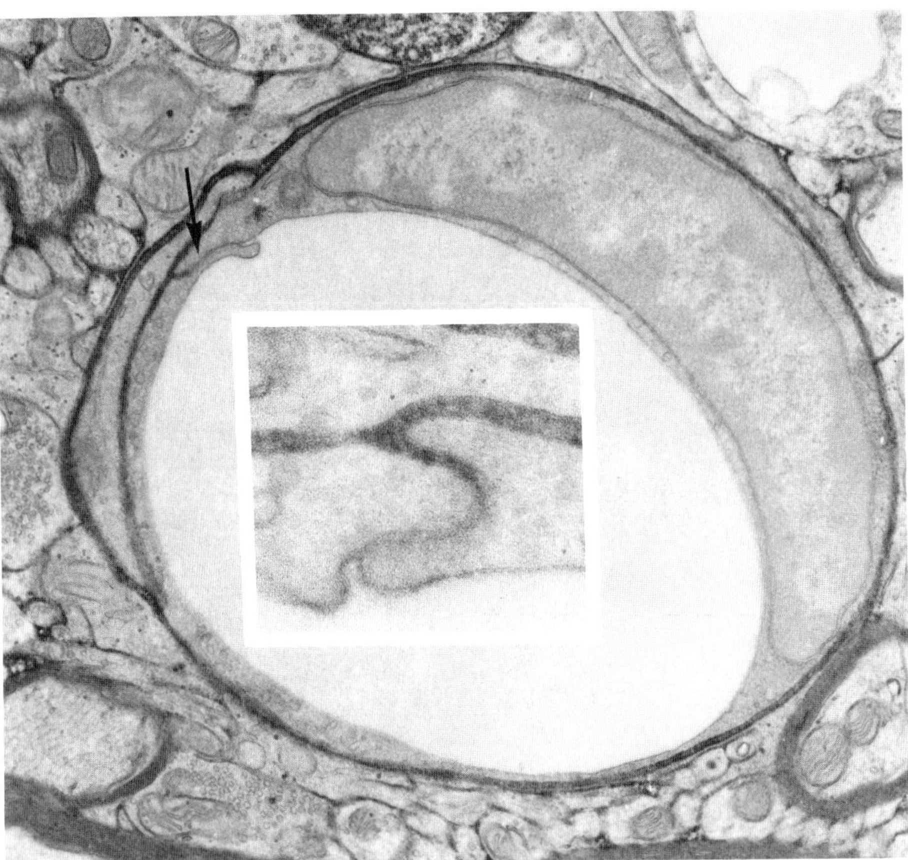

Figure 13.2. Horseradish peroxidase administered into the lateral ventricle is not prevented from reaching the abluminal surface of blood-brain barrier endothelia extracellularly but is precluded from entering the blood by interendothelial tight junctions (*arrow* and *inset*). Although the abluminal surface of these endothelia can be exposed to the tracer for extended periods of time, demonstrable endocytosis of the protein into the endothelia is virtually nonexistent at the abluminal plasmalemma (see Fig. 13.4).

potential of representing a global event, occurring in the absence of receptor binding. Receptor-mediated transcytosis is a highly specific event involving the recognition of a ligand (e.g., iron bound transferrin, insulin, etc.) by a receptor. The time course and intracellular pathway for receptor-mediated transcytosis through BBB endothelia may be abbreviated compared to those associated with adsorptive transcytosis (23).

As with other cell membranes, the cerebral endothelium is permeable to low molecular weight, nonpolar, lipid-soluble substances such as oxygen, carbon dioxide, and anesthetics. The endothelium is highly selective in its permeability to water-soluble substances (12). Most metabolic substrates and inorganic ions enter the brain through the endothelium by carrier-mediated mechanisms and energy-dependent pumps associated with the endothelial plasmalemma. The cerebral endothelium appears polarized with regard to structure and function; it harbors Na^+-K^+ pumps on the abluminal surface and specific receptor proteins on the luminal plasmalemma (9). This polarization allows the endothelium to transport water, solutes, and the like in particular directions, a property the cerebral endothelial cell shares with specialized epithelia such as that of the choroid plexus. An additional polarization of the BBB is demonstrated with electron dense tracers (23, 30). Native HRP is

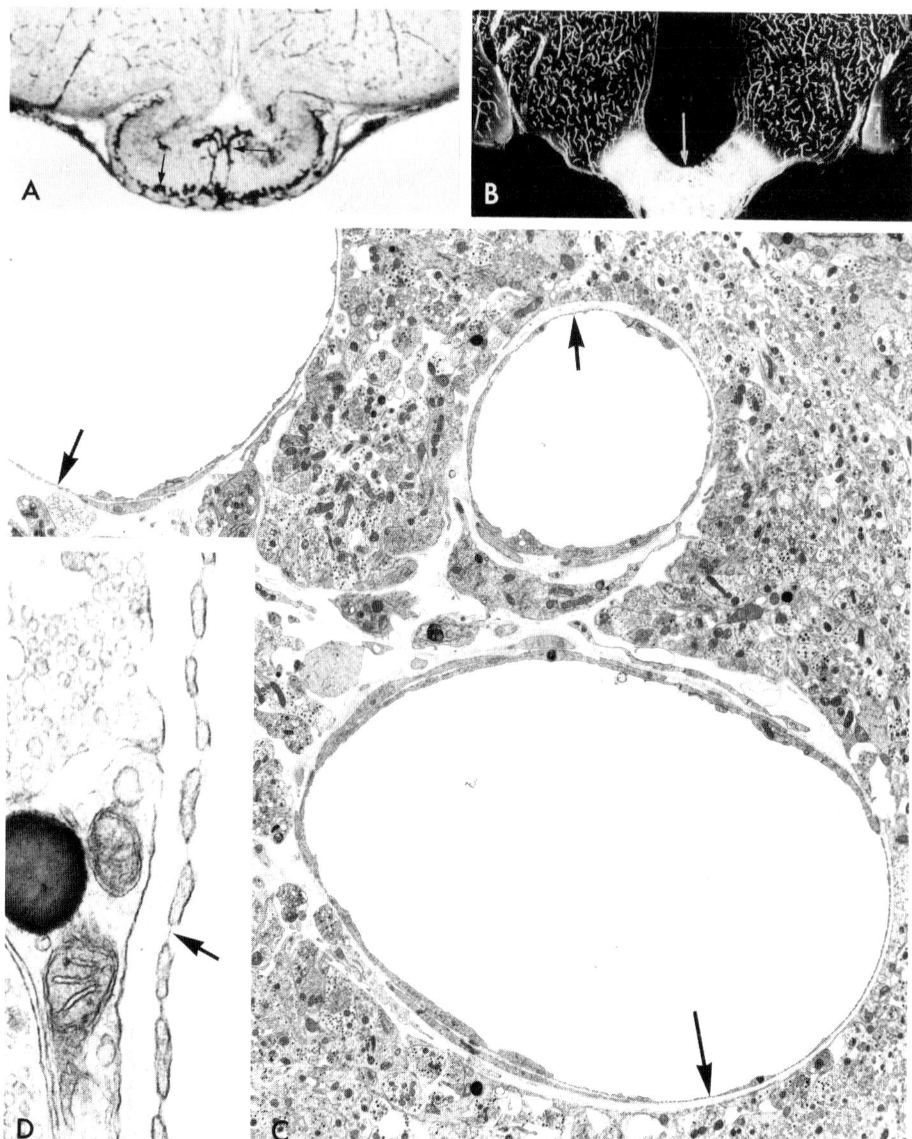

Figure 13.3. The mammalian median eminence (*A–D*), located at the floor of the third ventricle, represents one of a half dozen circumventricular organs that possesses fenestrated endothelial cells and, therefore, lies outside the blood-brain barrier. These endothelia are visualized readily at the light microscopic level in brain sections fixed by immersion and incubated to reveal the endogenous peroxidase activity inherent to red cells trapped within the vessel lumen (*A, arrows*). Blood-borne peroxidase escapes the fenestrated blood vessels as seen in *B* (*arrow*); in this figure, note that blood-brain barrier vessels in CNS parenchyma above the median eminence are labeled with peroxidase reaction product. The fenestrated characteristic of endothelia supplying the median eminence is appreciated at the ultrastructural level (*C* and *D, arrows*).

endocytosed avidly from the luminal side of the cerebral endothelium, whereas HRP and lectin-conjugated HRP delivered intraventricularly to the abluminal endothelial surface fail to undergo endocytosis (Fig. 13.2, 13.4, and 13.5). These data suggest two significant characteristics of the BBB endothelium concerning its membrane behavior: First, the endothelial cell appears polarized with regard to the internalization of cell surface membrane and the endocytosis of macromolecules; second, the proc-

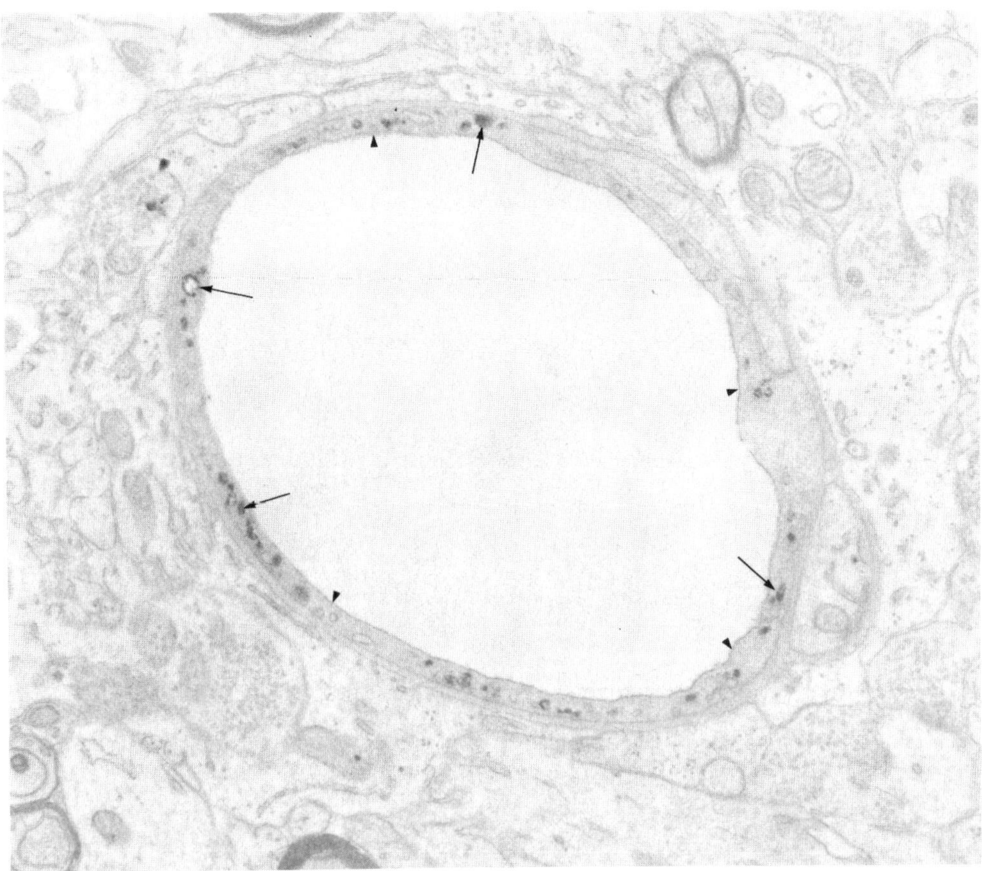

Figure 13.4. Blood-borne peroxidase exposed to the luminal plasmalemma of blood-brain barrier endothelia is endocytosed avidly. Within 5 minutes postinjection of the tracer intravenously, reaction product coats the luminal surface membrane (*arrowheads*) and is evident within endothelial endocytic vesicles, endosomes (vacuoles rimmed internally with reaction product), multivesicular bodies, and dense bodies (*arrows*). Note the absence of reaction product within the perivascular clefts and extracellular spaces of the neuropil.

ess of transcytosis through the BBB is vectorial, from blood to brain but not from brain to blood. Differences in the membrane events observed on the luminal and abluminal faces of the BBB support the concept that the BBB is not absolute; however, its counterpart, the brain-blood barrier, may well be (22, 23).

The absence of demonstrable endocytic activity at the abluminal surface of the nonfenestrated cerebral endothelium is an enigma if transcytosis of blood-borne macromolecules through the BBB is significant. Endocytosis, which entails the retrieval or internalization of cell surface membrane, represents a compensatory response to exocytosis and necessarily involves the addition of exocytic (secretory) vesicle membrane to the plasmalemma. Exocytosis and endocytosis are complimentary events in the process of secretion and together ensure that the overall surface area of the cell remains static with each exocytic event. How transcytosis through the BBB occurs in the absence of endocytosis at the abluminal surface remains to be clarified (23).

The interface between blood and brain includes, in addition to the endothelial cell, a surrounding investment of astrocytic end feet, a basal lamina, and perivascular phagocytes (e.g., microglia, macrophages, pericytes). Since protein tracers injected into the ventricle reach the abluminal surface of BBB endothelia without difficulty, the tracers clearly must pass through the ground substance and intercellular clefts among as-

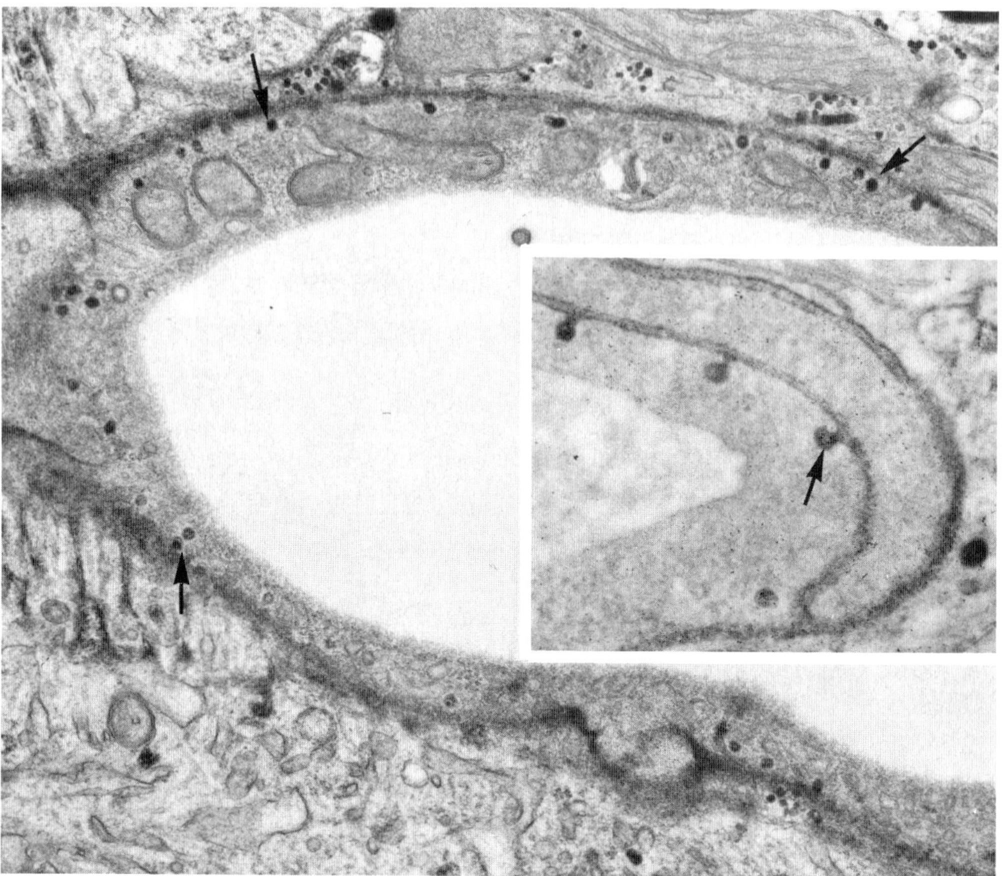

Figure 13.5. The abluminal plasma membranes of blood-brain barrier endothelia frequently are studded with pits or invaginations (*arrows*) that fill with peroxidase that has reached the perivascular clefts from the blood through a physically compromised blood-brain barrier or, as in this preparation, following ventriculocisternal perfusion of the tracer. These pits easily are misinterpreted in random thin section analysis as vesicles engaged in transcytosis from blood to brain or from brain to blood. Serial thin sections reveal the presumptive "transporting vesicles" are in continuity with the abluminal plasma membrane (*inset*). Note the absence of peroxidase-labeled organelles comparable to those seen in Figure 13.4. The data, therefore, suggest that the blood-brain barrier is polarized with regard to the endocytosis of macromolecules and the internalization of its cell surface membranes. This polarization further suggests that the transcytosis of macromolecules through blood-brain barrier endothelia is vectorial, from blood to brain but not from brain to blood (24).

trocytic processes and perivascular phagocytes; hence, the investing cell processes do *not* contribute a barrier comparable to that of the nonfenestrated cerebral endothelium (16, 17). From the perspective of the BBB, the perivascular phagocytes may serve as a final cellular defense once blood-borne proteins have succeeded in escaping enzymatic degradation within BBB endothelia or when they have circumvented the barrier extracellularly (6, 23, 26, 33). Blood-borne macromolecules reaching the abluminal surface of BBB endothelia are endocytosed by perivascular phagocytes for subsequent lysosomal degradation (6, 23, 26, 33).

Blood-borne proteins undergoing adsorptive or receptor-mediated transcytosis through the BBB are confronted by perivascular phagocytes (23, 26). Blood-borne proteins entering BBB endothelia by the nonspecific process of fluid phase endocytosis (e.g., native HRP) likewise become sequestered within perivascular phagocytes (6, 23, 25, 27, 31, 33); although these proteins experience lysosomal degradation within the endothelium and fail to be transported through the endothelium, they can enter the mammalian CNS by circumventing the BBB extracellularly. The extracellular routes involve the circumventricular organs, such as the median eminence and area postrema, and the pial surface (6, 23, 25, 27). Our current belief is that the large vessels inhabiting the Virchow-Robbins spaces at the pial surface do not have interendothelial tight junctions, thus permitting blood-borne protein, including endogenous serum proteins, to escape through the pial surface and perivascular clefts. Once the latter is reached, the pulsatile activity of the arterioles in the live animal move the extracellular protein deeper into the CNS for eventual phagocytosis by perivascular cells. In the subarachnoid space, macrophages serve to cleanse the pial surface of contamination by blood-borne protein.

Although the glial investment on the basal lamina surrounding the abluminal surface of BBB endothelia may not contribute specifically to the functional BBB, astrocytes are believed to play a role in the induction and maintenance of the barrier (8, 63). In vitro studies suggest that the development of nonfenestrated endothelia and/or of interendothelial tight junctional complexes depends on the surrounding astrocytes (4, 63, 100).

The recent development of techniques for the isolation and culture of endothelial cells has provided considerable insight to the properties inherent to the BBB endothelium and to those related to endothelial cell interaction with other cell types (51). In isolated capillaries, enzymes such as alkaline phosphatase and alpha-glutamyl transpeptidase are distributed equally between the luminal and abluminal surfaces; 5^1-nucleotidase and Na^+-K^+-ATPase are located only on the abluminal side (9). These observations are consistent with the movement of D-glucose and essential large neutral amino acids bidirectionally across the BBB by transport carriers and the active pumping of small neutral amino acids and potassium from brain into blood (51, 52). Endothelial cells grown in culture possess tight junctional complexes, and the morphology of these cells and their permeability to [^{14}C]-sucrose are altered by exposure to calcium free media and to 1.6 M arabinose (13). When cultured cerebral endothelia are grown on one side of a filter and C6 glial cells on the other, the intracellular transport of [^{3}H] α-methylaminoisobutyric acid is more rapid from the glial side, suggesting an influence of the glial cells on the polarity of the barrier (8). The test substance in this particular experiment is a Na^+-dependent (A-system) amino acid, the transport of which has been localized to the abluminal membrane. When transport of this amino acid is tested in the absence of the glial cells, no difference between the two directions is observed. The uptake of glucose by capillary endothelial cells has been studied extensively in culture and demonstrates the characteristics of carrier-mediated transport systems (104). Other enzymes involved in glucose metabolism have been localized in situ (32).

Although the structure and some properties of BBB endothelia have been defined more fully, elucidating the role the barrier plays in brain homeostasis remains difficult. Certainly, the BBB contributes to the precise control of the neuronal environment and perhaps to the ionic composition of the cerebrospinal and interstitial fluids of the brain (39). The BBB regulates the access of necessary substrates involved in the energy-dependent and structural processes of the neuron and restricts the exposure of the nervous system to toxins and some elements of the immune system. Comparative studies of BBB morphology and function among vertebrate and invertebrate animals surely will provide further insights to the function of the BBB (38).

ALTERATION OF THE BARRIER IN DISEASE

An increase in the permeability of the human BBB to protein-bound and water-soluble contrast agents is responsible for enhanced visualization of inflammatory conditions, infections, and vascular diseases with computed tomography and magnetic resonance imaging. Acute hypertension produced in rats by aramine results in an increased permeability of BBB endothelia to blood-borne peroxidase. This increased permeability was initially attributed a priori to transendothelial vesicular transport (109); however, this interpretation is not without criticism (see above). The alternative possibilities of endothelial cell damage or compromised tight junction integrity are more likely (20, 23, 84, 86).

With cerebral artery occlusion, permeability alterations occur in the distribution of the vessel. Endothelial permeability to HRP is proportional to the duration of ischemia in experimental animals. In cats subjected to transorbital occlusion of the middle cerebral artery (MCA), disruption of the BBB detected by leakage of Evans blue dye is evident at 3–9 hours following occlusion but is undetected by CT contrast enhancement during the first 24 hours (65). Thrombosis of the middle cerebral artery (MCA) induced in rats by laser irradiation and platelet aggregation results in HRP permeability after 15 minutes of ischemia (42). This form of alteration in barrier permeability is so diffuse that the release of chemical substances or neurohumoral factors after endothelial cell damage is hypothesized. Conceivably, oxygen free radicals could be the mediators of the observed damage. In dogs MCA infarctions produced by the embolization of silicone pellets into the internal carotid artery yield a threefold increase in the number of endocytic vesicles without discernible change in the tight junctions (61).

The pathophysiology of BBB alteration after subarachnoid hemorrhage (SAH) also is likely to be complex, since hypertension, ischemia and chemical mediators are present. Blood injected into the subarachnoid space of rats produces an increased extravasation of Evans blue dye and [^{14}C] sucrose as early as 3 hours following SAH with an immunohistochemically defined increase in albumin as early as 30 minutes (43). Ultrastructurally, an increased number of endocytic vesicles is observed at 6 hours, and the mitochondria become swollen; opening of some tight junctions also is evident. The release of vasoactive substances from the breakdown products of extravasated blood is speculated to affect the microvessels directly. Opening of tight junctions to HRP is seen in major cerebral arteries after experimental SAH in the dog; the effect of elevated intracranial pressure (ICP) in this particular instance cannot be discounted (93).

The increase in BBB permeability related to meningitis has been studied with intracisternal injections of meningeal pathogens in the rat. An increase in endocytic vesicles and compromised junctional complexes have been reported as early as 4 hours following meningitis induction (82). In response to infections and demyelinating disorders such as multiple sclerosis, the concentration of immunoglobulins is increased in the CSF. The increase does not appear to be related to an enhanced secretory activity of the choroid plexus (2); hence, immunological participation in the origin of and response to brain tumors may require antibody entry through BBB defects. Considerably less information is available concerning the pathophysiology of BBB alteration in other disease states. Both electrically induced and metrazol induced seizures initiate intracerebral extravasations of blood-borne HRP. Whether these results can be attributed directly or indirectly to hypertension or hypervolemia (58) as opposed to some intrinsic mechanism is difficult to state unequivocally.

IS THERE A BARRIER IN TUMORS?

Radioiodinated serum albumin (RISA) was introduced in 1951 for the diagnosis and localization of human brain tumors. Protein-bound RISA thereafter was localized within cavities containing high-protein concentrations (e.g., tumor cysts and subdural collections); however, little evidence was available at that time to explain the localization of the tracer within the tumor itself. Was the increased uptake due to increased blood flow, and did the tracer occupy the extracellular or the intracellular space? The localization of RISA as well as contrast agents for CT and MRI scanning depends on the relative leakiness of brain tumor endothelial cells.

The first electron microscopic study of two astrocytomas after the administration of RISA suggested that tumor capillaries demonstrate an increased rate of endocytosis (83). In this report, the subject of the

BBB was addressed only briefly. In 1970, Long (68) presented an ultrastructural analysis of the capillaries in 19 human malignant brain tumors and compared their structure to that of normal brain. The most striking and frequent abnormalities were found in the endothelial "tight" junctions, some of which were patent and lacked the pentalaminar structure found in normal brain capillaries. A normal glial investiture was absent consistently, and many of the capillary cells demonstrated vesicular formation as well as attenuation and irregularities of the cells, especially in areas of endothelial hyperplasia. Long concluded that one was "more correct to speak of an absence rather than a breakdown of the blood-brain barrier in human brain tumors." This variety of abnormalities was confirmed by others (56, 81, 105). Fenestrations have been described as especially prominent in the endothelial cells of ependymomas (102). Metastatic tumors to the brain may demonstrate different alterations, some of which are based on the parental tissue of origin. For example, metastatic renal carcinoma is known to possess endothelial cells with the characteristic fenestrae of renal vasculature (57). In a study of 14 human brain tumors, the uptake pattern of ^{99m}Tc-pertechnetate correlated with the absence of tight junctions and not with the presence of fenestrations (7). This important observation is supported by the fact that opening of the tight junctions is the most frequent mechanism underlying experimental methods for increasing blood-brain barrier permeability (20, 84, 85, 86).

Many of the ultrastructural abnormalities described in human brain tumors are observed in the surrounding brain tissue. Blood vessels in the peritumoral environment assume characteristics of leaky vessels in the absence of contact with tumor cells, a consequence attributed to the diffusion of induction factors (97). In addition to an increase in open junctions and vesicle density in peritumoral endothelia, a decrease in the number of pericytes compared to normal tissue is observed. In the zone of tumor infiltration, the endothelial cells become progressively thinner and develop villous processes on their luminal surface. These immature capillaries are more similar to the endothelial buds found in the center of the tumor than to normal capillary endothelia in the surrounding parenchyma (108). None of these studies is consistent with the observation that the brain adjacent to tumor (BAT) may be less permeable to water-soluble tracers or that delivery of such agents to some model brain tumors may depend on a tumor-to-BAT diffusion (66).

Experimental brain tumors demonstrate many of the same abnormalities as human tumors. The canine glioma induced by intracerebral inoculation of avian sarcoma virus (ASV) or by serial transplantation of the tumor cells demonstrates endothelia exhibiting interendothelial gap junctions and fenestrae (90, 103). Permeability to HRP is demonstrated for the ASV model in rodents as well as for a variety of other model brain tumors (41, 53, 54). A high degree of variability exists in the permeability demonstrated by different types of tumors, within a given tumor, and between tumors of the same type grown in different animals. The marginal zone is usually the most permeable, as confirmed by the radiographic appearance of the canine glioma model in which contrast enhancement on CT scans occurs in a ring-like pattern (91). In the ethylnitrosourea (ENU)-induced rat brain tumor, HRP penetration is seen around sinusoidal and venule-like microvessels; the endothelial cells do not demonstrate increased endocytic vesicles but possess fenestrations and gap junctions (77). These changes are associated with a statistically significant decrease in the number of mitochondria and an increase in the amount of rough endoplasmic reticulum (ER).

The permeability of capillaries in model brain tumors also is demonstrated by pharmacologic means (40). In the rat ASV model, measurements of the blood-to-tissue transfer constant (K) and the tissue blood flow are accomplished by application of double-label quantitative autoradiography (11). The K values do not appear to correlate with tumor size, although other workers have observed that the permeability of model tumors increases during the development and growth of the lesion

(110). In all studies, the K value is highly variable from area to area within the tumor. Nevertheless, increases in the K value may not be sufficient to deliver adequate amounts of water-soluble drugs with short plasma half-lives to tumor tissue, partially because of the effect of capillary surface area. These issues in human brain tumors can be studied by positron emission tomography (PET). For example, the permeability of tumor capillaries to small hydrophilic molecules is decreased by the administration of corticosteroids in humans (64).

CAN THE BARRIER BE MODIFIED?

Breakdown of the BBB in humans and experimental animals is demonstrated in a wide variety of pathological conditions, including cerebral edema, hypertension, seizures, concussion, hypoxia, ischemia, inflammation and neoplasm. Increased permeability usually is ascribed to a combination of effects including alteration of the tight junctional complex, an increase in transcellular vesicular transport, formation of parajunctional channels, and a failure in metabolically dependent processes such as carrier systems and ionic pumps. Although permeability of the BBB can be increased by pathological means, the effect is not localized necessarily to a given region of the brain and is described more properly as a type of damage or injury with permanent alteration of barrier function. A number of laboratories currently are active in the development of methods by which the BBB can be altered in a local and potentially reversible manner.

Physical techniques applied to modify barrier permeability have been studied widely, particularly the delivery of hyperosmotic agents into the carotid artery, a method pioneered by Rapoport (20, 86). In adult rats, hyperosmotic arabinose (1.4 M) infused as a bolus into the internal carotid artery over a period of 30 seconds results in the exudation of blood-borne HRP and lanthanum around cerebral arterioles (44). The ionic lanthanum is found in extracellular pools, presumably after passing through successive layers of tight junctions. Although open junctional complexes are difficult to discern, bona fide evidence supporting transcellular transport is unavailable; the ionic lanthanum appears localized to pits and vesicles that are primarily abluminal in location (44). These observations are consistent with the earlier reports of HRP entry to the rabbit brain following exposure to hypersomotic urea (20).

Whether or not the hyperosmotic technique improves the distribution of drug entry to a model brain tumor as opposed to normal brain remains the subject of considerable debate. The effect of hyperosmotic mannitol on the BBB has been evaluated when coadministered with Evans blue dye-albumin (MW 68,000), HRP (MW 40,000) and 5-fluorouracil (MW 130). After hyperosmotic mannitol delivery, penetration of Evans blue-albumin and HRP is increased demonstrably in the normal brain but not in the tumor. Although a slight increase in the concentration of 5-fluorouracil within the tumor was identified, the increase in tumor-free regions of the brain appears significantly greater. Thus, the intracarotid administration of hyperosmotic mannitol may increase neurotoxicity rather than increase the efficacy of brain tumor chemotherapy. Albumin immunoreactivity and serum extravasation in normal rat brain are seen 30 minutes after mannitol infusion and remain prominent for 48 hours; small but definite foci of infarction are evident in 38% of the animals and delayed ischemic neuronal death is demonstrated in 25% of the animals sacrificed 4–6 days after infusion (99). Failure of hyperosmotic solutions to alter capillary permeability in model brain tumors is confirmed in a number of systems. In the ENU-induced rat brain tumor, neither the penetration of Evans blue-albumin nor bromodeoxyuridine uptake (BrdU) appears to be altered by hyperosmotic mannitol; however, the penetration of Evans blue-albumin into the normal brain is increased dramatically (59). Negative results with the hyperosmotic approach have been obtained after quantitative autoradiography of [^{14}C]methotrexate delivery in both RG-2 and ENU-induced gliomas (74, 94, 107).

Hyperthermia represents an additional approach investigated intensively as a physical means by which the BBB can be opened reversibly. Just as the tonicity of a hyperosmolar solution must reach a concentration threshold before its effect on the BBB becomes manifest, so too the level of heat must exceed a threshold level of approximately 43°C for 30–60 minutes. Early studies of the effect of hyperthermia on the BBB failed to reach this threshold or were beset by numerous other methodological problems. Preston (80) was unable to open the BBB to [^{14}C]sucrose or [^{125}I]albumin in the rat after whole-body heating with an infrared lamp or with 2450-MHz microwave irradiation; in this experiment, the core-body temperature (i.e., not brain temperature) failed to exceed 42°C. In another report, the BBB was opened inconsistently to [^{125}I]albumin when extremely long hyperthermia exposures (2–5 hours) were conducted at relatively low temperatures (i.e., 41°C); the investigator incorrectly concluded that the duration of exposure rather than the absolute temperature is the important variable (72). However, nearly all effects of hyperthermia on the brain are the result of the product of both the amplitude and duration, as one would expect for a physical modality (90). Furthermore, nonionizing or microwave radiation is frequently used to produce hyperthermia and interpretational problems are possible based on incorrect thermometry. Since metal heats in a microwave field and this results in hot spots, ordinary thermistors and thermometers should not be used in microwave experiments. Although all of the biological effects of microwaves at ordinary power are related to hyperthermia per se, early studies often ascribed the biological changes to microwave application.

Oscar and Hawkins (78) employed the double indicator technique of Oldendorf and exposed rats to 1.3 GHz energy from external applicators. Permeability increases for [^{14}C]mannitol and [^{14}C]inulin were observed immediately after exposure and at 4 hours but not at 24 hours after exposure. The effect was believed reversible; however, brain and body temperatures were not measured. In another study, transfer of fluorescein at 1.2 GHz or [^{14}C] mannitol at 1.3-GHz radiation was not confirmed unless the rats were warmed in a 43°C environment for 30 minutes; the authors concluded that "the brain must be made hyperthermic for microwave induced changes in the permeability of the barrier to occur" (70). In this pioneering study, brain temperatures were measured by a conventional thermistor after microwave irradiation had been terminated; hence, no conclusions could be drawn with regard to the heating profile within the brain. Similarly, temperatures were not measured in another study which failed to demonstrate BBB opening to 2.8 GHz microwaves as measured by the permeability-capillary surface area product for [^{14}C]sucrose (55).

The issue of hyperthermia effects on BBB permeability also has been assessed morphologically. Low level exposure of Chinese hamsters to microwaves at 2.45 MHz results in an increase in permeability of the BBB to horseradish peroxidase immediately after treatment; the effect is reported as less noticeable at 1 hour and absent at 2 hours, supporting the authors' claim for reversibility (1). Since "compromised" endothelial tight junctions filled with peroxidase reaction product were not identified, the authors assumed the increased endothelial permeability to blood-borne HRP was due to transendothelial vesicular transport. None of the photographs in the report provides convincing evidence for such transport and no temperatures were measured. The authors most likely misinterpreted HRP-filled abluminal pits as transporting vesicles (see above discussion and 5, 7, 23, 30). In yet another study, Wistar rats were exposed to 2450-MHz microwaves for 20 minutes, and brain temperatures were measured with nonfield-perturbing thermistors; extravasation of Evans blue was used as the indicator for BBB alteration (67). The authors showed the effect was reversible after 30 minutes and occurred with brain temperatures greater than 44°C. These results are consistent with an approximate threshold of 45°C administered for 60 minutes. When a single microwave antenna operating at 2450 MHz is implanted into the rabbit brain and a temperature of 45°C is achieved for 60 minutes, the extent of Evans blue-albumin staining exactly corresponds to the diameter of the hyperthermia field (Fig. 13.6). In

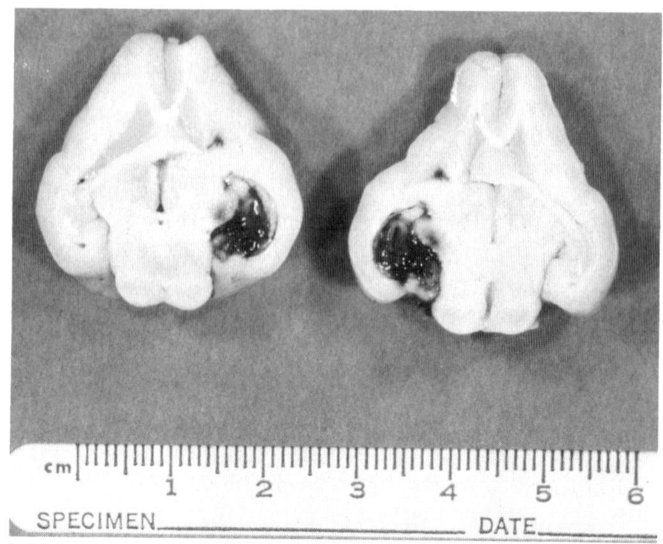

Figure 13.6. Blood-brain barrier opening after microwave hyperthermia in the rabbit. Evan's blue dye was administered immediately after microwave heating with an implanted 2450-MHZ antenna at 43° for 60 minutes; the diameter of dye leakage is approximately equal to the diameter of the field of maximal heating.

recent experiments we likewise have shown that penetration of HRP into the brain depends on the point of maximum microwave power deposition (Fig. 13.7); these two variables can be isolated by employing a water-cooling jacket around the microwave antenna (71).

A number of chemical and biological agents have been investigated for their effect on BBB permeability. The normal capillary endothelium of the rat has a negative charge that binds colloidal iron after the brain has been perfused with a buffer to clear it of blood. Protamine sulfate markedly decreases binding of the positively charged iron and increases the penetration of HRP into the brain (73). The effects of protamine can be reversed through the co-administration of heparin. The cytoplasm of some capillaries is flooded with HRP after protamine administration, indicating the technique is not viable for reversibly altering barrier function. The negative charge on the luminal surface appears to be due to the carboxyl groups of sialic acid which may play a role in maintaining normal capillary function.

Transient and permanent opening of the BBB after systemic administration of dimethyl sulfoxide (DMSO) in concentrations of 20–30% also has been reported (29, 34); the effect may be a consequence of nonspecific damage and/or generalized epileptiform shaking (5). The intracarotid administration of dehydrocholate is shown to open reversibly the BBB to Evans blue, sodium fluorescein and [^{99m}Tc]diethylenetriaminepentaacetic acid (DTPA); prolonged disruption could be maintained for over 3 days (96). Seizures were experienced by these animals, and no morphological studies were carried out to determine the possible toxic effects and locus of action for this bile salt.

Arachidonic acid is released rapidly from cell membrane phospholipids after pathological insults associated with brain edema; subsequent changes in BBB permeability most likely are related to the development of vasogenic edema. Arachidonic acid administration to rat brain slices results in the formation of superoxide free radicals and lipid peroxides. When arachidonic acid is injected directly into the rat brain, parenchymal staining with Evans blue is increased dramatically as is the ^{125}I-labeled albumin space 24 hours after injection (37). The lipoxygenase metabolism of arachidonic acid results in the formation of leukotrienes, and their injection into rat brain also produces Evans blue extravasation (10). The BBB effect of arachidonic acid in these experiments is blocked by the administration of a lipoxygenase inhibitor. Interleukin-2 has been shown to increase the transfer constant for ^{14}C-labeled ami-

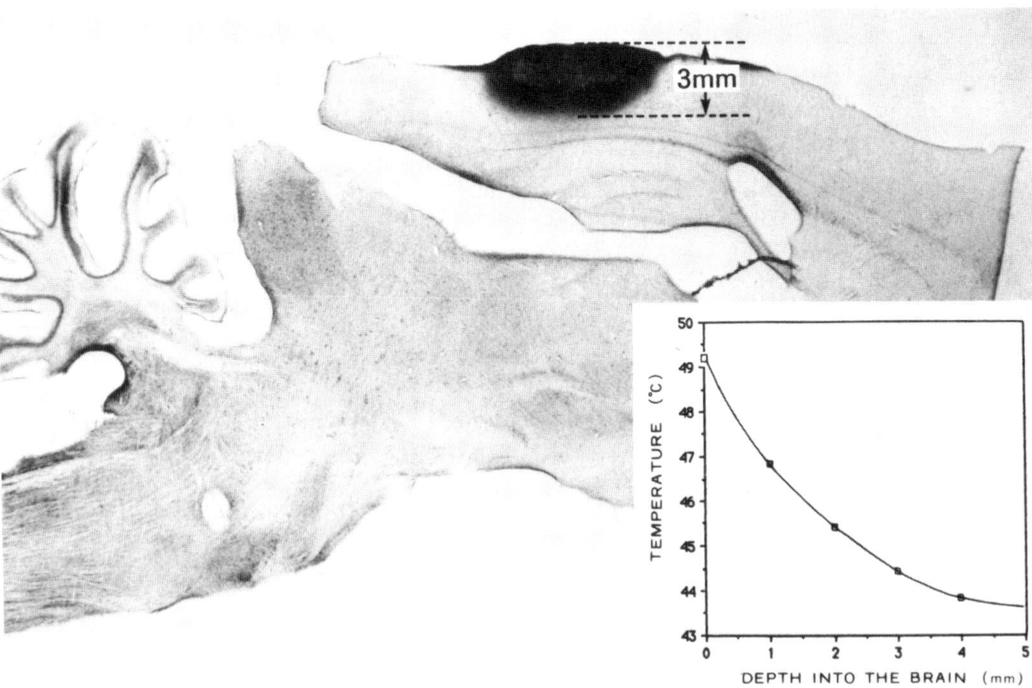

Figure 13.7. Blood-brain barrier opening after microwave hyperthermia in the rat. An antenna operating at 2450-MHZ was placed on the surface of the cortex perpendicular to the plane of section and horseradish peroxidase (HRP) infused at the end of the heating; note that the extent of barrier opening indicated by leakage of the tracer is less than 3 mm–the depth at which the thermal field was less than 44°C (see *inset*).

noisobutyric acid (AIB) in the peritumoral tissue of rats bearing the 9L gliosarcoma (3); this finding is of interest because of the markedly increased cerebral edema often observed in brain tumor patients after such therapy.

Only corticosteroids have been shown consistently to protect barrier function and reverse the effect of methodologies designed to provoke barrier disruption. The normal BBB may be responsive to both neural and hormonal influences, and these systems may play a role in maintaining homeostasis within the central nervous system (69). Adrenalectomy, but not adrenal demedullation, increases the permeability of ^{125}I-labeled albumin in rat brain; these effects are reversed with corticosterone replacement (55). In glioma-bearing rats, pretreatment with dexamethasone reduces the delivery of methotrexate after osmotic opening of the BBB by two-thirds in tumor tissue and somewhat less so in brain distant to the tumor (76). The new 21-aminosteroid, U-74006F, which has antioxidant and antilipolytic activity, can reduce or prevent the Evans blue extravasation seen after experimental subarachnoid hemorrhage in rats (111). In this study, the 21-aminosteroid also reduced the Evans blue extravasation after the administration of either arachidonic acid or $FeCl_2$. U-74006F inhibits in vitro iron-dependent lipid peroxidation with a potency that equals that of the antioxidant γ-tocopherol and surpasses that of the iron chelator deferoxamine. Adrenal glucocorticoids are inhibitors of phospholipase A_2, the enzyme that helps hydrolyze membrane phospholipids to form arachidonic acid and other lipid compounds.

Tissue transplantation in the brain represents a recently explored methodology for manipulation of the BBB (98). Solid grafts of peripheral tissues (e.g., anterior pituitary gland, autonomic ganglia, muscle) from adult, neonatal, or fetal donors when placed intracerebrally within adult hosts (Figs. 13.8*A* and *B*) fail to exhibit a BBB to blood-borne proteins (21, 24, 25, 27, 28, 31, 89, 106). Cell suspensions of PC12 cells (18, 62) and canine glioma model tumor (28, 46, 92) likewise do not manifest barrier properties to circulating protein, despite the fact that these suspensions are vascularized with host cerebral vessels that initially are of the BBB type (Fig. 13.9). Solid grafts of fetal/neonatal CNS tissue (Figs. 13.8*C* and *D*) (21, 24, 25, 27, 28, 31) and cell suspensions of neurons, type I astrocytes, and oligodendroglia (28, 46) are vascularized with endothelia expressing BBB properties to blood-borne macromolecules. In solid grafts of peripheral and CNS tissues, blood vessels indigenous to the grafts are sustained and anastomose with host vessels predominantly at the host-graft interface (21, 24, 25, 27, 28). The data indicate that a "window" in the BBB of the host is created by intracerebrally placed solid grafts of peripheral origin and tumor cell suspension grafts. This "window" can permit the unimpeded entry of blood-borne therapeutics and the like into the host brain parenchyma. A similar window should exist in the intracerebral adrenal medullary grafts used in the clinical treatment of Parkinson's disease. Whether or not such a "window" in the host BBB can be utilized successfully for the intracerebral delivery of blood-borne therapeutics remains to be seen. Although intracerebral grafting is unlikely to be of importance in

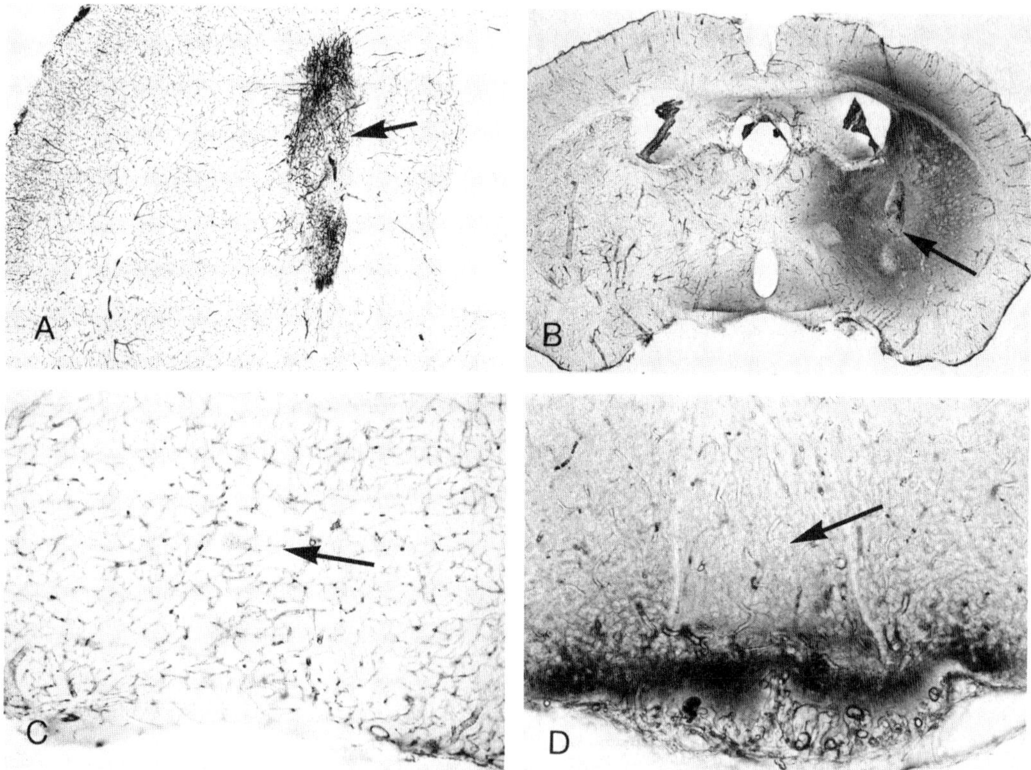

Figure 13.8. Solid peripheral tissue (e.g., anterior pituitary gland) allografts (*A* and *B, arrows*) placed into the striatum of adult hosts appear well-vascularized in sections from host brains fixed by immersion and incubated to reveal the endogenous peroxidase activity in red cells trapped within the vessels (*A*). These vessels supplying peripheral tissue grafts are leaky to peroxidase administered intravenously to the host (*B*). CNS allografts (*C* and *D, arrows*) placed into the third ventricle of the host brain express a blood-brain barrier to horseradish peroxidase delivered intravenously to the host. In *D* blood-borne peroxidase is evident in the host median eminence but is absent in the graft.

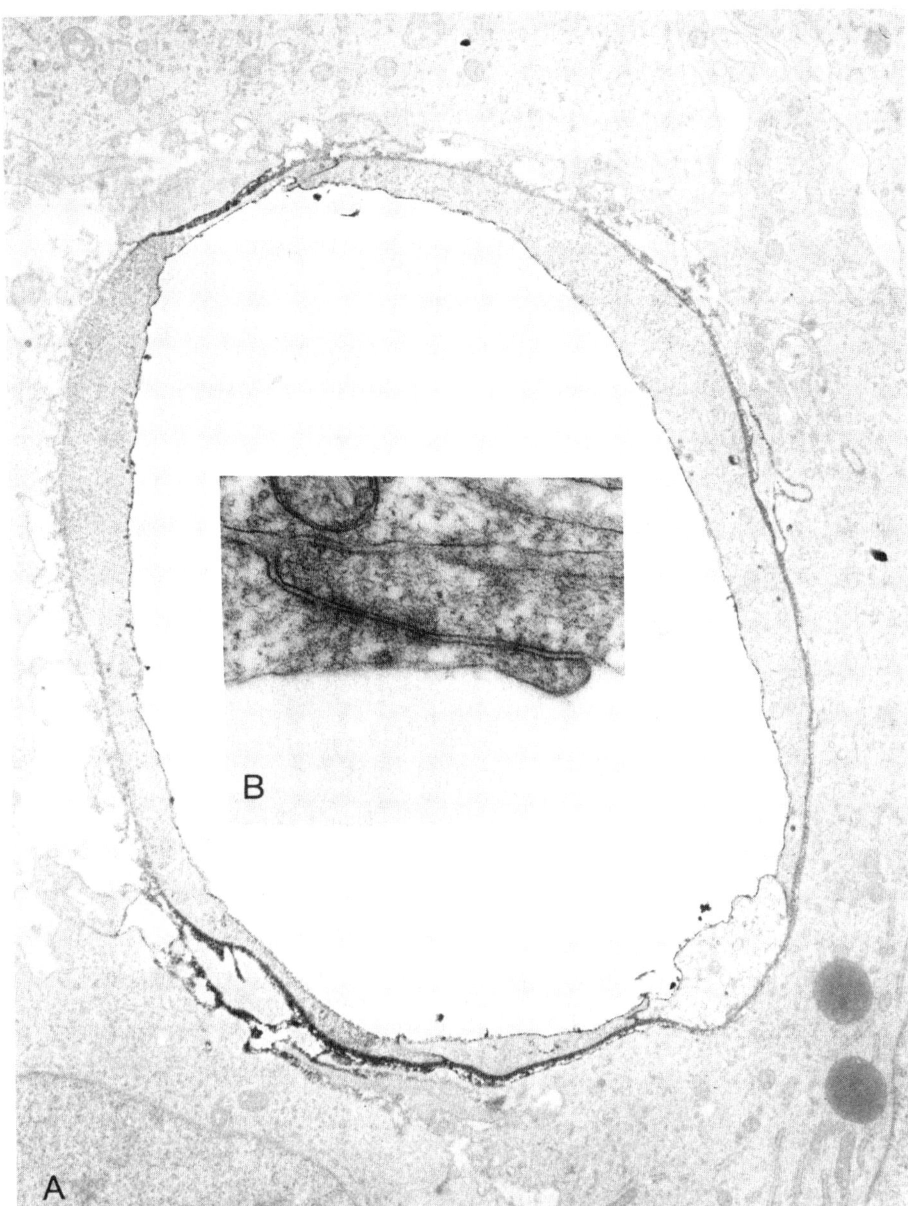

Figure 13.9. A glioma model dog tumor cell suspension delivered into the stratum of athymic mice becomes vascularized with host CNS vessels which now are leaky to horseradish peroxidase delivered intravenously (*A*). The junctional complex between contiguous endothelia supplying the tumor cell suspension is not tight and represents a patent intercellular cleft between the lumen and perivascular space (*B*).

brain tumor therapy, lessons learned from the study of barrier function within intracerebral grafts may well prove critical to the eventual success of neural transplantation in general, since tissue survival is dependent upon rapid vascularization.

WILL BARRIER MODIFICATION BE USEFUL IN BRAIN TUMOR THERAPY?

No definitive answer to this question is possible at the present time. The arguments for and against barrier modification in the treatment of brain tumors are summarized in Table 13.1. The majority of naturally occurring and experimental primary brain tumors possess a variable degree of barrier incompetency as demonstrated by morphological techniques, the uptake of radiological contrast agents, and the measurement of radiolabelled pharmaceuticals. Leakiness of the capillary endothelium within tumors is at least as geographically heterogenous as any other morphologic or biologic parameter of these highly complex lesions. Some metastatic tumors may demonstrate a more uniform impermeability based on an absence of connectivity with the vasculature of the surrounding parenchyma. When hypertonic solutions are used to open the barrier transiently in tumor bearing animals, the heterogenic distribution of water-soluble and ionic tracers does not appear to change significantly (60, 74, 94). Similar negative findings are obtained when protein-bound tracers are used as the test substance (59). Exposure of the normal nontumor bearing brain to potentially toxic substances is increased dramatically (60, 74) and may account for seizures, small infarcts and respiratory abnormalities seen in many animals after hyperosmotic barrier disruption (34, 99). Proponents of the hyperosmotic approach have demonstrated the neurotoxicity of 5-fluorouracil, Adriamycin, *cis*-platinum, and bleomycin given in association with osmotic barrier disruption (75). Furthermore, the intraarterial delivery of chemotherapeutic agents without barrier disruption has resulted in significant clinical morbidity. Nevertheless, future active substances may be developed with differential effects on the tumor and the surrounding brain that can only be achieved at increased concentration in the tumor. Since drugs now can be chemically engineered to cross the BBB (47) (e.g., AZQ and spirohydantoin mustard), their failure in clinical trials indicates the specific resistance of the tumor to the agent under study as well as the simplicity of the notion that a single chemotherapeutic agent is capable of eradicating a lesion as complex and protean as a glioblastoma. Drug delivery is but one component of the complex array of interacting factors that must be considered in the design of successful chemotherapy for brain tumors (Fig. 13.10).

TABLE 13.1.
Arguments for and against BBB Modification in Brain Tumor Therapy

For

1. Transfer constants for drugs vary in model tumors.
2. Uptake of contrast is modified after BBB reversal in humans.
3. Uptake of drugs and tracers is increased after BBB reversal in animals.
4. Transfer of antibiotics, enzymes, and other agents to whole brain is desirable.

Against

1. The normal BBB is not absolute.
2. Human and animal tumors have leaky capillaries.
3. Opening of the BBB exposes only normal brain to toxic drugs.
4. New agents can be engineered to cross the BBB (e.g., AZQ, spirohydantoin mustard).
5. Immunoglobulin fragments may cross the BBB.

CONCLUSIONS

The blood-brain barrier is a unique property of the cerebral endothelium by which the specific internal milieu of the brain is controlled. The barrier consists of the presence of circumferential belts of tight junctions between adjacent endothelial cells and a relative absence of vesicular transport across the cells. The barrier appears to be polarized such that rates of endocytosis, ion extrusion and carrier-mediated transport are different when comparing the abluminal and luminal faces of the endothelium. Human brain tumors and experimental tumors in animals do not exhibit normal barrier function; permeability to protein-bound tracers is increased by defects in tight junctions and the presence of fenestrated cell membranes. Permeability also is increased in a variety of other pathological conditions including hypervolemia, hypertension, convulsions, subarachnoid hemorrhage, ischemia and trauma. Dysfunction of the barrier is an important contributing factor to the development of vasogenic edema. The normal barrier can be circumvented by a number of physical and chemical means including ionizing radiation, hyperthermia and the intracarotid

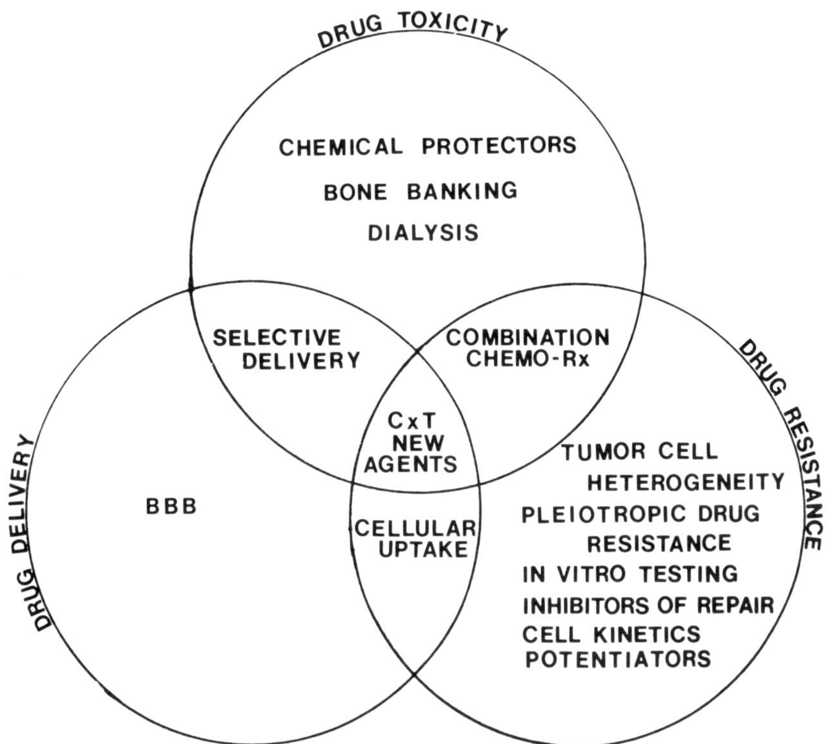

Figure 13.10. Venn diagram of factors important to successful chemotherapy. Note that the blood-brain barrier and other issues related to drug delivery represent but a small part of the problem of developing successful chemotherapy for brain tumors. Other issues such as drug resistance and drug toxicity are even more important and in some cases overlap. (C × T is the concentration over time profile of drug administration).

delivery of hyperosmotic solutions. The ability of arachidonic acid and the leukotrienes to open the barrier may be related closely to the mechanism of barrier failure observed in nonneoplastic conditions. The barrier also can be bypassed with tissue transplantation. Although barrier modification is unlikely to be important in the chemotherapy of most primary brain tumors, barrier function will remain a subject of critical concern to students of neuroimmunology, neural transplantation and neurooncology.

REFERENCES

1. Albert, E.N. and Kerns, J.M. Reversible microwave effects on the blood-brain barrier. Brain Res., *230:*153–164, 1981.
2. Aleshire, S.L., Hajdu, I., Bradley, C.A., *et al.* Choroid plexus as a barrier to immunoglobulin delivery into cerebrospinal fluid. J. Neurosurg., *63:*593–597, 1985.
3. Alexander, J.T., Saris, S.C., and Oldfield, E.H. The effect of interleukin-2 on the blood-brain barrier in the 9L gliosarcoma rat model. J. Neurosurg., *70:*92–96, 1989.
4. Arthur, F.E., Shivers, R., and Bowman, P.D. Astrocyte-mediated induction of tight junctions in brain capillary endothelium: an efficient in vitro model. Dev. Brain Res., *36:*155–159.
5. Balin, B.J., Broadwell, R.D., and Salcman, M. Tubular profiles do not form transendothelial channels through the blood-brain barrier. J. Neurocytol., *16:*721–725, 1987.
6. Balin, B.J., Broadwell, R.D., Salcman, M., *et al.* Avenues for entry of peripherally administered protein to the central nervous system in mouse, rat and squirrel monkey. J. Comp. Neurol., *251:*260–280, 1986.
7. Bar-Sella, P., Front, D., Hardoff, R., *et al.* Ultrastructural basis for different pertechnetate uptake patterns by various human brain tumors. J. Neurol. Neurosurg. Psychiatry, *42:*924–930, 1979.
8. Beck, D.W., Vinters, H.V., Hart, M.N., *et al.* Glial cells influence polarity of the blood-brain barrier. J. Neuropathol. Exp. Neurol., *43:*219–224, 1984.

9. Betz, A.L., Firth, J.A., and Goldstein, G.W. Polarity of the blood-brain barrier: distribution of enzymes between the luminal and antiluminal membranes of brain capillary endothelial cells. Brain Res., *192*:17–28, 1980.
10. Black, K.L. and Hoff, J.T. Leukotrienes increase blood-brain barrier permeability following intraparenchymal injections in rats. Ann. Neurol., *18*:349–351, 1985.
11. Blasberg, R., Molnar, P., Groothuis, D., *et al.* Concurrent measurements of bloodflow and transcapillary transport in avian sarcoma virus-induced experimental brain tumors: implications for chemotherapy. J. Pharm. Exp. Ther., *231*:724–735, 1984.
12. Blasberg, R.G. Pharmacodynamics and the blood-brain barrier. Natl. Cancer Inst. Monogr., *46*:19–27, 1977.
13. Bowman, P.D., Ennis, S.R., Rarey, K.E., *et al.* Brain microvessel endothelial cells in tissue culture: a model for study of blood-brain barrier permeability. Ann. Neurol., *14*:396–402, 1983.
14. Bradbury, M.W.B. and Segal, M.B. Transport of potassium at the blood-brain barrier. In: *Proceedings of the Wates Foundation, Symposium on the Blood-Brain Barrier*, pp. 143–149. Oxford, Truex Press, 1970.
15. Bradbury, M.W.B. The structure and function of the blood-brain barrier. Fed. Proc., *43*:186–190, 1984.
16. Brightman, M.W. Morphology of blood-brain interfaces. In: The ocular and cerebrospinal fluids. Exp. Eye Res., 25 (suppl): 1-25, 1977.
17. Brightman, M.W. The intracerebral movement of proteins injected into blood and cerebrospinal fluid of mice. in: *Progress in Brain Research*, Vol. 29, edited by A. Lajtha and D. H. Ford. Amsterdam, Elsevier Publishing, 1968.
18. Brightman, M.W. and Reese, T.S. Junctions between intimately apposed cell membranes in the vertebrate brain. J. Cell Biol., *10*:648–677, 1969.
19. Brightman, M.W. The anatomic basis of the blood-brain barrier. In: *Implications of the Blood-Brain Barrier and Its Manipulation*, edited by E. H. Neuwelt, pp. 53–83. New York, Plenum Press, 1988.
20. Brightman, M.W., Hori, M., Rapoport, S.I., *et al.* Osmotic opening of tight junctions in cerebral endothelium. J. Comp. Neurol., *152*:317–326, 1973.
21. Broadwell, R.D. Addressing the absence of a blood-brain barrier within transplanted brain tissue. Science, *24*:473, 1988.
22. Broadwell, R.D. Movement of macromolecules across the blood-brain barrier. In: *16th Princeton Conference on Cerebrovascular Diseases*, edited by M. Ginsburg and W. D. Dietrich, pp. 411–416. New York, Raven Press, 1989.
23. Broadwell, R.D. Transcytosis of macromolecules through the blood-brain barrier. A critical appraisal and cell biological perspective. Acta Neuropathol., *79*:117–128, 1989.
24. Broadwell, R.D. Origins of blood vessels in allogeneic neural grafts. In: *Pathophysiology of the Blood-Brain Barrier: Longterm Consequences of Barrier Dysfunction for the Brain*, edited by B. B. Johansson, C. H. Owman, and H. Widner, pp. 561–572. Amsterdam, Elsevier Publishing, 1990.
25. Broadwell, R.D. Cell biology of the blood-brain barrier in normal and transplanted brain-immunological consequences. In: *Peripheral Signaling of the Brain. Role in Neural-Immune Interactions and Learning and Memory*, edited by R. C. A. Frederickson, J. L. McGaugh, and D. L. Felton. Hogrefe and Huber, in press, 1990.
26. Broadwell, R. D., Balin, B.J., and Salcman, M. Transcytosis of blood-borne protein through the blood-brain barrier. Proc. Natl. Acad. Sci., *85*:632–636, 1988.
27. Broadwell, R.D., Charlton, H.M., Ganong, W.F., *et al.* Allografts of CNS tissue possess a blood-brain barrier. I. Grafts of medial preopic area in hypogonadal mice. Exp. Neurol., *105*:135–151, 1989.
28. Broadwell, R.D., Charlton, H.M., Ebert, P., *et al.* Angiogenesis and the blood-brain barrier in solid and dissociated cell grafts within the CNS. Prog. Brain Res., *82*:95–101, 1990.
29. Broadwell, R.D., Salcman, M., and Kaplan, R.S. Morphologic effects of DSMO on the blood-brain barrier. Science, *217*:164–166, 1982.
30. Broadwell, R.D., Balin, B.J., Salcman, M., *et al.* Brain-blood barrier? Yes and no. Proc. Natl. Acad. Sci., *80*:7352–7356, 1983.
31. Broadwell, R.D., Charlton, H.M., Balin, B.J., *et al.* Angio-architecture of the CNS, pituitary gland, and intracerebral grafts revealed with peroxidase cytochemistry. J. Comp. Neurol., *260*:47–62, 1987.
32. Broadwell, R.D., Cataldo, A.M., and Salcman, M. Cytochemical localization of glucose-6-phosphatase activity in cerebral endothelial cells. J. Histochem. Cytochem., *31*:818–822, 1983.
33. Broadwell, R.D. and Salcman, M. Expanding the definition of the blood-brain barrier to protein. Proc. Natl. Acad. Sci. U.S.A., *78*:7820–7824, 1981.
34. Bullard, D.E. and Bigner, D.D. Blood-brain barrier disruption in immature Fischer 344 rats. J. Neurosurg., *60*:743–750, 1984.
35. Bundgaard, M. Pathways across the vertebrate blood-brain barrier: morphological viewpoints. Ann. NY Acad. Sci., *481*:7–19, 1986.
36. Bundgaard, M. Vesicular transport in capillary endothelium: does it occur? Fed. Proc., *42*:2425–2430, 1983.
37. Chan, P.H. and Fishman, R.A. The role of arachidonic acid in vasogenic brain edema. Fed. Proc., *43*:210–213, 1984.
38. Cserr, H.F. and Bundgaard, M. Blood-brain interfaces in vertebrates: a comparative approach. Am. J. Physiol., *246*:R277–R288, 1984.

39. Davson, H. History of the blood-brain barrier concept. In: *Implications of the Blood-Brain Barrier and Its Manipulation*, edited by E. A. Neuwelt, pp. 27–52. New York, Plenum Press, 1988.
40. Deane, B.R., Greenwood, J., Lantos, P.L., *et al.* The vasculature of experimental brain tumors. Part 4. The quantification of vascular permeability. J. Neurol. Sci., *65:*59–68, 1984.
41. Deane, B.R., Papp, M.I., and Lantos, P.L. The vasculature of experimental brain tumors. Part 3. Permeability studies. J. Neurol. Sci., *65:*47–68, 1984.
42. Dietrich, W.D., Prado, R., Watson, B.D., *et al.* Middle cerebral artery thrombosis: acute blood-brain barrier consequences. J. Neuropathol. Exp. Neurol., *47:*443–451, 1988.
43. Doczi, T. The pathogenic and prognostic significance of blood-brain barrier damage at the acute stage of aneurysmal subarachnoid hemorrhage. Clinical and experimental studies. Acta. Neurochir., *77:*110–132, 1985.
44. Dorovini-Zis, K., Sato, M., Goping, G., *et al.* Ionic lanthanum passage across cerebral endothelium exposed to hyperosmotic arabinose. Acta. Neuropathol., *60:*49–60, 1983.
45. Duffy, K.R. and Pardridge, W.M. Blood-brain barrier transcytosis of insulin in developing rabbits. Brain Res., *420:*32–38, 1987.
46. Ebert, P., Broadwell, R.D., Wolf, A.L., *et al.* Intracerebral cell suspensions and the blood-brain barrier. Soc. Neurosci. Abstr., *15:*1371, 1989.
47. Egorin, M.J., Bellis, E.B., Salcman, M., *et al.* The pharmacology of diaziquone given in intravenous or intracarotid infusion to normal and intracranial tumor-bearing puppies. J. Neurosurg., *60:*1005–1013, 1984.
48. Ehrlich, P. Uber die Beziehungen von Chemische Constitution, Vertheilung, und Pharmakologischer Wirkung. In: *Collected Studies in Immunity*, pp. 567–595. (repr. and transl.), New York, John S. Wiley, 1906.
49. Fishman, J.B., Rubin, J.B., Handrahan, J.V., *et al.* Receptor-mediated transcytosis of transferrin across the blood-brain barrier. J. Neurosci. Res., *18:*299–304, 1987.
50. Goldmann, E.E. Vitalfarbung am Zentralnervensystem. Abh. Preuss. Akad. Wiss. Phys.-Math., *1:*1–60, 1913.
51. Goldstein, G.W., Betz, A.L., and Bowman, P.D. Use of isolated brain capillaries and cultured endothelial cells to study the blood-brain barrier. Fed. Proc., *43:*191–195, 1985.
52. Goldstein, G.W. and Betz, A.L. Recent advances in understanding brain capillary function. Ann. Neurol., *14:*389–395, 1983.
53. Groothuis, D.R., Fischer, J.M., Lapin, G., *et al.* Permeability of different experimental brain tumor models to horseradish peroxidase. J. Neuropathol. Exp. Neurol., *41:*164–185, 1982.
54. Groothuis, D.R., Fischer, J.M., Vick, N.A., *et al.* Comparative permeability of different glioma models to horseradish peroxidase. Cancer. Treat. Rep., *65(Supp 2):*13–18, 1981.
55. Gruenau, S.P., Oscar, K.J., Folker, M.T., *et al.* Absence of microwave effect on blood-brain barrier permeability to [^{14}C]sucrose in the conscious rat. Exp. Neurol., *75:*299–307, 1982.
56. Hirano, A. and Matsui, T. Vascular structures in brain tumors. Hum. Pathol., *6:*611–621, 1975.
57. Hirano, A. and Zimmerman, H.M. Fenestrated blood vessels in a metastatic renal carcinoma in the brain. Lab. Invest., *26:*465–468, 1972.
58. Horton, J.C. and Hedley-White, E.T. Protein movement across the blood-brain barrier in hypervolemia. Brain Res., *169:*610–614, 1979.
59. Inoue, T., Fukui, M., Nishio, S., *et al.* Hyperosmotic blood-brain barrier disruption in brains of rats with an intracerebrally transplanted RG-C6 tumor. J. Neurosurg., *66:*256–263, 1987.
60. Inoue, T., Tashima, T., Nishio, S., *et al.* Vascular permeability and cell kinetics of ethylnitrosourea (ENU)-induced rat brain tumors. Acta. Neurochir., *91:*67–72, 1988.
61. Inoue, M., Fukushima, M., Tsutsumi, K., *et al.* Freeze-fracture replica study of capillary endothelium after embolization in the dog. J. Neurosurg., *62:*737–742, 1985.
62. Jaeger, C.B. Fenestration of cerebral microvessels induced by PC12 cells grafted to the brain of rats. Ann. NY Acad. Sci., *481:*361–364, 1986.
63. Janzer, R.C. and Raff, M.C. Astrocytes induce blood-brain barrier properties in endothelial cells. Nature, *325:*253–257, 1987.
64. Jarden, J.O., Dhawan, V., Poltorak, A., *et al.* Positron emission tomographic measurement of blood-to-brain and blood-to-tumor transport of ^{82}RB: the effect of dexamethasone and whole-brain radiation therapy. Ann. Neurol., *18:*636–646, 1985.
65. Kuroiwa, T., Seida, M., Tomida, S., *et al.* Discrepancies among CT, histological, and blood-brain barrier findings in early cerebral ischemia. J. Neurosurg., *65:*517–524, 1986.
66. Levin, V.A., Freeman-Dove, M., and Landahl, H.D. Permeability characteristics of brain adjacent to tumors in rats. Arch. Neurol., *32:*785–791, 1975.
67. Lin, J.C. and Lin, M.F. Microwave hyperthermia-induced blood-brain barrier alterations. Radiat. Res., *89:*77–87, 1982.
68. Long, D.M. Capillary ultrastructure and the blood-brain barrier in human malignant brain tumors. J. Neurosurg., *32:*127–144, 1970.
69. Long, J.B. and Holaday, J.W. Blood-brain barrier: endogenous modulation by adrenal-cortical function. Science, *227:*1580–1583, 1985.
70. Merritt, J.H., Chamness, A.S., and Allen, S.J. Studies on blood-brain barrier permeability after microwave-radiation. Radiat. Environ.

Biophys., *15:*367–377, 1978.

71. Moriyama, E., Salcman, M., and Broadwell, R.D. Blood-brain barrier after microwave induced hyperthermia is purely a thermal effect. Part I. Temperature and power measurements. Surg. Neurol., submitted, 1990.
72. Mueller, S.M. Increased blood-brain barrier permeability during hyperthermia in the awake rat (abstr.). Ann. Neurol., *6:*150, 1979.
73. Nagy, Z., Peters, H., and Huttner, I. Endothelial surface charge: blood-brain barrier opening to horseradish peroxidase induced by the polycation protamine sulfate. Acta Neuropathol., (Suppl. VII)*:*7–9, 1981.
74. Nakagawa, H., Groothuis, D., and Blasberg, R.G. The effect of graded hypertonic intracarotid infusions on drug delivery to experimental RG-2 gliomas. Neurology, *34:*1571–1581, 1984.
75. Neuwelt, E.A., Glasberg, M., Frenkel, E., *et al.* Neuro-toxicity of chemotherapeutic agents after blood-brain barrier modification: neuropathological studies. Ann. Neurol., *14:* 316–324, 1983.
76. Neuwelt, E.A., Barnett, P.A., Bigner, D.D., *et al.* Effects of adrenal cortical steroids and osmotic blood-brain barrier opening on methotrexate delivery to gliomas in the rodent: the factor of the blood-brain barrier. Proc. Natl. Acad. Sci. U.S.A., *79:*4420–4423, 1982.
77. Nishio, S., Ohta, M., Abe, M., *et al.* Microvascular abnormalities in ethylnitrosourea (ENU)-induced rat brain tumors: structural basis for altered blood-brain barrier function. Acta Neuropathol., *59:*1–10, 1983.
78. Oscar, K.J. and Hawkins, T.D. Microwave alteration of the blood-brain barrier system of rats. Brain Res., *126:*281–293, 1977.
79. Pardridge, W.M. Mechanisms of neuropeptide interaction with the blood-brain barrier. Ann. NY Acad. Sci., *481:*231–249, 1986.
80. Preston, E. Failure of hyperthermia to open rat blood-brain barrier: Reduced permeation of sucrose. Acta Neuropathol., *57:*255–262, 1982.
81. Prokopanow, H. Capillary ultrastructure in gliomas of the central nervous system. Neuropathol. Pol., *18(1):*127–137, 1980.
82. Quagliarello, V.J., Long, W.J., and Scheld, W.M. Morphologic alterations of the blood-brain barrier with experimental meningitis in the rat: temporal sequence and role of encapsulation. J. Clin. Invest., *77(4):*1084–1095, 1986.
83. Raimondi, A.J. Localization of radio-labelled serum albumin in human glioma. An electron-microscopic study. Arch. Neurol., *11:*173–184, 1964.
84. Rapoport, S.I. Tight junctional modification as compared to increased pinocytosis as the basis of osmotically-induced opening of the blood-brain barrier. Further evidence of the tight junctional mechanism and against pinocytosis. Acta Neurol. Scand., *72:*107, 1985.
85. Rapoport, S.I. Osmotic opening of the blood-brain barrier. Ann. Neurol., *24:*677–680, 1988.
86. Rapoport, S.I., Hori, M., and Klatzo, I. Testing of a hypothesis for osmotic opening of the blood-brain barrier. Am. J. Physiol., *223:*323, 1972.
87. Reese, T.S. and Karnovsky, M.J. Fine structural localization of a bloodbrain barrier to exogenous peroxidase. J. Cell. Biol., *34:*207–217, 1967.
88. Rodriguez, L.A. Experiments on the histologic locus of the hemato-encephalic barrier. J. Comp. Neurol., 102:27–45, 1955.
89. Rosenstein, J.F. and Brightman, M.W. Circumventing the blood-brain barrier with autonomic ganglion transplants. Science, *221:* 879–881, 1983.
90. Salcman, M. and Samaras, G.M. Hyperthermia for brain tumors: biophysical rationale. Neurosurgery, *9:*327–335, 1981.
91. Salcman, M., Rao, C.V.G., Scott, E.W., *et al.* CT characteristics of a transplantable canine glioma model: preliminary kinetic analysis. Am. J. Neuroradiol., *4:*786–788, 1983.
92. Salcman, M., Scott, E.W., Schepp, R.S., *et al.* Transplantable canine glioma model for use in experimental neuro-oncology. Neurosurgery, *11:*372–381, 1982.
93. Sasaki, T., Kassell, N.F., Yamashita, M., *et al.* Barrier disruption in the major cerebral arteries following experimental subarachnoid hemorrhage. J. Neurosurg., *63:*433–440, 1985.
94. Shapiro, W.R., Voorhies, R.M., Hiesiger, E.M., *et al.* Pharmaco-kinetics of tumor cell exposure to (^{14}C)methotrexate after intracarotid administration with and without hyperosmotic opening of the blood-brain and blood-tumor barriers in rat brain tumors: a quantitative autoradiographic study. Cancer Res., *48:*694–701, 1988.
95. Smith, K.R. and Borchardt, R.T. Permeability and mechanism of albumin, cationized albumin, and glycosylated albumin transcellular transport across monolayers of cultured bovine capillary endothelial cells. Pharma. Res., *6:*466–472, 1989.
96. Spigelman, M.K., Zappulla, R.A., Malis, L.I., *et al.* Intracarotid dehydrocholate infusion: a new method for prolonged reversible blood-brain barrier disruption. Neurosurgery, *12:*606–612, 1983.
97. Stewart, P.A., Hayakawa, K., Farrell, C.L., *et al.* Quantitative study of microvessel ultrastructure in human peritumoral brain tissue. Evidence for a blood-brain barrier defect. J. Neurosurg., *67:*697–705, 1987.
98. Stewart, P.A. and Wiley, M.J. Developing nervous tissue induces formation of blood-brain barrier characteristics in invading endothelial cells: a study using quail-chick transplantation chimeras. Dev. Biol., *84:*183–192, 1981.
99. Suzuki, M., Iwasaki, Y., Yamamoto, T., *et al.*

Sequelae of the osmotic blood-brain barrier opening in rats. J. Neurosurg., *69:*421–428, 1988.

100. Tao-Cheng, J.H., Nagy, Z., and Brightman, M.W. Tight junctions of brain endothelium in vitro are enhanced by astroglia. J. Neurosci., *7:*3293–3299, 1987.

101. Triguero, D., Buciak, J.B., Yang, J., *et al.* Blood-brain barrier transport of cationized immunoglobin G: Enhanced delivery compared to native protein. Proc. Natl. Acad. Sci. U.S.A., *86:*4761–4765, 1989.

102. Uematsu, Y., Hirano, A., and Llena, J.F. Electron microscopic observations of blood vessels in ependymoma. Neurol. Surg. (Jpn), *16:*1235–1241, 1988.

103. Vick, N.A. and Bigner, D.D. Microvascular abnormalities in virally-induced canine brain tumors. Structural bases for altered blood-brain barrier function. J. Neurol. Sci., *17:*29–39, 1972.

104. Vinters, H.V., Beck, D.W., Bready, J.V., *et al.* Uptake of glucose analogues into cultured cerebral microvessel endothelium. J. Neuropathol. Exp. Neurol., *44:*445–458, 1985.

105. Waggener, J.D. and Beggs, J.L. Vasculature of neural neoplasms. Adv. Neurol., *15:*27–49, 1976.

106. Wakai, S., Meiselman, S.E., and Brightman, M.B. Muscle grafts as entries for blood-borne proteins into the extracellular space of the brain. Neurosurgery, *18:*548–554, 1986.

107. Warnke, P.C., Blasberg, R.G., and Groothuis, D.R. The effect of hyper-osmotic blood-brain barrier disruption on blood-to-tissue transport in ENU-induced gliomas. Ann. Neurol., *22:*300–305, 1987.

108. Weller, R.O., Foy, M., and Cox, S. The development and ultrastructure of the microvasculature in malignant gliomas. Neuropathol. Appl. Neurobiol., *3:*307–322, 1977.

109. Westergaard, E. The blood-brain barrier to horseradish peroxidase under normal and experimental conditions. Acta Neuropathol., *39:*181–187, 1977.

110. Yamada, K., Ushio, Y., Hayakawa, T., *et al.* Quantitative autoradiographic measurements of blood-brain barrier permeability in the rat glioma model. J. Neurosurg., *57:*394–398, 1982.

111. Zuccarello, M. and Anderson, D.K. Protective effect of a 21-aminosteroid on the blood-brain barrier following subarachnoid hemorrhage in rats. Stroke, *20:*367–371, 1989.

CHAPTER 14

Metabolic Studies of Brain Tumors in Vivo

PAUL L. KORNBLITH, M.D.

INTRODUCTION

The concurrent development of the modality of positron emission tomography (PET) and the discovery that 2-deoxyglucose could serve as a tracer for tumor metabolism has led to a detailed study of glucose metabolism in human brain tumors. In this research the regional hypothesis of Otto Warburg that neoplasms have a higher rate of aerobic metabolism has been used as a basis for evaluating metabolic activity in over 300 patients with malignant brain tumors (24, 25). In this chapter the basis of the metabolic studies and the implication for tumor diagnosis and therapy are discussed.

BASIS OF STUDIES OF GLUCOSE METABOLISM IN BRAIN TUMORS

Positron emission tomographic scanning utilizing [^{18}F]2-deoxyglucose (FDG-PET) permits the analysis of the overall glycolytic metabolic rates as well as regional metabolic patterns of brain tumors in situ (10, 21). In our studies of patients with glial tumors, we have observed that the FDG-PET-determined metabolic rates correlate well with the pathological grade of the tumor: the more malignant the tumor, the higher the metabolic rate (2, 3, 15). The differences in glucose metabolism seen within a single tumor, from one tumor to another, and from one pathological grade to another within the astrocytoma series, may be related to differences in vascular architecture, blood flow, or blood-to-brain transport. The differences, however, may also reflect biochemical variables intrinsic to the tumor cells themselves.

The availability of glioma-derived cell lines established in tissue culture from surgical tumor samples taken from patients who have also had an FDG-PET scan offered a valuable opportunity to clarify the basis of the observed differences in tumor metabolism.

The results of our studies of the correlation between the FDG-PET patient data and the in vitro glucose uptake data as well as the activities of enzymes regulating glycolytic flux (hexokinase, phosphofructokinase, glucose-6-phosphofructokinase, and glucose-6-phosphate dehydrogenase) appear to relate the cellular glycolytic metabolic processes directly to the clinical observations.

METHODS FOR BASIC METABOLIC STUDIES

At the time of surgery, tumor fragments or biopsies were obtained and placed in tissue culture medium. The tumor tissues were minced, and lines were derived from explant cultures as described previously (11). All culture stocks were routinely screened for the presence of mycoplasma infection and found to be negative.

For the experiments reported here, several glioma-derived lines were used at low passage (<15 in all cases) after initial explantation. Stock cultures were trypsinized (0.5% trypsin-EDTA, GIBCO), passed into 25 cm^2 flasks, and maintained in 5.0 ml of Ham's F10 + 10% fetal calf serum in a

37°C incubator. For the glucose consumption studies, flasks were refed with 2.0 ml of Eagle's MEM containing penicillin and streptomycin (20.0 ug/ml and 20.0 ug/ml, respectively). The initial concentration of glucose in Eagle's MEM is 4 mM.

Medium was buffered with 25 mM Hepes, pH 7.2. Flasks were maintained at 37°C throughout the experiment. At various times after the medium change, duplicate or triplicate cultures were removed from the incubator, the media was placed in test tubes and frozen at -70°C until use. Each flask was washed three times with ice cold phosphate-buffered saline, and 1.0 ml of 0.1 N NaOH was added to disrupt the cell monolayer.

Glucose was measured on 0.5–5-microliter aliquots of tissue culture medium by a fluorometric method described by Lowry and Passoneau (12). Protein content of each flask was determined on the NaOH solubilized material according to the procedure of Lowry et al. (13). The rate of glucose consumption was normalized against the protein content of the flask used in the experiment. Hexokinase, phosphofructokinase, and glucose-6-phosphate dehydrogenase were measured on crude homogenates by a coupled fluorometric assay.

EVALUATION AND CORRELATION OF BASIC METABOLIC DATA

Based on our studies of a series of primary cerebral tumors, a clear grouping into two major categories—high FDG uptake (astrocytomas III and IV) and low FDG uptake (astrocytomas I and II)—is possible. In order to make a comparison of metabolic rates 48 patients were evaluated; 20 had high-grade tumors; the other 28 had low-grade tumors.

The metabolic rate of the tumor in these cases of high-grade tumors ranged from 4.5 to 15.9 mg/100 g/min with a mean of 7.5 (SE ± 0.8). In each case the rate of glucose utilization in the tumor was higher than that in a comparable region of the opposite hemisphere. Each of this group of 20 neoplasms was proven to be a high-grade (III–IV) glioma. In 28 cases of low-grade tumor, metabolic rate in these cases ranged from 1.2 to 7.4 mg/10 g/min with a mean of 3.6 (SE ± 0.3). In each case the rate of glucose utilization in the tumor was lower than that in a comparable region of the opposite hemisphere. The diagnosis of low-grade gliomas (Grade I and Grade II) was made by biopsy in 10 cases and in 18 patients, who had no operations, on the basis of multiple clinical and neuroradiological criteria.

The relationship of glucose metabolism and tumor grade was demonstrated in that Grade IV gliomas showed a mean local cerebral metabolic rate ($LCMR_{glc}$) 1.6 fold greater than that of the contralateral normal brain. The $LCMR_{glc}$ in Grade III gliomas was near that of normal brain, and the low-grade tumors showed a somewhat depressed metabolic rate.

For the comparative studies of tumor glucose uptake measured in situ by the FDG-PET and biochemically in tissue culture lines obtained from the same tumor, seven lines obtained from six patients (two lines were derived from two sequential operations on a single patient) met our criteria of growth in culture, i.e., low passage number and known in situ glucose metabolic rate measured by FDG-PET. A direct correspondence between the in vitro glucose uptake and the $LCMR_{glc}$ measured by FDG-PET scans was found with a correlation coefficient *(r)* of 0.93. In normal cultured astrocytes and in cultures derived from low- and high-grade gliomas, both hexokinase and phosphofructokinase are significantly elevated while glucose-6-phosphate dehydrogenase is reduced in high-grade gliomas. The alterations in enzyme levels are consistent with the increased $LCMR_{glc}$ seen in high-grade gliomas.

CLINICAL EVALUATION OF TUMOR METABOLISM

In a series of clinical studies of tumor metabolism, patients were carefully evaluated using FDG-PET technique (4–6, 16–19). In one study, 100 cases were classified according to tumor grade. The classification into tumor grade was made as follows. The 15 cases of proven low-grade were diagnosed by biopsy as grades I or II. The 25 cases of suspected low-grade were not biopsied, but the patients' clinical condition, both prior to and subsequent to the PET scan, was stable and consistent with low tumor grade. The 49 cases of proven grade III and IV were all diagnosed by histology. Finally, the 11 miscellaneous high-grade lesions were classified according to several criteria. Cases 90–94 all had biopsies that either were ambiguous between III and IV, or they had other tumor classifications (oligodendroglioma, Case 91; pineocytoma, Case 94). Cases 95–100 were classified as high-grade because of deteriorating clinical condition, with at least two having died (Cases 95 and 100). In one case (Case 96) this classification was made despite a grade II biopsy report.

VISUAL APPEARANCE

In all of the high-grade lesions a visual hot spot was seen on PET, whereas only four hot spots were seen among the low-grade tumors.

The visual appearance of the tumor on PET is a far better guide to tumor grade than the absolute metabolic rate. This is not to say that visual diagnosis is easy. FDG images of the normal brain show a biphasic uptake, with high activity in gray matter areas (cortex, basal ganglia) and low activity in white matter areas (centrum semiovale, forceps major, forceps minor, etc.). The appearance of the tumor, therefore, depends on its location. A cold tumor within a white matter region will not stand out, but will be hypodense or, more likely, isodense with its surroundings. Sometimes the presence of the tumor may cause an expansion of the low activity area and perhaps a compression of adjacent structures. If a cold tumor invades a gray matter area such as the cortex, it appears as a cold spot within the area.

An example of the complexity involved is the apparent recurrence of tumor following surgery, radiation, and/or chemotherapy. In these patients there is frequently a large hypometabolic area associated with necrosis or metabolic suppression containing a small, faint focus of activity. This focus represents tumor recurrence which may be difficult to recognize because of its small size. These problems are instrumentational and may be further remedied as the resolving power of the scanners improves.

A remarkable consistency was found between FDG-PET and histology with no false-negative and only four false-positive results.

QUANTITATIVE RESULTS

The metabolic rates of the tumors are entered in Table 14.1, and a scatter plot for the different classifications is shown in Figure 14.1.

Note that the degree of overlap between high-grade and low-grade tumors based on absolute metabolic rate is much greater than for visual classification. This is caused by a multitude of physiologic and artifactual effects. For example, some patients who had radiation therapy preceding the PET scan exhibited low absolute metabolic rates not only in the tumor but throughout the entire brain; these are indicated by “” in Figure 14.1 and Table 14.1. In addition, there is the normal interpatient variability of about ±20%, even in rescans of the same patient. Whether this is due to undetected errors in the method or to actual variation in day-to-day brain metabolism is not clear.

Finally there is the partial volume artifact—the quantitative aspect of the spatial resolution problem. That is, when the malignancy is confined to a small volume, as with rim tumors, the measured metabolic rate is really the average of tumor rate with the surrounding tissue. Those high-grade tumors that exhibited low tumoral values because of this effect are indicated by 0 in Figure 14.1 and Table 14.1. Note that these two effects account for almost all of the anomalous low values within the high-grade groups. The partial volume artifact operates in both directions, i.e., small low-grade tumors embedded in normal gray matter will exhibit artifactually high metabolic rates, even though they still look “cold.” This is the explanation for high readings in Cases 13, 22, and 30 (in cortex) and Case 16 (in thalamus), and also for Cases 41, 51 of grade III. These cases are also indicated by 0.

Despite the above artifacts, we see a clus-

TABLE 14.1.
One Hundred Cases of Primary Cerebral Tumor[a]

			PET		CAT	
No.	Age	Sex	Glucose rate (mg/100 gm/min)	Visual focus	Attenuation	Enhancement
Verified low grade						
1	34	M	3.3	−	+	−
2	35	M	3.9	−	+ Ca	−
3	24	M	6.3	+	=	+
4	24	F	1.2	−	−	−
5	18	M	2.9	−	=	+
6	25	F	2.5	−	−	−
7	28	M	5.3	+	−	−
8	23	M	3.1	−	−	−
9	26	M	2.3	−	−	−
10	37	F	3.1	−	−	+
11	30	M	10.4	+	=	+
12	34	F	3.1	−	=	−
13	22	F	5.5[d]	−	−	−
14	46	M	4.1	−	+	−
15	57	F	[c]	−	+	+
Suspected low grade						
16	50	F	5.7[d]	−	+	−
17	30	M	3.9	−	−	−
18	65	F	2.9	−	+	−
19	23	F	1.9	−	−	−
20	26	M	2.5	−	−	−
21	27	M	1.3	−	−	−
22	36	M	5.2[d]	−	+	−
23	34	F	2.2	−	−	−
24	30	M	2.5	−	−	−
25	26	F	3.5	−	−	−
26	38	M	4.8	−	−	−
27	34	F	3.7	−	−	−
28	39	F	3.8	−	−	−
29	29	M	2.9	−	−	−
30	38	M	7.4[d]	−	+	−
31	58	F	3.7	−	+	−
32	48	M	[c]	−	+ Ca	−
33	74	M	3.6	−	=	−
34[b]	21	M	4.5	−	+	−
35	30	M	4.2	−	=	−
36	61	M	3.9	−	=	−
37	27	M	5.4	−	+ Ca	+
38	29	M	3.1	−	−	−
39[b]	56	M	1.0	−		+
40	54	M	5.1	+	−	−
Verified grade III						
41	28	M	11.6[d]	+	−	+
42	63	M	2.8[d]	+	−	+
43	28	F	2.1[d]	+	=	−
44	42	M	2.5[d]	+	−	+
45	35	F	5.7	+	=	+
46	53	M	3.0[e]	+	=	+
47	31	M	6.4	+	−	+
48	40	M	5.9	+	=	+
49	55	M	4.5	+	=	+
50	43	M	5.8	+	−	−
51	28	F	11.8[d]	+	−	−
52	28	M	3.4[d]	+	−	+

TABLE 14.1.—(*continued*)

			PET		CAT	
No.	Age	Sex	Glucose rate (mg/100 gm/min)	Visual focus	Attenuation	Enhancement
53[b]	35	M	4.8	+	+	−
54	49	M	7.4	+	+	+
55	53	M	3.3[e]	+	=	+
56	62	F	4.6	+	+ Ca	−
57[b]	63	F	4.9	+	=	+
58	27	F	6.7	+	−	+
59	37	M	4.2[d]	+	=	+
60	27	M	4.1[d]	+	−	+
61	32	M	[c]	+	=	+
62	19	F	8.4	+		+
Verified grade IV						
63	39	M	5.1	+	=	+
64	36	M	15.9	+	−	+
65	55	M	5.9	+	=	+
66	38	M	8.9	+	=	+
67	24	F	7.5	+	=	+
68	42	M	10.2	+	=	+
69	42	M	7.9	+	=	+
70	57	M	2.5[e]	+	−	+
71	27	M	14.9	+	=	+
72	40	M	3.3[d]	+	−	−
73	38	M	4.5[e]	+	=	+
74	59	F	3.2[d]	+	−	+
75	56	M	5.0	+	=	+
76	18	F	11.4	+	=	+
77	50	M	4.5[e]	+	=	+
78	56	M	4.2[e]	+	=	+
79	28	M	4.5[e]	+	=	+
80[b]	50	F	6.7	+	=	+
81	43	F	[c]	+	=	+
82[b]	66	M	2.0	+	=	+
83[b]	29	F	6.7	+	+ Ca	+
84	30	F	5.9	+	+	+
85	33	M	5.4	+	−	+
86	48	M	7.8	+	−	+
87	24	M	9.7	+		+
88[b]	31	M	11.2	+	=	+
89[b]	68	M	12.8	+	=	+
Suspected high grade (III-IV)						
90	65	M	7.1	+	=	+
91[b]	62	M	11.8	+	=	−
92[b]	64	F	7.3	+	=	+
93[b]	69	F	3.9[d]	+	+	−
94	34	F	7.4	+	+	−
95	43	F	5.0	+	=	+
96[b]	51	M	12.0	+	=	−
97	54	M	9.2	+	=	−
98	64	F	7.8	+	+	−
99[b]	58	F	4.9[d]	+		+
100	39	M	2.1[d,e]	+	=	

[a]Reprinted with permission from DiChiro, G., Brooks, R.A., Bairamian, D., *et al.* Diagnostic and prognostic value of positron emission tomography using [^{18}F]-fluoro-deoxyglucose in brain tumors. In: *Positron Emission Tomography,* pp. 291–309. New York, Alan R. Liss, Inc., 1985.
[b]Patients scanned with Neuro-PET.
[c]Metabolic rates not available because of difficulties with blood sampling or calibration.
[d]Partial volume artifact.
[e]Generally low metabolic rates following radiotherapy.

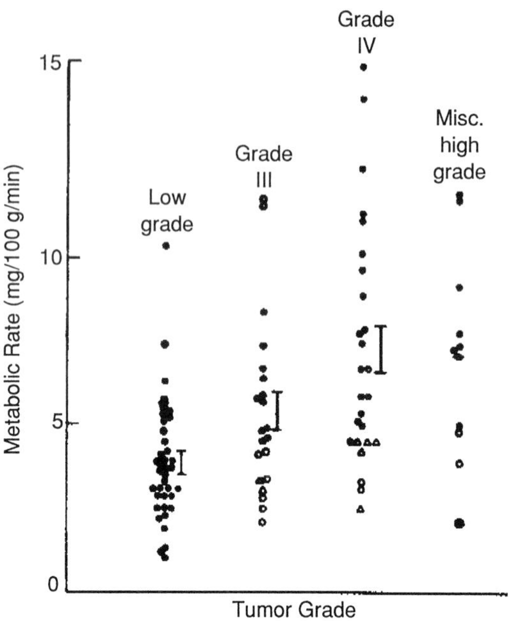

Figure 14.1. Plot of tumor metabolic rates according to tumor grade. The values labeled △ are cases in which not only the tumor rate but all cerebral metabolic rates are very low following radiotherapy. The values labeled O are altered by partial volume artifact: very low values can arise when a small hot tumor is in the midst of hypometabolic tissue, whereas artifactually high values can arise when a cold or warm tumor is in the midst of gray matter, which has a high metabolic rate. Error bars show standard error of the mean for each grade. (Reprinted with permission from DiChiro, G., Brooks, R.A., Bairamian, D., *et al.* Diagnostic and prognostic value of positron emission tomography using [^{18}F] fluoro-deoxyglucose in brain tumors. *Positron Emission Tomography,* pp. 291–309. New York, Alan R. Liss, Inc., 1985.)

tering of measurements for various grades about the following mean values:

	n	Mean (mg/100 gm/min)	SD (mg/100 gm/min)
All low-grade	38	3.8	1.8
All high-grade	58	6.6	3.3
Verified grade III	21	5.4	2.7
Verified grade IV	26	7.3	3.6

The difference in values between all low-grade and all high-grade tumors is significant at the 0.001 level, measured by Student's *t* test. Similarly, the difference in values between verified grade III and IV tumors is significant at the 0.05 level.

If we omit the high-grade cases with known artifact (Table 14.1) we obtain the following values:

	n	Mean (mg/100 gm/min)	SD (mg/100 gm/min)
Verified grade III	11	5.9	1.2
Verified grade IV	19	8.6	3.4

This difference is significant at the 0.01 level.

RATE CONSTANTS

Of the 100 tumor patients, 22 were scanned during the 30-min uptake period to determine the washout parameters k_1 and k_2, and also at 2.5–3 hr after injection to determine k_4. The mean results are shown below:

	k_1 (min^{-1})	k_2 (min^{-1})	k_4 (min^{-1})
Normal cortex	0.25	0.55	0.0083
Low-grade tumors	0.20	0.61	0.0099
High-grade tumors	0.19	0.72	0.0078

DISCUSSION AND CORRELATION OF BASIC AND CLINICAL DATA

High rates of glycolysis have been correlated with malignancy in non-CNS tumors (7, 14, 24, 25, 26, 27). Some evidence suggests that a similar relationship obtains in human cerebral gliomas (9, 20, 22, 28). The FDG-PET studies have shown a clear relationship between the $LCMR_{glc}$ and glioma pathological grade. FDG-PET scanning techniques do not, however, allow estimation of variables such as increased blood flow, increased vascularity or increased cellularity. Tissue culture methodology complements FDG-PET studies of human gliomas by permitting direct biochemical morphological and physiological examination of glioma cells. Thus, estimates can be made of the stable characteristics of glioma cells.

As shown in our data, a close relationship exists between the $LCMR_{glc}$ measured in situ and the glucose consumption rate measured in vitro for high-grade tumors. The comparability of this basic metabolic parameter in these very different milieus suggests that the glucose metabolism of gliomas is altered at the gene level even though differences in vascularity, blood flow and packing density undoubtedly contribute to the overall pathological picture (1, 8, 23). Tissue culture of gliomas may thus represent a useful model for examination of various aspects of glioma glycolysis.

With respect to regulatory mechanisms, altered levels of glycolytic enzymes are a common feature of certain non-CNS neoplasms (26). While the exact relationship of hexokinase and phosphofructokinase activity to glucose uptake rate is the subject of current study, it is clear that the two regulatory enzymes of glycolysis are increased 2–3 fold in high-grade gliomas. Enzymatic activities are also decreased in the phosphogluconate pathway in high-grade gliomas suggesting that pathways which decrease glycolytic intermediates are inactivated in the process of transformation.

The correlation of the FDG-PET observations with the in vitro glucose consumption data, in addition, serves to validate the utilization of FDG-PET for such studies. The validation of the FDG-PET method by the in vitro biochemical data suggests that application of the FDG-PET to tumor grading, follow-up after surgery, radiation therapy, and chemotherapy, may be valuable as a supplement to routine CT scanning. Further studies of glycolytic metabolism in malignant gliomas may, in addition, suggest new therapeutic approaches as they advance basic metabolic understanding of these tumors.

REFERENCES

1. Blasberg, R., Molnar, P., Horowitz, M., *et al.* Quantitative autoradiographic measurements of regional blood flow in the RT-9 brain tumor model. J. Neurosurg. *58:*863–873, 1983.
2. DiChiro, G., deLaPaz, R.L., Smith, B.H., *et al.* [^{18}F]-2-fluoro-deoxyglucose positron emission tomography of human cerebral gliomas. J. Cerebr. Blood Flow. Metab., *1:*11–12, 1981.
3. DiChiro, G., deLaPaz, R.L., Brooks, R.A., *et al.* Glucose utilization of cerebral gliomas measured by [^{18}F]-2-fluoro-deoxyglucose and positron emission tomography. Neurology, *32:* 1323–1329, 1982.
4. DiChiro, G., Oldfield, E.H., Bairamian, D., *et al.* Metabolic imaging of the brain stem and spinal cord: studies with positron emission tomography using [^{18}F]-2-deoxyglucose in normal and pathological cases. J. Comput. Assist. Tomogr., *7:*937–945, 1983.
5. DiChiro, G., Brooks, R.A., Patronas, N.J., *et al.* Issues in the in vivo measurement of glucose metabolism of human central nervous system tumors. Ann. Neurol., *15:*138–146, 1984.
6. DiChiro, G., Oldfield, E., Bairamian, D., *et al.* In vivo glucose utilization of tumors of the brain stem and spinal cord. In: *The Metabolism of the Human Brain Studied with Positron Emission Tomography,* edited by T. Greitz. St. Louis, C.V. Mosby, 1985.
7. Dickens, F. and Simer, F. The metabolism of the normal and tumor tissue. Biochem. J., *24:* 130–1326, 1930.
8. Fenstermacher, J.D., Blasberg, R.G., and Patlak, C.S. Methods for quantifying the transport of drugs across brain barrier systems. Pharmacotherapy, *14:*217–248, 1981.
9. Heller, I.H. and Elliott, K.H.C. The metabolism of normal brain and human gliomas in relation to cell type and density. Can. J. Biochem. Physiol., *33:*395–403, 1955.
10. Huang, S.C., Phelps, M.E., Hoffman, E.J., *et al.* Noninvasive determination of local cerebral metabolic rate of glucose in man. Am. J. Physiol., *238:*E69–E82, 1980.
11. Kornblith, P.L., and Szypko, P.E. Variation in response of human brain tumors to BCNU in vitro. J. Neurosurg., *48:*580–586, 1978.
12. Lowry, O.H., and Passoneau, J.V., (eds.) *A Flexible System of Enzymatic Analysis,* pp. 174, 177, 217. New York, Academic Press, 1972.
13. Lowry, O.H., Rosebrough, N., Farr, A.L., *et al.* Protein measurement with the Folin phenol reagent. J. Biol. Chem., *193:*265–275, 1951.
14. Macbeth, R.A.L. and Bekesi, J.G. Oxygen consumption and anaerobic glycolysis of human malignant and normal tissue. Cancer Res., *22:*244–248, 1962.
15. Patronas, N.J., DiChiro, G., Brooks, R.A., *et al.* Grading of cerebral gliomas by positron emission tomography (PET) using [^{18}F]-fluorodeoxyglucose (FDG). J. Nucl. Med., *23:*P6, 1982.
16. McKeever, P.E., Chronwall, B.M., Houff, S.A., *et al.* Glial and divergent cells in primate central nervous system tumors induced by JC virus isolated from human progressive multifocal leukoencephalopathy (PML). In: *Polyomavi-*

ruses and Human Neurological Diseases, edited by J. L. Sever and D. L. Medders, pp. 239–251. New York, Alan R. Liss, 1983.
17. Patronas, N.J., DiChiro, G., Brooks, R.A., *et al.* Work in progress: [^{18}F]-fluoro-deoxyglucose and positron emission tomography in the evaluation of radiation necrosis of the brain. Radiology, *144:*885–889, 1982.
18. Patronas, N.J., DiChiro, G., Smith, B.H., *et al.* Depressed cerebellar glucose metabolism in supratentorial tumors. Brain Res. *291:*93–101, 1984.
19. Patronas, N.J., DiChiro, G., Kufta, C., *et al.* Prediction of survival in glioma patients by means of positron emission tomography. J. Neurosurg., *62:*816–822, 1968.
20. Perria, L., Viale, G., Ibba, F., *et al.* Istocitochmica dei tumori endocranici. Neuropsich., *20:*419–532, 1964.
21. Sokoloff, L., Reivich, M., Kennedy, J.C., *et al.* The [^{14}C]-deoxyglucose method for the measurement of local cerebral glucose utilization: theory procedure and normal values in the conscious and anesthetized albino rat. J. Neurochem., *28:*897–916, 1977.
22. Timperley, W.R. Glycolysis on neuroectodermal tumors. In: *Brain Tumors, Scientific Basis, Clinical Investigation and Current Therapy,* edited by D.G.T. Thomas and D. I. Graham, pp. 145–167. London, Butterworth, 1980.
23. Vick, N.A. Brain tumor microvasculature. In: *Brain Metastasis,* edited by L. Weiss, H.A. Gilbert, and J.B. Posna, pp. 115–133. Boston, Hall, 1981.
24. Warburg, O. *The Metabolism of Tumors,* London, Arnold Constable, 1930.
25. Warburg, O. On the origin of cancer cells. Science, *123:*309–314, 1956.
26. Weber, G. Enzymology of cancer cells. N. Engl. J. Med., *296:*493–496;541–551, 1977.
27. Weinhouse, S. Glycolysis, respiration and anomalous gene expression in experimental hepatomas. Cancer Res., *32:*2007–2016, 1972.
28. Wollemann, M. Biochemistry of brain tumors. In: *Handbook of Neurochemistry,* edited by S. Lajtha, pp. 503–542. New York, Plenum Press, 1972.

CHAPTER 15

In Vivo Estimates of Kinetic Parameters

DAVID G. T. THOMAS, M.A., and MICHAEL SALCMAN, M.D.

Cerebral gliomas are the most common type of primary brain tumors. They are intracranial space-occupying lesions which may be rapidly fatal and which are, at present, incurable because of a relentless tendency to regrow in spite of surgery and other forms of treatment. The neuropathologist examines such tumors in vitro in the laboratory. Conventional neuropathological classification is based on the identification of the presumed cell type of origin of the neoplasm while grading of its malignancy is done by correlation of histological features with clinical experience typical of particular types of tumor. Thus, the recent WHO classification recognizes (*a*) Grade I ("benign"), (*b*) Grade II ("semi-benign"), (*c*) Grade III ("relatively malignant"), and (*d*) Grade IV ("highly malignant") gliomas. The principal features which are found to correlate with the degree of malignancy judged clinically are, increased cellularity, increased number and atypical appearance of mitotic figures, pleomorphism or anaplasia of individual cells, taken together with the presence of necrosis and hyperplasia of the vascular endothelium. It is implied that these static morphological features are correlated with variable cell kinetic and metabolic features to be found in life in different grades of glioma. It has become possible now to make estimates in vivo of these aspects of the behavior of brain tumors by application of single photon isotope and positron isotope scanning (positron emission tomography, PET), computerized axial tomography (CT) and magnetic resonance imaging (MRI). This chapter will discuss the way in which cell kinetics of brain tumors, their blood flow, their oxygen and glucose metabolism, as well as their blood-brain barrier permeability, can be measured in vivo as well as the ways in which the imaging methods may predict specific diagnoses and degree of malignancy in gliomas.

CELL KINETICS OF BRAIN TUMORS: IN VIVO MEASUREMENT OF TUMOR SIZE AND CELL KINETICS

Serial CT scanning has been used (50) to determine tumor doubling time (T_d) and to contrast this noninvasively measured parameter of cell kinetics with others derived from studies of tumor cells isolated from surgical specimens. Such studies need to be put in perspective in regard to the current general theoretical model of cell kinetics in solid tumors and in view of previous findings made by applying invasive studies to cell kinetics in human gliomas.

Before it was possible to measure cell kinetic parameters by laboratory methods in these tumors it was commonly assumed that all cells within a glioma were growing and that the rate of cell proliferation was fastest in the most malignant tumors. With the use of isotope labeling studies to measure nucleic acid synthesis in replicating cells in glioma, as well as in other types of solid tumor, a more complex model of tumor growth has emerged (48). The current cell kinetic model assumes pools of proliferating (i.e., the growth fraction, or GF) and nonproliferating cells which may be at rest before reentering the cell cycle and which may be sterile (G_0). There is some exchange between these pools and cells are constantly dying and being removed. Tumors increase in size because there is an increase in the proportion of proliferating cells (GF) and because cell death exceeds cell removal (cell loss factor, CLF), so that even dead cells contribute to the tumor bulk. The four critical stages of the mitotic cell cycle have been determined as a result of animal and human research and are defined in terms of the DNA content within the nucleus. The M phase or mitosis is visible under the microscope and consists of the distribution of previously synthesized paired chromosomes containing DNA to two daughter cells. The following postmitotic gap phase is called G_1. From this phase cells may move into the nonproliferating pool or proceed to a further cycle of cell division. In the latter case there is a period of synthesis of cell components and duplication of DNA termed S phase, to be followed by a short gap, G_2, prior to mitosis, during which further protein and RNA synthesis takes place. The period of time from one mitosis to the next is termed cell cycle time (T_c). Because the growth fraction is much less than 100% and because the further factor of cell loss (CLF) operates, the actual T_d is considerably longer than T_c.

When a tumor first begins to grow, cell loss and population pressures are so low that virtually all cells are actively dividing, the growth fraction is close to 100% and the T_d may indeed approach the T_c. This situation is virtually never observed clinically but is quite often seen in tissue culture or in the early growth phase of an experimental neoplasm. Such explosive growth in a cell population has been termed "exponential" and obeys the same first order kinetic law that governs bacterial multiplication. The kinetic behavior of an experimental canine brain tumor has been examined both in tissue culture and by CT in the early days following its implantation in the brains of adult mongrel dogs (45, 46). The in vitro T_d is on the order of 24 hours and this compares with in vivo calculations of 1.6–1.9 days in the first week of tumor growth in the animal (45). As the tumor begins to enlarge further, areas of necrosis and decreased viability appear. The factors of cell loss and decreased growth fraction then serve to moderate or brake the growth of the tumor mass and the T_d becomes much longer than the T_c. Indeed, even in the canine model tumor, T_d slowed down to 5–8 days within the second week after implantation.

The cell kinetics of human glioma have been studied by Hoshino and colleagues (24) using invasive techniques of administering isotopically labelled precursors of DNA prior to surgical biopsy, coupled with autoradiographic study of the tumor sections. More recently, this group has employed flow microfluorometric techniques (25), which can analyze biopsy material without requiring prior isotope administration to the patient. The measured growth fraction (GF) of human malignant gliomas has been in the range of 15–40%. In Grade IV gliomas the T_c is 48–72 hours, the S phase is 7–10 hours, with a GF of 30–40% and CLF of 80–85%. In Grade II–III gliomas S phase is also 7–8 hours with probably a slightly longer T_c and lower GF. After partial removal of the mass of a malignant glioma, G_0 cells may rapidly move into the proliferating pool to repopulate the tumor. However, in less malignant gliomas, movement of G_0 cells into the small proliferating pool is less significant. Therapy by partial surgical removal or partial tumor killing by radiotherapy is potentially therefore much more beneficial in this lower grade tumor.

Hirakawa and co-workers have investigated the relationship between tumor doubling time in vivo by CT scan and cell cycle time as determined by DNA quantification in vitro (23, 50). Tumor doubling time was estimated by comparing two or more CT scans where tumor volume could be measured at time intervals ranging from 2 months to 5 years. It is possible to calculate the tumor doubling time according to the formula:

$$T_d = \frac{\log 2}{\log (V_b/V_a)} \times t$$

where V_b/V_a is the ratio of two CT estimates of the tumor volume, t is the interval in days between the two observations and T_d is the doubling time, also in days (55). It is also possible to estimate the cell cycle time from such data if values for the growth fraction (GF) are either assumed or measured and the following simple formula is employed:

$$T_c = \frac{\log(1 + \mathrm{GF}) \times t}{\log(V_b/V_a)}$$

In order to estimate the growth fraction, these workers carried out a DNA analysis on cells recovered and separated from paraffin embedded sections and stained for DNA using the acriflavine Feulgen nuclear reaction. Nonspecific dye reaction was blocked by azocarmine-G staining. The samples were postirradiated to remove primary fluorescence and to stabilize the specific nuclear fluorescence. The number of cells in each phase of cell division was determined by fluorocytometry and the cell kinetics were derived from the frequency distribution using the cumulative phase index obtained from the histogram.

Nine malignant gliomas and one cerebellar astroglioma were studied in this way. A T_d as short as 2 weeks was observed in a cerebral glioma. In this case the number of cells in GF was high and the patient's life short. By contrast, tumors with a T_d of over 1 month showed significantly smaller GF and longer survival. This information is summarized in Table 15.1 (50).

Two examples of medulloblastoma were also studied by this method and illustrate the resulting in vivo estimate of kinetics in individual cases and the discrepancy with corresponding cell kinetics measured in vitro. In one child who first developed symptoms at 3 years 9 months but who did not deteriorate and come to surgery until the age of 5 years and 4 months, it was found that the tumor doubling time was 69 days (23) with a growth rate of 0.01, and a time of tumor inception at 14–23 weeks gestational age, assuming a single tumor cell diameter of 14–17 μ. The in vitro data of the DNA histogram showed a G_0/G_1 phase of 66.79%, an S phase of 26.23%, and a G_2M phase of 6.68%, giving a calculated cell uptake time using the cumulated phase index of 16–41 hours. The cell loss factor was calculated to be 49%. In a second case with initial symptoms and CT scan at 2 months and further scan and surgery at 4 months the tumor doubling time was found to be 9.4 days with a growth rate of 0.074 and a calculated time of inception at 16.3–17.4 weeks' gestational age. The in vitro data revealed a G_0/G_1 phase of 62.0%, S phase of 27.0%, and G_2M phase of 11.0%, with a cell cycle time of 16.5–42.9 hours and cell loss factor of 46%. It has been proposed that medulloblastoma arises from the fetal external granular layer (43) and that the oncogenic process occurs at a critical time of cell differentiation and migration. The growth rate and cytokinetic data fit this hypothesis well, with the implied oncogenic event occurring at 14–23 weeks gestational age, despite the clinical differences in age and speed of disease progression. The in vivo and in vitro results show a discrepancy between growth in tumor size and cell cycle

TABLE 15.1.
Cell Kinetics of Glioma: Correlation of GF and CT[a]

	Case	S Phase Cells (GF) (%)	T_d (days)	Survival (mos)
Malignant glioma	1	26%	14	12
	2	25%	17	13 (alive)
	3	21%	17	12
	4	23%	12	3
	5	14%	74	25 (alive)
	6	21%	45	15
	7	17%	55	15
	8	16%	175	22
	9	22%	178	22
Cerebellar astrocytoma	1	71%	84	24 (alive)

[a] Modified from Suzuki, K., Yoshimo, E., Ueda, S., *et al.* CT DNA histogram. Prog. Comput. Tomogr., *3(6)*:687–692, 1981.

time. The two cases showed widely varying tumor T_d but similar T_c and it is assumed that differences in GF and CLF account for these differences and for resulting differences in clinical behavior. The same group of workers have also studied the regional variation in the relationship between CT and cell kinetics and have attempted to correlate the CT appearance of the tumor edge with malignancy. The edge of the enhanced region of malignant gliomas on CT contained many S phase cells, while the center of the enhancing area contained polyploid cells (56). The CT enhancement correlated better with vascularity and tumor necrosis than the DNA content (49).

Salcman and colleagues (45) have employed sequential CT scanning in a dog brain tumor model in similar ways. This allows experimental examination of the hypotheses and the formulae used in the Japanese human studies to predict T_c from T_d. These studies confirm the extreme sensitivity of noninvasive kinetic analysis to the time of observation and its relationship to the total growth history of the tumor. As indicated above, the kinetic parameters of the tumor change with time and with the size of the lesion. Estimates of growth fraction based on sampling of selected tissue blocks must invariably suffer from the extreme heterogeneity of the total tumor mass. Visualization of the tumor by CT is also sensitive to changes that occur with progressive growth of the lesion; Yamada and his colleagues have shown that the blood-brain barrier properties of model tumors change in a predictable fashion with continued growth of the lesion (53). Thus, small tumors well within the spatial resolution of CT fail to enhance with contrast and cannot be used in kinetic analysis.

SPECIFIC DIAGNOSIS OF TUMOR TYPE AND ITS DEGREE OF MALIGNANCY BY IMAGING METHODS IN VIVO

The CT scanner was first reported by Ambrose and Hounsfield in the early 1970s (2) and rapidly entered clinical neuroradiology (1). It rapidly became the most accurate single method for revealing the presence of a cerebral lesion until the development of MRI. The plain CT scan, supplemented by scanning after intravenous contrast enhancement if necessary, shows an abnormality in 98% of intracerebral tumors at first examination (12). By contrast, the older noninvasive neuroradiological method of isotope scanning with pertechnetate has a positive detection rate of about 90% in malignant gliomas (36, 52), and 60% in low-grade gliomas. The newer method of MRI, which does not require ionizing radiation, rivals and in some cases may even surpass CT because it has both the capacity to depict cross-sectional anatomy easily in multiple planes and the potential to show changes in tissue more subtle than those revealed by CT (9).

CT SCANNING AND GLIOMAS

The displayed CT scan image is the result of calculated values of relative density of different tissues to the transmitted x-ray beam. Water has a radiodensity value of 0 Hounsfield units (HU). Tissue attenuation depends on the atomic number of the elements in a picture volume unit, or voxel, specific gravity and the tissue density relative to the hardness of the x-ray beam in kVp. The x-ray attenuation characteristics of tissue may be deliberately altered by administration of contrast enhancement. In clinical practice, the substances which have sufficient total mass to be useful as enhancing agents at the effective x-ray energies applied in CT are iodine compounds, administered by injection, or the rare gas xenon, which is administered by inhalation. Routine intravenous enhancement of CT is done with salts of monomeric compounds, diatrizoate, metrizoate, or iothalmate, which contain three iodine atoms. A typical amount of intravenous contrast is 60 ml containing 25 gm of iodine given by bolus injection to cause a blood level of 1.5–2.5 mg/ml of iodine at the time of scanning. In the normal brain the large iodine containing organic molecules are excluded by the blood-brain barrier, but elsewhere the contrast distributes in both intra- and extravascular spaces. The blood volume of normal brain is 2–5%, and this causes a small degree of enhancement of 2–4 HU. Larger cerebral arteries and veins may be visualized, and the meninges and orbital and cranial muscles enhanced. Brain lesions show a variable degree of enhancement, proportional to the amount of contrast they contain, which is mainly dependent on the degree to which the blood-brain barrier has broken down and become permeable, rather than on blood volume changes. There is a small risk of severe idiosyncratic reactions to the contrast of about 1 in 14,000 (4).

Information may be deduced from a CT scan of a tumor by assessing the apparent deformity of normal anatomy, the nature of tissue attenuation, and the intensity and extent of enhancement. Some deformity, due to mass effect, is present with most brain tumors but it is not specific and occurs also in inflammatory lesions, stroke and head injury. Abnormal tissue attenuation in a tumor may be due to characteristics of the tumor itself or to calcification, hemorrhage, necrosis, or cystic changes. Peritumoral edema and ischemic changes in brain related to tumor also can alter attenuation. Overall, CT is abnormal in over 98% of patients with intracerebral tumors (12). However, in a recent series, 1–5% of supratentorial gliomas were not detected by initial CT and 6–5% of gliomas were wrongly diagnosed as benign (31).

Malignant gliomas (astrocytomas Grades III and IV, glioblastoma) are of mixed attenuation on plain CT in about 60%, the remainder being of increased (15%), isodense (15%), or decreased (10%) attenuation when compared to normal brain (Fig. 15.1) (30). Calcification, which may be recognized by attenuation greater than 100 HU, is present in fewer than 10%. Contrast enhancement takes place in 98% and is characteristically of irregular outline, forming a ring in about 50%. However, in some cases the enhancement is regular and homogeneous. It is possible that areas of low attenuation are due to necrotic or cystic components, and that high attenuation is related to hemorrhagic areas with persisting high hemoglobin levels (the characteristic attenuation of clotted blood is 45–55 HU) while the enhancing ring reflects altered vascularity and varied permeability. By comparison, CT of grade 1 gliomas usually is of low attenuation, although they may be isodense. Calcification on CT is evident in about 30%, and enhancement is minimal or absent. Grade 2 tumors have low attenuation in 40%, with others being of mixed or isodense attenuation and calcification is less frequent overall. Enhancement is usually present and may be either irregular or homogeneous or, when associated with a cyst, appears as a fairly circular ring. Over 70% of oligodendrogliomas show calcification, with the

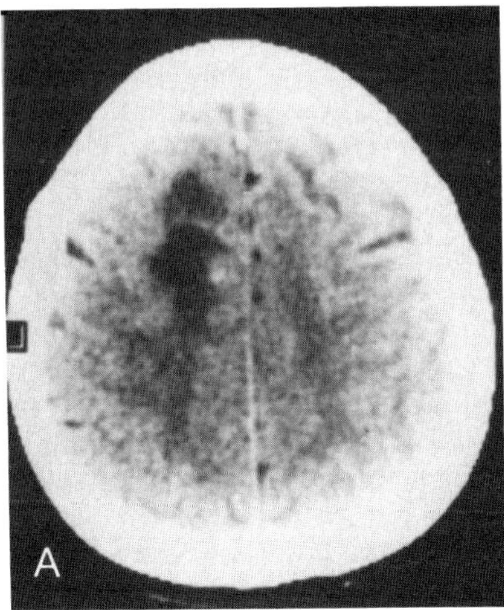

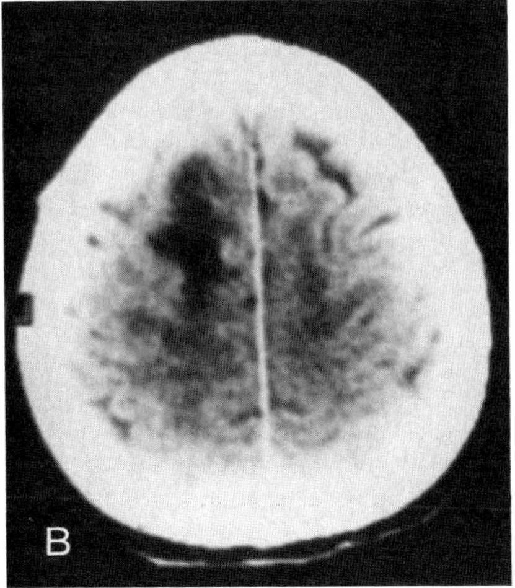

Figure 15.1. CT scan of cerebral glioma (low-grade). *A*) nonenhanced. *B*) enhanced (no change in tremor).

noncalcified areas generally being of low attenuation. Irregular enhancement is common, but 10% show no enhancement. In anaplastic oligodendroglioma enhancement may be irregular (70%) or homogeneous (30%).

Peritumoral edema is common around malignant gliomas, and tends to spread along fiber tracts in the white matter with well demarcated edges. It is less prominent in low-grade tumors, but may be even more extensive in the presence of meningioma or metastasis.

Cysts in cerebellar astrocytoma or in hemangioblastoma may have an attenuation very similar to CSF. In general, however, the fluid in tumor cysts is highly proteinaceous so that the specific gravity of the fluid and the x-ray attenuation both increase in relation to the protein content and deviate from that seen with CSF (44). Above protein concentrations of 300 mg/dl, there is almost a linear relationship between protein concentration and mean attenuation if the region of measurement is large enough to provide statistically meaningful attenuation values. Very low attenuation, in the range 0–50 HU may be found in lipomas and in some dermoids and epidermoids, which contain fatty material.

None of these CT features are pathognomic of tumor type, except the last mentioned, and they do not conclusively estimate the grade of the individual tumor in vivo. Modifications to CT enhancement techniques have been made to gain more information in vivo about tumor physiology in specific circumstances.

High dose (80 gm iodine) intravenous contrast with delayed scanning at 2–3 hours in some cases causes enhancement of tumors not brought about by conventional methods (20). It may also give special information about the nature of an individual lesion. For example, where there has been peripheral enhancement in solid and microcystic tumors on an early scan, slow diffusion of contrast may take place to opacify the entire lesion on a delayed scan. Similar enhancement in cystic or necrotic tumors may appear as fluid layers, indicating clearly the liquid nature of the center of the lesion.

Xenon enhancement of CT may also be used to define tumor cysts. Atoms of xenon and iodine behave similarly in absorbing amounts of x-radiation and cause similar attenuation changes in CT scanning. They differ radically in other respects. Xenon is a chemically inert, nontoxic gas which in concentrations of over 50% induces anesthesia. It is usually administered for scanning by an anesthetist through an endotracheal tube in a mixture of 70% xenon 30% oxygen in a closed circuit. It diffuses freely through the blood-brain barrier (BBB) and is 2–3 times more soluble in brain than water, and twice as soluble in white as in grey matter. The very low xenon uptake in cyst fluid or in a necrotic area (59) may allow definition of vascularity and definitive diagnosis of a cyst. It may also be useful in distinguishing between tumor and recent infarction, the latter having generally lower perfusion. However, the difference in xenon uptake in various tumors has not proved useful in differential diagnosis.

Changes in intensity and extent of contrast enhancement may change with time. Thus, in serial scans enhancement in gliomas may increase in intensity and extent while in infarcts it diminishes and eventually disappears (51). Permeability of the blood-brain barrier may be altered by steroid administration (13) and by in vivo manipulation of the barrier by intracarotid mannitol or as a result of radiation.

Dynamic CT scanning (22) utilizes rapid intravenous bolus injection of contrast followed by rapid serial 3-second CT scans with interscan times of only 1 second, from which the data are reprocessed to create 12 serial images covering the 35 seconds immediately following contrast injection. The studies provide high resolution cerebral perfusion images, which in the normal brain are usually symmetrical with respect to the two hemispheres. Blood transit time, blood volume and distribution as well as abnormal leakage through the blood-brain barrier are recognized by constructing iodine wash-out curves. This method gives a crude indication of blood flow, although it has not been calibrated with other methods. Several types of abnormal perfusion pattern have been found in brain tumors

(18), while infarction is associated with absent perfusion and carotid stenosis with delayed and diminished perfusion.

In a study of 14 brain tumors (18) including 9 gliomas, it was found that the time to peak in the time density curve was not useful in tumor evaluation. However, the magnitude of the peak increase of tumor enhancement did correlate with the degree of tumor vascularity assessed angiographically. Furthermore, the residual enhancement of the main tumor area at the end of the rapid series of scans was universally increased compared to normal brain, presumably due to altered BBB characteristics (Table 15.2). The method proved useful in distinguishing intra- from extracerebral tumors by making it easier to visualize the tumor boundaries.

ISOTOPE SCANNING AND GLIOMAS

The uptake of single photon emitting isotopes, like ^{99}Tc-pertechnetate into tumors is similar to that of the enhancement observed with iodine containing compounds by CT. The vascular component is useful for the detection of highly vascular lesions with a rapid circulation. Capillary permeability changes to technetium are in general similar to those to iodine compounds. Technetium uptake can be detected in 90% of anaplastic astrocytomas, but only 60% of more benign gliomas (36, 52).

In malignant gliomas, the isotope uptake is often intense, with heterogeneous density and irregular outline. Low-grade astrocytomas, when positive, tend to have less uptake. Dynamic methods of isotope scanning using rapid serial isotope scanning have been applied to brain tumor diagnosis and grading (7). The highest rate of correct tumor type diagnosis (86%) was in high-grade glioma where radionuclide angiography by early serial scans showed decreasing activity from arterial to venous distribution. Later scans showed moderate increase in tumor uptake with changes in the outline of the area of abnormality. In low–grade gliomas the method was successful in histological diagnosis in only 46%. Here, in positive cases, radionuclide angiography tended to show moderate increase from arterial to venous distribution with later accumulation in a regularly shaped tumor outline.

Recently, antibody enhanced isotope scanning has been employed (16). However, it is not yet clear whether this will be efficient in tumor type diagnosis.

PLAIN SKULL X-RAY, ANGIOGRAPHY AND GLIOMAS

Plain x-rays in malignant glioma may show calcification in about 5% of cases. In Grade I and II gliomas, the proportion of calcification is about 20%, and in oligodendrogliomas about 60% (29). However, it is not pathognomic for tumor type or grade.

Angiography can show changes pathognomonic of malignancy in about one in three anaplastic astrocytomas and glioblastomas (30). Such features include increased irregular vessels with large early draining veins. Another one-third of cases show moderate or slight increase in vascularity and the remainder are avascular masses. Lower grade gliomas generally do not have obvious vascularity.

MRI SCANNING AND GLIOMAS

MRI imaging was first proposed in the early 1970s (15, 34) and practical prototype scanners were subsequently developed (3, 20, 35). Currently, with commercial availability of the method, its use is rapidly increasing (8), and its utility in evaluation of brain tumors is rapidly being assessed.

TABLE 15.2.
Mean Increase in Attenuation Coefficient for Tumor Area and Normal Gray Matter in Nine Gliomas

	Peak	Residual
Tumor	11.2 HU (SD ± 6.2)	8.6 HU (SD ± 3.5)
Gray matter	10.4 HU (SD ± 2.4)	4.0 HU (SD ± 1.6)

[a] Modified from Dubois, P.J., Drayer, B.P., Heinz, E.R., *et al.* Rapid serial cranial computed tomography for tumour diagnosis. Neuroradiology, *21*:79, 1981.

In a comparative study of patients with brain tumors using MRI and CT it was possible to compare tumor evaluation in 93 cases. MRI was thought to be more valuable in 41%, equal to CT in 32%, and less useful in 27% (60).

MRI imaging relies on the administration of sequences of radiofrequency pulses to the patient in the presence of a carefully controlled magnetic field in order to produce images of cross sections of the body at any anatomical site. The physical basis of the scan is the distribution and behavior of hydrogen nuclei, that is, protons, during this process.

Human tissues as visualized on MRI scans have high contrast due to three basic parameters: proton density, T_1, and T_2. T_1 is the time constant which characterizes spin-lattice or longitudinal relaxation, while T_2 is the constant for spin-spin or transverse relaxation. The proton density, the mean values, the complexities and the frequency dependencies of the two main relaxation processes may all vary in different normal and diseased tissues. Bone, which has few protons, gives a low signal on the MRI scan. The absence of bone artifact is useful in the diagnosis of acoustic neuroma (57) and other posterior fossa tumors. Tissues with long T_1 appear dark on inversion recovery sequences (IR) while those, like fat, with short T_1 are light by this method. White matter has a short T_1 and appears white; the grey matter, with longer T_1 appears dark. Thus IR scans give good grey-white matter discrimination (Fig. 15.2*A*). On spin echo (SE) scans, tissues with a long T_2 appear light, while those with a short T_2 appear dark. Brain tumors tend to have prolonged T_1 and T_2 constants (Table 15.3) but brain edema tends to have similar prolonged values. Thus, it is difficult to distinguish tumor from peritumoral edema. (Fig. 15.2*A* and *B*).

The optimum combination of spin sequence is required to bring out the best contrast in proton density and relaxation times in brain parenchyma and in glioma tissue (14). In SE images the tumor and surrounding edema are highlighted against a relatively featureless brain. IR images give greater anatomical detail of the surrounding brain. By increasing the scan time and interpulse intervals the separation between tumor and edema may be brought out in tumors with a very long T_1. Unlike CT, small areas of calcification in a tumor cannot be

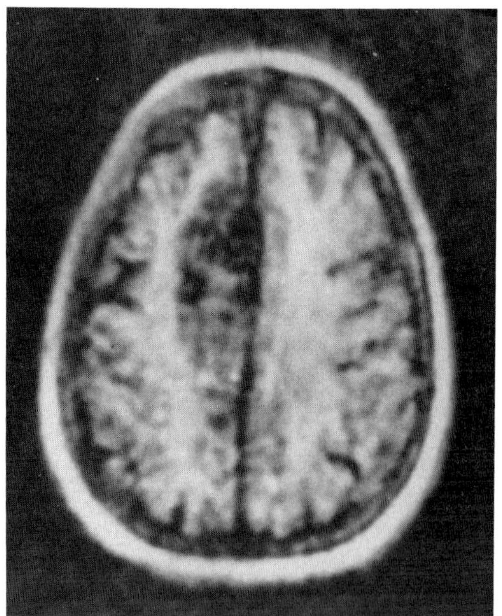

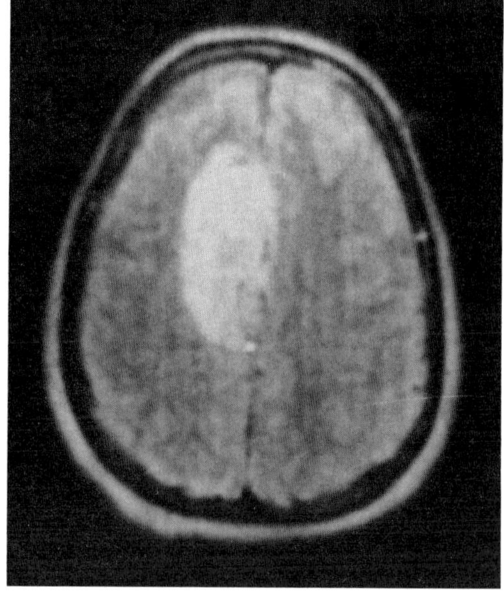

Figure 15.2. MRI scan, same case as Figure 15.1. *A*) T_1, IR sequence. *B*) T_2, SE sequence.

TABLE 15.3.
T_1 Values by MRI in Brain Tumors[a]

	T_1 in milliseconds
Glioma	750–1520
Metastasis	510–1370
Meningioma	520–600
Acoustic neuroma	
Solid	570–700
Cystic	1070

[a] Modified from Bydder, G.M., Steiner, R.E., Young, I.R., *et al.* Clinical NMR imaging of the brain: 140 cases. Am. J. Radiol., *139*:215, 1982.

seen. In general, malignant tumors show a greater increase in T_1 and T_2 than benign ones. There are also situations where tumors have short T_1 and T_2. These include fat containing tumors, tumors where there has been hemorrhage and melanoma metastases which contain paramagnetic free radicals.

SE images of 26 primary intracranial tumors were compared with corresponding CT scans. In most cases, T_1 and T_2 were prolonged in the tumors and separation from edema was possible in some (5). In 16 of 26 cases information not obtained by CT was available on MRI. The differences included detection of altered tissue characteristics, where CT showed only mass effect, as well as more accurate definition of tumor site and extent, in some cases, by MRI. However, MRI did not reveal two cases of calcification.

Methods of changing tissue contrast in MRI have been sought and the most effective enhancing agent at present is gadolinium which causes a marked decrease in T_1 and T_2. Gadolinium is a paramagnetic ion which may be given intravenously at a dose of 0.1 mg/kg in vivo as a chelated compound, gadolinium diethylene triaminine pentacetic acid (Gd-DTPA) (10). The unpaired electrons in Gd^{3+} give it a large magnetic moment allowing it to interact with protons and speeding up their return to equilibrium after the perturbation caused by the radiofrequency pulses during MRI imaging. This agent has been found to cause enhancement of cerebral tumors with improved definition of the tumor-edema boundary.

In an early study, contrast enhancement was seen in all 12 patients with cerebral tumor, of which 3 were histologically verified malignant gliomas, studied by MRI before and after intravenous Gd-DPTA (11). The most frequent pattern found was ring enhancement, in seven cases, but homogeneous central, linear, patchy and diffuse enhancement was also seen, both with IR and SE sequences. In eight cases the tumor enhancement on MRI appeared greater than on CT, in three it was similar by both methods and in one case it was less by MRI.

At present, in vivo tumor type differentiation by MRI as with other neuroradiological methods, is based on correlation of MRI information with such general considerations as patient age and tumor site and extent. Tissues with similar x-ray density on CT may differ in their proportions of water and other constituents, differences which can be detected by MRI.

One of the early hopes for MRI (15) was that it would allow better tumor type prediction than CT because the in vitro T_1 and T_2 of neoplastic tissues were prolonged compared to corresponding normal tissue. There is in practice an overlap of relaxation times between neoplastic and normal tissue (Table 15.3). However, by changing the scan parameters the optimum specificity may be obtained, and tissue identification may become possible (37). A biochemical hypothesis (58) is that water in tumors is less well-ordered than in normal tissue. In the ordered phase the motion of water molecules is more reduced by interaction with macromolecules (38). Most of the MRI signal comes from water in tissue, and it is possible that these differences are the basis for increased T_1 and T_2 in tumors. However, cellular lipids, containing protons, must also be important in this respect.

PET SCANNING AND GLIOMAS

PET scanning can be used to study the pathophysiology of brain tumor metabolism in vivo (39, 41). Positron emitting radioisotopes exist of biologically important elements like oxygen, nitrogen and carbon, so that labeled biological tracers can be imaged using the positron computed tomograph. The physical basis of the scan is that positrons emitted in tissue rapidly encounter some of the very much more numerous negatively charged electrons. With this encounter the particles are annihilated and replaced by two photons, traveling in opposite directions along a straight line from the point of impact. Coupled detectors, placed diametrically opposed around the patient's head, detect such paired photons and the algorithm of the tomograph's computer calculates the site in space of the annihilation event. Calibration to allow for tissue attenuation is made by conventional transmission CT using a static ring source of radiation. The spatial resolution of the method is less than CT or MRI (a typical current instrument may resolve pixels 14 mm × 14 mm in the tomographic plane with a slice with thickness of 16 mm). However, in spite of these constraints, the PET scan is a unique method of quantitating the distribution of radioactive tracer deep in the brain in vivo relatively noninvasively. Appropriate mathematical models have been developed for the fate of several labeled tracers in the brain and it is therefore possible to use PET scanning not only to image brain tumors but also to evaluate quantitatively their metabolic activity in vivo in respect to cerebral blood flow, oxygen utilization, glucose utilization and blood-brain barrier permeability, as well as to qualitatively follow the distribution of amino acids (27) and chemotherapy drug uptake in the tumors (54).

BLOOD FLOW AND OXYGEN UTILIZATION

The blood volume corrected, oxygen-15 (^{15}O) steady state inhalation method was used to produce the results illustrated in Figure 15.3 and Table 15.4 (19, 33). ^{15}O has a half-life of 2.1 minutes and is produced by a cyclotron adjacent to the PET tomograph. It is used as a tracer when the patient inhales through a face mask sequentially $C^{15}O_2$, $^{15}O_2$ followed by a minute quantity of carbon-11 (half-life 20.1 minutes) labeled ^{11}CO. The theoretical basis of the method and its practical limitations have been examined in detail (32). Values are obtained for regional cerebral blood flow (rCBF) and oxygen utilization ($rCMRO_2$) together with the fraction of oxygen extracted in the brain from arterial blood (rOER) as well as regional blood volume (rCBV). In cerebral glioma it has been found that rCBF can be very variable between individual tumors and within different areas of a single tumor (28), with the mean lying close to that found in contralateral, presumably normal white matter. However, every glioma studied in this way has consistently shown low $rCMRO_2$ and low rOER, implying that these neoplasms have more than adequate blood supply to meet their metabolic demand for oxygen; that is, they are not ischemic. Moreover, there was no significant correlation between tumor perfusion, as indicated by CBF, and tumor vascularity, as indicated by CBV. The physiology of surrounding and remote areas of brain was generally consistently altered so that rCBF and $rCMRO_2$ were lower in regions of peritumoral edema than in contralateral brain, while rOER remained normal or became lower than normal. This finding indicates either coupled or reduced oxygen utilization in peritumoral areas, with no indication of ischemia. The ipsilateral cerebral cortex had depressed rCBF and $rCMRO_2$ compared to normal cortex. It has been possible to use serial PET studies as an in vivo measure of the effect of therapy on cerebral metabolism. Thus, 12–24 hours after administration of dexamethasone to patients with brain tumors there appears to be a further fall in rCBF and rCBV in cerebral cortex. By contrast, decompression by surgery partially reverses the depression of rCBF and $rCMRO_2$ noted in contralateral cortex. In the early phase at completion of therapy, the effects of the external beam radiation treatment of malignant glioma have been an increase in rCBF in normal cortex with maintained constant $rCMRO_2$, and therefore reduced rOER. There is an increase in rCBV which parallels rCBF. However, three or more months later, a fall in rCBF and rCBV is found in irradiated normal brain with maintained $rCMRO_2$ and therefore increased rOER, although there is no significant ischemia. In response to radiation treatment, the brain tumor itself shows a progressive drop in rCBF, rOER, $rCMRO_2$ and rCBV, changes which may possibly be correlated with tumor cell killing.

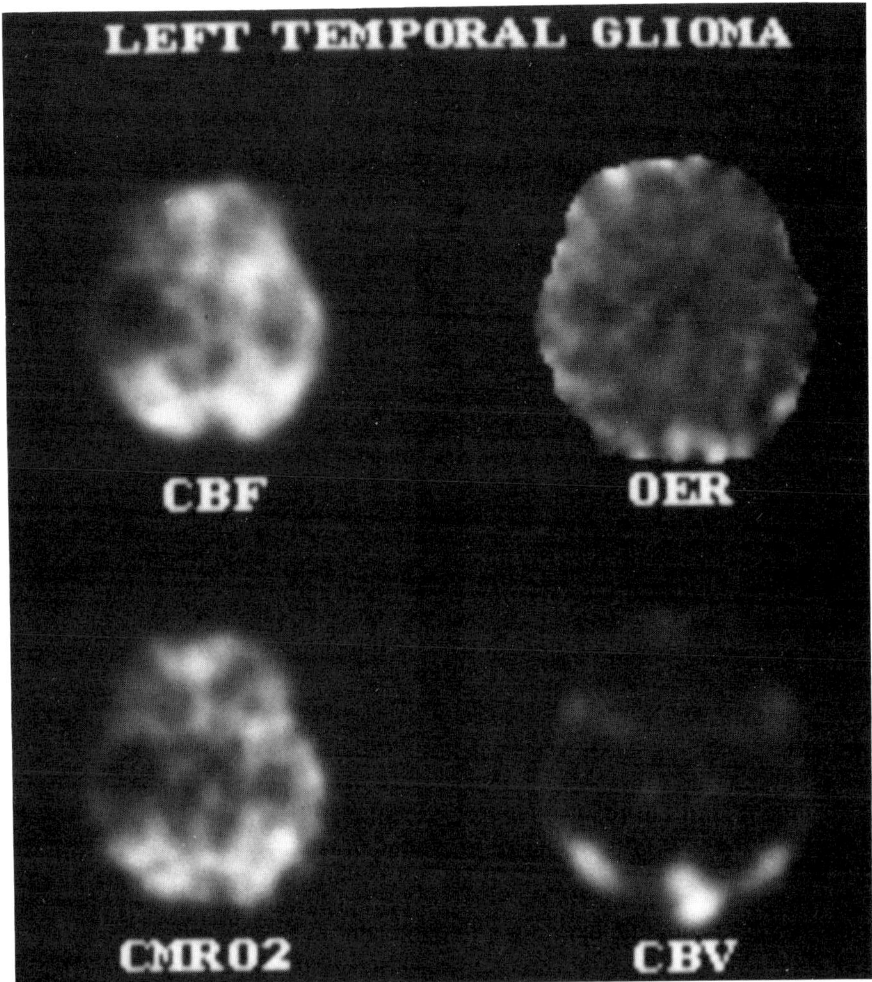

Figure 15.3. PET scan of cerebral glioma. *CBF, CMRO$_2$, OER*, and *CBV* are shown.

GLUCOSE METABOLISM

There is no positron emitting isotope of hydrogen but fluorine-18 (^{18}F, half-life 109 minutes) can be used as a radioisotopic label for compounds of biological interest like glucose. A method of determining regional cerebral glucose utilization (rCMRGlu) in vivo is based on the intravenous injection of ^{18}fluorodeoxyglucose (^{18}FDG), using principles modified (40) from the autoradiographic technique developed by Sokoloff (47) using ^{14}C-deoxyglucose in experimental animals.

TABLE 15.4.
Metabolic Parameters in Cerebral Glioma Measured by PET (Seven Cases)[a]

		Tumor Area	Contralateral Cortex
CBF	(ml/100 ml/min)	32.0 (SD ± 9)	32.0 (SD ± 5)
OER	(CBF:CMRO$_2$)	0.21 (SD ± 0.07)	0.47 (SD ± 0.05)
CMRGlu	(mg/100 ml/min)	4.8 (SD ± 1.4)	5.4 (SD ± 1.1)
GER	(CBF:CMRGlu)	0.16 (SD ± 0.03)	0.17 (SD ± 0.04)

[a] Modified from Rhodes, C.G., Wise, R.J.S., Gibbs, J.M., *et al.* In vivo disturbance of the oxidative metabolism of glucose in human cerebral gliomas. Ann. Neurol., *12(6)*:614, 1982.

The labeled tracer ^{18}FDG analogue competes in the brain with authentic glucose for facilitated transport into brain cells, and once inside the cell, for hexokinase-mediated phosphorylation. Once inside the cell, phosphorylated ^{18}FDG is effectively trapped because it cannot proceed further in the normal glycolytic pathways, nor can it readily reverse its path. This biochemical phenomenon is the basis of the mathematical model (42) which may be used to derive by PET quantitative values for rCMRGlu in normal and diseased brain by relating the tissue levels of ^{18}FDG recorded by the PET tomograph to the plasma curves of ^{18}FDG and glucose measured in rapid serial blood samples after bolus injection of the tracer. Of course, there are differences in the properties of ^{18}FDG and normal glucose, such as the rate constants for transport, phosphorylation and dephosphorylation for example. A lumped constant is incorporated into the tracer model equation which is intended to accommodate such differences. The lumped constant can be checked experimentally for whole brain but not for individual diseased areas of brain. It remains controversial as to whether brain tumor tissue should be treated as having the same lumped constant as normal brain (26). In spite of this, several findings of interest have been made.

Di Chiro and co-workers have established a direct correlation between glucose utilization and grade in primary brain tumors (17). The peak rCMRGlu found in Grades III and IV gliomas was higher than that in Grades I and II. rCMRGlu in areas of cortex connected to the tumor region by fiber tracts as well as peritumoral white matter was generally depressed. Cerebellar diaschisis, that is, reduced rCMRGlu in the contralateral cerebellar cortex, was also demonstrated. A further, clinically useful, distinction was that areas of radiation necrosis of brain showed low rCMRGlu, in contrast to recurrent tumor where rCMRGlu was high.

Combined studies applying both the ^{18}FDG method and the ^{15}O steady state inhalation method in the same patient have allowed a detailed in vivo analysis of oxidative metabolism of glucose in gliomas summarized in Table 15.4 (42). In a given tumor rOER is generally depressed while regional glucose extraction (rGER) is maintained. In normal brain rOER and rGER are tightly coupled. The implication of the PET findings is that gliomas have increased nonoxidative metabolism of glucose, where aerobic metabolism of glucose is the norm, probably by aerobic glycolysis.

BLOOD-BRAIN BARRIER

Rubidium-82 (^{82}Rb, half-life 1.2 minutes) is a positron emitting isotope similar in its permeability to the potassium ion. The normal blood-brain barrier is highly impermeable to potassium ions. It is possible to quantitate ^{82}Rb extraction by PET scanning during constant intravenous infusion of the isotope and to relate this to rCBF and rCBV obtained by the methods described above, as well as to the degree of contrast enhancement on CT scan following intravenous injection of iodine compounds, noted previously (6). The distribution of ^{82}Rb correlates well with the enhanced CT area (Table 15.5) implying that these two methods indicate to a similar

TABLE 15.5.
Rb Extraction in 14 Brain Tumor Patients[a]

		rCBF (ml/100 ml/min)	rCBV (ml/100 ml)	Rb Extraction (%)
Enhancing on CT (n = 11)	Tumor	17 (SD ± 9)	2.8 (SD ± 1.4)	29 ± 13
	Peritumoral edema	15 (SD ± 3)	2.6 (SD ± 0.4)	1.4 ± 0.3
	Contralateral brain	27 (SD ± 7)	3.9 (SD ± 0.9)	2.4 ± 1.6
Nonenhancing on CT (n = 3)	Tumor	30 (SD ± 7)	3.1 (SD ± 0.6)	1.3 ± 1.1
	Contralateral brain	39 (SD ± 2)	4.9 (SD ± 1.6)	2.3 ± 0.6

[a] Modified from Young, I.R., Burl, M., Clarke, G.J., *et al.* Magnetic resonance properties of hydrogen: imaging the posterior fossa. Am. J. Radiol., *137*:895–901, 1981.

extent the blood-brain barrier disruption. Areas of presumed peritumoral edema do not have increased ^{82}Rb uptake.

The volumes of tissue studied in vivo by all the methods outlined above are macroscopic and, compared to the techniques of the neuropathologist, the resolution of such methods in estimating the kinetic parameters of brain tumors is inevitably limited. However, these methods may be applied in life rather than requiring biopsy or autopsy. Moreover, it is inherently unlikely that uniquely malignant metabolic properties which are qualitatively totally different from normal tissue will ever be picked up by imaging techniques. The currently established techniques rest on quantitative differences in behavior between neoplastic cells and normal brain as well as between neoplastic cells of different grades of malignancy, so that some overlap must necessarily occur.

REFERENCES

1. Ambrose, J. Computerized transverse axial scanning (tomography). Part 2. Clinical application. Br. J. Radiol., *46:*1023–1047, 1973.
2. Ambrose, J. and Hounsfield, G. Computerized transverse axial tomography. Br. J. Radiol., *46:*148–149, 1973.
3. Andrew, E.R. NMR imaging of intact biological systems. Philos. Trans. R. Soc. Lond. [Biol]., *289:*471–481, 1980.
4. Ansell, G. Adverse reactions to contrast agents. Scope of problem. Invest. Radiol., *5:*374–391, 1970.
5. Brandt-Zawadzki, M., Badormi, J.P., Mills, C.M., *et al.* Primary intracranial tumor imaging: a comparison of magnetic resonance and CT. Radiology, *150:*435–440, 1984.
6. Brooks, D.J., Beanev, R.P., Lammertsma, A.A., *et al.* Quantitative measurement of blood-brain barrier permeability using rubidium-82 and positron emission tomography. J. Cereb. Blood Flow. Metab., *4:*535–545, 1984.
7. Büll, U., Niendorf, H.P., Kazner, E., *et al.* Computerized transaxial tomography and cerebral serial scintigraphy in intracranial tumors: rates of detection and tumour-type identification: concise communication. J. Nucl. Med., *19:*476, 1978.
8. Bydder, G.M. Nuclear magnetic resonance imaging of the brain. Br. Med. Bull. *40:*170–174, 1984.
9. Bydder, G.M., Steiner, R.E., Young, I.R., *et al.* Clinical NMR imaging of the brain: 140 cases. Am. J. Radiol., *139:*215–236, 1982.
10. Carr, D.H. The use of iron and gadolinium chelates as NMR contrast agents: animal and human studies. Physiol. Chem. Phys. Med. NMR, *16:*137–144, 1984.
11. Carr, D.H., Bydder, G.M., Brown, J., *et al.* Intravenous chelated gadolinium as a contrast agent in NMR imaging of cerebral tumors. Lancet, *1:*484–486, 1984.
12. Claveria, L.E., Kendall, B.E., and du Boulay, G.H. Computerized axial tomography in supratentorial gliomas and metastases. In: *First European Seminar on Computerized Axial Tomography in Clinical Practice*, edited by G.H. du Boulay and I.F. Moseley. Berlin, Springer-Verlag, 1977.
13. Crocker, E.F., Zimmerman, R.A., Phelps, M.E., *et al.* Effects of steroids on the extravascular distribution of radiographic contrast materials and technetium pertechnetate in brain tumours as determined by CT. Radiology, *119:*471–474, 1976.
14. Crooks, L.E., Mills, C.M., Davis, P.L., *et al.* Visualization of cerebral and vascular abnormalities by NMR imaging. The effects of imaging parameters on contrast. Radiology, *144:*843–852, 1982.
15. Damadian, R. Tumor detection by nuclear magnetic resonance. Science, *171:*1151–1153, 1971.
16. Davies, G., Coakham, H., Richardson, R., *et al.* Radioimmunolocalisation of human brain tumours using monoclonal antibody (abstr.). J. Neurooncology, *2*(3):273, 1984.
17. DiChiro, G., De La Paz, R.L., Brooks, R.A., *et al.* Glucose utilization of cerebral gliomas measured by ^{18}F-fluorodeoxyglucose and positron emission tomography. Neurology, *32:*1323–1329, 1982.
18. DuBois, P.J., Drayer, B.P., Heinz, E.R., *et al.* Rapid serial cranial computed tomography for tumour diagnosis. Neuroradiology, *21:*79–86, 1981.
19. Frackowiak, R.S.J., Lenzi, G.L., Jones, T., *et al.* Quantitative measurement of regional cerebral blood flow and oxygen metabolism in man using ^{15}O and positron emission tomography: theory, procedure and normal values. J. Comput. Assist. Tomogr., *4:*727–736, 1980.
20. Hawkes, R.C., Holland, G.N., Moore, W.S., *et al.* Nuclear magnetic resonance (NMR) tomography of the brain: a preliminary clinical assessment with demonstration of pathology. J. Comput. Assist. Tomogr. *4:*577–586, 1980.
21. Hayman, A.L., Evans, R.A., and Hinck, V.C. Delayed high dose contrast computed tomography. Cranial neoplasms. Radiology, *136:*677–684, 1980.
22. Heinz, E.R., Dubois, P., Osbourne, D., *et al.* Dynamic computed tomography study of the brain. J. Comput. Assist. Tomogr., *3:*641–649, 1979.
23. Hirakawa, K., Suzuki, K., Ueda, S., *et al.* Cytokinetics and growth rate of medulloblastoma, Abstract 64. San Francisco, Proceedings of American Association of Neurological Surgeons, 1984.
24. Hoshino, T., Barker, M., Wilson, C.B., *et al.* Cell

kinetics of human gliomas. J. Neurosurg., *37:*15–26, 1972.
25. Hoshino, T., Nomura, K., Wilson, C.B., *et al.* The distribution of nuclear DNA from human brain-tumour cells. Flow cytometric studies. J. Neurosurg., *49:*13–21, 1978.
26. Huang, S.C., Phelps, M.E., Hoffman, E.J., *et al.* Noninvasive determination of local cerebral metabolic rate of glucose in man. Am. J. Physiol. *238:*E69–82, 1980.
27. Hubner, K.F., Purvis, J.T., Mahaley, S.M., *et al.* Brain tumour imaging by positron emission computed tomography using "C-labelled amino acids. J. Comput. Assist. Tomogr., *6:*544–550, 1982.
28. Ito, M., Lammerstma, A.A., Wise, R.J.S., *et al.* Measurement of regional cerebral blood flow and oxygen utilisation in patients with cerebral tumours using ^{15}O and positron emission tomography: analytical techniques and preliminary results. Neuroradiology, *23:*63–74, 1982.
29. Kalan, C. and Burow, E.H. Calcification in intracranial gliomata. Br. J. Radiol., *35:*589, 1962.
30. Kendal, B. Neuroradiology. In: *Brain Tumors, Scientific Basis, Clinical investigation and Current Therapy,* edited by D.G.T. Thomas and D.I. Graham. London, Butterworths, 1980.
31. Kendall, B.E., Jakubowski, J., Pullicino, P., *et al.* Difficulties in diagnosis of supratentorial gliomas by CAT scan. J. Neurol. Neurosurg. Psychiatry, *42:*485–492, 1979.
32. Lammertsma, A.A., Jones, T., Frackowiak, R.S.J., *et al.* A theoretical study of the steady-state model for measuring regional cerebral blood flow and oxygen utilization using oxygen-15. J. Comput. Assist. Tomogr., *5:*544–550, 1981.
33. Lammertsma, A.S., Wise, R.J.S., Heather, J.D., *et al.* Correction for the presence of intravascular oxygen-15 in the steady state technique for measuring regional oxygen extraction ratio in the brain. 2. Results in normal subjects and brain tumour and stroke patients. J. Cereb. Blood Flow Metabol., *3:*425–431, 1983.
34. Lauterbur, P.C. Image formation by induced local interactions: examples employing nuclear magnetic resonance. Nature, *242:*190, 1973.
35. Moore, W.S. and Holland, G.N. Nuclear magnetic resonance imaging. Br. Med. Bull., *36:*297–299, 1980.
36. Moreno, J.B. and de Laud, F.H. Brain scanning in the diagnosis of astrocytomas of the brain. J. Nucl. Med., *12:*107–111, 1971.
37. Orr, J.S., Bydder, G.M., Pennock, J.M., *et al.* Nuclear magnetic resonance (NMR) in neoplastic disease. J. Pathol., *141:*297–307, 1983.
38. Packer, K.J. The dynamics of water in heterogeneous systems. Philos. Trans. R. Soc. Lond. [Biol], *278:*59–87, 1977.
39. Phelps, M.E., Hoffman, E.J., Mullani, N.A., *et al.* Application of annihilation coincidence detection by transaxial reconstruction tomography. J. Nucl. Med., *16:*210–224, 1975.
40. Phelps, M.E., Huang, S.C., Hoffman, E.J., *et al.* Tomographic measurement of local cerebral glucose metabolic rate in humans with (F-18) 2-fluoro-2-deoxy-D-glucose: validation of method. Ann. Neurol., *6:*371–388, 1979.
41. Phelps, M.E., Mazziota, J.C., and Huang, S.C. Study of cerebral function with positron computed tomography. J. Cereb. Blood Flow Metab., *2:*113–162, 1982.
42. Rhodes, C.G., Wise, R.J.S., Gibbs, J.M., *et al.* In vivo disturbance of the oxidative metabolism of glucose in human cerebral gliomas. Ann. Neurol., *12(6):*614, 1982.
43. Russell, D.S. and Rubinstein, L.J. *Pathology of Tumours of the Nervous System,* ed. 4. London, Edward Arnold, 1977.
44. Salcman, M. In vivo correlation of absorption coefficients with intracranial fluid protein concentrations and specific gravities. Neurosurgery, *5:*16–20, 1979.
45. Salcman, M., Rao, K.C., Scott, E.W., *et al.* CT characteristics of a transplantable canine glioma model: preliminary kinetic analysis. Am. J. Neuroradiol., *4:*786–788, 1983.
46. Salcman, M., Scott, E., Schepp, R.S., *et al.* A transplantable canine glioma model for use in experimental neurooncology. Neurosurgery, *11:*373–381, 1982.
47. Sokoloff, L., Reivich, M., Kennedy, C., *et al.* The [^{14}C] deoxyglucose method for the measurement of local cerebral glucose utilization: theory, procedure, and normal values in the conscious and anaesthetised albino rat. J. Neurochem., *28:*897–916, 1977.
48. Steel, G.C. Growth kinetics of brain tumors. In: *Brain Tumors, Scientific Basis, Clinical Investigations, and Current Therapy,* edited by D.G.T. Thomas and D.I. Graham, p. 10. London, Butterworths, 1980.
49. Suzuki, K., Nakagawa, Y., Ueda, S., *et al.* Prognostic significance of contrast enhancement in supratentorial astrocytoma. Morphological studies and DNA histograms. Prog. Comput. Tomogr., *4(3):*299, 1982.
50. Suzuki, K., Yoshimo, E., Ueda, S., *et al.* CT DNA histogram. Prog. Comput. Tomogr., *3(6)* :687–692, 1981.
51. Weisberg, L.A. and Nice, C.N. Intracranial tumors simulating the presentation of cerebrovascular syndromes. Am. J. Med., *63;*517–524, 1977.
52. Witcofski, R., Maynard, C.D., and Roper, T.H. A comparative analysis of the accuracy of the technetium-99m pertechnetate brain scan: follow-up 1000 patients. J. Nucl. Med., *8:*187, 1967.
53. Yamada, K., Yukitaka, U., Hayakawa, T., *et al.* Quantitative autoradiographic measurements of blood-brain barrier permeability in the rat glioma model. J. Neurosurg., *57:*394–398, 1982.
54. Yamamoto, Y.L., Diksio, M., Sano, K., *et al.*

Pharmacokinetic and metabolic studies in human malignant glioma. In Magistratti, P.L.: *Functional Radionuclide Imaging of the Brain*, p. 327. New York, Raven Press, 1983.
55. Yamashita, T. Estimation of the growth rate of malignant gliomas by CT scanning. Calculation of the actual tumor doubling times and clinical application of the growth rate of malignant gliomas. Yokahama Med. J., *32*:469–479, 1981.
56. Yoshimo, E., Suzuki, K., Ueda, S., *et al.* Significance of contrast enhancement in malignant glioma. Relation between contrast enhancement and nuclear DNA content of tumour cells. Prog. Comput. Tomogr., *3(2)*:149, 1981.
57. Young, I.R., Burl, M., Clarke, G.J., *et al.* Magnetic resonance properties of hydrogen: imaging the posterior fossa. Am. J. Radiol., *137*:895–901, 1981.
58. Zent-Györgyi, A. *Bioenergetics*. New York, Academic Press, 1957.
59. Zilhka, E., Ladurner, G., Iliff, L.D., *et al.* Computer subtraction in regional cerebral blood volume measurements using the EMI scanner. Br. J. Radiol., *49*:330, 1976.
60. Zimmerman, R.A., Bilaniuk, L.T., Grossman, R.I., *et al.* Cerebral NMR: diagnostic evaluation of brain tumors by partial saturation technique with resistive NMR. Neuroradiology, *27*:9–15, 1985.
61. Zülch, K.J. (in collaboration with pathologists in 14 countries). *Histological Typing of Tumours of the Central Nervous System.* International Histological Classification of Tumours No. 21. Geneva, World Health Organization, 1979.

CHAPTER 16

Prognostic Factors in Patients with Brain Tumors

ROGER J. PACKER, M.D.

INTRODUCTION

Brain tumors are a heterogeneous group of neoplasms with varying histologies, sites of origin, growth rates and patterns of growth (19, 92). Over the past two decades, the length and rate of survival have improved for some forms of primary central nervous system neoplasms (19). As more effective means of treatment become available, there is increasing need to identify those factors which impact on survival. Identification of such predictive factors results not only in a better understanding of the disease process for the patient, family members and physicians, but also in better selection of those patients who require more aggressive therapy and, in contradistinction, those patients who might do as well with a reduction in potentially neurotoxic therapy. For tumors in which total surgical removal impacts favorably on survival, knowledge of such a relationship may convince the surgeon to attempt a more radical surgical resection even at the risk of increased neurologic damage. For other neoplasms, in which the extent of resection is not as important a determinant of survival, less aggressive surgery with potentially less postoperative neurologic morbidity may be warranted. Similarly, for tumors with a high likelihood of leptomeningeal dissemination at diagnosis, the use of presymptomatic craniospinal radiation may result in an improved rate of cure, whereas the use of similar radiation for tumors which rarely, if ever, spread from their site of origin would lead to a needlessly increased risk of radiation damage to the nervous system. In the planning of clinical studies, stratification of patients into different treatment arms based on prognostic factors allows for more rational treatment plans. An understanding of factors which impact on outcome is also needed to evaluate the efficacy of any treatment, since outcome may be as much a factor of initial patient characteristics as it is of the treatment employed.

GLIAL TUMORS

Tumors of neuroglial origin are composed of cells which show great variation in their degree of maturation (92). There are inherent difficulties in reliably correlating certain features of glial tumors to outcome. These tumors tend to be infiltrating and are rarely amenable to total surgical resection (92). Portions of the tumor removed at surgery may not be representative of all the tumor, making cellular histology, at times, an unreliable predictor of outcome (92). If at rebiopsy or at postmortem examination a more malignant process is seen than on the initial biopsy, this may represent initial sampling error or dedifferentiation of the tumor. In addition, due to the infiltrative nature of glial tumors, determination of tumor margins and the extent of surgical resection at the time of surgery are relatively arbitrary. Computed tomography is a more objective measure of postoperative tumor extent. Even with this technique, the leading edges of gliomas are often difficult to delineate and the separation of postoperative changes from residual tumor may be impossible. Magnetic resonance imaging

(MRI), especially when used with gadolinium, may be more sensitive in this regard. However, it has yet to be conclusively proven that MRI can distinguish between infiltrating tumor and edema.

Different classification systems have been employed for tumors of glial origin. It seems clear that independent of the location of the tumor within the neuroaxis the distinction between low-grade lesions and anaplastic or malignant lesions is of prognostic significance (19, 92). Within the low-grade tumors, there have also been attempts to relate outcome to the cell type present. For purposes of this review, glial tumors will be initially separated on the basis of their location in the neuroaxis and then subclassified based on their histological features.

CORTICAL ANAPLASTIC (MALIGNANT) GLIOMAS

Malignant gliomas are the most common form of primary central nervous system tumor. Over the past decade, multiinstitutional, randomized clinical trials have identified factors predictive of the duration and rate of survival. Two of the most comprehensive evaluations have been performed by the Brain Tumor Study Group (BTSG) and Radition Therapy Oncology Group — Eastern Cooperative Oncology Group (RTOG-ECOG) (15, 116). Large, single institution retrospective studies have also supplied useful prognostic information.

Clinical features have been proven to be of prognostic importance. Gehan and Walker reporting on the BTSG evaluation of 225 patients found that younger age at diagnosis, higher performance status at diagnosis, and seizures or cranial nerve dysfunction at the time of diagnosis were all favorably related to length of survival (39). Sex and duration of symptoms prior to diagnosis were not significantly related to survival. Chang *et al.*, for the RTOG-ECOG study of 535 evaluable patients, reported that younger age at diagnosis was the single, most predictive clinical factor associated with improved outcome (15). A better performance status at the time of diagnosis, more than 4 months of symptoms prior to diagnosis, normal mental status at diagnosis, the presence of seizures, and complaints of diplopia or speech impairment were all predictive of longer median time of survival and a higher 18-month survival rate. An additional factor that has been related to survival is the patient's blood type, as for unknown reasons patients with blood type O have a significantly better survival rate (96).

In the BTSG study, patients with occipital tumors survived longest, whereas those with parietal tumors had the shortest survival (39). In this study, few patients had tumors of the basal ganglia, thalamus or cerebellum; however, in those patients survival was likewise short. The location of the tumor was not found to be prognostically important in the RTOG-ECOG study (15).

In both the BTSG and RTOG-ECOG studies, the degree of surgical resection was related to survival (15, 39). Patients who underwent a biopsy had a shorter median length of survival and lower rate of survival than those who underwent a subtotal or total resection. Median length of survival was 6.8 months and 18-month survival was 15% for patients who underwent biopsy in the RTOG-ECOG study, as compared to 12 months and 34% for patients who had a total resection. In these studies, the extent of resection was not strictly defined by postsurgical CT findings. In a report of the experience at the University of San Francisco, Levin *et al.* found that patients with larger residual tumors on CT had a poorer prognosis (60).

Determination of the effect of histological features on prognosis in patients with anaplastic gliomas has been limited by the failure of neuropathologists to agree on one grading system, the subjectivity of the determinations made, and the possibility of sampling error (especially when small portions of tumor are removed at surgery). Nelson *et al.* for the RTOG-ECOG group found that the presence of one or more foci of coagulation necrosis was highly predictive of survival, as patients with malignant neoplasms without necrosis had a median survival of 28 months, as compared to 8 months for patients with malignant neoplasms with necrosis. They concluded that necrosis was a "reliable, decisive prognostic factor" while grading by the Kernohan system (grades I through IV, with Grade IV glioblastoma multiforme) "was of limited value in assessing prognosis" (70). Even when adjustments were made for age, performance status at diagnosis, and extent of surgery, survival was significantly better in patients with anaplastic gliomas without necrosis (70).

Davis *et al.* described a separate grading system for anaplastic gliomas which separated the tumors into glioblastoma multiforme, gemistocytic astrocytoma, highly anaplastic astrocytoma, moderately anaplastic astrocytoma, mildly anaplastic astrocytoma, and nonanaplastic astrocytoma subgroups (24). In this report of 258 patients, there was a good correlation between these individual subtypes and outcome. The prognostic significance of DNA quantification was shown by Hirakawa *et al.* who found that the percentage of S-phase cells and the percentage of polyploid cells were predictive of outcome, as patients with more rapidly dividing tumors fared less well (45). Utilizing bromodeoxyuridine labeling as an index of mitotic activity, Hoshino *et al.* found, not surprisingly, that patients with less rapidly dividing tumors fared better (47).

Postoperative radiation therapy increases survival in patients with malignant gliomas, as compared to treatment with surgery alone. In the BTSG study, median survival for patients treated without radiation therapy was 14 weeks, as compared to 35 weeks for those who received radiation (116). Although a partial dose response relationship exists between the total dose of radiation therapy and median survival, even at doses near normal brain tolerance, long-term tumor control is not achievable for most patients (117). In addition, it is unclear whether the volume of radiation given (whole brain radiation versus local radiation therapy) influences survival. The use of radiation potentiator drugs has not improved outcome (15). Other means to increase the amount or effectiveness of radiation without increasing neurotoxicity, such as hyperfractionation radiation therapy and superfractionation therapy are presently being evaluated and preliminary results suggest some efficacy (101).

Chemotherapy alone (BCNU) has a small beneficial effect on length of survival, as compared to treatment with surgery alone. The addition of chemotherapy (BCNU) to radiation therapy did not result in an improved rate of survival in patients in the BTSG study. In the RTOG-ECOG study, the addition of either BCNU or methyl CCNU and DTIC after radiaton resulted in a significantly improved survival rate (15, 116). The benefit of chemotherapy was seen primarily in patients between 40 and 60 years of age at diagnosis and was independent of ambulatory status of the patient prior to treatment or the histologic features of the tumor (15).

Summary

Multiple factors have been associated with survival in patients with anaplastic gliomas (or at least longer median length of survival) (see Table 16.1). The factors which seem most related to a favorable outcome include a younger age at diagnosis, an improved performance status at the time of diagnosis, extensive resection at the time of initial surgery, histological absence of necrosis, the use of radiation therapy, and possibly the addition of adjuvant chemotherapy. Newer means of evaluation, such as DNA quantification and labeling indices, may be found to be even more predictive in the future.

TABLE 16.1.
Anaplastic Gliomas: Factors Associated with Improved Survival

Clinical	Age less than 40 at diagnosis
	Higher performance rating at diagnosis
	? Seizures at the presentation of illness
Histological	Absence of necrosis
Treatment	Extensive resection
	Radiation therapy

CORTICAL LOW-GRADE ASTROCYTOMA

Patients with low-grade astrocytomas of the cerebral cortex fare better than patients with malignant lesions in similar areas of the brain (19, 92). The age of the patient at diagnosis is the most important clinical variable relating to outcome. In a retrospective review by Laws *et al.* of 461 patients, 15-year survival was over 80% for patients under age 19 at diagnosis, as compared to less than 40% for older patients (57). Other clinical variables associated with increased survival include lack of major preoperative neurological deficit, longer duration of symptoms prior to surgery, seizures at presentation of illness, and lack of major postoperative neurological deficit.

The prognostic significance of histology for patients with low-grade lesions is not well-documented. Elvidge separated astrocytomas into piloid, gemistocytic, and diffuse cell types and found that long-term survival was best for the piloid astrocytoma, although long-term survival also occurred with the other types of astrocytoma (34). Leibel *et al.* found that patients with Grade I lesions had a 58% 5-year survival, while those with Grade II lesions had a 25% survival (59). Similar differences between Grade I and Grade II lesions were not found by Stage and Stein (105) or Laws *et al.* (57). As in high-grade tumors, Hoshino and co-workers found an association between the Budr labeling index of individual tumors and outcome, as even some histologically low-grade lesions had an elevated rate of mitotic activity and poorer outcome (48).

The location of the tumor, extent of surgical resection, and the employment of radiation therapy seem to be important but not mutually exclusive prognostic factors. Leibel *et al.* found that patients with deep seated lesions treated with surgery alone fared better than those with cortical tumors (10-year survival of 33% with deep-seated tumors *vs.* 15% with cerebral tumors) and that this difference was even more striking (10-year survival of 50% for deep lesions *vs.* 24% for cerebral tumors) when radiation was added (59). This was found, despite some of the cortical lesions being "completely resected," again highlighting the difficulty in determining the extent of resection for glial tumors. Fazekas found that patients with grossly resected tumors had an excellent 90% survival rate at 5 years, but this fell to 25% at 10 years (35). In this study, 5-year survival rate was improved by radiation in patients with subtotally resected tumors, but at 10 years this difference was much less marked as survival rates of less than 20% were found in both irradiated and nonirradiated patients (48). Laws *et al.* found that gross surgical resection was related to improved survival and that radiation was primarily of benefit in patients over age 40 (57).

Summary

Factors which relate to improved survival in patients with low-grade gliomas are primarily younger age at diagnosis, better neurologic status prior to and after surgery, and seizures at the onset of illness. The histology of the tumor, the extent of surgical resection, and the use of radiation therapy may impact on survival. Based on these multiple parameters, Laws *et al.* have suggested a point scale that is predictive of survival, with good risk patients having greater than a 50% predicted 15-year survival, as compared to 16% survival for the average patient with a low-grade glioma (57) (see Table 16.2; Fig. 16.1).

GLIOMAS OF THE THALAMUS AND HYPOTHALAMUS

Gliomas of the hypothalamus and thalamus are a heterogeneous group of tumors. Overall, outcome is dependent primarily on the histological type of tumor with higher grade anaplastic tumors having a less favorable prognosis than low-grade tumors (9). In one study of patients less than 18 years of diagnosis, all 20 patients with malignant tumors died a mean of 1.1 years after diagnosis, while in contradistinction, the mean survival of children with benign lesions was 5.3 years and 8 of 11 patients were alive 7.2 years following diagnosis (9). Children with tumors of the diencephalon

TABLE 16.2.
Scoring System for Low-Grade Hemispheric Gliomas[a]

Score[b] = Age at Diagnosis x 0.072 plus	
0	+1
Surgery after 1949	Surgery prior to 1949
No personality change	Personality change
Normal consciousness	Altered consciousness
Total resection	Partial resection
Site other than frontal or temporal lobe	Frontal or temporal lobe
Mild postoperative neurological deficit	Moderate-to-severe postoperative neurological deficit

[a]Adapted from Laws, E. R., Taylor, W. F., Clifton, M. B., *et al.* Neurosurgical management of low-grade astrocytoma of the cerebral hemispheres. J. Neurosurg. *6*:665–673, 1984.
[b]For survival correlation, compare computed score to Figure 16.1.

fare better than adults (9, 39). Conflicting statements about the prognostic significance of different factors in these tumors is due to the tendency to treat them without histological confirmation because of their location (9).

Radiation therapy may be of benefit in prolonging the length and rate of survival in patients with such neoplasms, but because of the forementioned problems of determining the histologic type of the tumors, its efficacy is difficult to document (9). In adults and children with documented high-grade lesions, local radiation rarely results in long-term disease control (9, 39).

There is clearly an overlap between low-grade hypothalamic tumors of childhood and low-grade chiasmatic gliomas. Once again, many patients with presumed low-grade tumor are treated without histological confirmation, but overall, radiation has been reported to increase the length of survival and survival rates of up to 50% are reported for radiated patients, as compared to the few long-term survivors in children treated without radiation (9, 35).

CHIASMATIC GLIOMAS

Gliomas of the chiasm exist primarily in two forms. The childhood form of chiasmatic glioma tends to be a histologically low-grade (most often pilocytic) astrocytoma which at the time of diagnosis involves the optic nerve, chiasm, optic tracts, hypothalamus, diencephalon, and/or optic radiation (67, 76). In contradistinction, optic gliomas of adulthood are rarer than in childhood and are primarily malignant neoplasms. The adult form of chiasmatic

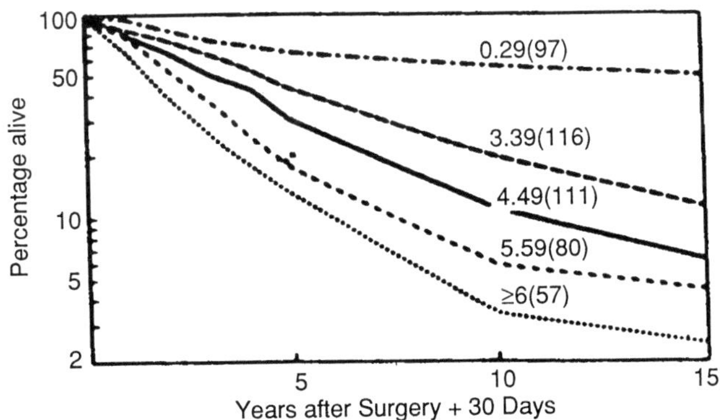

Figure 16.1. Survival related to score for low-grade astrocytoma. The score range and the number of patients are given for each curve. (Reprinted with permission from Laws, E. R., Taylor, W. F., Clifton, M. B., *et al.* Neurosurgical management of low-grade astrocytoma of the cerebral hemispheres. J. Neurosurg., *61*:665–673, 1985.)

glioma is almost always fatal and the benefit of radiation is at best only temporary (49).

The age of the patient at diagnosis has not been clearly related to outcome in children with chiasmatic gliomas. However, in our experience, younger patients tend to have more extensive disease at diagnosis and suffer an increased incidence of residual neurologic and visual morbidity after treatment than do older children (76). Approximately 10 to 20% of patients with chiasmatic glioma of childhood have neurofibromatosis. The presence of neurofibromatosis has been related to a more favorable outcome in some series; however, other series have not found an association with outcome (23, 73, 76).

Based on clinical symptoms, signs, and tomographic and pneumoencephalographic criteria, patients with chiasmatic gliomas have been separated into anterior tumors (involving solely the optic chiasm with or without involvement of the optic nerves) and posterior tumors (which in addition to infiltrating the chiasm, involve the optic tracts, hypothalamus or third ventricular structures). Miller *et al.* found that anterior lesions had a very favorable prognosis with nearly 100% survival excluding postoperative deaths, while those with posterior tumors fared less favorably (67). In fact, there was some suggestion that anterior lesions represented hamartomatous masses and required little specific therapy (67). Packer *et al.* suggested that both anterior and posterior lesions were potentially aggressive tumors and that there was no clearcut difference in prognosis between these two types of neoplasms, as deaths secondary to tumor growth occurred in both groups of patients (76). Furthermore, with the advent of CT scanning, it has been shown that these tumors are more extensive than clinically believed and that so-called anterior chiasmatic gliomas, with involvement of only the chiasm, are relatively uncommon (76). Most lesions involve the hypothalamus, diencephalon or optic tracts at the time of diagnosis. For this reason, Packer *et al.* suggested that characterization of chiasmatic gliomas as anterior and posterior lesions was arbitrary and probably meaningless (76).

There is no consensus on the impact of treatment on outcome for these lesions. Radiotherapy has been reported to improve both the quality of vision and the survival rate of children with these lesions; 5-year survival rates of nearly 100% after radiation treatment have been reported (23, 111). However, others have found no clearcut benefit to radiotherapy and 10-year survival rates of only 50% in radiated patients (44, 63, 73, 76). Recently, chemotherapy with actinomycin-D and vincristine has been reported to be as efficacious as radiotherapy for short-term disease control in young children with progressive lesions and possibly to result in a lower treatment related morbidity (75).

BRAIN STEM GLIOMAS

Brain stem gliomas are infiltrating lesions that constitute 8 to 10% of primary childhood brain tumors (83). With refinements in neuroradiographic techniques, diagnosis has become more exact and lower rates of survival (between 0 and 10% at 3 years) are being reported (1, 74). However, others have reported a higher 50% rate of survival at 5 years after standard radiotherapy (1, 61). The reasons for these differing reported rates of survival are probably due to the inclusion or exclusion of different subsets of patients with infiltrating brain stem lesions.

The patient's age at diagnosis and sex are not associated with differing survival rates (7). A shorter duration of symptoms prior to diagnosis has been found to be predictive of a poorer response to radiotherapy and shorter overall survival in some series, but not in others (1, 7, 61, 74). Albright *et al.* in a review of 87 consecutive patients treated at the University of Pittsburgh and Children's Hospital of Philadelphia, found that a variety of factors correlated with long-term survival after radiotherapy (1). Patients with tumors on CT scanning which diffusely involved the brain stem and/or patients who presented with multiple cranial nerve deficits, rarely survived after radiotherapy. In contradistinction, patients with more localized tumors on computed tomography without cranial nerve palsies at diagnosis had a better rate of survival. Within the group of patients with diffuse tumors, histology was not statistically predictive of survival. However, in the subset of patients with more localized tumors and in those without cranial neuropathies at diagnosis, the presence of anaplasia on biopsy denoted a less than 10% chance of survival at 3 years, whereas greater than 50% of patients were alive 3 years after diagnosis if their biopsies were low-grade. Stroint *et al.*, reporting the experience at Toronto Sick Children's Hospital, used a different classification system for brain stem gliomas (106). This study also found that patients with diffuse tumors fared poorly. However, patients with more localized exophytic tumors, especially those occurring at the cervicomedullary junction, had a much better prognosis after treatment with standard radiotherapy or in some cases after treatment with surgery alone. In Hoffman's classification system, which categorized brain stem gliomas into four different types, histology was not found to be predictive of outcome. The studies of Albright *et al.* and Hoffman *et al.* both utilized CT scanning to designate the location and extent of the brain stem lesions. Since MRI scanning often shows these lesions to be much more extensive than is appreciated on CT scanning it is unclear whether the findings of these studies are directly applicable to MRI evaluated lesions.

As stated previously, the role of surgical biopsy for patients with brain stem gliomas is questionable. It is true that essentially no patient with a malignant tumor on biopsy will survive with conventional means of management (1). Patients with low-grade tumors have been reported to have better 5-year survival rates, but this may pertain mainly to patients with more localized lesions. Since open surgical biopsy results in increased neurologic morbidity in up to one-third of patients, obtains inadequate tissue for diagnosis in up to another one-third of patients, and is limited by sampling error, its prognostic utility is far from ideal (87). CT-guided and MRI-guided stereotactic procedures may improve upon these results, but may also introduce sampling errors.

Treatment has not dramatically altered outcome for patients with brain stem gliomas. Conventional doses of local radiotherapy (5500 cGy of radiation therapy given in daily fractions of 180 cGy to 200 cGy) do increase the length of survival and probably the overall survival rate of patients with brain stem gliomas as compared to patients who have not been treated (58). There is some evidence that the length and rate of survival is greater with increasing doses of radiation therapy, although a clear cut dose-response curve does not exist. Recent work has suggested that hyperfractionated radiotherapy, where radiotherapy is given in smaller daily fractions at least twice daily to a higher total dose, may be of some utility. Doses in the range of 7200 cGy have been reported to improve survival. However, it is not yet clear whether this is so for all patients with brain stem gliomas or rather is of benefit only to patients with more localized lesions. Adjuvant chemotherapy, to date, has not favorably affected either the length or rate of survival (88).

CEREBELLAR GLIOMAS

Cerebellar gliomas have the best prognosis of all childhood brain tumors. Unlike most forms of glial tumors, the most common form of cerebellar glioma, the cerebellar astrocytoma, tends to be a well-circumscribed and surgically removable lesion with a long-term survival rate of nearly 100% (42, 48).

The microscopic appearance of cerebellar gliomas is of prognostic importance. Gjerris and Klinken divided tumors into two groups based on microscopic anatomy: (*a*) the classical juvenile cerebellar astrocytoma consisting of compact areas of strongly fibrillary fusiform cells alternating with loose areas of nonfibrillated stellate astrocytes with microcysts; and (*b*) the diffuse astrocytoma with equal distribution of glial fibrils, uniform cells, and small evenly dispersed cavities (41). The classical juvenile form was usually found in children under 10 years of age and overall made up 70% of patients with cerebellar astrocytomas. These patients had a cumulative 25-year survival rate of 94%. In comparison, patients with the diffuse form of cerebellar astrocytoma, found more often in children over age 10, had a survival rate of 38% (41).

In this study, the presence of macroscopic cysts in portions of the tumor did not impact on survival.

Gilles *et al.* evaluated the prognostic importance of 15 microscopic characteristics in 145 patients with cerebellar gliomas (40). In this detailed study, multiple features were identified which correlated with outcome. A multivariate analysis was performed and two major clusters of microscopic findings were delineated. Cluster A consisted of tumors containing one or more of four cytological findings including microcysts, leptomeningeal deposits, Rosenthal fibers, or oligodendroglia. Cluster B contained tumors with perivascular pseudorosettes or one or more of the following features: high cell density, necrosis, mitosis or calcifications. The 10-year survival in patients with cluster A findings was 94% as compared to 29% for patients in cluster B. Within each cluster of patients, the presence of more than one factor affected outcome (i.e., the more cluster B features present, the poorer the outcome). The presence of cysts correlated with an improved survival rate. In this study, as in some others, the presence of pleomorphism, endothelial proliferation, and hypervascularity did not influence survival.

Both of these studies discuss a group of patients selected over many years who were not treated homogeneously. The effect of treatment, including the extent of resection or the use of radiation, on any of these subtypes of cerebellar astrocytoma is difficult to determine. However, it does appear that astrocytomas of the Gilles' cluster B type and possibly the diffuse type of cerebellar astrocytoma may be less surgically resectable and at higher risk for recurrence.

Although a focus of oligodendroglioma was found to be a good prognostic factor in Gilles' study, Packer *et al.* reported that in three of four patients with cerebellar gliomas with large areas of oligodendroglioma there was dissemination to the leptomeninges after subtotal resection and local radiation therapy (80). This is similar to the findings of Salazar who found that anaplastic gliomas of the posterior fossa frequently disseminate after partial resection and local radiation therapy (94).

The extent of surgical resection impacts greatly on outcome for the child with a classical juvenile astrocytoma. With complete surgical removal of the tumor, a nearly 100% cure rate is achievable (42, 48, 88). Local recurrence may occur after subtotal resection, although, for reasons which are not clear, even partial resection of the classical cerebellar astrocytoma has been associated with prolonged disease-free survival (48).

The effect of radiation therapy on this tumor is questionable. Improved survival rates have been reported in children with partially resected cerebellar astrocytomas after local radiation therapy (11, 42). As stated previously, in children with anaplastic gliomas and oligodendrogliomas of the cerebellum, radiation therapy is recommended, though the influence of partial *vs.* complete resection in these tumors is unclear (94). Also, the appropriate volume of radiation therapy to be employed is unknown; in the patients with anaplastic gliomas reported by Salazar and Packer *et al.* the use of craniospinal radiation therapy improved outcome (80, 94).

Summary

The classical juvenile astrocytoma carries an excellent prognosis if totally resected. For the patient with a cerebellar astrocytoma with anaplastic features, it seems that radiation therapy may improve outcome; however, it is unclear whether this is true for all patients or only in patients with subtotally resected lesions. Likewise, it is unclear in patients with astrocytomas with unfavorable histological features whether the extent of surgery or the use of radiation therapy is the most important determinant of outcome.

OLIGODENDROGLIOMAS

Oligodendroglioma occurs primarily in the cerebral hemispheres of adult patients. Outcome in this tumor is extremely variable and the analysis of the impact of various factors on survival has been limited by the inconsistent clinical picture.

The age of patients at the time of diagnosis has not been found to be an important predictor of outcome. Dohrmann *et al.*

found no difference in survival in their series of 12 cases of oligodendroglioma occuring in childhood as compared to survival figures reported in adults (27). Since the vast majority of tumors occur in the cerebral hemispheres, information concerning outcome for oligodendrogliomas in other sites is difficult to obtain. However, in one series by Packer *et al.* oligodendrogliomas in the posterior fossa of childhood were highly malignant lesions, as three of four patients developed leptomeningeal dissemination (80).

Histologic features have been unreliable predictors of outcome except for the grading system proposed by Smith based on the presence of endothelial proliferation, necrosis, nuclear/cytoplasmic ratio, cell density, and pleomorphism (30, 92, 104). Of these five factors, only pleomorphism was independently and significantly related to survival, as patients whose tumors contained pleomorphism had a median survival of 24 months as compared to 46 months in patients without pleomorphism (104).

Extent of surgery was found to be prognostically important by Roberts and German, as the average duration of survival was 13 years for grossly resected tumors, compared to 3.3 years for partially resected lesions (89). The efficacy of radiaton therapy remains controversial. Sheline *et al.* in their review of 37 adult patients found that patients treated with local radiaton therapy had a 5-year survival of 85%, while those treated with operation alone had a 31% survival (100). Although the median survival was longer for irradiated patients, the 10-year survival was not significantly different in irradiated and nonirradiated patients.

EPENDYMOMAS

Ependymomas constitute 5 to 10% of all primary CNS neoplasms in all age groups. Factors predictive of outcome in patients with these tumors are far from established (19, 92). This tumor may occur both in the supratentorial and infratentorial space, and survival rates varying between 10 and 70% have been reported (26, 37, 50, 85, 95, 100, 110).

The age of the patient at diagnosis and the location of the tumor are somewhat interrelated and impact on outcome. Supratentorial lesions are more common in adults, and although these lesions are often more histologically malignant than infratentorial masses, the duration of postoperative survival is longest for adults with cortical lesions (100). Survival in children with ependymomas varies tremendously, but as a whole, reported survival rates are lower in children than adults, possibly in part because of the more common posterior fossa location in childhood (26, 85). Pierre-Kahn *et al.* found that children under 2 fared worse than older children (66% 5-year survival vs. 41% 5-year survival) (85). The extent of thc tumor at diagnosis (as evaluated by cerebrospinal fluid cytology) has not yet to be shown of prognostic value, since few, if any, lesions are disseminated at diagnosis (78).

There is no consensus concerning the impact of the histological features of these neoplasms on outcome. It is clear that ependymoblastoma, often classified as a subtype of ependymoma, is highly aggressive and carries a very poor prognosis (64, 85). While some consider this lesion a malignant form of ependymoma (64, 85), others consider it a subvariety of primitive neuroectodermal tumor (90). Grading systems have been used to correlate histology with outcome in patients with ependymomas. Liu *et al.* separated ependymomas into well-differentiated, intermediate, and malignant grades and found outcome to be highly correlated with the degree of cytologic differentiation and anatomical location (64). They found most supratentorial ependymomas to be more histologically aggressive and to carry a poorer prognosis. The infratentorial ependymomas in this series were better differentiated and prognosis was good when complete surgical resection could be accomplished. Although others have not found as direct a relationship between location, histology, and outcome, in general, most studies have found that better differentiated tumors carry a more favorable prognosis (26, 37, 50, 85, 95, 100, 110).

The impact of the degree of surgical resection on outcome has not been well-demonstrated. However, at least in the studies by Lui *et al.* and Barone *et al.*, more extensive (gross total) resection was related to improved outcome, especially in well-differentiated tumors (64, 100). The effectiveness of radiation therapy and the optimal amount and volume of radiation required for disease control is not well-documented. There is no consensus as to how often ependymomas disseminate throughout the neuroaxis and whether craniospinal radiation therapy is more efficacious than local radiation therapy in prolonging survival. Frequency of cerebrospinal fluid dissemination varies in the literature from 0 to 60% and seems to depend in part on the histological malignancy of the tumor and especially whether ependymoblastomas are included in the group of patients with malignant ependymomas (26, 37, 50, 85, 95, 100, 110). Making interpretation even more difficult is the failure of most studies to discuss the timing of dissemination (78).

Radiation therapy has been reported to improve the rate and length of survival in patients with ependymomas, although Barone *et al.* have reported long-term survival in both totally and subtotally resected patients treated by surgery alone (100). In general, survival has been greater when higher doses of radiation therapy have been used; 5-year survival rates of over 40% are reported when 4500 rad is delivered locally as compared to less than 20% in those patients receiving less radiation. In addition, the best survival rates have been reported in series using craniospinal radiation therapy, although in these studies higher local doses of radiation were also used (19, 93, 95).

Summary

It seems that histology is an important determinant of outcome in patients with ependymomas and that the extent of surgical resection is likewise important, especially in low-grade lesions. Radiation therapy seems to be of benefit in prolonging and increasing the rate of survival with this tumor, although the optimal volume of radiation needed is unclear.

PRIMITIVE NEUROECTODERMAL TUMORS; *MEDULLOBLASTOMA*

Primitive neuroectodermal tumors are primarily malignancies of childhood. Disagreement exists concerning the proper classification of such tumors (90, 92). For purposes of this discussion, all tumors composed primarily of undifferentiated neuroepithelial cells, regardless of their location in the neuroaxis, will be considered as primitive neuroectodermal tumors (90). Included are tumors which have been termed medulloblastoma, pineoblastoma, primitive neuroectodermal tumors of the cerebral cortex, ependymoblastoma, and central or cerebral neuroblastoma. Prognostic factors will be discussed for this group of tumors as a whole, although the variables are best worked out for those tumors arising in the posterior fossa.

The age of the patient at the time of diagnosis is an extremely important predictor of outcome in children with primitive neuroectodermal tumors of the posterior fossa. Younger children, especially those under age 5 at diagnosis, do less well than older patients (2, 3, 28, 82). A high percentage of the patients who are less than 5 years of age at diagnosis have disseminated disease. Allen and Epstein found that leptomeningeal dissemination at diagnosis occurred in 9 of 14 (64%) patients 5 years of age or younger as compared to 2 of 16 (13%) patients older than 5. Packer *et al.* reported that patients with primitive neuroectodermal tumors who had leptomeningeal spread were significantly younger (median age 2 years) than patients who did not have leptomeningeal disease at diagnosis (78). However, in a multivariate analysis on the latter group of patients, age, even when corrected for the extent of dissemination at diagnosis, was of independent prognostic value (82). Evans *et al.* also found that age was independently associated with survival and reported that 5-year survival was 32% for children under age 4 at diagnosis, as compared to 70% for older patients (2).

The impact of the location of the tumor on prognosis is not totally clear. Overall, primitive neuroectodermal tumors which are grossly resected and have not disseminated at the time of diagnosis respond more favorably to therapy than disseminated lesions, independent of their location in the neuroaxis. Most primitive neuroectodermal tumors which occur in the cerebral cortex are not amenable to gross total surgical resection (28). However, Berger *et al.* reported 11 patients with undifferentiated primitive neuroectodermal tumors, two of which were totally resectable (28). They found that cortical tumors which were cystic responded best to therapy, as all six patients with cystic lesions (including the two patients for whom gross total resection was possible) were free of recurrent tumor at 26 to 109 months after surgery and radiation therapy. Primitive neuroectodermal tumors (pineoblastomas) which occur in the pineal region are frequently disseminated at the time of diagnosis, are often not amenable to extensive surgical resection, and long-term survival is unusual (78, 81).

The posterior fossa is the most common site for PNET, and in this location, the size of the tumor and its extent at the time of diagnosis are prognostically important. The Chang staging system has been extensively used to describe the size and extent of tumor at diagnosis and is predictive of outcome (16) (Table 16.3). It was designed as a preoperative staging system, based primarily on the surgeon's intraoperative impression. Patients with Chang tumor stage T_1 or T_2 fare better than patients with T_3 or T_4 lesions (2, 82). It is unclear how the degree of surgical resection impacts on the utility of this preoperative staging system. Brain stem involvement is a particularly poor prognostic factor; in one series, 5-year survival was 34% for patients with brain stem involvement as compared to 54% for patients without brain stem involvement (16).

The presence of tumor dissemination at diagnosis is an even more important prognostic factor. In a prospective study performed by the Children's Cancer Study Group and Radiation Therapy Oncology Group (CCSG-RTOG) reviewed by Evans *et al.* patients without metastasis at diagnosis had a 5-year event-free survival of 58% as compared to 32% for those with metastasis (2). This was found to be true even though cerebrospinal fluid cytology was assayed in only 45% of the patients who were evaluated and myelographies were performed in only 10% (2). In series reported by Allen *et al.* and Packer *et al.* including

TABLE 16.3.
Chang Staging System for Posterior Fossa Medulloblastoma[a]

Stage	Definition
Tumor Stage	
T-1:	Tumor less than 3 cm in diameter and limited to the midline position in the vermis, the roof of the fourth ventricle, and less frequently to the cerebellar hemispheres.
T-2:	Tumor more than 3 cm in diameter, further invading one adjacent structure or partially filling the fourth ventricle.
T-3:	(Divided into T-3a and T-3b)
T-3a:	Tumor invading two adjacent structures or completely filling the fourth ventricle with extension into the aqueduct of Sylvius, foramen of Magendie, or foramen of Luschka, thus producing marked internal hydrocephalus.
T-3b:	Tumor arising from the floor of the fourth ventricle or brain stem and filling the fourth ventricle.
T-4:	Tumor further spreading through the aqueduct of Sylvius to involve the third ventricle or midbrain or tumor extending to the upper cervical cord.
Metastasis Stage	
M-0:	No evidence of gross subarachnoid or hematogenous metastasis.
M-1:	Microscopic tumor cells found in cerebrospinal fluid.
M-2:	Gross nodule seedings demonstrated in the cerebellar, cerebral subarachnoid space, or in the third or lateral ventricles.
M-3:	Gross nodule seedings in the spinal subarachnoid space.
M-4:	Extraneuroaxial metastasis.

[a]Adapted from Chang, C. H., Housepian, E. M., Herbert, C. Jr., *et al.* An operative staging system and a megavoltage radiotherapeutic technique for cerebellar medulloblastomas. Radiology *93:*1351–1359, 1969.

only patients who were evaluated for dissemination at the time of diagnosis, median length of survival was much shorter for patients with dissemination (3, 82). In the latter series, 4 of 19 (21%) patients with leptomeningeal disease at diagnosis were alive, as compared to 26 of 48 (54%) patients without dissemination at diagnosis (82). Myelography was necessary to confirm the presence of disseminaton in up to one-third of patients (25, 78).

Histological features are also of prognostic importance for patients with primitive neuroectodermal tumors, although the separation of primitive neuroectodermal tumors of the posterior fossa into classical medulloblastoma and desmoplastic types is of unreliable prognostic value (5, 17). Kopelson *et al.* separated tumors on the basis of the presence of cytoplasmic processes, necrosis, mitosis, desmoplasia, and location of tumor (52). Based on these parameters, patients could be placed into favorable, intermediate, and poor-risk groups. Rorke has outlined a system which separates PNETs on the basis of their degree of cellular differentiation (90) (Fig. 16.2). Packer *et al.*, utilizing this classification, found that patients with tumors of the posterior fossa which showed no evidence of cellular differentiation had a 4-year event-free survival of 70% compared to 32% for those lesions which showed differentiation along glial and/or ependymal and/or neuronal lines (82). Caputy *et al.* utilizing different histologic criteria have found the opposite result: patients with more differentiated tumors fared better (13). Both these reports utilized primarily light microscopy to determine the extent of cellular differentiation. However, as newer immunohistochemical techniques become available to better characterize cellular differentiation, this issue will need to be restudied.

The effects of cellular differentiaton, age, and extent of tumor are all interrelated. In the group of patients reported by Packer *et al.* patients who had differentiated tumors were more likely to be younger at the time of diagnosis and have more extensive disease at diagnosis (82). In addition, younger patients and patients with differentiated tumors were also less likely to have tumors which could be completely resected at the time of diagnosis. In this study, the effect of differentiation was prognostically significant independent of any other factor.

The extent of surgical resection is an important determinant of outcome. However, it is unclear whether extent of resection is an independent prognostic variable or a function of the extent of disease at the time of diagnosis. Norris *et al.* and Park *et al.* found the extent of resection to be an extremely important determinant of outcome (16, 71). In the series reported by Park, 5-year survival was 59% for totally resected

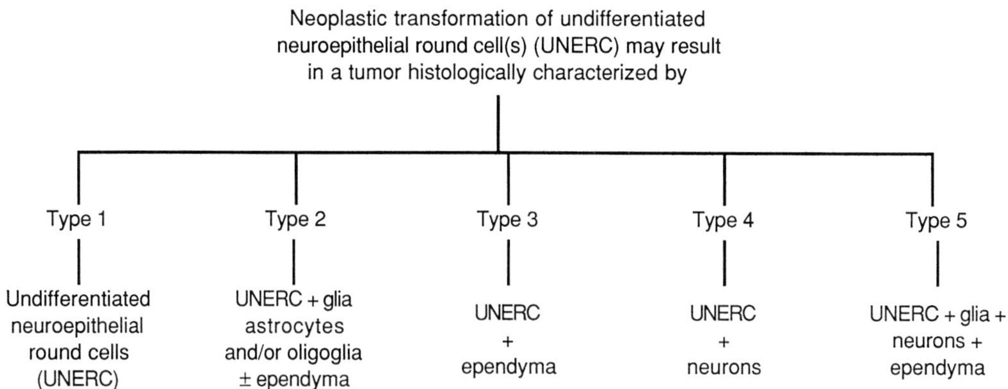

Figure 16.2. Classification of primitive neuroectodermal tumors (including medulloblastoma) of childhood. (Derived from Rorke, L. B. The cerebellar medulloblastoma and its relationship to primitive neuroectodermal tumors. J. Neuropathol. Exp. Neurol., *42*:1–15, 1983.)

tumors as compared to 30% for tumors which were partially removed (16). Norris *et al.* reported a 4-year relapse-free survival of 84% for patients with gross total resection as compared to 38% for patients who were subtotally resected or biopsied (13). Evans *et al.* could find no statistical difference in patients with complete resection versus those who underwent a subtotal resection; however, patients who underwent only a biopsy fared less well (2). Interpreting many of these studies is difficult because the means for determining the extent of resection varied. In the study by Evans *et al.* a postoperative computed tomography scan was not required to confirm the degree of surgical resection but was used in all patients in the Norris *et al.* series (13).

Of all the advances which have impacted favorably on the outcome for patients with primitive neuroectodermal tumors of the posterior fossa, the most important has been the addition of presymptomatic craniospinal radiation therapy (55, 66, 103). With local radiation therapy alone, long-term survival is uncommon in patients with medulloblastoma. Patients treated with presymptomatc craniospinal radiation therapy and local boost therapy have 5-year survival rates of greater than 50% (2, 55, 66, 71, 103). Although there does seem to be a partial dose-response curve in patients with primitive neuroectodermal tumors, as patients who receive greater local doses of radiation therapy seem to do better, there is no consensus over whether a dose response curve is present for the craniospinal portion of the radiation therapy (2, 55, 66, 71, 103).

The effect of adjuvant chemotherapy for all patients with primitive neuroectodermal tumors on outcome is unclear. Although there have been reports of unstaged patients having a somewhat higher rate of survival if treated with adjuvant chemotherapy, most of these studies report relatively few patients without a concurrent and comparable control group (32). In the prospective, randomized study performed by the CCSG-RTOG, patients with more extensive disease at the time of diagnosis benefited from the addition of chemotherapy (methylCCNU and vincristine) (2). Five-year event-free survival in patients with T_3-T_4 stage tumors was 59% as compared to 41% for patients treated with radiation alone (2). More recently, a study by Packer *et al.* demonstrated a greater than 90% per 12-month survival for patients with "poor-risk" posterior fossa primitive neuroectodermal tumors after treatment with radiotherapy and adjuvant CCNU, cisplatinum, and vincristine (77).

Summary

Multiple factors are of prognostic importance in patients with primitive neuroectodermal tumors. These include the age of the patients at diagnosis, the location of the tumor, and extent of tumor dissemination at the time of diagnosis, possibly the extent of surgical resection, the volume and dose of radiation therapy used, and possibly the addition of adjuvant chemotherapy. It is our feeling that based on this information, patients can be separated into prognostic groups at the time of diagnosis (Table 16.4). In this way, a more rational approach to treatment selection and evaluation is possible.

GERM CELL TUMORS

Germ cell tumors primarily occur in the pineal and suprasellar regions (19, 92). Within this category of tumors, there are

TABLE 16.4.
Stratification of Patients with Primitive Neuroectodermal Tumors of the Posterior Fossa

	Good Risk	Average Risk (One or More)
Age at diagnosis	Greater than 3 years of age	Less than 3 years of age
Extent of disease	Chang stage T_1 or T_2/M_0	Chang stage T_3 or T_4 or any T with M_1–M_4
Extent of resection	Gross total	Partial (especially biopsy)
Histological features	Undifferentiated	Differentiated

multiple different tumor types including germinomas, endodermal sinus tumors, embryonal cell carcinomas, choriocarcinomas, and mixed germ cell tumors. The most predictive factor of outcome is the histology of the tumor at the time of diagnosis (81).

Since these tumors are often treated without biopsy, interpretation of most series discussing pineal region tumors is impossible. Surgically confirmed germinomas carry the best prognosis and 5-year survival as high as 80% with current means of treatment is possible (118). Embryonal cell carcinomas, choriocarcinomas, and mixed germ cell tumors carry a poor prognosis, with few if any survivors after conventional therapy (79). Embryonal cell carcinomas and choriocarcinomas secrete markers into the cerebrospinal fluid which are useful in following the course of disease. However, the presence of the markers at diagnosis and the degree of their elevation has not been shown to be of prognostic value. Elevation of CSF markers after a treatment-related decline does correlate with tumor recurrence and progressive disease (79).

The location of the tumor at the time of diagnosis may be of prognostic value. Wara *et al.* reported that germinomas occurring in the pineal region carried a more favorable prognosis than tumors of the suprasellar region (118). This has not been our experience at Children's Hospital of Philadelphia since patients with suprasellar germinomas have done as well as those with pineal region masses.

The extent of disease at diagnosis may be of prognostic importance. These tumors, especially the germinoma, may metastasize to the leptomeningeal space, and patients with disseminated tumors probably fare worse than those with localized lesions (78).

It is clear that radiation favorably affects the outcome in patients with pineal region germinomas, as survival rates as high as 80% have been reported in patients receiving radiation (118). Treatment failure may occur outside of the primary site and a dose-response curve and consensus on the need for craniospinal radiation therapy for patients with this tumor does not exist. Recently, preradiation chemotherapy with high-dose cyclophosphamide has been shown to be effective in the treatment of disseminated germ cell tumors (4).

PITUITARY ADENOMAS

The past two decades have witnessed tremendous improvement in the understanding and treatment of pituitary adenomas (120). The classical histological classification of adenomas on the basis of light microscopy has been essentially replaced by a classification system based on the hormones these tumors secrete (120). Since 1969, a modern transphenoidal surgical approach has been used to treat these lesions and because of this and the introduction of microscopic techniques preserved pituitary function has been possible (43). In general, outcome is dependent on the type of tumor present and possibly the size of tumor at diagnosis. Pituitary adenomas occur primarily in adulthood; however, in at least one report, onset of disease during puberty was associated with a high risk of the tumor becoming invasive after treatment (38).

Prolactin secreting tumors make up the largest group of pituitary tumors. Wilson found in his surgical series of 100 female patients without prior surgery or radiation therapy that the best outcome occurs in those with estrogen-related tumors (i.e., those occurring after prior pregnancy or while on oral contraceptives) (120). Patients with lower preoperative prolactin levels, shorter duration of symptoms prior to diagnosis, and microadenomas fared better (120). Long-term remission after transsphenoidal surgery alone occurred in 93 percent of patients with microadenomas and 88% of patients with suprasellar extension. Lateral extension of the tumor at the time of diagnosis predicted a less favorable outcome (120). Bromocriptine (6, 113) and pergolide mesylate (51) have been shown by other studies to produce significant shrinkage of prolactin secreting pituitary tumors. These drugs are not cytotoxic and thus are not curative but may be of benefit as a preoperative adjunct to shrink prolactinomas (6). The use of bromocriptine preoperatively was not associated with a higher long-term control rate in Wilson's series and there was some suggestion that prior treatment with this drug made surgical treatment more difficult (120). Wilson recommended radiation therapy only for tumors which recurred postoperatively with mass effect or evidence of invasion (120).

As concerns growth hormone secreting tumors, Wilson once again reported excellent outcome in patients treated with surgery alone and related prognosis to the size of the tumor and its extent at the time of diagnosis (120). In patients with growth hormone secreting tumors, he found no correlation between outcome and sex, preoperative duration of symptoms, or age of the patient at the time of treatment. The best response rate was found in patients undergoing surgery as first treatment, as compared to patients who were previously treated with radiation therapy. Laws *et al.*, in a series of 82 consecutive acromegalic patients operated on transphenoidally, divided patients into those with microadenomas, diffuse adenomas, and invasive adenomas (56). Patients with more extensive tumors had higher preoperative prolactin levels. "Cures" were reported in 87.5% of patients with macroadenomas, but only 68% of those with diffuse adenomas and 54% of those with invasive lesions. Eastman *et al.* suggested that conventional irradiation alone is as effective as transphenoidal surgery or more aggressive forms of irradiation for long-term control of acromegaly (31). However, patients were not as carefully characterized in this series as in others. Bromocriptine and pergolide have also been used to treat acromegalic patients (51, 112), but their efficacy has been questioned (6) and how these drugs impact on outcome when combined with radiation and/or surgery is unclear.

Evaluation of factors influencing outcome with ACTH-secreting adenomas is made more difficult by the uncertainty of diagnosis in some patients (120). Prognosis may depend on where in the pituitary the adenoma arises, as tumors arising in the intermediate lobe may be less likely to respond to microsurgery than anterior lobe tumors (54). Wilson reports lasting remissions in over 90% of patients in whom total adenomectomy is possible transphenoidally (10, 120). No correlation was found between histological characteristics, the size or location of the tumor or the duration of symptoms and outcome, except for lateral extension which predicted an adverse result (10). A subgroup of patients, those under age 20 at the time of surgery, fared worse than older patients in Wilson's series, as 4 of 13 suffered a recurrence. Conventional irradiation is also effective in the management of Cushing's disease (99), although the rate of "cure" has not been as high as reported in surgical series. However, children seem to fare well when treated with pituitary irradiation (18).

In contrast to the study reported by Wilson, Ciric *et al.* concluded that the most important predictor of outcome for macroadenomas (independent of the type of tumor present) was the extent of suprasellar extension at the time of diagnosis (18). Patients with tumors which extended greater than 2 cm above the sella at the time of diagnosis fared worse than patients with smaller lesions. In this study, lateral extension of the tumor or invasion of the tumor into the sinus at the time of diagnosis was not a predictor of poor outcome. Ciric *et al.* also reported that the best results in the series of macroadenomas occurred when patients were given radiation therapy, independent of the degree of resection.

MENINGIOMAS

Meningiomas are the second most common tumor in adults. They are generally benign, slow-growing tumors with a relatively good prognosis (22, 86, 92). Mirimanoff in a review of 225 patients with meningiomas found that the sex of the patient, the age of the patient at the time of diagnosis, and the duration of symptoms prior to diagnosis were not predictive of outcome (68). Although children are more likely to have tumors of the lateral ventricle, cystic tumors, tumors without dural attachment, and sarcomatous lesions (97), their outcomes, if treated aggressively, were not worse than adults with tumors in similar locations (98). In 101 patients with suprasellar meningiomas, Symon and Rosenstein found that a duration of symptoms of less than 2 years prior to diagnosis was associated with lower surgical morbidity and better visual outcome (91, 108). Also, patients with suprasellar lesions had better long-term visual function, if there was less than 50% visual loss preoperatively or normal optic discs on funduscopic examination (91).

Histology has not been a reliable prognostic factor. Earl *et al.* found histology a poor predictor of outcome in a review of 243 patients with meningiomas (29). The presence of sarcomatous elements or mitotic figures were not predictive factors in either Earl's study or the study by Schut *et al.* (98). In fact, mitotic figures have been found in as high as 45% of meningiomas (21). The presence of a papillary pattern has been purported as an indication of malignancy, especially in childhood (62). Angioblastic meningiomas may metastasize at a somewhat higher rate than other forms of meningiomas, but there is no absolute relationship between the histologic pattern (115) and dissemination. Simpson found no relationship between histology and the incidence of recurrence (102), while others have found some histologic factors, including high cellularity, numerous mitoses, and cortical invasion predictive of a higher rate of recurrence (21).

The location of the tumor is an important factor in outcome, as convexity and parasagittal meningiomas are less likely to recur than parasellar meningiomas. Sphenoid ridge and olfactory groove meningiomas have the highest risk of recurrence (68). In the study by Mirimanoff, the higher rate of recurrence for sphenoid ridge meningiomas was believed to be because this tumor was less amenable to total surgical resection (68). However, olfactory groove meningiomas had a higher probability of local recurrence despite total resection. Patients with suprasellar lesions less than 3 cm in size have a better rate of survival and visual outcome (108).

The most important determinant of survival has been the extent of surgical resection. Mirimanoff reported 5-, 10-, and 15-year survivals of 93%, 80%, and 68% for totally resected tumors, independent of the site of origin. In contrast, the 5-, 10-, and 15-year rates of survival were 63%, 45%, and 9%, respectively for subtotally resected tumors (68). Simpson found a similar relationship between extent of resection and recurrence-free survival (102). Radiotherapy is of benefit in subtotally resected tumors. Wara *et al.* reported, in a series of 82 partially resected patients, that 43 of 54 patients treated with surgery alone developed recurrent tumor while 10 of 34 patients treated with radiation therapy recurred (119).

CRANIOPHARYNGIOMAS

Craniopharyngiomas are the most common non-neuroglial tumor occurring in childhood and may also arise in adults (19, 92). Prognosis in patients with craniopharyngiomas has dramatically changed over the past 30 years primarily because of improved postoperative care including the use of adrenocorticosteroids (19).

Onoyama *et al.* found age to be of prognostic importance, as patients who were under 25 at the time of diagnosis had a 5-year survival rate of 80% while older patients only had a slightly greater than 30% chance of survival at 5 years (31). This study also found that female patients did better than males.

The major controversies concerning the outcome for patients with craniopharyngiomas are the importance of the extent of resection and the efficacy of radiation therapy (72). Matson and Crigler, reporting on results in 74 patients, concluded that the best results were obtained with total or at least radical excision (65). In recent series, a nearly 100% short-term disease-free survival in childhood was reported after total excision and a less than 50% disease-free survival when subtotal excision was performed (12, 46). Sweet *et al.* reported an overall success rate of 69% in 37 patients, including both adults and children, treated with radical surgery alone (107). In a recent (primarily adult) series, Symon and Sprich reported a 5.5% recurrence rate in patients followed for a mean of 3.1 years (109). Patients with totally excised tumors are said to have better vision, neurologic function, and possibly better residual endocrinologic function than patients treated with subtotal excision and radiation (12). Neuroradiographic findings prior to the time of surgery, including the presence of calcification or cystic areas, extension into the third ventricle, and hydrocephalus, did not affect the extent of resection possible or the outcome (12).

Series of patients treated with subtotal resection followed by local irradiation also report impressive survival figures. Bloom found an 81% 3-year survival in mainly pediatric patients treated with radiotherapy after subtotal resection (109). Kramer *et al.* found that 9 of 10 patients were alive and well greater than 5 years after treatment with subtotal excision and radiation therapy (53). Cavazzuti *et al.* reporting on 95 patients who underwent treatment between 1959 and 1982, concluded that subtotal resection followed by primary radiation was associated with a lower morbidity and better neuropsychological outcome than treatment with extensive tumor resection alone (14). Unfortunately, the patients treated by gross total resection and those treated with subtotal resection and cranial radiation were not completely comparable in this series; the majority of patients treated with resection alone underwent operation before 1972 and included patients with recurrent disease undergoing multiple operations, while all of the patients treated with radiation and conservative surgery had been evaluated after 1972. In a separate report of a subgroup of 37 children treated at the same institution between 1972 and 1981, radiation therapy after conservative operation was found to be "equally, if not more, effective" than attempted total excision in controlling subsequent tumor growth and it "is inferred that conservative operations combined with radiation therapy offers less risk for psychosocial impairment than does attempted tumor excision" (36). However, this was not a controlled, randomized study; some patients had been treated elsewhere prior to entry into the study, and patients undergoing radical resections were younger and more frequently had hydrocephalus than conservatively treated patients. Criteria used to choose one treatment over another were not stated and there were only eight patients in whom a "total" removal was achieved. The mean length of follow-up was 4 years for the conservatively treated group and 5 years for those treated with radical resection; the differences in outcome were not statistically significant.

CONCLUSIONS AND PERSPECTIVES FOR THE FUTURE

There is a marked disparity between the identification of prognostic factors for some tumors as compared to others. This is due in part to the rarity of some types of central nervous system neoplasms and also, the relative lack of carefully controlled studies in patients with brain tumors. Factors predictive of survival are best worked out for malignant astrocytomas of the cerebral cortex in adults, childhood brain stem tumors, and primitive neuroectodermal (especially posterior fossa) tumors in childhood. These factors have often been elucidated during carefully performed multicenter clinical trials. Better agreement concerning the classification of brain tumors is needed so that more useful studies can be performed. Newer techniques, such as the characterization of tumors with specific monoclonal antibodies, immunohistochemical staining, genetic techniques, and nuclear magnetic resonance, will undoubtedly contribute to our understanding of the prognostic factors important in the survival of patients with brain tumors.

ACKNOWLEDGMENTS

I would like to thank Lisa Gray and Linda Cella for their secretarial assistance; Kathy R. Siegel for her help in collecting and analyzing the data; and Peter H. Berman and Audrey E. Evans for reviewing the manuscript. Supported in part by the Foerderer Fund for Excellence and Children's Cancer Research Center Grant 14489.

REFERENCES

1. Albright, A.L., Guthkelch, A.N., Packer, R.J., *et al.* Prognostic factors in pediatric brain-stem gliomas. J. Neurosurg., *65:*751–755, 1986.
2. Allen, J.C. Childhood brain tumors: current status and clinical trials in newly diagnosed patients and recurrent disease. Pediatr. Clin. North Am., *32:*633–681, 1985.
3. Allen, J.C. and Epstein, F. Medulloblastoma and other primary malignant neuroecto-

dermal tumors of the CNS. The effect of patients' age and extent of disease on prognosis. J. Neurosurg., *57*:446–451, 1982.
4. Allen, J.C., Kim, J.H., and Packer, R.J. Neoadjuvant chemotherapy for newly diagnosed primary CNS germ cell tumors. J. Neurosurg., *67*:65–70, 1987.
5. Bailey, P. and Cushing, H. Medulloblastoma cerebelli. A common type of midcerebellar glioma of childhood. Arch. Neurol. Psychiatry, *14*:192–224, 1925.
6. Barrow, D.L., Tindall, G.T., Kovacs, K., *et al.* Clinical and pathological effects of bromocriptine on prolactin-secreting and other pituitary tumors. J. Neurosurg., *60*:1–7, 1984.
7. Berger, M.S., Edwards, M.S.B., LaMasters, D., *et al.* Pediatric brain stem tumors: Radiographic, pathological and clinical correlations. Neurosurgery, *12*:298–302, 1983.
8. Berger, M.S., Edward, M.S., and Wara, W.M., *et al.* Primary cerebral neuroblastoma. J. Neurosurg., *59*:418–423, 1983.
9. Bernstein, M., Hoffman, H.J., Halliday, W.C., *et al.* Thalamic tumors in children. Long-term follow-up and treatment guidelines. J. Neurosurg., *61*:649–656, 1984.
10. Bogan, J.E., Tyrell, J.B., and Wilson, C.B. Transphenoidal microsurgical management of Cushing's disease. J. Neurosurg., *59*:195–200, 1983.
11. Bouchard, J. and Peirce, C.B. Radiation therapy in the management of neoplasms of the central nervous system with a special note in regard to children. Twenty years' experience, 1939–1958. Am. J. Roentgenol., *84*:610–628, 1960.
12. Bruce, D.A., Schut, L., and Rorke, L. Craniopharyngiomas in a capsule. Concepts Pediatr. Neurosurg., *1*:29–35, 1981.
13. Caputy, A.J., McCullough, D.C., and Manz, H.J. A review of the factors influencing the prognosis of medulloblastoma. The importance of cell differentiation. Cancer, *66*:80–87, 1987.
14. Cavazzuti, V., Fischer, E.G., Welch, K., *et al.* Neurological and psychological sequelae following different treatments of craniopharyngioma in children. J. Neurosurg., *59*:409–471, 1983.
15. Chang, C.H., Horton, J., Schoenfeld, D., *et al.* Comparison of postoperative radiotherapy and combined postoperative radiotherapy and chemotherapy in the multidisciplinary management of malignant gliomas. Cancer, *52*:997–1007, 1983.
16. Chang, C.H., Housepian, E.M., and Herbert, C. Jr. An operative staging system and a megavoltage radiotherapeutic technique for cerebellar medulloblastomas. Radiology, *93*:1351–1359, 1969.
17. Chatty, E.M. and Earle, K.M. Medulloblastoma: a report of 201 cases with emphasis on the relationship of histologic variants to survival. Cancer, *28*:977–983, 1971.
18. Ciric, I., Mikhael, M., and Stafford, T. Transphenoidal microsurgery of pituitary macroadenomas with long-term follow-up results. J. Neurosurg., *59*:395–401, 1983.
19. Cohen, M.E. and Duffner, P.K. *Brain Tumors in Children. Principles of Diagnosis and Treatment.* New York, Raven Press, 1984.
20. Concannon, J.P., Kramer, S., and Berry, R. The extent of intracranial gliomata at autopsy and its relationship to technique used in radiation therapy of brain tumors. Am. J. Roentgenol., *84*:99–107, 1960.
21. Crompton, M.R. and Gautier-Smith, D.C. The prediction of recurrence in meningiomas. J. Neurol. Neurosurg. Psychiatry, *33*: 80–87, 1970.
22. Cushing, H. and Eisenhardt, L. *The Meningiomas.* Springfield, IL, Charles C Thomas, 1938.
23. Danoff, B.F., Kramer, S., and Thompson, N. The radiotherapeutic management of optic gliomas in children. Int. J. Radiat. Oncol. Biol. Phys., *6*:45–50, 1980.
24. Davis, R.L., Lui, H.C., Vestys, P., *et al.* Correlation of survival and diagnosis in supratentorial malignant gliomas (abstr.). J. Neurooncol., *2*:267, 1984.
25. Deutsch, M. and Reigel, D.H. The value of myelography in the management of childhood medulloblastoma. Cancer, *45*:2194–2197, 1980.
26. Dohrmann, G.J., Farwell, J.R., and Flannery, J.T. Ependymomas and ependymoblastomas in children. J. Neurosurg., *45*:273–283, 1976.
27. Dohrmann, G.J., Farwell, J.R., and Flannery, J.T. Oligodendrogliomas in children. Surg. Neurol., *10*:21–25, 1978.
28. Duffner, P.K., Cohen, M.E., Heffner, R.R. *et al.* Primitive neuroectodermal tumors of childhood. An approach to therapy. J. Neurosurg., *55*:376–381, 1981.
29. Earle, K.M. and Richany, S.F. Meningiomas: a study of the histology, incidence and biologic behavior of 243 cases from the Frazier-Grant collection of brain tumors. Med. Ann. District Columbia, *38*:353–358, 1969.
30. Earnest III, F., Kernohan, J.W., and Craig, W. McK. Oligodendrogliomas: a review of 200 cases. Arch. Neurol. Psychiatry, *63*:964–976, 1950.
31. Eastman, R.C., Gordon, P., and Roth, J. Conventional supervoltage irradiation as an effective treatment for acromegaly. J. Clin. Endocrinol. Metab., *48*:931–940, 1979.
32. Edwards, M.S., Levin, V.A., and Wilson, C.B. Brain tumor chemotherapy: an evaluation of agents in current use for Phase 2 and 3 trials. Cancer Treat. Rep., *64*:1179–1205, 1980.
33. Edwards, M.S.B., Wara, W.W., and Urtasan, R.C. Hyperfractionated radiation therapy for brainstem gliomas: a phase I-II trial. J. Neurosurg., *70*:691–700, 1989.
34. Elvidge, A.R. Long-term survival in the astrocytoma series. J. Neurosurg., *28*:399–404, 1968.
35. Fazekas, J.T. Treatment of Grade 1 and 2 brain

astrocytomas: the role of radiotherapy. Int. J. Radiat. Oncol. Biol. Phys., *2*:661–666, 1977.
36. Fischer, E.G., Welch, K., and Belli, J.A. Treatment of craniopharyngiomas in children: 1972–1981. J. Neurosurg., *62*:496–501, 1985.
37. Fokes, E.C. Jr. and Earle, K.M. Ependymomas: clinical and pathological aspects. J. Neurosurg., *30*:585–594, 1969.
38. Fraiole, B., Ferrante, L., and Celli, P. Pituitary adenomas with onset during puberty. J. Neurosurg., *60*:590–595, 1983.
39. Gehan, E.A. and Walker, M.D. Prognostic factors for patients with brain tumors. In: *Modern Concepts in Brain Tumor Therapy: Laboratory and Clinical Investigations,* edited by J.C. Bailar and E.K. Weisberger. National Cancer Institute Monograph, No. 46, pp 189–195, 1977.
40. Gilles, F.H., Winston, K., Fulchiero, A. *et al.* Histologic features and observational variation in cerebellar gliomas in children. J. Natl. Cancer Inst., *58*:175–181, 1977.
41. Gjerris, F. and Klinken, L. Long-term prognosis in children with benign cerebellar astrocytoma. J. Neurosurg., *49*:179–184, 1978.
42. Griffin, T.W., Beaufait, D., and Blasko, J.C. Cystic cerebellar astrocytomas in childhood. Cancer, *44*:276–280, 1979.
43. Hardy, J. Transphenoidal microsurgery of the normal and pathological pituitary. Clin. Neurosurg., *16*:185–217, 1969.
44. Heiskanan, O., Raitta, C., and Torsti, R. The management and prognosis of gliomas of the optic pathways in children. Acta. Neurochir., *43*:193–199, 1978.
45. Hirakawa, K., Suzuki, K., Ueda, S., *et al.* Multivariate analysis of factors affecting postoperative survival in malignant astrocytoma. J. Neuro-oncol., *2*:331–340, 1984.
46. Hoffman, H.J., Hendrich, E.B., and Humphreys, R.P. Management of craniopharyngiomas in children. J. Neurosurg., *47*:218–227, 1977.
47. Hoshino, T., Nagashima, J.A., Murovic, J.A. *et al.* In situ cell kinetics studies on human neuroectodermal tumors with bromodeoxyuridine labeling. J. Neurosurg., *64*:453–459, 1986.
48. Hoshino, T., Rodriguez, L.A., Cho, K.G., *et al.* Pronostic implications of the proliferative potential of low-grade astrocytomas. J. Neurosurg., *69*:839–842, 1988.
49. Hoyt, W.F., Meskel, L.G., Lessell, S., *et al.* Malignant optic glioma of adulthood. Brain, *96*: 121–132, 1973.
50. Kernohan, J.W. and Fletcher-Kernohan, E.M. Ependymomas: a study of 109 cases. A Res. Nerv. Ment. Dis. Proc., *16*:182–209, 1973.
51. Kleinberg, D.L., Boyet, A.E., and Wardlow, S. Pergolide for the treatment of pituitary tumors secreting prolactin or growth hormone. N. Engl. J. Med., *309*:704–708, 1983.
52. Kopelson, G., Linggood, R.M., and Klienman, G.M. Medulloblastoma. The identification of prognostic subgroups and implications for multimodality management. Cancer, *51*: 312–319, 1983.
53. Kramer, S., Southard, M. and Mansfield, C.M. Radiotherapy in the management of craniopharyngioma. Further experiences and late results. Am. J. Radiol., *103*:44–52, 1968.
54. Lamberts, S.W.J., de Lange, S.A., and Stefanko, S.Z. Adenocorticotropin-secreting pituitary adenomas originate from the anterior or intermediate lobe in Cushing's disease: differences in the regulation of hormone secretion. J. Clin. Endocrinol. Metab., *54*:286–291, 1982.
55. Landberg, T.G., Lindgren, M.L., Cavallin-Stahl, E.K., *et al.* Improvements in the radiotherapy of medulloblastoma, 1946–1975. Cancer, *45*:670–678, 1980.
56. Laws, E.R., Prepgras, D.G., Randall, R.V. *et al.* Neurosurgical management of acromegaly. J. Neurosurg., *50*:454–461, 1979.
57. Laws, E.R., Taylor, W.F., Clifton, M.B., *et al.* Neurosurgical management of low-grade astrocytoma of the cerebral hemispheres. J. Neurosurg., *61*:665–673, 1984.
58. Lee, F. Radiation of infratentorial and supratentorial stem tumors. J. Neurosurg., *43*:65–68, 1975.
59. Leibel, S.A., Sheline, G.E., Wara, W.M., *et al.* The role of radiation therapy in the treatment of astrocytomas. Cancer, *35*:1551–1557, 1975.
60. Levin, V.A., Wilson, C.B., and Vestrys, P.S. Primary intracranial gliomas: clinical studies and treatment. Regimen of the Brain Tumor Research Center, University of California, San Francisco 1979, Cancer Treat. Rep., *65*(Suppl. 2):83–88, 1981.
61. Littman, P., Jarrett, P., Bilaniuk, L., *et al.* Pediatric brain stem gliomas. Cancer, *45*:2787–2792, 1980.
62. Ludwin, S.K., Rubenstein, L.J., and Russell, D.L. Papillary meningioma: a variant of meningioma. Cancer, *36*:1363–1373, 1975.
63. Lowes, M., Bojsen-Moller, M., Vorre, P., *et al.* An evaluation of gliomas of the anterior visual pathway. A ten year survey. Acta Neurochir., *43*:34–41, 1978.
64. Lui, M., Boggs, J., and Kidd, J. Ependymomas of childhood. Child's Brain, *2*:92–110, 1976.
65. Matson, D.D. and Crigler, J.F. Management of craniopharyngioma in childhood. J. Neurosurg., *30*:377–390, 1969.
66. McFarland, D.R., Horowitz, H., Saenger, E.L., *et al.* Medulloblastoma. A review of prognosis and survival. Br. J. Radiol., *42*:198–214, 1969.
67. Miller, N.R., Illif, W.J., Green, W.R. Evaluation and management of gliomas of the anterior visual pathway. Brain, *97*:743–754, 1975.
68. Mirimanoff, R., Dosoretz, D.E., Linggood, R.M., *et al.* Meningioma: analysis of recurrence and progression following neurosurgical resection. J. Neurosurg., *62*:18–25, 1985.

69. Myles, S.T. and Murphy, S.B. Gliomas of the optic nerve and chiasm. Can. J. Ophthalmol., *8*:508–514, 1973.
70. Nelson, J.S., Tsukada, Y., Schoenfeld, D., *et al.* Necrosis as a prognostic criterion in malignant supratentorial, astrocytic glioma. Cancer, *52*:550–554, 1983.
71. Norris, D.G., Bruce, D.A., Byrd, R.I., *et al.* Improved relapse-free survival in medulloblastoma utilizing modern techniques. Neurosurgery, *9*:661–664, 1981.
72. Onoyama, Y., Ono, K., Yabumoto, E., *et al.* Radiation therapy of craniopharyngioma. Radiology, *125*:799–803, 1977.
73. Oxenhandler, D.C. and Sayers, M.P. The dilemma of childhood optic gliomas. J. Neurosurg., *48*:34–41, 1978.
74. Packer, R.J., Allen, J.C., and Deck, M., *et al.* Brain stem glioma: clinical manifestations of meningeal gliomatosis. Ann. Neurol., *14*: 177–182, 1983.
75. Packer, R.J., Rosenstock, J.G., Bilaniuk, L.T., *et al.* Chiasmatic/hypothalamic/thalamic gliomas in childhood: efficacy of treatment with chemotherapy alone (abstr.) Ann. Neurol., *168*: 402, 1984.
76. Packer, R.J., Savino, P.J., Bilaniuk, L.T., *et al.* Chiasmatic gliomas of childhood: a reappraisal of natural history and effectiveness of cranial irradiation. Child's Brain, *10*:393–403, 1983.
77. Packer, R.J., Siegel, K.R., Sutton, L.N., *et al.* Efficacy of adjuvant chemotherapy for patients with poor-risk medulloblastoma: a preliminary report. Ann. Neurol., *24*:503–508, 1988.
78. Packer, R.J., Siegel, K.R., Sutton, L.N., *et al.* Leptomeningeal dissemination of primary central nervous system tumors of childhood. Ann. Neurol., *18*:217–222, 1985.
79. Packer, R.J., Sutton, L.N., Rorke, L.B., *et al.* Intracranial embryonal cell carcinoma. Cancer, *54*:142–146, 1984.
80. Packer, R.J., Sutton, L.N., Rorke, L.B., *et al.* Oligodendroglioma of the posterior fossa in childhood. Cancer, *56*:195–200, 1985.
81. Packer, R.J., Sutton, L.N., Rosenstock, J.G., *et al.* Pineal region tumors of childhood. Pediatrics, *74*:97–103, 1984.
82. Packer, R.J., Sutton, L.N., Rorke, L.B., *et al.* Prognostic significance of cellular differentiation in primitive neuroectodermal tumors (medulloblastoma) of childhood. J. Neurosurg., *6*:296–301, 1984.
83. Panitch, M.S. and Berg, B.O. Brain stem tumors of childhood and adolescence. Am. J. Dis. Child, *119*:465–472, 1970.
84. Paterson, E. and Farr, R.F. Cerebellar medulloblastoma: treatment of the whole central nervous system. Acta Radiol., *39*:323–336, 1953.
85. Pierre-Kahn, A., Hirsch, J.F., Roux, F.X., *et al.* Intracranial ependymomas in childhood — survival and functional results of 47 cases. Child's Brain, *10*:145–156, 1983.
86. Quest, D.Q. Meningiomas: an update. Neurosurgery, *3*:219–225, 1978.
87. Reigel, D.H., Scarff, T.B., and Woodford, J.E. Biopsy of pediatric brain stem tumors. Child's Brain, *5*:329–340, 1979.
88. Ringertz, N. and Nordenstam, H. Cerebellar astrocytoma. J. Neuropathol. Exp. Neurol., *10*:343–367, 1951.
89. Roberts, M. and German, W.J. A long-term study of patients with oligodendrogliomas: follow-up of 30 cases including Dr. Harvey Cushing's series. J. Neurosurg., *24*:697–700, 1966.
90. Rorke, L.B. The cerebellar medulloblastoma and its relationship to primitive neuroectodermal tumors. J. Neuropathol. Exp. Neurol., *42*:1–15, 1983.
91. Rosenstein, J. and Symon, L. Surgical management of suprasellar meningioma. Part 2: prognosis for visual function following craniotomy. J. Neurosurg., *61*:642–648, 1984.
92. Rubinstein, L.J. Tumors of the Nervous System. Atlas of Tumor Pathology, Second Series, Fascicle 6, Armed Forces Institute of Pathology, Bethesda, MD, 1972.
93. Salazar, O.M. A better understanding of CNS seeding and a brighter outlook for postoperatively irradiated patients with ependymomas. Int. J. Radiat. Oncol. Biol. Physiol., *9*:1231–1234, 1983.
94. Salazar, O.M. Primary malignant cerebellar astrocytomas in children: a signal for postoperative craniospinal irradiation. Int. J. Radiat. Oncol. Biol. Physiol. *7*:1661–1665, 1981.
95. Salazar, O.M., Rubin, P., Bassano, D., *et al.* Improved survival of patients with intracranial ependymomas by irradiation: dose selection and field extension. Cancer, *35*:1563–1573, 1975.
96. Salcman, M., Machado, E., Montgomery, E., *et al.* Prognostic factors for long-term (>24 mo) survival in malignant astrocytoma. J. Neuro-Oncol., *2*:274, 1984.
97. Sano, K., Wakai, S., Ochai, C., *et al.* Characteristics of intracranial meningiomas in childhood. Child's Brain, *8*:98–106, 1981.
98. Schut, L., Canady, A., Sutton, L., *et al.* Meningeal tumors in children. Concepts Pediatr. Neurosurg., *4*:335–347, 1983.
99. Sheline, G.E. Conventional radiation therapy in the treatment of pituitary tumors. In: *Clinical Management of Pituitary Disorders,* edited by G.E. Tindall and W.F. Collins, pp. 287–314. New York, Raven Press, 1979.
100. Sheline, G.E., Boldrey, E.B., Karlsberg, P., *et al.* Therapeutic considerations in tumors affecting the central nervous system. Oligodendroglioma. Radiology, *82*: 84–89, 1964.
101. Shin, K.H., Muller, P.J., and Geggie, P.H. Superfractionation radiation therapy in the treatment of malignant astrocytoma. Cancer, *52*:2040–2043, 1983.
102. Simpson, D. The recurrence of intracranial meningiomas after surgical treatment. J. Neurol. Neurosurg. Psychiatry, *20*:22–39, 1957.

103. Smith, C.E., Long, D.M., Jones, T.K. Jr., *et al.* Experiences in treating medulloblastoma at the University of Minnesota hospitals. Radiology, *109:*179–182, 1973.
104. Smith, M.T., Ludwig, C.L., Godfrey, A.D., *et al.* Grading of oligodendrogliomas. Cancer, *52:*2107–2114, 1983.
105. Stage, W.S. and Stein, J.J. Treatment of malignant astrocytomas. Am. J. Roentgenol. Radiat. Therapy Nucl. Med., *120:*7–18, 1974.
106. Stroink, A.R., Hoffman, H.J., Hendrick, E.B., *et al.* Diagnosis and management of pediatric brain-stem gliomas. J. Neurosurg., *65:*745–750, 1986.
107. Sweet, W.H. Radical surgical treatment of craniopharyngioma. Clin. Neurosurg., *23:*52–79, 1976.
108. Symon, L. and Rosenstem, J. Surgical management of suprasellar meningioma. Part 1: the influence of tumor size, duration of symptoms and microsurgery on surgical outcome in 101 consecutive cases. J. Neurosurg., *61:* 633–641, 1984.
109. Symon, L. and Sprich, W. Radical excision of craniopharyngioma. J. Neurosurg., *62:*174–181, 1985.
110. Svien, H., Mabon, R.F., Kernohan, J.W., *et al.* Ependymomas of the brain: pathologic aspects. Neurology, *3:*1–15, 1953.
111. Taveras, J.M., Mount, L.A., and Wood, E.H. The value of radiation therapy in management of gliomas of optic nerves and chiasm. Radiology, *66:*518–528, 1956.
112. Thorner, M.O., Chart, A., Aitkes, M., *et al.* Bromocriptine treatment of acromegaly. Br. Med. J., *1:*299–303, 1975.
113. Thorner, M.O., Martin, W.H., Rogol, A.D., *et al.* Rapid regression of pituitary prolactinomas during bromocriptine treatment. J. Clin. Endocrinol. Metab., *51:*438–445, 1980.
114. Tym, R. Piloid gliomas of the anterior optic pathways. Br. J. Surg., *49:*322–331, 1961.
115. Tytus, J.S., Lasersohn, J.T., and Reefel, E. The problem of malignancy in meningiomas. J. Neurosurg., *27:*551–557, 1967.
116. Walker, M.D., Alexander, E., Hunt, W.E., *et al.* Evaluation of BCNU and/or radiotherapy in the treatment of anaplastic gliomas. J. Neurosurg., *49:*333–343, 1978.
117. Walker, M.D., Strike, A., and Sheline, G.E. An analysis of dose-effect relationship in the radiotherapy of malignant gliomas. Int. J. Radiat. Oncol. Biol. Phys., *5:*1725–1731, 1979.
118. Wara, W.M., Jenkins, R.D.T., Evans, A., *et al.* Tumors of the pineal and suprasellar region: children cancer study group treatment results, 1960–1975. Cancer, *43:*698–701, 1979.
119. Wara, W.M., Sheline, G.E., Newman, H., *et al.* Radiation therapy of meningiomas. Am. J. Radiol., *123:*453–458, 1975.
120. Wilson, C.B. A decade of pituitary microsurgery: the Herbert Olivecrano lecture. J. Neurosurg., *84:*814–833, 1984.
121. Wong, I.G. and Lubow, M. Management of optic glioma of childhood — a review of 42 cases. In: *Neuro-Ophthalmology Symposium of University of Miami and Bascom Plamer Eye Institute, vol.* VI, pp. 51–60, St. Louis, Mosby, 1972.

PART IV

Therapeutic Rationale and Modes of Treatment

CHAPTER 17

Ionizing Radiation

JAMES E. MARKS, M.D.

VALUE

Any treatment that improves *neurological function* in the host, causes *regression* or *disappearance* of the tumor, lengthens the *interval* between treatment, and subsequent neurological deterioration or lengthens *survival* can be said to have value. Ionizing radiation by itself or in addition to surgery significantly reduces the tumor, improves the condition of the host, and prolongs survival of patients with a variety of primary neoplasms of the central nervous system. Some neoplasms like the suprasellar germinoma are very sensitive to radiation and are therefore curable, while others like glioblastoma multiforme are relatively resistant, temporarily shrink and invariably regrow within 24 months. Others like the low-grade astrocytoma or oligodendroglioma also respond to ionizing radiation, shrink slowly on serial computed tomography scans, and regrow after longer intervals than the glioblastoma multiforme. The very cytologically benign glioma like the optic nerve glioma and cerebellar astrocytoma are thought by many to be hamartomatous self-limiting malformations that do not need treatment. Nonetheless, some are relatively aggressive, damage the adjacent central nervous system, lead to significant neurologic impairment and do respond to ionizing radiation. The problem is to select the optic nerve glioma and the cerebellar astrocytoma which might benefit from irradiation and to observe those that can be successfully extirpated or that seldom progress after years of follow-up. Some cytologically benign neoplasms of the central nervous system like the craniopharyngioma and meningioma do respond to ionizing radiation and are not as resistant as previously thought. Ionizing radiation has value for the incompletely removed or unresectable craniopharyngioma and the incompletely removed or unresectable meningioma. Indeed, there are a spectrum of neoplasms in the central nervous system with a range of responses to ionizing radiation from complete to partial and which are lasting or temporary depending on the radiosensitivity, growth rate, and total number of clonogenic cells in the tumor. The local invasiveness, propensity for spread to parts of the central nervous system distant from the site of origin, and the biological behavior of primary brain tumors vary enormously and correlate with histopathology. Similarly, outcome after treatment by surgery, radiation, and chemotherapy varies greatly and primarily reflects the nature of the tumor under consideration. The remainder of this chapter will be devoted to elucidating the effects of ionizing radiation on tumors and normal tissues of the central nervous system, documenting the value of ionizing radiation in the treatment of particular types of CNS tumors, and exploring newer methods of using ionizing radiation that might result in a therapeutic gain.

RADIATION MODALITIES

Radiation is electromagnetic or particulate and is produced by decaying isotopes or machines. Electromagnetic radiations most commonly used to externally irradiate patients with brain tumors are gamma photons from cobalt 60-sources and x-rays from betatrons and linear accelerators. The most common particulate radiation used to irradiate the central nervous system is the electron beam from betatrons and linear accelerators. These machines, along with cobalt-60, replaced kilovoltage machines in the late 1940s and early 1950s, and marked the end of the kilovoltage era and the beginning of the megavoltage era. The energy of megavoltage beams produced by Cobalt-60 sources, betatrons, and linear accelerators is measured in millions of electron volts (MeV) instead of thousands of electron volts (keV) and improved the ability of the radiotherapist to localize the radiation in the region of the tumor with relative sparing of the surrounding brain and transit tissues between the surface and the tumor. Megavoltage gamma photon and x-ray beams were more penetrating and sharply defined, and affected scalp, cranial soft tissues and cranium less than kilovoltage beams. Consequently, there were fewer observable acute effects on the scalp and late complications such as bone exposure and loss of craniotomy flaps. Because the acute effects on the scalp and cranial soft tissues were less limiting with megavoltage than kilovoltage beams, there developed a tendency to deliver greater doses to the tumor and surrounding normal brain thereby increasing the risk of damage to the normal brain. The problem faced by the radiotherapist has been to exploit the favorable physical characteristics of megavoltage beams without over irradiating intervening normal brain.

X-rays and gamma photons enter one side of the head and exit the other while electrons penetrate a limited distance before attenuation is complete. This distance increases with increasing energy of the electron beam and makes it possible to confine radiation to one side of the cerebrum and to spare the other (Fig. 17.1). X-rays, gamma photons and electrons are attenuated by the processes of photoelectric effect, Compton scattering, and pair production. Megavoltage beams in the range of 1 to 10 MeV are largely attenuated by Compton scattering and depend on the electronic density of the tissue they traverse. Above 10 MeV pair production becomes relatively more important than the other processes of attenuation.

These radiation beams are termed ionizing because they produce energetic charged particles that ionize molecules in the absorbing medium. X-rays, gamma photons, and electrons are *sparsely* ionizing, while particulate radiations such as neutrons and heavy ions are *densely* ionizing because they have lower velocity, greater mass, and charge. Densely ionizing radiations dissipate their energy over a shorter path length, cause more damage in biologic mediums, and are said to have a higher linear energy transfer (LET) than sparsely ionizing radia-

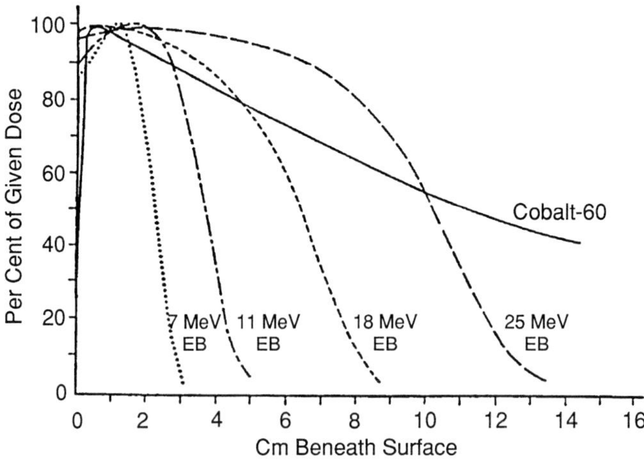

Figure 17.1. Percentage of maximum dose as a function of depth in water for Cobalt-60 and electron beams (10 × 10 cm fields).

tions. Particulate radiations being studied on an experimental basis are neutrons, protons, and heavy ions such as pi-mesons, Helium and Neon nuclei. Boron capture of slow neutrons that results in the emission of destructive alpha particles or Helium nuclei has also been utilized to treat brain tumors. Once a radiation beam interacts with tissue it is possible to quantitate the amount of energy deposited per unit mass of medium by using ionization chambers, photographic emulsions, Lithium fluoride dosimeters, and calorimeters. One rad equals 100 erg/gm of absorbing medium and 1 Gray (Gy), the new international unit of absorbed dose, is equivalent to 100 rad.

Interstitial irradiation of brain tumors was initially promulgated by Mundinger who inserted active Cobalt-60 sources into malignant gliomas using stereotactic technique (60). Interstitial implantation of brain tumors has been practiced more in recent years than ever before but the tendency has been to use *afterloading* instead of active loading of radioactive sources to avoid exposure to personnel involved in the procedure. The tumor is implanted with hollow plastic tubes in the operating room under stereotactic guidance or in radiology using computed tomography (CT) control. Films and CT scans are taken for radiation dosimetry and the catheters are then loaded with a variety of isotopes that are temporarily left and removed or permanently left until they have emitted the prescribed dose to the periphery of the tumor. These same hollow plastic tubes also accommodate coaxial microwave antennae that may be used to interstitially heat the tumor (49). The isotopes used most commonly to interstitially irradiate brain tumors are Iodine-125 and Iridium-192 (35). The gamma photons emitted by Iridium-192 are more energetic than the soft characteristic x-rays emitted by Iodine-125 and consequently result in greater exposure to personnel than Iodine-125. Rupture of an Iodine-125 seed, on the other hand, is a possibility that does not exist for Iridium-192 which is in the form of wire. Other isotopes used to implant brain tumors are the beta emitting isotope Gold-198 and the neutron-emitting isotope Californium-252 (59).

Interstitial implants have been used primarily for brain tumors recurrent after previous surgery, external irradiation, and chemotherapy and more recently as part of the initial treatment by surgery and external irradiation. Gutin has reported tumor regression in 53% (18 of 34) of recurrent gliomas implanted with removable high activity Iodine-125 sources (26). Five patients required second craniotomy for the removal of focal radionecrosis of the brain and each of these patients improved after the craniotomy. Half of the patients with recurrent glioma were living after a median follow-up of 9 months. Further follow-up and comparison with patients whose recurrence is untreated are required to document the value of interstitial implantation for recurrent gliomas.

The Brain Tumor Study Group is currently conducting a trial to determine the value of interstitial implantation in addition to craniotomy, BCNU, and external irradiation for previously untreated malignant gliomas. No results have been reported, but it is hoped that interstitial boost will result in the cure of some malignant gliomas. Gutin cautions that focal radionecrosis may occur in a significant number of these cases, but is usually surgically manageable (26).

Efforts are underway to standardize the implantation procedure. A variety of approaches have been utilized. Some have subjected patients to two craniotomies, one for placement of catheters and a second for their removal. Others have implanted the tumor percutaneously under general anesthesia using a dedicated CT scanner to guide placement of the catheters. Most, however, have used a stereotactic frame to guide placement of the catheters. The problem has been to integrate the use of the frame with CT scanning to preplan the placement of the catheters and then to document their placement afterward for computerized dosimetry. Coffey and Friedman report a method whereby available computed tomographic imaging software is used with a standard radiotherapy treatment planning computer and the Brown-Roberts-Wells stereotactic system for preoperative imaging, brachytherapy catheter placement, and postoperative confirmation of radiation dosimetry (16).

BIOLOGICAL INTERACTIONS

Sparsely ionizing radiations such as gamma photons and x-rays interact with biological mediums to produce fast-moving electrons and free radicals while densely ionizing radiations such as neutrons interact with "knock on" protons. The production of free radicals by sparsely ionizing radiation is oxygen dependent while the production of "knock on" protons by neutrons is not. Free radicals, fast-moving electrons and "knock on" protons interrupt chemical bonds between the base pairs of DNA to damage the reproductive capacity of individual cells or clonogens. Once damaged, the individual cell or clonogen expresses lethality in one of three ways (*a*) immediate death, (*b*) postmitotic death or (*c*) giant cell formation. Cells undergoing mitosis are the most sensitive to radiation and experience immediate lysis or interphase death while those in nonmitotic phases of the cell cycle continue functioning and cycle once or several times before undergoing postmitotic death. A few undergo nuclear, but not cytoplasmic division, to form giant cells, a telltale sign that tissue has been irradiated. Since postmitotic cell death predominates there is a correlation between the rate of tumor regression and doubling time of the tumor, the latent period for the development of radiation injury, and the turnover rate of cells in the target tissue. Some rapidly dividing glioblastomas and sensitive germinomas regress quickly while the more slowly dividing low-grade astrocytomas and oligodendrogliomas shrink slowly for many months after irradiation. Some, like the cerebellar astrocytoma, show no observable change in size for many years after irradiation. Radiation damage to rapidly dividing epithelium of scalp and hair follicles becomes apparent during irradiation and is classified as an acute effect while damage to the slowly dividing oligodendroglia and endothelium of blood vessels results in radionecrosis of brain 12 to 24 months or many years after irradiation and is known as a late effect.

The development of in vitro clonogenic cell assays and the growth of human gliomas in the subcutaneous tissues of immune deficient mice permit quantitative measurements of clonogenic cell kill by radiation and drugs. In vitro studies of the biological effects of radiation on normal and neoplastic cells in the central nervous system have been hampered because of limited ability to culture these cells. The clonogenic capacity or mean colony forming efficiency ranges from 1.5% for meningiomas to 0.643% for malignant gliomas to 0.0165% for well-differentiated astrocytomas (65). Once the cells of a glioma are cultured in vitro or grown in vivo it should be theoretically possible to predict clinical response and provide rational guidance for the treatment of an individual tumor. Kornblith developed a microtoxicity assay (41) that predicted lack of response in five of five and response in six of nine patients whose gliomas were treated by radiation and 1,3-*bis*(2-chloro-ethyl)-1-nitrosourea (BCNU) (42). Because of the time required to complete the assay, the results were not available soon enough in the clinical course to be of value. Nonetheless, these assays have greatly increased our understanding of the biological effects of radiation and drugs on cells and tissues under normal and altered conditions. It is clear that (*a*) cell killing is logarithmic instead of linear, (*b*) each mammalian cell system has a characteristic survival curve whose individual parameters vary, (*c*) synchronized cells respond differently depending on the part of the division cycle they are in at the time of radiation or drug exposure, (*d*) cell killing by sparsely ionizing radiation is greater in the presence than the absence of oxygen, and (*e*) the shape of the survival curve and the degree of cell killing depend on the type of radiation. Such studies have also elucidated the processes of repair, regeneration, redistribution, and reoxygenation during fractionated radiotherapy.

The majority of gliomas persist after fractionated irradiation with or without chemotherapy and hence cell kill can be estimated by volumetric quantification of tumor on serial CT scans (50). Only the 25% of gliomas that disappear completely have clinically unquantifiable numbers of cells remaining. As many as 10^6 cells may remain when a tumor has disappeared and it is this clinically inapparent cell burden that accounts for the inevitable regrowth of most gliomas. Serial measurements of polyamines in cerebrospinal fluid have some value in predicting regrowth of medulloblastomas and measurement of serum antibodies to gliomas using the same microtoxicity assay used to predict clinical response to drugs may have some value in quantifying response to treatment. Even in the absence of a satisfactory marker to accurately quantitate cell kill in the host it is obvious that the degree of logarithmic cell killing by radiation and chemotherapy is insufficient to prevent the regrowth of most gliomas.

Study of individual parameters of radiation cell survival curves have provided clinically useful insights. An individual glioblastoma is composed of a heterogeneous population of clonogens (68) which have a radiosensitivity (Do) and capacity to repair sublethal radiation injury (Dq) that vary. Hence, the cells that remain after full-course irradiation are less radiosensitive and more capable of repairing sublethal injury than those that have been killed by radiation. Other agents that modify sublethal repair and enhance radiation injury or kill the cell by different mechanisms are needed.

Alteration of cells by various methods of synchronization led to the discovery that cells in the G2-M phase of the cell cycle are generally more sensitive to radiation than cells in the S or DNA synthetic phase while Go cells in resting phase are relatively unaffected by radiation and drugs. In vivo tritiated thymidine studies of recurrent glioblastomas have shown a cell cycling time of 2 to 3 days and a tumor doubling time of 4 to 7 days (31). The time it takes for 100 tumor cells to produce another 100 cells is longer than the cell cycle time would suggest because only about one-third of the tumor cells are actively proliferating at any one time. Strategies to selectively synchronize cycling cells and irradiate them at the "right time" along with methods of recruiting resting cells into the actively proliferating phase of the cell cycle would enhance and improve the efficiency of radiation cell kill.

The failure of radiation to eradicate gliomas has been largely presumed to be due to the oxygen effect, or the demonstration that cell killing by sparsely ionizing radiation is two and one-half to three times greater in the presence than the absence of oxygen. Oxygen is necessary for the production of free radicals which cause 60 to 70% of DNA strand breaks by sparsely ionizing radiation. The central necrosis of glioblastomas and the dictum that rapidly growing tumors outgrow their blood supply has long been observed, but only recently have direct measurements of decreased oxygen utilization been confirmed by positron emission tomography. Understanding that foci of hypoxic cells in tumors can limit their curability by x-rays has led to the development of a variety of clinical strategies including irradiation of patients under hyperbaric oxygenation, the use of chemical modifiers such as electron affinic hypoxic cell sensitizers, and densely ionizing radiations such as heavy ions and neutrons.

Cell killing is greater and repair of sublethal radiation injury and dependence on oxygenation is less with densely ionizing neutrons than sparsely ionizing x-rays and Cobalt-60 gamma photons. Presumably, densely ionizing radiations cause more direct irreparable damage to DNA than sparsely ionizing radiations. Indeed neutrons have eradicated many more glioblastomas than conventional photons but have failed to prolong the life of the host (45). Pathologic studies of brains irradiated by neutrons have shown central necrosis in the region of the major tumor mass, a few residual glioblastoma cells, and some edema and radiation effect in the surrounding brain. Demyelinization, apparent to some, has not been easy to identify because the oligodendroglia, although damaged, remain intact. They only die if the host lives long enough for them to divide and undergo postmitotic death. Original estimates of radiobiologic effect (RBE), the ratio of dose of 250 kVp x-rays to dose of fast neutrons to produce the same biological effect, were probably underestimates. Hornsey in a recent study of RBE for the central nervous system using neutrons from the Hammersmith cyclotron found an RBE of 5.2 instead of 3.0 to 3.5 used in previous clinical trials (30). She thought it likely that neutron doses in most clinical trials were above the tolerance of the normal brain. Estimates of RBE for these trials were obtained in biological systems other than the central nervous system such as skin and soft tissue. The amount of fat and hydrogenous content of these tissues is less than the central nervous system, and it is therefore not surprising that neutrons had a relatively greater effect on the fat-laden brain and spinal cord than on the tissues used to estimate RBE. Neutrons are attenuated by "knock on" protons and preferentially absorbed by fatty tissues with a high hydrogenous content.

Historical experience has taught us that maximum depopulation of a tumor with acceptable toxicity can best be achieved by giving sparsely ionizing radiation in small amounts over a long period. By using small daily doses and protracting the time to deliver the total dose it is possible to avoid acute desquamation of the scalp and achieve significant cell killing in gliomas. During fractionated irradiation of a tumor a number of important processes are simultaneously ongoing. While normal and neoplastic cells are damaged by radiation and die some undergo enzymatic repair of broken DNA cross-links and continue to divide and live. The enzymatic repair of sublethal damage occurs within a fairly short period, a matter of 3 to 4 hours after radiation is given. While cells in the more sensitive parts of the cell cycle are being damaged by radiation others continue to cycle and redistribute themselves into more sensitive phases of the cell cycle. If too much time is allowed to lapse between fractions of radiation, cells regenerate and tumor and normal tissues progressively repopulate, a phenomenon that is desirable for the normal tissues but not for the tumor. As a tumor shrinks during radiation hypoxic components are reoxygenated as the cell-to-capillary distance diminishes and they no longer reside beyond the physical limits of oxygen perfusion. Understanding just how the processes of repair, redistribution, regeneration, and reoxygenation operate to depopulate a tumor without damaging normal tissues is complex. The success of radiotherapy cannot be explained by a greater radiosensitivity of tumor cells than normal cells nor by a greater capacity for normal cells to repair sublethal injury than tumor cells because the Dos and Dqs of normal and neoplastic cells are comparable. It may be that fractionated radiation exploits differences in the kinetics of the cell populations being irradiated and depopulates the tumor more than the normal tissues or it may be that there are simply more normal cells than tumor cells. If that were the case, tumor cell kill might be the same or less than the normal tissue cell kill, and the total numbers of normal cells within and at the periphery of the radiation field would regrow to repopulate the normal tissues after radiation is complete. The tumor can regrow also if one or more clonogenic cells remain at completion of radiation. Such is the case with most gliomas.

FRACTIONATION

Division of the total dose of radiation into small daily increments is termed fractionation. Conventional fractionated radiotherapy delivers 1.8 to 2.0 Gy per day and 9.0 to 10 Gy per week to total doses of 50 to 60 Gy over 5 to 7 weeks. Unconventional forms of fractionation deliver the same total dose in shorter periods of time or deliver greater amounts of dose over the same period as conventional fractionation. *Hyperfractionation* delivers a total dose 10 to 20% greater than conventional fractionation over the same period using 2 to 4 daily fractions that are smaller than conventional fractions. *Accelerated fractionation* delivers the same total dose as conventional fractionation over a shorter period of time using 2 to 3 daily fractions of conventional size.

Accelerated fractionation is one strategy that would seem appropriate for a rapidly dividing tumor such as glioblastoma. With this strategy a total of 50 Gy might be delivered to the central nervous system in 14 treatment days over a period of 3 weeks using 2 daily fractions of 1.8 Gy each. Each daily fraction would be separated by an interval of 4 hours or greater to allow some repair of sublethal damage inflicted on rapidly dividing target cells such as scalp epithelium. The shorter interval between fractions reduces the opportunity for tumor cells to proliferate but might exacerbate the acute effects of radiation on the scalp and cause desquamation. Simpson conducted one of the earliest comparisons of conventional, hyperfractionated, and accelerated radiotherapy in glioblastomas (76). The patients were treated in a step-wise fashion using progressively higher doses over shorter periods of time and were monitored carefully for radionecrosis. The outcome of his dose and time-seeking study suggested an advantage for accelerated fractionation but was inconclusive because of the small numbers of patients in each fractionation category (Table 17.1). A number of fractionation studies have been compared to conventional fractionation since Simpson's original studies but none have used accelerated fractionation in the purest sense. The trials that have delivered the same total dose over shorter periods of time have used multiple daily fractions smaller than conventional size.

Hyperfractionation is another strategy that has theoretical advantages for glioblastoma. In this strategy the total radiation dose is 10 to 20% greater and is given in the same overall treatment time using 2 to 3 daily fractions that are smaller than conventional fractions. Radiation delivered in this manner is more likely to kill rapidly dividing tumor cells that redistribute themselves into more sensitive portions of the cell cycle than slowly dividing tumor cells that linger in less sensitive phases of the cell cycle. Unfortunately, the theoretical advantages of hyperfractionation have not been proven for glioblastoma. The Brain Tumor Study Group compared 1.1 Gy twice daily, 5 days/week to a total of 66 Gy in 6 weeks to 60 Gy in 30 to 35 conventional fractions over 6 weeks and found no difference in survival between the two groups (23). Both groups had craniotomy with debulking of tumor and BCNU in addition to radiation.

Payne compared conventional fractionation (50 Gy in 5 weeks, 2 Gy/day) to a hybridized form of hyper- and accelerated fractionation (36 to 40 Gy over 2 weeks using 4, 1-Gy fractions/day 3 hours apart) and found no difference in survival (63). All patients received CCNU (1-(2-chloroethyl)-3-cyclohexyl-1 nitrosourea) and hydroxyurea.

Shin compared conventional fractionation (50 Gy in 5 weeks, 2 Gy/day) to superfractionation (40 Gy in 3 weeks, 1 Gy 3 times daily plus a boost of 10 Gy in 5 fractions in 1 week) and found an advantage to superfractionation (73). One and 2-year actuarial survival rates were 54% and 21% for

TABLE 17.1.
Glioblastoma Multiforme One-Year Survival as Related to Fractionation[a]

Type of Fractionation	No. of Patients	Dose (Gy)	Time (Days)	Number	Fraction Size (Gy)	One-Year Survival (%)
Conventional	13	30	21	21	1.43	21
Hyper-	11	30	21	63	0.48	25
Accelerated	14	30	7	21	1.43	37
Conventional	7	40	28	28	1.43	0
Hyper-	9	40	28	84	0.48	12
Accelerated	11	40	9⅓	28	1.43	47
Conventional	23	40	21	21	1.90	18
Hyper-	22	40	21	63	0.63	28
Accelerated	24	40	7	21	1.90	44

[a]Reprinted with permission from Simpson, W.J. and Platt, M.E.: Fractionation study in the treatment of glioblastoma multiforme. Int. J. Radiat. Oncol. Biol. Phys., *1*:639–644, 1976.

the superfractionation group and 32% and 10% for the conventional fractionation group. Both treatment groups received CCNU. This trial is thus the first to confirm Simpson's original study showing an advantage to giving the total dose of radiation over shorter periods of time using multiple daily fractions.

VOLUME AND DOSE

When a radiotherapist sees a patient with a biopsy proven brain tumor he has to decide how much radiation to give and what to irradiate. The volume to be irradiated depends on whether the tumor is localized, multifocal or spreads to parts of the central nervous system distant from the site of origin. Most gliomas and well-differentiated tumors remain localized. Even the malignant astrocytomas and glioblastomas are generally localized. Only a small proportion, roughly 3% of glioblastomas are multifocal and require whole brain irradiation. It is now generally accepted that CT scans provide a reasonably accurate assessment of the gross and microscopic extent of glioblastoma. Hochberg found that CT scans correlated with the pathologic extent of glioblastomas at autopsy with a margin of 2 cm in 29 of 35 patients evaluated (28). The major source of error in the remaining patients was unsuspected subependymal spread. It is also known that magnetic resonance images provide the radiotherapist with an accurate assessment of tumor extent. Kelly has performed serial stereotactic biopsies of a variety of histopathologic types of glioma and correlated the presence of gross or infiltrating tumor with CT and magnetic resonance images (36). Necrosi, with foci of tumor are found in the central necrotic zone on CT; solid tumor is found in the zone of contrast enhancement on CT and infiltrating tumor between bundles of axons is seen in the edematous zone or region of decreased density around the tumor (17).

Kelly also demonstrated that tumor cells infiltrated to the periphery of the T2-weighted magnetic resonance image (36). He showed that the volume of the T2-weighted magnetic resonance image was significantly greater than the tumor volume defined by CT (Table 17.2). This finding has practical significance for the radiotherapist who has to define target volume. Magnetic resonance images generally demonstrate greater tumor extent than CT images and should be used whenever available to plan radiation fields. Generous local fields with 2 to 3 cm margins around a magnetic resonance image of the tumor are surely adequate for most gliomas, even the very malignant glioblastoma. Whole-brain irradiation should not any longer be considered mandatory for glioblastomas since most are localized and well-demonstrated by CT and MR images and since few are multifocal.

Those tumors that have a propensity to seed the subarachnoid space and implant in sites distant from the site of origin are generally poorly differentiated neuroecto-

TABLE 17.2.
Tumor Volume as Defined by Computed Tomography and Magnetic Resonance Images of Untreated Brain Tumors

Histopathology	Mean Calculated Tumor Volume (mm^3)		
	CT-CE	CT Hypodensity	T_2MRI
Grade 4 astrocytoma	27,768	63,264	71,853
Grade 3 astrocytoma	12,196	31,776	41,359
Grade 2 astrocytoma		16,252	47,038
Grade 4 mixed oligoastrocytoma	28,914	66,016	65,753
Grade 3 mixed oligoastrocytoma	22,776	34,221	55,619
Grade 2 mixed oligoastrocytoma		15,916	42,261
Grade 3 oligodendrogliomas	2,058	11,416	85,921
Grade 2 oligodendrogliomas		22,193	36,677
Grade 1 oligodendrogliomas		13,378	58,734
Mean	19,519	28,299	52,969

dermal tumors that primarily or secondarily involve the ventricular system. These include the medulloblastoma, ependymoblastoma, pineoblastoma, the suprasellar and pineal germinoma, the primitive yolk sac tumor, and the cerebellar glioblastoma. All of these tumors require craniospinal irradiation which is performed with multiple spliced fields or a single field at an extended distance from the source of radiation. Controversy surrounds the use of craniospinal irradiation for well-differentiated ependymomas and pineal tumors other than the pineoblastoma, the yolk sac tumor, and germinoma. The well-differentiated ependymoma, pinealoma, pineal teratoma, or glioma seldom seed and do not require prophylactic craniospinal irradiation. Pathologic documentation of tumor type is critical if the radiotherapist is to decide whether craniospinal irradiation is needed for all tumors in general and pineal tumors, in particular (53).

The radiation dose selected depends on the dose-response of the tumor and normal brain and is largely limited by the radiation tolerance of the normal brain. The maximum dose that can be safely delivered to the surrounding normal brain without risking radionecrosis is 54 to 55 Gy in 6 weeks (51). The radiotherapist should be conservative and not exceed these dose limits in patients with a good prognosis who are likely to live longer than 3 years, the period required for the majority of brain necroses to appear (43). Patients with low-grade astrocytomas, mixed gliomas, and oligodendrogliomas are likely to live a long time and should, therefore, be irradiated conservatively while patients with glioblastoma or an anaplastic glioma have a poor prognosis and might benefit as a group from more aggressive irradiation. It seems clear that the survival of glioblastoma patients is prolonged with increasing doses of radiation (82), (67) (Table 17.3) and it may also be true that accelerated fractionation prolongs the survival of patients with malignant gliomas (73). The best dose-response information available is for the patient with glioblastoma (82) since it is these patients that have been studied more extensively by clinical trial. Similar dose-response information needs to be accrued for a variety of intracranial neoplasms to enhance our understanding of how much radiation dose is necessary for tumor control in a sensitive neoplasm like the germinoma and how much will lead to an optimum outcome of maximum survival with acceptable toxicity in the remainder.

ACUTE AND LATE EFFECTS

An understanding of the acute and late effects of radiation on the transit tissues between the point of entry and the tumor is important because it is these effects that limit the delivery of radiation and determine how much can be safely given to the patient. The time it takes to develop an effect from radiation depends on the turnover rate of the target cell population, and the fact that postmitotic cell death is the predominant form of cell death. It is not until the cell cycles and tries to divide that lethality or radiation effect is noted. Hence, the effects of radiation on rapidly dividing cell populations such as scalp epithelium are noted acutely during the course of radiation while the effects on slowly dividing cell populations such as oligoden-

TABLE 17.3.
Glioblastoma Multiforme Median Survival as a Function of Radiation Dose

Author & Year	Median Dose (Gy)	Median Survival (wks)
Walker *et al.*, 1979	0	18
Walker *et al.*, 1979	32.5	13.5
Walker *et al.*, 1979	50	28.5
Walker *et al.*, 1979	55	36
Walker *et al.*, 1979	60	42
Salazar *et al.*, 1979	75	56

droglia are noted later after a period of months or years.

The acute effects of conventionally fractionated radiation on the scalp and cranial soft tissues are usually tolerated and seldom are severe enough to require interruption of treatment. Patients usually experience a dry red desquamation of the scalp, with epilation and occasionally experience swelling of cranial soft tissues on the side of the craniotomy, folliculitis, suturosis, swelling of ears, otitis externa, and/or otitis media (4). External irradiation can exacerbate swelling of brain around a tumor, cause headache, and require exogenous steroids to reduce swelling and pressure. Approximately 10% of patients with gliomas become steroid dependent and require steroids in the postirradiation period (50).

The acute and permanent effects of radiation on the scalp and cranial soft tissues can be reduced by using high energy x-rays alone or in combination with lower energy megavoltage beams. The use of high energy x-rays significantly reduces radiation dose to the superficial transit tissues which are located in the region of electronic build-up and, therefore, receive less than the maximum deposition of energy. Depending on the amount of high energy x-rays used and the reduction in dose-achieved, regrowth of hair after temporary epilation ranges from partial to complete. This reduction in dose can also significantly reduce the incidence of serious late effects on cranial soft tissues such as necrosis of scalp, bone exposure, and loss of the craniotomy skull flap. In one study, the systematic use of high energy x-rays to reduce dose to cranial soft tissues reduced the incidence of serious late effects from 21 to 9%. (56).

Acute swelling of brain is worse with large than small daily radiation doses and is best avoided by the use of steroids and radiation fractions in the usual therapeutic range of 1.8 to 3 Gy/day. Fractions of 6 Gy/day, several times weekly for melanoma are tolerated when given with steroids, but fractions greater than 6 Gy/day may cause severe swelling of brain and risk tentorial herniation of supratentorial contents.

In one study, 2 daily doses of 7.5 Gy caused headaches, nausea, vomiting, and temperature elevation in half the patients (86); in another study a single dose of 10 Gy caused five deaths in 54 patients within 2 to 7 days despite the concurrent use of steroids (27).

The late effects of radiation on the normal brain surrounding a tumor depend on total dose, fraction size, and the time over which the radiation is given. In a study of 337 patients who received 45 Gy or greater the risk of cerebral radionecrosis increased rapidly above a threshold dose of 54 Gy in 30 fractions over 42 days (55). The incidence of radionecrosis was 6% for a dose biologically equivalent to 60 Gy in 35 fractions over 49 days and 13% for a dose biologically equivalent to 60 Gy in 30 fractions over 42 days. The observed incidence of 13% for a dose of 60 Gy in 30 fractions exceeded the previously estimated incidence of 5 percent (43) for this dose and fractionation. In this same study the incidence of cerebral radionecrosis was reduced from 5 to 0% by reducing the dose to the brain an average of 7% from the early to the later part of the study (56). The brain is a sensitive biological dosimeter and should not receive more than 54 Gy in 30 fractions if the patient is likely to live 1 to 3 years, the period required for radionecrosis to appear. Suspicion of radionecrosis should be high in any patient who has received a high dose of radiation, neurologically deteriorates and develops a lesion adjacent to or distant from the site of the original tumor on CT scan. When the zone of necrosis is localized, repeat craniotomy and removal of the necrotic brain may improve and stabilize the patient's neurological condition, but when the necrosis is extensive, most patients irreversibly deteriorate, require nursing home care and ultimately die.

RESPONSE

Glioblastoma Multiforme

The value of ionizing radiation for glioblastoma multiforme is proven by clinical trial and observation. Neurological function after craniotomy and radiation improves in roughly half the patients, remains the same in 40% and worsens in approximately 10% (Table 17.4) (54). Serial CT scans after surgery and radiation correlate

TABLE 17.4.
Neurologic Function after Craniotomy and Radiation

Glioblastoma Multiforme		
Improved	Same	Worse
39/85 (46%)	34/85 (40%)	23/85 (14%)
Astrocytoma		
Improved	Same	Worse
22/39 (57%)	13/39 (33%)	4/39 (10%)

well with the patient's neurologic status, that is, if the patient improves, the CT scan generally shows regression or no change in lesion size (50). In the 10% of patients who neurologically deteriorate during radiation, CT scans invariably show enlargement of the tumor, edema, and mass effect. Altogether, craniotomy and radiation cause regression and improve neurologic function in the majority of patients. In the Scandinavian Study Group Trial, roughly three-quarters of all patients treated by surgery, radiation, and/or chemotherapy were able to care for themselves after the treatment and 23 of 80 (28%) were able to return to work (44). Two major clinical trials, one by the Brain Tumor Study Group (BTSG) (81) and the other by the Scandinavian Glioblastoma Study Group (SGSG) (44) showed that median survival was doubled by the addition of radiation to surgery (Table 17.5). The doses delivered to the whole brain were 45 Gy by the SGSG and 60 Gy by the BTSG. The tumors of all patients in the Scandinavian trial and roughly 85% of those in the BTSG trial were classified as glioblastoma multiforme; the remaining 15% in the BTSG trial had anaplastic astrocytomas. In each trial, age and functional status were comparable for the treatment groups and steroids were carefully monitored. Since these two carefully controlled studies obtained similar results, it seems safe to conclude that radiation doubles median survival and has significant value for patients with glioblastoma multiforme as well as for those with anaplastic astrocytoma.

Low-Grade Astrocytoma

The value of ionizing radiation for low-grade astrocytomas of the cerebrum, though unproven by clinical trial, is proven by clinical observation and comparison of irradiated patients with unirradiated historical controls. As with glioblastomas, ionizing radiation improves neurologic function in the majority of patients (Table 17.4) and causes regression of the majority of tumors on serial CT scans (54). Only a few patients, approximately 10%, deteriorate during treatment and exhibit increasing edema and mass effect on CT scans.

At Washington University, patients with astrocytoma were seldom referred for radiation after craniotomy before 1965, since most of the referring neurosurgeons doubted the value of radiation in addition to surgery (21). As the value of radiation in addition to surgery gained acceptance, patients with astrocytomas of the cerebrum were referred in greater numbers and it then became possible to compare those treated by surgery only with those treated by surgery and irradiation. Both the Washington University (21) and University of California, San Francisco (UCSF) series (47) showed that the addition of radiation to surgery doubled median survival (Table 17.6) and was most beneficial for those patients whose tumor was subtotally removed. At the 10-year point, however, the survival of the patients treated by surgery only and those treated by surgery plus radiation was equivalent (21) and thus it would appear that radiation does nothing more than delay regrowth of the tumor. The hypothesis that all low-grade astrocytomas eventually regrow is apparently incorrect since a cohort of 10 to 15% survive beyond

TABLE 17.5.
Glioblastoma Multiforme Median Survival after Surgery Alone (SA) and Surgery Plus Radiation (S & R)

	SA	S&R	*p* Value
BTSG	14 weeks	36 weeks	0.001
SGSG	5.2 months	10.8 months	

TABLE 17.6.
Astrocytoma of the Cerebrum: Five-Year Survival after Surgery Alone (SA) and Surgery Plus Radiation (S & R)

Reference		SA(%)	S & R(%)
(47)	UCSF	19	46
(21)	WASH U.	21	50

15 years from the time of diagnosis and parallel the survival of an age-matched normal population (46). Thus, it seems that radiation has a significant but temporary effect that lasts no more than 10 years for most patients with low-grade astrocytomas of the cerebrum while a small cohort of patients live for longer periods after treatment by surgery and radiation.

Young patients with low-grade astrocytomas of the cerebrum or those less than 20 years of age have a better prognosis than those who are older (46). Radiation should be used judiciously and cautiously in these patients since its value is unproven by clinical trial and since there is risk of radiation damage to the brain (57). Radiation should probably be avoided in the patient with the very well differentiated pilocytic astrocytoma of the cerebrum and the patient with a mural nodule of astrocytoma in a cyst that has been completely removed.

Oligodendroglioma (Mixed Glioma)

The value of ionizing radiation for mixed glioma, a tumor with a neoplastic mixture of glial elements usually astrocytic, oligodendrocytic and ependymal, is controversial, somewhat anecdotal and unproven by clinical trial. These are a very slowly growing group of tumors which exhibit a long interval between onset of symptoms (usually seizures) and diagnosis. After surgery and radiation, the median survival for mixed gliomas is on the order of 7 to 8 years while the median survival of 8 to 9 years for oligodendrogliomas is even longer (58). As might be expected, the slow rate of growth parallels a slow rate of regression following irradiation. There is little or no published information about the effect of radiation on the neurologic function and performance status of patients with mixed gliomas. The addition of radiation to surgery improved 5-year survival from 80 to 100% in one study (15) and from 31 to 85% in another (69). Another more recent study, however, did not show any improvement in survival with the addition of radiation to surgery for the slowly growing oligodendroglioma (10). The value of radiation for slowly growing tumors like the mixed glioma and oligodendroglioma is difficult to document because the tumors are uncommon, regress slowly, and require long periods of observation to document effect or change in rate of death. As with low-grade astrocytomas, which are more common and thoroughly studied than either mixed glioma or oligodendroglioma, radiation probably delays regrowth of the tumor.

Medulloblastoma

The value of ionizing radiation in addition to surgery for medulloblastoma is accepted and proven by one historically controlled study (32). The medulloblastoma is a primitive neuroectodermal tumor that grows rapidly, requires immediate neurosurgical intervention and postoperative radiation to prevent regrowth. These tumors frequently seed the subarachnoid space of the central nervous system distant from the site of origin and, therefore, require irradiation of the entire central nervous system. Only one study has compared local-field to craniospinal axis irradiation and that study showed a clear survival benefit to those who received extended-field irradiation of the central nervous system (32). Irradiation of these patients is technically difficult, requires great attention to detail, and careful monitoring of the patient. Postsurgical and preirradiation myelography has shown subarachnoid spinal seeding in approximately one-quarter of patients (19). These patients probably require a greater dose to the spine than those with undocumented subarachnoid seeding. It is critical to deliver the most radiation to the site of tumor origin in the posterior fossa since this is the region where most documented recurrences occur (6,75). Very seldom does tumor appear distant from the site of origin in the absence of recurrent tumor in the posterior fossa.

Ependymoma

The value of ionizing radiation for ependymoma is accepted but unproven. Ependymomas are unusual tumors that originate above and below the tentorium. Those above the tentorium seldom involve the ventricles and are predominantly parenchymal in location. Those below the tentorium often originate in the ventricle and frequently involve the cerebellum. The pathologic incidence of subarachnoid seeding is low (0 to 15%) and the clinical incidence is lower yet (4%) (52). Subarachnoid seeding occurs more commonly from ependymomas of the posterior fossa than ependymomas of the cerebrum probably because the posterior fossa ependymomas more commonly involve the ventricle and shed cells into the circulating cerebrospinal fluid. Poorly differentiated ependymomas or the rare ependymoblastoma more commonly seed than do the well-differentiated tumors which exhibit rosette formation by light microscopy (71). Hence, local field irradiation is all that is required for the majority of ependymomas and craniospinal axis irradiation need only be utilized for those with a propensity to seed. Regression of tumor and improvement in neurologic function are poorly documented and no historically controlled or published clinical trials show that radiation improves survival. Five-year survival is 35% for ependymomas of the cerebrum and 59% for posterior fossa ependymomas treated by surgery and irradiation (52).

Pineal Region Tumors

The value of ionizing radiation for pineal region tumors is accepted but unproven by clinical trial comparing observation to treatment by irradiation. Pineal tumors are histologically a diverse group of tumors, some of which shed cells into the adjacent third ventricle and spread to other parts of the central nervous system. The tumors that have a propensity for subarachnoid seeding are the germinomas which comprise approximately one-half of pineal tumors, the very primitive yolk sac tumor, and pineoblastoma (53). It is these tumors that require craniospinal irradiation, while all the better differentiated pineocytomas, teratomas, and gliomas do not. Now that the mortality of operating on pineal tumors has been reduced to acceptable levels, it is important to biopsy them and obtain a tissue diagnosis to determine which require craniospinal axis irradiation and which do not (14). A tissue diagnosis is preferable to a short trial of irradiation and a repeat scan to determine rate of regression in order to decide to do craniospinal irradiation for those that regress rapidly and to do local-field irradiation for those that do not. Irradiation causes regression of tumor and neurologic improvement in the majority of cases, but this anecdotal observation needs better documentation. Many pineal region tumors, particularly the germinoma, are cured by radiation while 5-year survival for all histologies taken together ranges from 60 to 70% (33).

Suprasellar Germinoma

The value of ionizing radiation for suprasellar germinoma is proven by clinical observation. Clinical trial is unnecessary since the majority of these patients are cured of their tumor by craniospinal irradiation (66). Sung documented that 57% of histologically documented germinomas seeded the spinal subarachnoid space following local field irradiation (78). Consequently, craniospinal irradiation should be used in all cases. Germinomas are very sensitive to irradiation and probably require no more than 45 Gy over a 5-week period. One recently published series of nine patients treated in the same institution over a 10-year period documented tumor control with doses that did not exceed 45 Gy (20). Further dose-seeking studies to establish the lower limits of radiation dose required to cure this tumor are needed. Ionizing radiation causes complete regression of suprasellar germinomas and improves or stabilizes neurologic function in the host. The more extensive germinomas frequently result in endocrine and electrolyte imbalances that may be life threatening if not monitored closely during the follow-up period.

Cerebellar Astrocytoma

The value of ionizing radiation for cerebellar astrocytoma is unproven by clinical trial or observation. As a group, these are very slow growing neoplasms that have been characterized as benign, self-limiting malformations when, in fact, a few do regrow following surgical removal and result in the demise of the host. To determine which cerebellar astrocytomas are likely to regrow and require irradiation, a long-term study of 96 cerebellar astrocytomas treated between 1928 and 1976 at Barnes Hospital was undertaken (21a). On the average, those that regrew did so 8.5 years after surgical extirpation. A study of those followed a minimum of 8.5 years showed that the risk of tumor regrowth was greatest among those who had incomplete removal of a solid cerebellar astrocytoma. Those who had complete removal of a solid tumor or those who had incomplete or total removal of a cystic tumor seldom regrew (Table 17.7). A second and third craniotomy with removal of additional tumor frequently improved or stabilized the patient's neurologic condition and added many additional years of life. Long-term survival of those with incompletely removed solid tumors was significantly worse than the remaining patients with completely removed solid tumors or cystic tumors. A few patients with incompletely removed or recurrent tumors were irradiated, but in no instance was it possible to document that radiation caused regression or delayed regrowth of tumor or improved the neurologic condition of the host.

Brain Stem Glioma

The value of ionizing radiation for brain stem glioma is accepted, proven by clinical observation and unproven by clinical trial. Brain stem gliomas are seldom biopsied since they are diffusely infiltrating and attempts at removal are associated with significant mortality. The patients instead are referred to radiotherapy and irradiated based on their clinical presentation and radiographic evidence of a brain stem lesion. Pneumoencephalography was still required for the diagnosis of some brain stem gliomas, even after the advent of noninvasive computed tomography. Only with the advent of magnetic resonance imaging has it been possible to eliminate pneumoencephalography and to selectively demonstrate brain stem lesions with a high degree of accuracy. Generous local field irradiation is sufficient and whole brain irradiation is not required even though half of these patients are ultimately proven at autopsy to harbor a high-grade malignant glioma (37). Radiation improves neurologic signs and symptoms in three-quarters and leads to long-term survival in one-third of the patients (24). The subset of patients with pontine lesions fare somewhat worse than those with brainstem lesions and children do worse than adults.

TABLE 17.7.
Regrowth of Cerebellar Astrocytoma according to Morphology of Tumor and Degree of Surgical Removal (39)

Regrowth	Subtotal Solid	Subtotal Cystic	Total Solid	Total Cystic
No	20	6	12	27
Yes	11	3	0	1

Thalamic Glioma

The value of ionizing radiation for thalamic gliomas is also accepted and proven by clinical observation. Thalamic gliomas like brainstem gliomas are generally referred to radiotherapy unbiopsied and irradiated on the basis of clinical findings and radiographic evidence of a thalamic lesion. The contralateral weakness that results from involvement of the corticospinal fibers in the adjacent internal capsule generally improves during the course of irradiation. Neurologic improvement coincides with regression of tumor on serial CT scans in the majority of cases and approximately 40% of patients survive 5 years and beyond (24). The outcome of irradiating thalamic gliomas, therefore, is somewhat better than it is for brainstem gliomas.

Optic Nerve Gliomas

The value of ionizing radiation for optic nerve gliomas is controversial but supported by some clinical observations. Some optic gliomas are histologically benign, very slow growing, and respond poorly to irradiation. Others are more aggressive, rapidly growing, and destructive. Generally speaking, those associated with von Recklinghausen's disease that have produced minimal fusiform swelling of the optic nerves and chiasm can be safely observed and may not require treatment. The more rapidly growing optic gliomas that obtain significant size, however, should be treated to preserve vision and stabilize neurologic function. Extirpation of bulky gliomas of the prechiasmatic portion of the optic nerves is unnecessary as irradiation frequently causes regression of tumor, reduces proptosis, and stabilizes vision. Partial extirpation of bulky optic gliomas originating from the chiasm is advised along with postoperative irradiation for residual glioma to preserve remaining vision and stabilize neurologic function. The rare optic tract glioma also responds well to irradiation. Preirradiation cerebral arteriography is advised, particularly in children with von Recklinghausen's disease, as these patients often have associated arterial malformations (Moya-Moya disease) that predispose them to vascular thrombosis, rupture and cerebral hemorrhage. Irradiation is beneficial for optic gliomas, but needs to be used cautiously and given in small amounts over long periods since many of the patients are children and are more susceptible to radiation injury than adults.

Pituitary Adenomas

The value of ionizing radiation for pituitary adenomas is proven by clinical observation and historically controlled studies, but unproven by clinical trial. Pituitary adenomas are a very slow growing group of benign tumors which gradually destroy the sella turcica and compress the optic nerves and adjacent central nervous system. These tumors may or may not secrete a variety of polypeptide hormones which act systemically to produce well-recognized clinical syndromes such as acromegaly and Cushing's disease. Other nonsecreting adenomas selectively destroy the ability of the normal pituitary to secrete baseline levels of hormones required for normal bodily functions resulting in various degrees of hypopituitarism. Microadenomas of the pituitary may be removed by transphenoidal procedures and require nothing more than observation (9). Larger pituitary adenomas that are incompletely removed or require transcranial surgery for their removal are generally referred for postoperative irradiation. Very few of these regrow after doses of 45 to 50 Gy in 5 to 5.5 weeks and if they do, they require many years to do so. Grigsby reported that the median time to recurrence after surgery and radiation for large pituitary adenomas was 10 years (25). Acromegalics who have persistent elevation of growth hormone following surgery are often referred for postoperative irradiation. Radiation effectively reduces the output of growth hormone over a 2- to 3-year period in 80% of patients (70). Radiation is also effective for the intact or incompletely removed ACTH secreting adenoma; hypercortisolism is corrected in 50% of adults (62) and 80% of children (34). Radiation seems less effective against the intact or partially removed prolactinoma than other secreting adenomas; prolactin levels are reduced to the normal range in only one-third of these patients (72). Besides reducing hormonal secretion, radiation also improves or stabilizes vision in three-quarters of patients who present with visual deficit (25). Vision seldom returns to normal, however, unless surgery has been performed before the radiation. Patients who have undergone surgery and radiation develop hypopituitarism in 60 to 80% of cases and require exogenous thyroxin, cortisone, and testosterone. Radiation alone seems just as effective as surgery and radiation for those patients with secreting or nonsecreting adenomas who either refuse or are unable to undergo surgery (70). Long-term studies have shown that the survival of nonacromegalic patients with pituitary adenoma is equivalent to the survival of age-matched controls following treatment by radiation and/or surgery (25). Acromegalic patients do not survive as long as age matched controls and there is no evidence thus far that treatment by surgery and radiation improves their survival though it is clear that diabetes and other systemic manifestations of acromegaly are easier to manage.

Craniopharyngioma

The value of ionizing radiation is proven by clinical observation for selected patients with craniopharyngioma and unproven by clinical trial. External beam irradiation, though it may cause temporary regression of an intact craniopharyngioma is generally unable to eradicate one of these very slowly growing benign tumors. If the craniopharyngioma can be totally removed, then radiation, in addition to surgery, is not required (3). If, on the other hand, a craniopharyngioma is incompletely removed, the use of radiation significantly delays or prevents regrowth of the tumor. Rather than attempt total removal in all cases, and risk irreversible neurologic damage to the visual system and adjacent hypothalamus and significant mortality, many neurosurgeons remove as much tumor as is safely possible and then give postoperative irradiation. Conservative surgical removal and postoperative external beam irradiation significantly reduce mortality, improve neurological outcome and effectively control these tumors just as well as total removal (8). Installation of P-32 into a recurrent craniopharyngioma cyst is occasionally successful.

Meningioma

The value of ionizing radiation for incompletely removed, recurrent, and malignant meningiomas has been proven by clinical observation, but not by clinical trial. The more aggressive meningiomas, the angioblastic and malignant variants, tend to recur, despite gross surgical removal and should be routinely irradiated. There is an intermediate group which exhibits pleomorphism, some necrosis, and mitotic activity that is sometimes classified as an atypical variant; these tumors are more aggressive than benign meningotheliomatous, transitional, psammomatous, and fibroblastic variants of meningioma and recur if incompletely removed. Incomplete removal is more common for those located in the olfactory groove, sphenoid ridge, parasellar region, floor of the middle cranial fossa, parasagittal region, and tentorium. The addition of radiation following incomplete removal of a benign meningioma reduces the recurrence rate from 60 to 32% (5). Long-term follow-up is required as these are slowly growing tumors that take considerable time to regrow. A few unresectable meningiomas have been preoperatively irradiated and later resected (85). Carella has presented serial CT scans before and after irradiation that showed regression of some meningiomas and growth arrest of others (11). Information such as this has clearly demonstrated the value of irradiation for incompletely removed, recurrent, and malignant meningiomas.

CHEMICAL ADDITIVES

Chemotherapeutic agents, like radiation, exert cell kill, shrink malignant gliomas, and delay their regrowth. The degree of cell killing and prolongation of the progression-free interval is less with drugs than radiation. Nonetheless, it is clear that chemotherapeutic agents, in particular, the nitrosoureas, benefit patients whose gliomas have regrown after surgery and radiation and provide marginal benefit to patients when initially given in addition to surgery and radiation. Response rates of 25 to 40% are noted when nitrosoureas are given to patients with gliomas, persistent or recurrent, following surgery and radiation. The nitrosoureas, in addition to surgery and radiation, have been shown by clinical trial to extend life on the order of several weeks (83). This achievement, though significant, is much less than radiation which doubles survival when given in addition to surgery (Table 17.8). Neither modality alone or in combination is capable of eradicating all of the clonogens that remain after craniotomy for a malignant glioma. The amounts of radiation and chemotherapeutic agents that may be safely given to the host are limited by the tolerance of the normal brain in the case of radiation and the tolerance of the hematopoietic system, liver, lungs, and kidneys in the case of chemotherapeutic agents. The use of hydroxyureas and autologous marrow transplantation has not effectively extended life and has merely defined the dose limits for organ systems other than the bone marrow (29).

Some chemotherapeutic agents, like hydroxyurea have been shown to modify the response of cells in vitro to the effects of radiation (77). Hydroxyurea impairs the ability of cells to repair sublethal injury to irradiation, but has yet to show clinical benefit for patients with malignant gliomas. The one clinical trial performed by Levin *et al.* showed a marginal, but insignificant benefit when hydroxyurea was given in addition

TABLE 17.8.
Malignant Glioma Trials

Group	Treatment	Patients	Median Survival Rate
BTSG (81)	Supportive	222	14 weeks
	BCNU		19 weeks
	Radiation		36 weeks
	Radiation and BCNU		35 weeks
BTSG (83)	Me CCNU	467	31 weeks
	Radiation		37 weeks
	Radiation and BCNU		49 weeks
	Radiation and methyl CCNU		43 weeks
BTSG (22)	Radiation and BCNU	609	50 weeks
	Radiation and procarbazine		43 weeks
	Radiation and methylprednisone		41 weeks
	Radiation, BCNU, and methylpred.		41 weeks
RTOG (13)	60 Gy in 6–7 weeks	626	9.9 months
	70 Gy in 7–8 weeks		8.4 months
	60 Gy and BCNU		10.0 months
	60 Gy, Methyl CCNU, and DTIC		9.8 months
NCOG (48)	Radiation and BCNU	99	31 weeks
	Radiation, BCNU, and hydroxyurea		41 weeks

to radiation and BCNU (48). The study was probably inconclusive due to the limited number of patients entered. The ability of some chemotherapeutic agents to potentiate the effects of radiation in vitro has yet to be demonstrated in the host. It is likely that the marginal benefit we see with the use of chemotherapeutic agents is due to additive cell kill.

PHYSICAL AND CHEMICAL MODIFIERS

Hyperbaric Oxygen

Cell killing by sparsely ionizing radiation is clearly oxygen dependent, and this fact was the basis for the hyperbaric oxygen trial performed by Chang *et al.* at Columbia Presbyterian Hospital in New York (12). The study was logistically difficult to perform because the patients had to be irradiated while in a hyperbaric chamber. The experimenters initially used fewer and larger size radiation fractions and later used conventional fractionation. Median survival of those irradiated in the hyperbaric chamber was significantly greater than for control patients, but ultimately, the survival curves came together and no long-term benefit was realized. In the end the malignant glioma overcame an heroic technical effort to cure it.

Hypoxic Cell Radiosensitizers

In 1963, Adams and Dewey published experimental results showing that the nitroimidazoles were able to replace oxygen and sensitize hypoxic cells to the effects of radiation (1). These compounds are electron-affinic radiosensitizers that enhance the effects of radiation by factors ranging from 1.3 to 1.7. They reach peak serum levels within a period of 2 to 3 hours and equilibrate with the central nervous system within 4 to 6 hours of administration. Biopsies of normal brain and gliomas have demonstrated levels that are 80 to 90% of serum levels (80). The principle side effects are peripheral neuropathy, gastrointestinal disturbance, and occasionally central nervous system toxicity manifested by convulsions and psychosis. Dose-seeking studies have established that the incidence of peripheral neuropathy becomes unacceptable when the dose of misonidazole exceeds 12 gm/m^2 (84). To take advantage of a drug which may be given in limited amounts on a weekly or biweekly basis, most investigators have designed unconventional fractionation regimens and have utilized large fractions concurrently with the nitroimadazole (Table 17.9). Unfortunately, many of the studies are flawed because conventional instead of unconventional fractionation was utilized for the control arm; thus it is not possible to determine if any observed differences were due either to the unconventional fractionation or to the addition of the radiosensitizer. To avoid the effects of large fractions of irradiation on the central nervous system investigators have utilized multiple small doses of misonidazole combined with conventional fractionated radiotherapy (2). This approach avoids the risk of radiation injury to the brain, but may not demonstrate the value of the radiosensitizer due to the natural reoxygenation that occurs during multifractionated irradiation (18).

Metronidazole was the first radiosensitizer reported to be effective for malignant astrocytomas (79). The median survival of 15 weeks reported for the control arm was unusually short and not at all comparable to the usual median survival of 36 to 40 weeks that results after surgery and conventional fractionated radiotherapy. Nonetheless, the administration of metronidazole 4 hours before a large fraction of radiation (3.35 Gy) 3 times weekly over a period of 3 weeks significantly improved median survival.

Misonidazole is a more effective radiosensitizer than metronidazole on an equal molar basis and has, therefore, been used in most clinical trials. The fractionation schedules utilized for the experimental and control arms and the outcome of the misonidazole trials are shown in Table 17.9. Aside from the Vienna Trial, no group has been able to demonstrate a significant improvement in survival with the addition of misonidazole (40). The improved result in the Vienna trial may have been due to an unequal distribution of prognostic variables between treatment groups.

Halogenated Pyrimadines

Bromodeoxyuridine (BUdR) and iododeoxyuridine (IUdR) are known to enhance the effects of radiation on bacteria and are theoretically capable of enhancing the effects of radiation on tumor cells. Phase I and II trials have investigated the best method of administration. Continuous infusion with doses of 1.5 gm/m^2 over 24 hours have resulted in thrombocytopenia, leukopenia, and a maculopapular rash (64). Doses of 1 gm/m^2 over 24 hours have been better tolerated and can be given over a period of 2 weeks (38). Intraarterial administration is particularly attractive since high concentrations of the drug can be delivered directly to the central nervous system. Clinical trials testing the value of the halogenated pyrimadines have yet to be performed.

SUMMARY

To date, no modality of treatment, including ionizing radiation has proven more effective against tumor than normal cells. Both neoplastic and normal cells are affected simultaneously and the amount of the treatment modality given is limited by its effect on the normal tissues. Consequently, one is unable to totally depopulate a tumor without irreversibly damaging the normal tissues. In the case of radiation, it is the brain that limits delivery of curative doses and in the case of chemical additives, it is other organ systems, such as bone marrow, liver, lung, kidneys, and peripheral nerves. The amounts of sparsely and densely ionizing radiation that can be given with safety have been documented with a fair degree of accuracy as have the doses of the nitrosoureas, nitroimadazoles, and other chemical additives. Interstitial implantation of the brain with radioactive sources and the generation of heat with microwave antennae are likewise limited by the tolerance of the normal brain to the effects of radiation and heat. Thus the major obstacle in the treatment of malignant gliomas is our inability to preferentially affect the tumor with the modalities available. Current methods of localizing ionizing radiation, drugs, and heat are crude and need to be developed to the point that it is possible to directly target the neoplastic cell without affecting so many of the adjacent normal cells.

TABLE 17.9.
Summary of Randomized Trials to Study the Value of Misonidazole for Malignant Gliomas

Group	Fractionation: Control (M W F)	Fractionation: Misonidazole (M) (M W F(M))	Dose (gm/m²)	Median Survival Controls vs. Misonidazole
Cambridge (7)	2.94 Gy 2.94 Gy 5.0 Gy 43.52 Gy 12 F/4 weeks 2.02 Gy M, Tu, W, Th, F 56.56 Gy 28 F5.5 weeks M (M)Th	2.94 Gy 2.94 Gy 5.0 Gy 43.52 Gy 12 F/4 weeks M (M)Th	12	31 weeks vs. 39 weeks 38 weeks vs. 39 weeks
Vienna (40)	1, 2, 8 weeks 4.0 Gy 4.00 Gy 3–7 weeks 1.7 Gy ×5 66.50 Gy 31 F/8 weeks	1, 2, 8 weeks 4.0 Gy 4.00 Gy 3–7 weeks 1.7 Gy × 5 66.50 Gy F/8 weeks M (M) T Th F	13.5	8.7 months vs. 15.5 months
RTOG (61)	1.7 to 2 Gy/day × 5 60 Gy/30–35 F/6–7 weeks BCNU days 3, 4, and 5 8 weeks	4.0 Gy 1.5 Gy 1.5 Gy 1.5 Gy 1.8 Gy × 5 7th week 60 Gy/29 F/7 weeks BCNU days 3, 4, and 5 q. 8 weeks M(M) T W Th(M) F	15	55 weeks vs. 46 weeks
BTSG (23)	1.7 to 2 Gy/day × 5 60 Gy/30–35 F/6–7 weeks BCNU 3, 4, and 5 q. 8 weeks	1.7 to 2 Gy/day × 5 60 Gy/30–35 F/6–7 weeks BCNU 3, 4, and 5 q. 8 weeks	18	40 weeks vs. 40 weeks
(74)	58 Gy/30 F/6 weeks 61.41 Gy/69 F/4.5 weeks (0.89 Gy 3 × daily) CCNU at recurrence	61.41 By/69 F/4.5 weeks (0.89 Gy 3 × daily) CCNU at recurrence		27 weeks vs. 49 weeks 57 weeks vs. 49 weeks

REFERENCES

1. Adams, G.E. and Dewey, D.L. Hydrated electrons and radiobiological sensitization. Biochem. Biophys. Res. Commun., *12:*473–477, 1963.
2. Ang, K.K., Van Der Schueren, E., Notter, G. *et al.* Split course multiple daily fractionated radiotherapy schedule combined with misonidazol for the management of grade III and IV gliomas: a pilot feasibility study of the radiotherapy group of the EORTC. Int. J. Radiat. Oncol. Biol. Phys., *8:*1657–1664, 1982.
3. Amacher, A.L. Craniopharyngioma: the controversy regarding radiotherapy in children. Child's Brain, *6:*57–64, 1980.
4. Baglan, R.J. and Marks, J.E. Soft tissue reactions following irradiation of primary brain and pituitary tumors. Int. J. Radiat. Oncol. Biol. Phys., *7:*455–459, 1981.
5. Barbaro, N.M., Gutin, P.H., Wilson, C.B. *et al.* Radiation therapy in the treatment of partially resected meningiomas. J. Neurosurg., *20 (4):*525–528, 1987.
6. Berry, M.P., Jenkin, R.D.T., Keane, T.W. *et al.* Radiation treatment for medulloblastoma: a 21-year review. J. Neurosurg., *55:*43–51, 1981.
7. Bleehan, N.W., Wiltshire, G.R., Plowman, P.N., *et al.* A randomized study of misonidazol and radiotherapy for grade 3 and 4 cerebral astrocytoma. Br. J. Cancer, *43:*436–442, 1981.
8. Bloom, H.J.G. Intracranial tumors: response and resistance to therapeutic endeavors. Int. J. Radiat. Oncol. Biol. Phys., *8:*1083–1113, 1982.
9. Boggan, J.E., Tyrrell, J.B., and Wilson, G. Transphenoidal microsurgical management of Cushing's disease: report of 100 cases. J. Neurosurg., *59:*195–200, 1983.
10. Bullard, D., Rawlings, C.E., Phillips, B. *et al.* Oligodendroglioma: an analysis of the value of radiation therapy. Cancer, *60:*2179–2188, 1987.
11. Carella, R.J., Ransohoff, J., and Newall, J. Role of radiation therapy in the management of meningioma. J. Neurosurg., *10:*332–339, 1982.
12. Chang, C.H. Hyperbaric oxygen as a radiation sensitizer in treatment of malignant gliomas. In: *Tumors of the Central Nervous System. Modern Radiotherapy in Multidisciplinary Management,* edited by C.H. Chang and E.M. Housepian, pp. 23–30. New York, Mason Publishing, 1982.
13. Chang, C.H., Horton, J., Schoenfeld, D., *et al.* Comparison of postoperative radiotherapy and combined postoperative radiotherapy and chemotherapy in the multidisciplinary management of malignant gliomas—a joint radiation therapy oncology and eastern cooperative oncology group study. Cancer, *52:*997–1007, 1983.
14. Chapman, P.H. and Linggood, R.M. The management of pineal tumors: a recent reappraisal. Cancer, *46:*1253–1257, 1980.
15. Chin, H.W., Hazel, J.J., Kim, T.H., *et al.* Study of oligodendrogliomas. Cancer, *45:*1458–1466, 1980.
16. Coffey, R.J. and Freidman, W.A. Interstitial brachytherapy of malignant brain tumors using computed tomography-guided stereotaxis and available imaging software: technical report. J. Neurosurg., *20:*4–7, 1987.
17. Daumas-Duport, C., Scheithauer, B.W., and Kelly, P.J. A histologic and cytologic method for the spatial definition of gliomas. Mayo Clin. Proc. *62:*435–449, 1987.
18. Denekamp, J., McNally, N.J., Fowler, J.F., *et al.* Misonidazol in fractionated radiotherapy: are many small fractions best? Br. J. Radiol., *53:*981–990, 1980.
19. Deutsch, M. and Reigel, D.H. Myelography and cytology in the treatment of medulloblastoma. Int. J. Radiat. Oncol. Biol. Phys. *7:*721–725, 1981.
20. Fields, J.V., Fulling, K.H., Thomas, P.R.M., *et al.* Suprasellar germinomas: radiation therapy. Radiology *164:*247–249, 1987.
21. Garcia, D., Fulling, K., and Marks, J.E. The value of radiation therapy in addition to surgery for astrocytomas of the adult cerebrum. Cancer *55:*917–919, 1985.
21a. Garcia, D.M., Marks, J.E., Latifi, H.R., and Kliefoth, A. Childhood cerebellar astrocytomas: is there a role for post-operative irradiation? Int. J. Radiat. Oncol. Biol. Phys., *18:*815–818, 1990.
22. Green, S.B., Byar, D.P., Walker, M.D., *et al.* Comparisons of carmustine, procarbazine, and high-dose methylprednisolone as additions to surgery and radiotherapy for the treatment of malignant glioma. Cancer Treat. Rep. *67:* 121–132, 1983.
23. Green, S.B., Byar, D.P., Strike, T.A., *et al.* Randomized comparisons of BCNU, streptozotocin, radiosensitizer, and fractionation in the postoperative treatment of malignant glioma (study 7702). Proc. Am. Soc. Clin. Oncol. *3:*260 (Abstr)1984a.
24. Grigsby, P.W., Thomas, P.R.M., Schwartz, H.G., *et al.* Irradiation of primary thalamic and brainstem tumors in a pediatric population: a thirty-three year experience. Cancer *60:*2901–2906, 1987.
25. Grigsby, P.W., Stokes, S., Marks, J.E., *et al.* Prognostic factors and results of radiotherapy alone in the management of pituitary adenomas. Int. J. Radiat. Oncol. Biol. Phys., *15:*1103–1110, 1988.
26. Gutin, P.H., Phillips, T.L., Wara, W.M., *et al.* Brachytherapy of recurrent malignant brain tumors with removable high-activity iodine-125 sources. J. Neurosurg., *60:*61–68, 1984.
27. Hindo, W.A., DeTrana, F.A. III, Lee, M.S., *et al.* Large dose increment irradiation in treatment of cerebral metastases. Cancer *26:*138–141, 1970.
28. Hochberg, F.H. and Pruitt, A. Assumptions in the radiotherapy of glioblastoma. Neurology *30:* 907–911, 1980.

29. Hochberg, F.H., Parker, L.M., Takoorian, T., *et al.* High dose BCNU with autologous bone marrow rescue for recurrent glioblastoma multiforme. J. Neurosurg. *54:*455–460, 1981.
30. Hornsey, S., Morris, C.C., Myers, R., *et al.* Relative biological effectiveness for damage to the central nervous system by neutrons. Int. J. Radiat. Oncol. Biol. Phys. *7:*185–189, 1981.
31. Hoshino, T., Wilson, C.B., Rosenblum, M.L., *et al.* Chemotherapeutic implications of growth fraction and cell cycle time in glioblastomas. J. Neurosurg. *43:*127–135, 1975.
32. Jenkin, R.D.T. Medulloblastoma in childhood: radiation therapy. Can. Med. Asso. J. *100:*51–53, 1969.
33. Jenkin, R.D.T., Simpson, W.J.K., and Keen, C.W. Pineal and suprasellar germinomas: results of radiation treatment. J. Neurosurg. *48:*99–107, 1978.
34. Jennings, A.S., Liddle, G.W., and Orth, D.N. Results of treating childhood Cushing's Disease with pituitary irradiation. N. Eng. J. Med. *297:*957–962, 1977.
35. Kelly, P.J., Olson, M.H., and Wright, A.W. Stereotactic implantation of iridium-192 into CNS neoplasms. Surg. Neurol. *10:*349–354, 1978.
36. Kelly, P.J., Shapiro, J.R., Daumas-Dupport, C., Kispert, D.B., *et al.* Image-based stereotaxic serial biopsies in untreated intracranial neoplasms. J. Neurosurg. *66:*865–874, 1987.
37. Kim, T.H., Chin, H., Pollan, S., *et al.* Radiotherapy of primary brain-stem tumors. Int. J. Radiat. Oncol. Biol. Phys. *6:*51–57, 1980.
38. Kinsella, T.J., Russo, A., Mitchell, J.B., *et al.* The use of prolonged constant intravenous infusions of bromodeoxyuridine (BUdR) as a radiosensitizier. J. Clin. Oncol. *2:*1144–1150, 1984.
39. Deleted in proof.
40. Kogelnik, H.D., Karcher, K.H., Szepsi, T., *et al.* High dose irradiation and misonidazol in the treatment of malignant gliomas: a preliminary report. In: *Progress in Radio-oncology II,* edited by K.A. Karcher, pp. 189–195. New York, Raven Press, 1982.
41. Kornblith, P.L., Pollock, L.A., Coakham, H.B., *et al.* Cytotoxic antibody responses in astrocytoma patients. J. Neurosurg. *51:*47–52, 1979.
42. Kornblith, P.L., Smith, B.H., Leonard, L.A. Response of cultured human brain tumors to nitrosoureas: correlation clinical data. Cancer, *46:*255–265, 1981.
43. Kramer, S., Southard, M.E., and Mansfield, C.M. Radiation effect and tolerance of the central nervous system. Front. Radiat. Therapy Oncol. *4:*332–345, 1972.
44. Kristiansen, K., Hagen, S., Kollevold, T., *et al.* Combined modality therapy of operated astrocytomas Grade III and IV, confirmation of the value of postoperative irradiation, and lack of potentiation of bleomycin on survival time. Cancer *47:*649–652, 1981.
45. Laramore, G.E., Griffin, T.W., Gerdes, A.T., *et al.* Fast neutron and mixed (neutron/photon) beam teletherapy for Grades III and IV astrocytomas. Cancer *42:*96–103, 1978.
46. Laws, E.R., Taylor, W.F., Clifton, M.B., *et al.* Neurological management of low-grade astrocytomas of the cerebral hemispheres. J. Neurosurg. *61:*665–673, 1984.
47. Leibel, S.A., Sheline, G.E., Wara, W., *et al.* The role of radiation therapy in the treatment of astrocytomas. Cancer *35:*1551–1557, 1975.
48. Levin, V.A., Wilson, C.B., Davis, R., *et al.* A phase III comparison of BCNU, hydroxyurea, and radiation therapy to BCNU and radiation therapy for treatment of primary malignant gliomas. J. Neurosurg. *51:*526–532, 1979.
49. Lyons, B.E., Britt, R.H., and Strohbehn, J.W. Localized hyperthermia in the treatment of malignant brain tumors using an interstitial microwave antenna array. IEEE Trans. Biomed. Eng., *31:*53–62, 1984.
50. Marks, J.E. and Gado, M. Serial computed tomography of primary brain tumors following surgery, irradiation and chemotherapy. Radiology *125:*119–125, 1977.
51. Marks, J.E., Baglan, R.J., Prasad, S.C., *et al.* Cerebral radionecrosis: incidence and risk in relation to dose, time, fractionation, and volume. Int. J. Radiat. Oncol. Biol. Phys. *7:*243–252, 1981.
52. Marks, J.E. and Adler, S.J. A comparative study of ependymomas by site of origin. Int. J. Radiat. Oncol. Biol. Phys. *8:*37–43, 1982a.
53. Marks, J.E. and Thomas, P.R.M. Prophylactic central nervous system irradiation. In: *Modern Radiation Oncology,* edited by A. Gilbert. Philadelphia, Harper & Row, Vol. II, pp. 217–235.
54. Marks, J.E. and Sheline, G.E. The value of radiation for brain tumors. In: *The Radiological Society of North America's Categorical Course on Therapy of CNS Tumors,* edited by J.E. Marks and M.L. Griem, pp. 418A/2–418A/30. Chicago, Radiological Society of North America, 1983.
55. Marks, J.E. and Wong, J. The risk of cerebral radionecrosis in relation to time dose and fractionation. Prog. Exp. Tumor Res., *29:*210–218, 1985.
56. Marks, J.E., Baglan, R.J., and Wong, J. Radiation damage to brain and cranial soft tissues: outcome and incidence before and after reduction in dose. In: *Biology of Brain Tumor,* edited by M.D. Walker and D.G.T. Thomas, pp. 325–339. Netherlands, Martinus Nijhoff, 1986.
57. Marsa, G.W., Probert, J.C., Rubinstein, L.J., Radiation therapy in the treatment of childhood astrocytic gliomas. Cancer, *32:*646–655, 1973.
58. Marsa, G.W., Goffinet, D.R., Rubinstein, L.J., *et al.* Megavoltage irradiation in the treatment of gliomas of the brain and spinal cord. Cancer, *36:*1681–1689, 1975.
59. Maryuyama, Y., Chin, H.W., Young, A.B., *et al.* Works in progress: 252-Co neutron brachytherapy for hemispheric malignant glioma. Radiology, *145:*171–174, 1982.
60. Mundinger, F. The treatment of brain tumors

with interstitially applied radioactive isotopes. In: Wang, Y., Paoletti, P., (eds): *Radionuclide Applications in Neurology and Neurosurgery,* pp. 199–265. Springfield, IL., Charles C Thomas, 1970.

61. Nelson, D.F., Schoenfeld, A., Weinstein, A.S., *et al.* A randomized comparison of misonidazol sensitized radiotherapy plus BCNU for treatment of malignant glioma after surgery. Preliminary results of an RTOG study. Int. J. Radiat. Oncol. Biol. Phys., *9:*1143–1151, 1983.
62. Orth, D.N. and Liddle, G.W. Results of treatment in 108 patients with Cushing's syndrome. N. Engl. J. Med., *285:*243–248, 1973.
63. Payne, D.G., Simpson, W.J., Keen, C., *et al.* Malignant astrocytoma: Hyperfractionated and standard radiotherapy with chemotherapy in a randomized clinical trial. Cancer, *52:*2301–2306, 1982.
64. Phuphanich, S., Levin, E., and Levin, V. Phase I study of intravenous bromodeoxyuridine used concurrently with radiation therapy in patients with primary malignant brain tumors. Int. J. Radiat. Oncol. Biol. Phys., *10:*1769–1772, 1984.
65. Rosenblum, M.L., Vasquez, D.A., Hoshino, T., *et al.* Development of a clonogenic cell assay for human brain tumors. Cancer, *41:*2305–2314, 1978.
66. Rubin, P. and Kramer, S. Ectopic pinealoma: a radiocurable neuroendocrinologic entity. Radiology, *85:*512–523, 1965.
67. Salazar, O.M., Rubin, P., Feldstein, M.L., *et al.* High dose radiation therapy in the treatment of malignant gliomas: final report. Int. J. Radiat. Oncol. Biol. Phys., *5:*1733–1740, 1979.
68. Shapiro, J.R. and Shapiro, W.R. The subpopulations and isolated cell types of freshly resected high grade human gliomas: their influence on the tumor's evolution in vitro. Cancer Metastasis Rev., *4(2):*107–124, 1985.
69. Sheline, G.E., Boldrey, E., Karlsberg, P., *et al.* Therapeutic considerations in tumors affecting the central nervous system: oligodendrogliomas. Radiology, *82:*84–89, 1964.
70. Sheline, G.E. Treatment of chromophobe adenomas of the pituitary gland and acromegaly. In: Kohler, P.O., Ross, G.T. (eds): *Excerpta Medica.* pp. 201–216. Amsterdam, 1973.
71. Sheline, G.E. Radiation therapy of tumors of the central nervous system in childhood. Cancer *35:*957–964, 1975.
72. Sheline, G.E., Grossman, A., Jones, A.E., *et al.*. Radiation therapy for prolactinomas. In: Black, P.M., Zervas, N.T., Ridgeway, E. *et al.* (eds): *Secretory Tumors of the Pituitary Gland.* pp. 93–108. New York, Raven Press, 1984.
73. Shin, K.H., Muller, P.J., Geggie, P.H.S. Superfractionation radiation therapy in the treatment of malignant astrocytoma. Cancer *52:*2040–2043, 1983.
74. Shin, K.H., Urtasun, R.C., Fulton, D. *et al.* Multiple daily radiation and misonidazole in the management of malignant astrocytoma: a preliminary report. Cancer, *56:*758–760, 1985.
75. Silverman, C.L., and Simpson, J.R. Cerebellar medulloblastoma: the importance of posterior fossa dose to survival and patterns of failure. Int. J. Radiat. Oncol. Biol. Phys., *8:*1869–1876, 1982.
76. Simpson, W.J. and Platt, M.E. Fractionation study in the treatment of glioblastoma multiforme. Int. J. Radiat. Oncol. Biol. Phys., *1:*639–644, 1976.
77. Sinclair, W.K. The combined effect of hydroxyurea and x-rays on Chinese hamster cells in vitro. Cancer Res., *28:*198–206, 1968.
78. Sung, D.I., Harisiadis, L., and Chang, C.H. Midline pineal tumors and suprasellar germinomas: highly curable by irradiation. Radiology *128:*745–751, 1978.
79. Urtasun, R.C., Band, P., Chapman, J.D., *et al.* Radiation and high dose metronidazole in supratentorial glioblastomas. N. Engl. J. Med. *294:*1364–1367, 1976.
80. Urtasun, R.C., Band, P., Feldstein, M.L., *et al.* Clinical phase I study of the hypoxic cell radiosensitizer RO-07-0582, a 2-nitroimidazole derivative. Radiology *122:*801–804, 1977.
81. Walker, M.D., Alexander, E., Hunt, W.E., *et al.* Evaluation of BCNU and/or radiotherapy in the treatment of anaplastic gliomas. J. Neurosurg. *49:*333–343, 1978.
82. Walker, M.D., Strike, T.A., and Sheline, G.E. An analysis of dose-effect relationship in the radiotherapy of malignant gliomas. Int. J. Radiat. Oncol. Biol. Phys. *5:*1725–1731, 1979.
83. Walker, M.D., Green, S.B., Byar, D.P., *et al.* Randomized comparisons of radiotherapy and nitrosoureas for the treatment of malignant glioma after surgery. N. Engl. J. Med. *303:*1323–1329, 1980.
84. Wasserman, T.H., Phillips, T.L., Johnson, R.J., *et al.* Initial United States clinical and pharmacologic evaluation of misonidazole (RO-07-0582): a hypoxic cell radiosensitizer. Int. J. Radiat. Oncol. Biol. Phys. *5:*775–786, 1979.
85. Wara, W., Sheline, G.E., Neuman, H., *et al.* Radiation therapy of meningiomas. Am. J. Roentgenol. Radium Ther. Nucl. Med. *123:*453–458, 1978.
86. Young, D.F., Posner, J.B., Chu, F., *et al.* Rapid course radiation therapy of cerebral metastases: results and complications. Cancer, *34:*1069–1076, 1974.

CHAPTER 18

Chemotherapy of Brain Tumors

STUART A. GROSSMAN, M.D.

CHEMOTHERAPEUTIC AGENTS: BASIC PRINCIPLES

Historical Perspective

Advances in the treatment of bacterial diseases in the early 1900s provided a paradigm for the development of antineoplastic agents (100). Erlich demonstrated that infectious diseases could be cured in rodents and that animal models predicted effectiveness in humans. The development of bacterial resistance to antibiotics was noted and combinations of active drugs were found to be more effective than single agents. Dosing schedules were also identified to be of major importance.

In the early 1960s Skipper and colleagues used a rodent leukemia model to develop a series of important principles in cancer chemotherapy (137–139). These have had a major influence on the evolution of treatment for malignant diseases using chemotherapeutic agents and can be summarized as follows:

(a) A single clonagenic malignant cell can ultimately lead to the death of the host and the interval between the injection of these cells and the death of the host is dependent on the number of clonagenic tumor cells present and the doubling time of the cells.

(b) In contrast to antimicrobial chemotherapy, where the immune system plays a major role in the cure of infections, immunologic responses appear to be much less important in the therapy of malignant disease.

(c) Cell kill by antineoplastic agents follows first order kinetics. In other words, a constant percentage of tumor cells, not a fixed number of cells, are killed by the administration of chemotherapy. Patients with advanced malignancies may have a total body tumor burden of 1 kg (10^{12} cells). Chemotherapy which kills 99.99% of the tumor would reduce the total tumor burden resulting in a clinical remission. However, any one of the many remaining tumor cells with clonagenic potential could ultimately lead to a relapse of the cancer.

Agents Available and Mechanisms of Action

From the inception of the National Cancer Institute's drug screening program in 1955, through 1975, agents with activity against the murine L1210 leukemia were gradually phased into clinical trials (77). More recently, agents active against the chemosensitive rodent P388 mouse leukemia are tested against a panel of animal tumors and xenographed human tumors in athymic mice. Skipper and Schabel noted that the product of the drug concentration and the time of exposure (C × T) yields similar degrees of cytotoxicity in different species (127, 138). This has made it possible to convert doses of drugs in animals into estimated doses for humans. The past 3 decades of animal and clinical testing have resulted in a continually increasing number of clinically effective antineoplastic agents available for general clinical use (Fig. 18.1).

Almost all antineoplastic agents share two properties: *(a)* They work by affecting

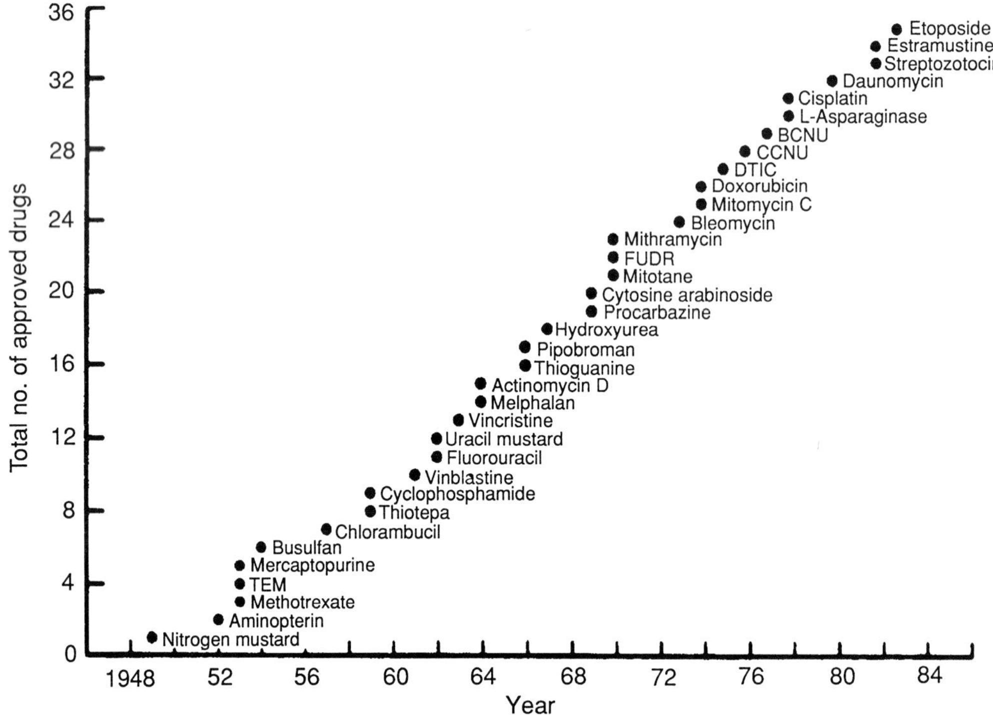

Figure 18.1. The development of clinically available chemotherapeutic agents. (Reprinted with permission from DeVita, V.T. *Cancer: Principles & Practice of Oncology,* edited by V.T. DeVita, S. Hellman, and S.A. Rosenberg. Philadelphia, J.B. Lippincott, 1985.)

DNA synthesis or function and *(b)* they usually do not kill resting cells unless such cells are destined to divide soon after exposure to the agent. The mechanisms of action of selected antineoplastic agents are shown in Figure 18.2. Many of these agents act at specific phases of the cell cycle and are most effective in killing dividing cells. As a result, the best therapeutic results with chemotherapy in human malignancies are seen in tumors with a large number of cells in the process of division. Burkitt's lymphoma is an excellent example. This is a rapidly growing tumor with over half of the cells synthesizing DNA at any time and a growth fraction approaching 100%. It is responsive to a variety of chemotherapeutic agents which now cure over 50% of children requiring systemic therapy for this malignancy. Similarly, many normal tissues proliferate rapidly and can be severely affected by antineoplastic agents. The most common dose limiting toxicities of these drugs are a result of their effects on normal bone marrow and intestinal mucosa.

Most human solid tumors have a small number of cells either synthesizing DNA or actively cycling (the growth fraction). High-grade astrocytomas have a labelling index ranging from 0 to 10% and the clinical doubling time of these tumors is about 6 to 8 weeks (73). Many cells remain in Go for prolonged periods of time before entering the division cycle. As most antineoplastic agents act on processes such as DNA synthesis, transcription, or the mitotic spindle, it is not surprising that they are of limited utility in these slowly proliferating tumors.

Resistance to Chemotherapeutic Agents

In 1979 Goldie and Coldman applied principles of bacterial genetics to cancer chemotherapy (54). They postulated that nonrandom cytogenetic changes in human cancers would be associated with the capacity to resist the action of chemotherapeutic agents. Assuming a spontaneous mutation rate of 1 in 10^6 divisions, the likelihood of at least one resistant cell line is very high by the time the tumor is clinically

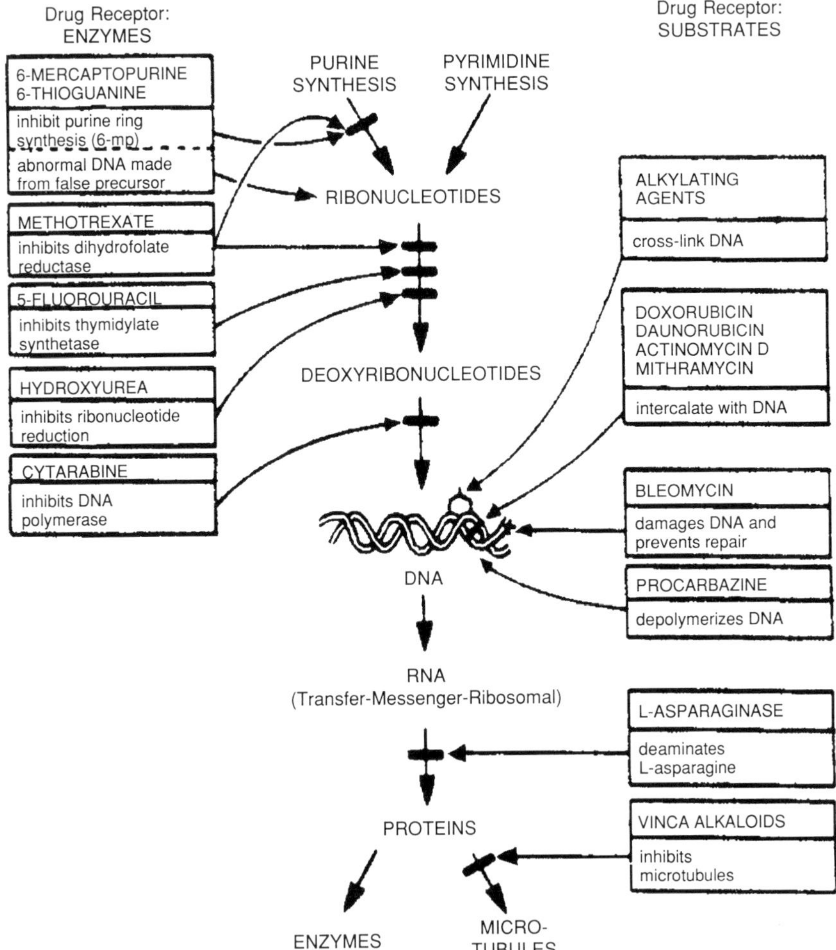

Figure 18.2. Mechanisms and sites of action of selected drugs used in cancer chemotherapy. (Reprinted with permission from Goodman and Gilman, *Pharmacology*. New York, Macmillan, 1985.)

detectable (54, 163). High rates of cell loss in many slow growing tumors further increase the probability of de novo chemotherapy resistant cells being present before antineoplastic treatments are initiated (30).

There are several mechanisms by which tumor cells exposed to chemotherapy can develop resistance to these agents (32). Examples of some of these are shown in Table 18.1. Agents within the same class of drugs may differ in their mechanism of entry into cells, activation by cellular enzymes, and in

TABLE 18.1.
Examples of Mechanisms by Which Tumor Cells May Acquire Resistance to Chemotherapeutic Agents

Mechanism	Example
Decreased drug uptake	Daunorubicin
Increased drug efflux	Vinca alkaloids
Increased drug inactivation	Cytosine arabinoside
Increased utilization of alternate biochemical pathways	Antimetabolites
Rapid repair of drug induced lesions	Alkylating agents
Gene amplification which increases the concentration of target enzymes	Methotrexate
Pleotropic drug resistance	Doxorubicin Vinca alkaloids

the nature of their reactive moieties. For this reason, tumors that develop resistance to one alkylating drug may still respond to a second from the same class of chemotherapeutic agents (18).

Recently, another type of drug resistance, called pleotropic resistance, has been described (32). This has been studied in Chinese hamster ovary cells exposed to colchicine. DNA from these cells appears to be able to transfer chemotherapy resistance to previously sensitive cell lines through a gene transmitted membrane effect. This affords another explanation for the observation that patients relapsing after exposure to one class of compounds may demonstrate resistance to a wide variety of other antineoplastic agents.

Doses and Schedules

In the clinical practice of oncology, the dose of chemotherapy is often reduced or the interval between treatments lengthened to minimize the toxicities of therapy. There is evidence that these changes may result in suboptimal therapeutic results. The dose-response curve for nearly all chemotherapeutic agents is steep for the desired effect and the toxicities of these drugs. In some rapidly growing animal tumors, reducing the dose by as little as 20% can result in a 50% reduction in cure (127). Clinical experience in oat cell carcinoma of the lung and childhood leukemias has demonstrated the same phenomenon (29, 116). The efficacy of therapeutic regimens in breast cancer and lymphomas has also been diminished by what appeared to be reasonable dose reductions (35, 74). Tumors which are marginally responsive to chemotherapy do not usually display as steep a dose-response relationship. Increasing the doses of ineffective agents is often associated with increased host toxicity without a corresponding increase in the efficacy of the administered agent.

Principles of Combination Chemotherapy

While choriocarcinoma and Burkitt's lymphoma can be cured using a single chemotherapeutic agent, these tumors remain the exception rather than the rule in clinical oncology. The use of combinations of agents began with the treatment of the leukemias and lymphomas when multiple effective drugs for these diseases became available. This approach is now used in the treatment of most chemotherapy responsive solid tumors. The design of a regimen using multiple agents should follow principles established for combination chemotherapy (35). Only agents which are known to be partially effective should be included in the regimen. Drugs with nonoverlapping toxicity profiles should be selected so that each agent can be administered at its optimal dose and schedule. Therapy with a combination of agents should adhere to a rigid schedule which is determined by the time required for recovery of normal tissues. The use of chemotherapy in this manner is designed to allow each agent to provide maximal cell kill with tolerable toxicity to the host. Combination chemotherapy should be more effective against a broad range of de novo resistant cell lines in a heterogeneous tumor population and should also prevent or slow the development of drug resistant cell lines.

SPECIAL PROBLEMS AND OPPORTUNITIES IN TREATING BRAIN TUMORS WITH CHEMOTHERAPY

Special Problems

Malignancies within the central nervous system pose unique problems to oncologists treating patients with chemotherapy (92, 131). The blood-brain barrier (BBB) is often considered a major factor limiting the penetration of antineoplastic drugs into brain tumors. The role of the BBB is discussed later in this chapter and in detail in Chapter 13 of this text. Rall and Zubrod, in 1962, determined that molecular weight, lipid solubility (often expressed as an octanol/water concentration ratio), and polarity were major criteria governing the passage of chemotherapeutic agents across an intact BBB (Table 18.2) (120). Blasberg and colleagues subsequently defined additional factors that influence the amount of drug which will passively diffuse from capillaries into brain tumors (11). These include the permeability of the capillaries with respect to the specific drug, the luminal surface area of the capillaries avail-

TABLE 18.2.
Molecular Weight and Lipid Solubility of Agents Used to Treat Primary Brain Tumors[a]

Agent	Molecular Weight	Solubility (log p)[b]
Hydroxyurea	76	Water[c]
5-FU	130	−0.95[c]
BCNU	214	1.53
Procarbazine	221	0.06
CCNU	233	2.85
Cytosine arabinoside	243	−0.79
Methyl CCNU	247	3.30
PCNU	262	0.37
Cisplatin	300	Water
Chlorambucil	304	−0.7
Melphalan	305	−1.7
Spirohydantoin Mustard	335	2.0
AZQ	364	0.50
Methotrexate	454	−2.52
Doxorubicin	580	−0.1
VM-26	656	Lipid[d]
Vincristine	923	2.8

[a]Data taken from Levin (91), Greig (59), Groothuis and Blasberg (60), Shapiro (131), and Blasberg and Groothuis (11).
[b] Log p = 1− octanol/water partition coefficient.
[c] Crosses BBB easily
[d] Crosses BBB poorly

able for exchange, blood flow to the tumor, the concentration of unbound drug in the plasma, and the length of time the drug circulates through the capillaries.

Quantitation of tumor response is also more difficult in brain tumors than it is in systemic cancers (63, 88, 162). Clinical criteria are difficult to use as neurological deficits may remain stable even in the face of significant tumor reduction. Computed tomographic (CT) and magnetic resonance (MR) brain scans, the most commonly used studies for response evaluation, do not permit actual "tumor" measurement. Mass effect, which represents the sum of the tumor size and adjacent peritumoral brain edema, is one factor which is evaluated on these scans. This may be altered by changes in peritumoral brain edema without affecting the size of the tumor. Another estimate of tumor size on CT and MR scans is the area of contrast enhancement. Brain tumors enhance because the abnormally permeable capillaries of the tumor allow the contrast agent to penetrate into the peritumoral region. Therefore, quantitative measurements of the area of contrast enhancement represent an estimate of BBB dysfunction which is only an indirect indication of tumor size. As a result of these difficulties in the accurate quantitation of the response of these neoplasms to therapy, results of brain tumor trials are usually reported in median time to progression and median survival time. The use of these parameters often makes investigational chemotherapy trials in patients with brain tumors difficult to interpret.

Several additional factors also pose unique problems for chemotherapists. The tumor mass, BBB disruption, peritumoral edema, absence of draining lymphatics, and the presence of a nondistensible skull all contribute to the development of increased intracranial pressure. These combine to complicate the administration of some chemotherapeutic agents. Certain antineoplastic drugs can exacerbate BBB dysfunction (44, 96, 115). Others, such as cisplatin and high dose cyclophosphamide, are administered with large quantities of fluids to protect the genitourinary tract from the known toxicities of these agents. Increases in BBB dysfunction or overhydration associated with chemotherapy can result in potentially catastrophic neurological events in these tenuously compensated patients.

Special Opportunities

There are also unique opportunities for the treatment of brain tumors with chemotherapy. These malignancies become apparent when the tumor burden is significantly lower than it is in most systemic malignancies. Brain tumors usually remain localized throughout the course of the patient's illness. Therefore, the patient's clinical course is not complicated by involvement of multiple organ systems. These tumors are often supplied by regional vessels which permit intraarterial chemotherapy to be considered. In addition, despite the concern that the BBB impairs chemotherapy entry, this barrier is selectively disrupted at the site of the malignant lesion (5, 10, 151). For this reason, the tumor will receive far higher doses of systemically or regionally administered chemotherapy than adjacent normal tissue. This favorable tumor to normal tissue distribution of antineoplastic agents is unique and should minimize the neurotoxicity of certain chemotherapeutic agents.

RESULTS OF CHEMOTHERAPY IN PATIENTS WITH BRAIN TUMORS

Nearly every antineoplastic drug active in systemic tumors has also been used in primary malignancies of the central nervous system (83). Unfortunately, median survival time and median time to progression are common end points of these trials. Many variables have been identified which have major impact on these parameters. Some include patient age, performance status, histopathologic classification of tumor, duration of symptoms, dose of radiation therapy administered, and aggressiveness with which repeated surgical resections and glucocorticoids are employed (37, 126, 155, 156). Many chemotherapy trials have not controlled for these variables which may have greater impact on survival than the agents being evaluated.

High-Grade Astrocytomas

The first randomized controlled prospective trial in the treatment of malignant astrocytomas was reported by members of the Brain Tumor Study Group in 1976 (153). Patients were randomized to receive mithramycin or no chemotherapy following surgical resection and radiotherapy. Although no benefit was found from mithramycin therapy, this study paved the way for a series of multiinstitutional prospective trials which have evaluated the role of chemotherapy in high-grade astrocytomas during the past decade.

The nitrosoureas are chemotherapeutic agents which were synthesized with characteristics which would allow them to penetrate the BBB. They are highly lipid soluble, small, and not ionized. BCNU (1-3-*bis*-2-chloroethyl-1-nitrosourea) was the first nitrosourea to be used clinically. The results of early Phase II studies using this agent were reported in 1970. Approximately half the patients treated intravenously with 240–300 mg/m^2 every 6 to 8 weeks demonstrated improvement (152, 161). However, responses lasted only 3 to 5 months. In the late 1970s, several large prospective randomized studies evaluated the role of BCNU given postoperatively and following cranial irradiation (Table 18.3) (56, 141, 154, 156). BCNU administered postoperatively extended the median survival of patients from 14 to 18 weeks while radiation therapy alone prolonged survival to approximately 35 weeks. The addition of BCNU to radiation therapy conferred only a minor survival advantage which was present at 18 months but disappeared shortly thereafter.

Other nitrosoureas were also tested in the postoperative setting and after radiation therapy (Table 18.3) (141). CCNU is a nitrosourea which can be administered orally. Several studies have noted that the results with this compound and with methylCCNU are no better than those with BCNU (156). Procarbazine and high dose glucocorticoids have also been studied (56). Procarbazine appears to be about as effective as BCNU. Corticosteroids do not demonstrate significant antitumor activity and do not add to the efficacy of the nitrosoureas.

Clinical investigators have also attempted treatment strategies for astrocytomas which have been successful in the management of systemic tumors. One of these is the use of combination chemotherapy. Unfortunately, the results of this approach in brain tumors are different than those in lymphomas, leukemias, and testicular cancer. The empiric combination of marginally effective agents in patients with astrocytomas has thus far failed to demonstrate a significant improvement over sin-

TABLE 18.3.
Selected Trials: Chemotherapy Drugs Used as Single Agents Postoperatively or Following the Administration of Radiotherapy In Postoperative Patients with Newly Diagnosed High-Grade Astrocytomas

Reference	No. of Evaluable Patients	with Glioblastoma	Treatment	Median Survival Time (weeks)
Walker *et al.* (155)	222	90%	Surgery alone	14
			BCNU	18.5
			XRT	35.0
			XRT + BCNU	34.5
Solero *et al.* (141)	102	100%	XRT	45
			XRT + BCNU	52
			XRT + CCNU	69
Walker *et al.* (156)	358	84%	Methyl CCNU	24
			XRT	36
			XRT + Methyl CCNU	42
			XRT + BCNU	51
Green *et al.* (56)	527	85%	XRT + Medrol	40
			XRT + procarbazine	47
			XRT + BCNU	50
			XRT + Medrol + BCNU	41

gle agent therapy (93). As a result, experimental approaches designed to increase the delivery of chemotherapeutic drugs to these tumors are currently being evaluated. The rationale and early results of high dose chemotherapy with autologous bone marrow rescue, intraarterial chemotherapy, and BBB disruption are discussed later in this chapter.

The results of chemotherapy used in an adjuvant setting with radiation therapy in high-grade astrocytomas in children are more encouraging. The median survival for these patients is approximately 20 months, but 25% survive for 5 years. The Children's Cancer Study Group has studied the combination of vincristine, CCNU and prednisone. The median disease free survival was 9 months with radiation therapy and 25 months with radiation and chemotherapy (40). More aggressive chemotherapy with the "8 in 1" regimen is now being studied by this cooperative group (12). Adjuvant studies of brainstem gliomas in children using similar agents have not had significant impact on survival. Several studies of chemotherapy given before radiation are now underway in an effort to delay the administration of radiation therapy and thereby reduce its toxic effects in young children (4).

Low-Grade Astrocytomas

Patients with low-grade astrocytomas have a median survival of 4 to 5 years. These tumors may remain indolent for long periods of time when few cells are actively proliferating and long doubling times are the rule. As a result, chemotherapy, which is most effective against rapidly growing neoplasms, is not usually administered to this patient population. Most data available on the efficacy of chemotherapy in low-grade astrocytomas has been obtained at the time of relapse following surgery and radiation therapy and is not controlled for major prognostic variables. Approximately 40% of these patients appear to transiently respond to the same agents which are used in the treatment of high-grade astrocytomas.

Oligodendrogliomas

Oligodendrogliomas account for less than 2% of all brain tumors and are not seen commonly enough to warrant separate clinical trials. These tumors tend to take on more of the histologic appearance and biologic characteristics of high-grade astrocytomas when they recur following surgery and radiation therapy. In these situations, chemotherapy is used in a manner identical to that employed for high-grade astrocytomas (123).

Meningiomas

Meningiomas are generally treated surgically. If they recur postoperatively, radiation therapy can be beneficial (48). In situations where additional surgery is hazardous and radiation therapy has already been administered, chemotherapy can be considered. Adriamycin or other regimens effective against systemic sarcomas are sometimes recommended because neoplastic degeneration often takes on a sarcomatous appearance.

Medulloblastomas

Medulloblastomas are primitive neuroectodermal tumors which arise from the roof of the fourth ventricle and cerebellar vermis. They are most common in young patients and may seed the cerebrospinal fluid (CSF) early in the course of their development. Approximately 30% of patients under 5 years of age with medulloblastomas have documented subarachnoid metastases and nearly 5% of all patients with medulloblastomas develop widespread systemic metastases (2, 82). Patients who recur generally do so at the original site of disease.

Current radiation therapy techniques result in an overall median survival of 5 years for patients with medulloblastomas (8). Although these tumors account for nearly one-fourth of all pediatric brain tumors, there are only about 250 new cases annually in the United States. Cooperative group efforts to study the efficacy of chemotherapy in this disease began in the mid 1970s. During the past decade, the Children's Cancer Study Group (CCSG), International Society of Pediatric Oncology (SIOP), and the Pediatric Oncology Group (POG) have placed over 580 patients with medulloblastomas on clinical research protocols utilizing chemotherapeutic agents (4). Preliminary results are available for the CCSG and SIOP trials. The overall 5-year disease free survivals were 50% in both studies. The addition of CCNU and vincristine added marginal benefit in both studies (59% *vs.* 49%, and 55% *vs.* 43% disease free survival at 4.5 years). The improvements were most pronounced in the highest risk patient groups: the very young and those with extensive tumor. As a result of the small numbers of these patients, the impact of chemotherapy on the entire study population was limited. POG and CCSG are evaluating craniospinal irradiation in good risk patients and radiation therapy combined with more aggressive chemotherapy ("8 in 1" chemotherapy) in the poorer risk patients. SIOP's poor risk protocol combines craniospinal irradiation with high dose methotrexate, procarbazine, vincristine, and CCNU.

Smaller uncontrolled studies have demonstrated that combination chemotherapy regimens such as procarbazine, CCNU, and vincristine (PCV), or nitrogen mustard, vincristine, procarbazine, and prednisone (MOPP) have activity in medulloblastomas. Crafts noted that 10 of 16 patients improved with PCV and Cangir demonstrated similar results in 8 of 10 patients using MOPP (24, 31). Several single agent chemotherapy studies have also demonstrated activity in this disease. Complete responses have been noted with cisplatin and the overall complete and partial response rate in the limited numbers of patients treated with this agent approaches 75% (157). Similar response rates have been found with "8 in 1" chemotherapy. This regimen combines methylprednisone, vincristine, BCNU, procarbazine, hydroxyurea, cisplatin, cytosine arabinoside, and cyclophosphamide (12).

Ependymomas

Ependymomas arise from ependymal lining cells and are most common in the posterior fossa. These tumors generally occur in younger patients and have a variable clinical course. They are difficult to completely remove surgically and often seed the cerebrospinal fluid. For these reasons, postoperative adjuvant therapy is generally employed. Radiation therapy clearly increases the duration of survival. Chemotherapy trials are currently underway. Most responses appear to be with nitrosoureas and cisplatin containing regimens (3, 128, 157).

Primary CNS Lymphomas

Primary CNS lymphomas are uncommon malignancies. They account for less than 2% of all nonHodgkins lymphomas and 1% of brain tumors (49, 140). These tumors are usually multifocal in origin and consist of a diffuse large cell lymphoma of

B cell lineage which has a predisposition for periventricular regions (50, 66, 80). CNS lymphomas are most commonly found in patients who are profoundly immunosuppressed. More than 50% of all lymphomas observed in patients who have undergone renal transplantation are primary CNS lymphomas (104, 114). This tumor also constitutes a significant problem for patients with the acquired immunodeficiency syndrome (AIDS). The incidence of CNS lymphoma in nonimmunosuppressed patients appears to be increasing for unknown reasons.

Patients with CNS lymphomas usually present with focal neurologic deficits, a change in mental status, or increased intracranial pressure. Lesions may appear multifocal on CT or MR scans and pathologically extend far beyond the areas of contrast enhancement. Stereotactic needle biopsy is often performed for diagnostic purposes as surgery does not prolong life (112). Special immunohistochemical studies can identify this tumor as one of B cell origin (150). One-third of patients have concomitant involvement of the cerebrospinal fluid.

Most series have demonstrated that primary CNS lymphomas are responsive to cranial irradiation. However, the overall survival of patients treated with surgery and radiation therapy is less than 50% at 1 year and less than 20% at 2 years (55, 94). Glucocorticoids have been shown to produce dramatic clinical and radiographic results which rarely last for a prolonged period of time (81, 147). Chemotherapy using agents which are effective against systemic large cell lymphomas has been attempted. Reports of patients treated with nitrosoureas, procarbazine, cytarabine, cyclophosphamide, bleomycin, and Adriamycin have shown modest results without significant prolongation of life (28, 51, 64). Several investigators have used high dose methotrexate with somewhat more encouraging results (41, 117, 136). Although response rates appear high, the duration of these responses is usually relatively brief. Preliminary results using chemotherapy following blood-brain barrier disruption are discussed later in this chapter.

Pineal Area and Germ Cell Neoplasms

Tumors originating in the region of the pineal gland and third ventricle usually present with visual symptoms or obstructive hydrocephalus. They occur most frequently near or around the time of puberty (78). Histologically, these tumors are most commonly astrocytomas, dysgerminomas, and teratomas. Pinealocytomas and pineoblastomas are rare. CSF levels of alpha-fetoprotein and the B-subunit of human chorionic gonadotropin and CSF cytology may be helpful in the diagnostic workup and follow-up of patients. Cranial irradiation or craniospinal irradiation result in nearly 60% of patients surviving 5 years (39, 143, 158).

There is only fragmentary evidence on the efficacy of chemotherapy for pineal tumors because of the rarity of this tumor and the heterogeneity of cell type. Adriamycin and vincristine were reported to markedly reduce the size of a recurrent pineal tumor in an adult (34). Combination chemotherapy regimens containing cisplatin and velban, which are effective in systemic germ cell neoplasms and brain metastases from these tumors, are also likely to be useful in primary CNS germ cell neoplasms (38).

EXPERIMENTAL APPROACHES TO DELIVER HIGHER CONCENTRATIONS OF CHEMOTHERAPY TO BRAIN TUMORS

The difficulties in delivering tumoricidal concentrations of chemotherapeutic agents to brain tumors are addressed elsewhere in this chapter. Evidence suggests that sublethal doses of antineoplastic agents will accelerate development of resistant cell lines. Human glioma cell lines in culture have been found to rapidly develop BCNU resistance when exposed to subtherapeutic doses of BCNU (130). As a result of these observations and the poor prognosis of patients with brain tumors treated in a conventional manner, experimental approaches designed to deliver higher concentrations of chemotherapy to brain tumors have been developed. Several of these will be briefly described below.

High Dose Chemotherapy with Autologous Bone Marrow Rescue

The dose limiting toxicity of most chemotherapeutic agents is the effect of these drugs on the normal bone marrow. The availability of donor bone marrow makes it possible to administer supralethal doses of chemotherapy and radiation in an attempt to kill a greater fraction of the malignant cells. Donor marrow reconstitutes the host's entire hematopoietic and immunologic system. This procedure has been shown to be of potential benefit in acute leukemia, chronic granulocytic leukemia, and in some patients with lymphomas refractory to conventional therapies (111, 146). The toxicities are considerable and include opportunistic infections, venoocclusive disease of the liver, graft-versus-host disease, and complications from immunologic incompetence. Some of these problems can be diminished by using an autologous marrow graft. Bone marrow is obtained from the patient under general or spinal anesthesia, cryopreserved, and reinfused after the patient has received high-dose antineoplastic therapy.

Autologous bone marrow rescue is now being widely explored in the treatment of a number of systemic malignancies. Hochberg and colleagues studied 11 patients with recurrent astrocytomas using this technique (70). Six hundred to 1400 mg/m^2 of BCNU were administered. CT scans on a stable dose of corticosteroids were improved in eight patients. The toxicity was considerable. Profound myelosuppression, sepsis, chemical hepatitis, pulmonary infiltrates and irreversible cortical damage were observed. Median survival time in this group of patients was only 7 months. While autologous bone marrow transplantation may be efficacious in rapidly growing, chemotherapy sensitive tumors, a single dose of chemotherapy in solid tumors with relatively low growth fractions appears unlikely to result in cure. The toxicity of this approach makes repeated administrations difficult.

Intraarterial Chemotherapy

The administration of chemotherapy into vessels directly supplying a tumor allows more drug to be delivered to the tumor without increasing the patient's overall exposure to the agent. This technique has been used with some success in the treatment of systemic malignancies and has been attempted in brain tumors since the 1960s (99). Fenstermacher and colleagues developed mathematical models which predicted that the intracarotid administration of chemotherapy would yield up to ten times more drug in the brain without changing systemic toxicity (42, 43). Data from the laboratory has supported these models. Levin and colleagues administered [^{14}C]-BCNU into the carotid artery of a squirrel monkey and demonstrated significantly higher concentrations in the infused hemisphere (89). Hiesiger et al. obtained similar results using quantitative autoradiographic techniques with methotrexate (67, 68).

Clinical trials with intraarterial BCNU in patients with primary and metastatic brain tumors demonstrated that responses could be obtained (23, 26, 57, 71, 98). In addition, metastatic lesions on the side of the infusion appeared to respond better than tumors in the contralateral hemisphere. The major limitation of initial attempts using intraarterial BCNU was toxicity to the ipsilateral eye resulting in severe pain, conjunctival irritation, and retinal damage which could result in blindness. Cisplatin has also been administered intraarterially (85, 142). This drug is associated with relatively little bone marrow suppression. Intraarterial cisplatin produced some responses but the toxicity above 75 mg/m^2 was considerable. Seizures, retinal damage, and motor weakness have been noted (72, 102, 142). Small uncontrolled trials and case reports using intraarterial BCNU, cisplatin, FUDR, and diaziquone continue to suggest some efficacy to this therapeutic approach (45, 58, 105, 149). In 1983, the Brain Tumor Cooperative Group initiated a large, well-controlled Phase III trial to compare intraarterial and intravenous BCNU therapy for primary brain tumors. This study failed to show an advantage to the intraarterial administration of BCNU and highlights the toxicities of this therapy

(132). Blindness and irreversible encephalopathy were prominent side effects of therapy.

Several investigators have tested catheters designed to deliver chemotherapeutic agents in the carotid artery above the takeoff of the ophthalmic artery (27, 36, 79, 101). While this reduces the incidence of eye toxicity, the supraophthalmic administration of BCNU appears to be toxic to the infused cerebral tissue. White matter changes were noted on CT scans in 20% of patients in one series (47). Pathologically, coagulative necrosis of white matter has been seen which is identical to the delayed changes that can follow radiation therapy (99).

The lack of consistent clinical efficacy and the neurotoxicity seen with intraarterial chemotherapy may be partially explained by studies of the streaming of intraarterially administered drugs in the carotid artery. Blacklock and colleagues evaluated the uniformity of the distribution of carbon-14-labelled iodopyrine administered in the carotid artery at different infusion rates in monkeys (9). They noted markedly heterogeneous drug deposition in the perfused hemisphere at infusion rates which are being used clinically. These investigators also developed an in vitro model of the cerebral circulation and were able to visualize streaming and confirm wide variations in drug delivery attributable to this phenomenon (95). Streaming of intraarterially administered agents can result in areas of the tumor receiving subtherapeutic levels of chemotherapy and areas of the normal brain receiving toxic concentrations of the drug. These observations make it difficult to interpret the results of clinical studies to date. Further advances in the delivery of regional chemotherapy will depend on the development of new catheters that minimize drug streaming.

Blood-Brain Barrier Disruption

The anatomic basis for the BBB appears to reside in the endothelial cells of the capillaries of the brain. These cells are unique in that they are joined by tight junctions which functionally restrict the passage of certain compounds. Agents which are water soluble, ionized, or over 200 daltons in size have difficulty entering the brain (120). As a result, many antineoplastic agents do not enter normal brain tissue in therapeutic concentrations. Within brain tumors, however, the BBB does not appear to be functionally intact. Tight junctions are distorted and in animal models large compounds such as horseradish peroxidase pass into brain tumor tissue (151). Clinically, BBB dysfunction results in the development of peritumoral brain edema and allows contrast agents and radioisotopes to enter the extracellular space making tumor visualization possible on brain scans. Antineoplastic agents also appear to enter malignant tissue within the brain as brain metastases have been shown to respond to the administration of systemic chemotherapy (124). However, these agents appear to be more effective against systemic tumors than against the same tumor metastatic to the brain in both animal and human studies (6).

Rapoport and colleagues demonstrated that the intracarotid infusion of hyperosmolar mannitol temporarily disrupts the BBB in the region of the infusion (121, 122). These investigators and others have demonstrated that the BBB within brain tumors is "partially" open in an inhomogeneous fashion that varies within lesions and from one lesion to another (10, 67). The barrier to drug entry within the tumor can be further disrupted with the administration of hyperosmolar mannitol. Neuwelt and colleagues have reported results of BBB disruption followed by chemotherapy administration in 38 patients with glioblastomas (106). All of these patients had prior surgery and radiation therapy. Barrier modification was achieved by an intracarotid or intravertebral artery infusion of mannitol. This was followed by intraarterial methotrexate, intravenous cyclophosphamide, and oral procarbazine. Tumor responses on the side of the infusion were occasionally accompanied by the development of new lesions in regions which were not disrupted prior to administration of chemotherapy. Neurologic complications of this procedure, which requires general anesthesia, included transient exacerbation of preexisting neurological deficits and a 15% incidence of seizures following BBB disruption. Three patients developed motor deficits following treatment. Neuwelt has also reported a series of 12 patients with primary CNS lymphomas treated in a similar fashion (107). The 75% 1-year survival noted in this study is approximately equal to the results seen with radiation therapy.

Considerable controversy exists regarding this approach to the treatment of CNS malignancies. Experiments in animal models demonstrate that BBB disruption followed by chemotherapy results in modest increases in chemotherapy levels within the tumor and major increases in levels in normal brain tissue where the BBB was previously intact (67). More research needs to be done to clarify the role of the BBB and of iatrogenic BBB disruption in the treatment of CNS malignancies.

Agents Specially Designed for CNS Malignancies

BCNU and AZQ are two of many antineoplastic agents synthesized to treat primary brain tumors. Although the results with these agents have been disappointing, several new drugs have recently been developed which may have promise in the therapy of CNS malignancies. Spirohydantoin mustard is one of a number of agents synthesized by Peng *et al.* in an attempt to provide improved agents for brain tumor therapy (113). This investigational drug is a lipophilic alkylating agent which combines a nitrogen mustard with a derivative of diphenylhydantoin. Plowman demonstrated that radiolabeled spirohydantoin mustard results in detectable CSF radioactivity when either the alkylating or phenytoin portions of the compound were labeled (118). This drug acts as a DNA cross-linking agent in the intracerebral rat 9L glioma model and in bone marrow (69). It does not appear to be a cell cycle specific agent. Its efficacy was tested against an intracranial ependymoblastoma model where it prolonged the life of animals harboring this tumor and in several other solid tumors (133). The primary toxicity noted in animals was myelosuppression. Neurotoxicity was seen at very high doses and consisted of seizures, ataxia, and tremors. Clinical trials demonstrated dose limiting CNS toxicity (20, 134, 135). Patients felt light-headed, confused, somnolent, or agitated, and mydriasis was observed. These symptoms were transient, usually subsiding 2 days following cessation of therapy. Physostigmine appeared to reverse the CNS toxicity and dividing the administered dose into smaller doses over a longer time period also diminished neurotoxicity. One adult with an astrocytoma was reported to have a complete response to therapy with this agent (33). However, the results seen in 16 patients with recurrent gliomas were discouraging (119). The Eastern Cooperative Oncology Group is currently conducting additional testing of spirohydantoin mustard in patients with primary and metastatic brain tumors.

The dihydropyridine-pyridinium salt redox delivery system is another potentially useful method to deliver drugs preferentially to the brain (13, 14, 15, 16). Most work to date using this system has focused on the delivery and sustained release of a variety of hormones in the brain. The structure of the 17-β(1,4-dihydrotrigonelline) ester of testosterone is shown in Figure 18.3. This lipid soluble compound crosses the BBB. Biologic oxidation in tissues results in the production of an ionic, hydrophilic quaternary derivative which is "locked" inside the BBB. In all other tissues this compound is excreted rapidly. Preliminary results with hormones linked to this redox system suggest that these agents may be released in the brain for weeks after a single intravenous injection. The feasibility of using this brain specific carrier delivery system for chemotherapy to treat CNS malignancies or glucocorticoids for peritumoral brain edema are currently under investigation (21).

Continuous Infusion Chemotherapy

The slow influx of compounds into brain tumors was first clinically appreciated in patients studied with radionuclide brain scans (75). Images of the brain are routinely obtained hours after the injection of the radioactive tracer because of the slow

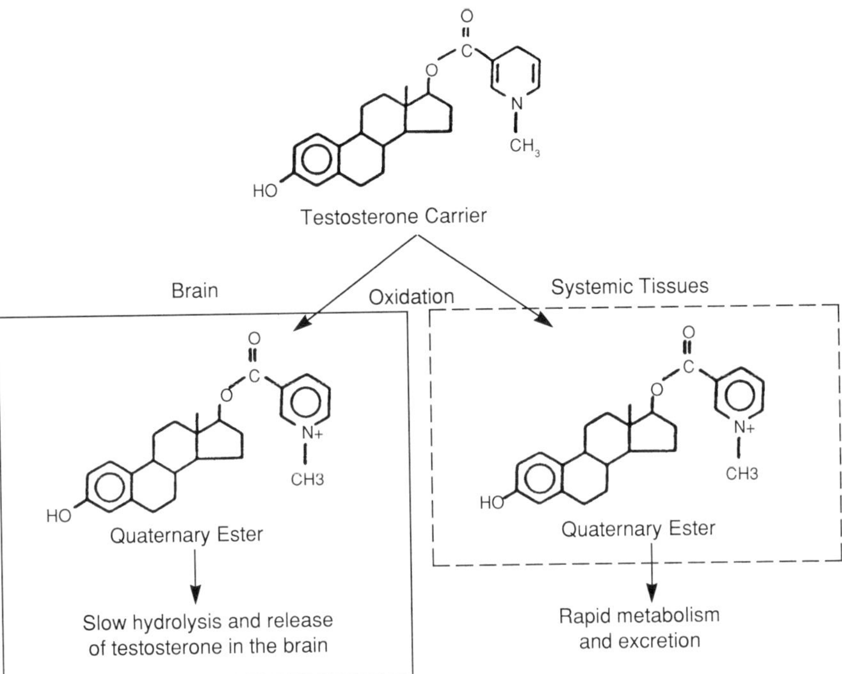

Figure 18.3. Brain-specific drug carrier system.

accumulation of tracers in brain tumors. In the 1970s, radiologists began using contrast agents to enhance CT brain scans. The outside "ring" of primary brain tumors appeared to enhance early after contrast administration while the "low density center" of the lesions often took hours to "fill in" (7, 22, 65, 108, 129, 144). Norman and colleagues postulated that the "low density center" represents a second compartment which equilibrates with intravascular and interstitial contrast material at a very slow rate (108). Similar observations have been noted in patients with metastatic brain tumors and in animal models (25, 129, 160). It is possible that the center of these lesions receives subtherapeutic levels of chemotherapy because most chemotherapeutic agents are given as a bolus and many have short half-lives. Sustained plasma levels of chemotherapeutic agents administered by continuous infusion may result in a more homogeneous distribution of the drugs within brain tumors. Few studies using this approach are reported. One trial using a continuous infusion schedule of 5FU reported that patients with low-grade astrocytomas lived longer than historical controls (90). A more recent study using BCNU and cisplatin has generated preliminary data suggesting that these agents have considerable activity when given by constant infusion (61). Additional clinical and laboratory work is needed to determine the efficacy of this approach in the treatment of brain tumors.

Topical Chemotherapy

Many investigators, in an attempt to improve therapy for this local malignancy, have instilled chemotherapy directly into brain tumors with little success (52, 125, 159). The drugs were usually injected into the tumor at a relatively rapid rate and a portion of these agents may have travelled out of the brain along the outside of the catheter. In addition, the distance these drugs were expected to traverse was probably unrealistic (84, 91).

New technologies are now being studied in an attempt to improve this therapeutic approach. Bouvier and colleagues stereotactically implanted 68 small catheters into a patient with a recurrent astrocytoma (17).

The catheters were spaced at 1 cm intervals. Each was attached to an osmotic minipump which delivered 12 μg of cisplatin per day (total dose 0.82 mg/day) for 10 days. No neurologic or systemic toxicity was reported and the patient's clinical condition and CT scan stabilized for 6 months following this procedure.

Negatively charged liposomes have also been studied as a means to deliver intratumoral chemotherapy. It has been demonstrated that certain liposomes can be injected intracerebrally in the mouse and rat without evident neurotoxicity (1, 46, 110). Studies using liposomes containing bleomycin demonstrated delayed clearance from the injection site when compared with the injection of free bleomycin. McKeran *et al.* have implanted Ommaya reservoirs into malignant astrocytomas and their preliminary data suggest that chemotherapy entrapped in liposomes may act as a depot preparation (97). No systemic or neurologic toxicities were noted in the small number of patients studied.

Another local depot chemotherapy delivery system employs bioerodable polymers which can be implanted at the time of surgical resection of a brain tumor. These polyanhydride compounds can be constructed to release drugs for months to years and appear to be quite biocompatible (19). The release kinetics of polymer loaded with BCNU, CCNU and methotrexate have been similar to those predicted. CCNU containing polymer placed in the peritoneal cavity of a mouse containing L1210 leukemia resulted in a 56% prolongation in life, demonstrating that active nitrosourea is released from the compounds (86, 87). Preliminary studies are now under way to determine the toxicity and feasibility of this approach in the treatment of brain tumors (62, 145).

CHEMOTHERAPY OF BRAIN TUMORS: THE FUTURE

The use of chemotherapy in the treatment of primary brain tumors has been explored in a preliminary manner in the past decade. To date, this approach has not yielded significant survival prolongation in adults following surgery for high-grade astrocytomas and adds little to radiation therapy in the same patient population. However, these agents appear to hold promise in the treatment of many childhood brain tumors.

New approaches to increase the amount of drug delivered to brain tumors are currently being evaluated. BBB disruption followed by chemotherapy appears to increase the concentration of chemotherapy in normal brain tissue more than it does in the tumor. Intraarterial chemotherapy and the topical administration of chemotherapy require further refinements and more evaluation. High dose systemic therapy with autologous marrow rescue is complicated by considerable systemic toxicity and the constraint of being able to treat patients with only one dose of therapy. Continuous infusions of chemotherapy, newly designed chemotherapeutic agents, and brain-specific carrier systems hold promise but have only been studied in a preliminary fashion.

It is evident from clinical efforts to deliver more drugs to these tumors that they are potentially responsive to chemotherapy. This provides optimism that refining currently available techniques or discovering new ones will result in improved response rates and prolonged survivals for patients with brain tumors. There are two major impediments which may make these improvements difficult. The first relates to the observation that the delivery of more drug results in better antineoplastic effect. Unfortunately, the delivery of high concentrations of chemotherapy is likely to be accompanied by increased neurotoxicity. At the present time there are few studies attempting to develop techniques to screen chemotherapeutic agents for neurotoxicity (53). Efforts in this area need to be expanded and refined so that future attempts to treat brain tumors with high doses of chemotherapy can be pursued using antineoplastic agents which are less neurotoxic.

The other potential difficulty in improving chemotherapeutic results in patients with brain tumors relates to the assessment of therapeutic response in these patients. Most brain tumor trials are reported using response criteria which are much more lenient than those used for other tumors (63, 88, 162). A partial response usually refers to an unspecified improvement in the CT scan or the patient's clinical condition on a stable dose of glucocorticoids. In contrast, a partial response using Eastern Cooperative Oncology Group criteria requires that the product of two perpendicular diameters of the lesion be reduced by 50% (109). Quantitative response measurements would be helpful in resolving differences in efficacy between chemotherapeutic regimens. Current technology permits "tumor" volumes to be calculated from CT scans and measurements of metabolic changes within the tumor appear possible using NMR spectroscopy and positron emission tomography (62, 76, 103, 148). Serial studies using these techniques may allow us to determine which agents are having a significant therapeutic effect on intracranial neoplasms.

The growing number of individuals committed to studying the chemotherapy of brain tumors, novel methods to increase the delivery of these agents to CNS malignancies, new imaging modalities which may improve quantitation of therapeutic responses, and a growing interest in the neurotoxicity of antineoplastic agents will determine progress in the treatment of brain tumors with chemotherapy during the next decade.

REFERENCES

1. Adams, D.H., Joyce, G., Richardson, I.J., *et al.* Liposome toxicity in the mouse central nervous system. J. Neurol. Sci., *31:*173–179, 1977.
2. Allen, J. and Epstein, F. Medulloblastoma and other primary CNS malignant neuroectodermal tumors: the effect of age and extent of disease on prognosis. J. Neurosurg., *57:*446–451, 1982.
3. Allen, J., Hancock, H., and Tan, C. A phase II trial of PCNU in recurrent primary CNS tumors in children: a negative study. Ann. Neurol., *12:*206, 1982.
4. Allen, J.C., Bloom, J., Ertel, I., *et al.* Brain tumors in children: current cooperative institutional chemotherapy trials in newly diagnosed and recurrent disease. Semin. Oncol. *13:*110–122, 1986.
5. Ausman, J.I., Levin, V.A., Brown, W.E. *et al.* Brain tumor chemotherapy. Pharmacological principles derived from a monkey brain-tumor model. J. Neurosurg. *46:*155–164, 1977.
6. Benjamin, R.S., Wiernik, P.H., and Bachur, N.R. Adriamycin chemotherapy—efficacy, safety, and pharmacologic basis of an intermittent single high dose schedule. Cancer *33:*19–27, 1974.
7. Bergvall, U. Temporal course of contrast medium enhancement in differential diagnosis of intracranial lesions with computer tomography. In: Salamon, G. (ed): *Advances in Cerebral Angiography*: pp. 346–348. Berlin, Springer-Verlag, 1975.
8. Berry, M., Jenkin, R., Keen, C., *et al.* Radiation therapy for medulloblastoma: a 21-year review. J. Neurosurg. *55:*43–51, 1981.
9. Blacklock, J.B., Wright, D.C., Dedrick, R.L., *et al.* Drug streaming during intraarterial chemotherapy. J. Neurosurg. *64:*284–291, 1986.
10. Blasberg, R.G., Groothuis, D., and Molnar, P. Application of quantitative autoradiographic measurements in experimental brain tumor models. Semin. Neurol. *1:*203–221, 1981.
11. Balsberg, R.G. and Groothuis, D.R. Chemotherapy of brain tumors. Physiological and pharmacokinetic considerations. Semin. Oncol. *13:*70–82, 1986.
12. Bleyer, W., Pendergrass, T., Millstein, J., *et al.* Eight drugs in 1 day chemotherapy for brain tumors: experience in 107 children and rationale for preradiation chemotherapy. J. Clin. Oncol., *5:*1221–1231, 1987.
13. Bodor, N., Shek, E., and Higuchi, T. Delivery of a quaternary pyridinium salt across the blood-brain barrier as its dihydropyridine derivative. Science *190:*155–156, 1975.
14. Bodor, N., Roller, R., and Selk, S. Elimination of a quaternary pyridinium salt delivered as its dihydropyridine derivative from the brain of mice. J. Pharmacol. Sci. *67:*685–687, 1978.
15. Bodor, N. and Brewster, M. Problems of drug delivery to the brain. Pharmacol. Ther. *19:*337–386, 1982.
16. Bodor, N. and Farag, H.H. Improved delivery through biological membranes XIV: brain specific, sustained delivery of testosterone using a redox chemical delivery system. J. Pharm. Sci. *73:*385–389, 1984.
17. Bouvier, G., Penn, R.D., Kroin, J.S., *et al.* Direct delivery of medication into a brain tumor through multiple chronically implanted catheters. J. Neurosurg. *20:*286–291, 1987.
18. Brockman, R.W. Circumvention of resistance: pharmacologic basis of cancer chemotherapy. 27th Annual Symposium on Fundamental Research, University of Texas, M.D. Anderson Hospital and Tumor Institute. Baltimore, Williams & Wilkins, 1975.
19. Brown, L.R., Wei, C.L., and Langer, R. In vivo and in vitro release of macromolecules from polymeric drug delivery systems. J. Pharm. Sci., *72:*1181–1185, 1983.

20. Brown, T.D., Ettinger, D.S., Donehower, R.C. A phase I clinical trial of spirohydantoin mustard. Proc. Am. Soc. Clin. Oncol. *3*:33, 1984.
21. Burch, P.A., Grossman, S.A., Brundrett, R., *et al.* Chlorambucil delivery and retention in brain using the brain specific chemical delivery system: a quantitative autoradiographic (QAR) study. Proc. Am. Assoc. Cancer Res. *29*:508, 1988.
22. Burman, S. and Rosenbaum, A.E. Rationale and techniques for intravenous enhancement in computed tomography. Radiol. Clin. North. Am. *20*:15–22, 1982.
23. Calvo, F.A., Pastor, M.A., Dy, C., *et al.* Intraarterial and intravenous chemotherapy for the treatment of malignant glioma. Preliminary results. Am. J. Clin. Oncol. *8*:200–209, 1985.
24. Cangir, A., VanEys, J., and Berry, D. Combination chemotherapy with MOPP in children with recurrent brain tumors. Med. Pediatr. Oncol. *4*:253–261, 1978.
25. Carson, B.S., Anderson, J.H., Grossman, S.A., *et al.* An improved rabbit brain tumor model amenable to diagnostic radiographic procedures. Neurosurg. *11*:603–608, 1982.
26. Cascino, T.L., Byrne, T.N., Deck, M.D., *et al.* Intraarterial BCNU in the treatment of metastatic brain tumors. J. Neurooncol. *1*:211–218, 1983.
27. Charnsangavej, C., Lee, Y., Carrasco, C.H., *et al.* Supraclinoid intracarotid chemotherapy using a flow-directed soft-tipped catheter. Radiology *155*:655–657, 1985.
28. Cohen, I.J., Vogel, R., Matz, S., *et al.* Successful nonneurotoxic therapy (without radiation) of a multifocal primary brain lymphoma with a methotrexate, vincristine, and BCNU protocol (DEMOB). Cancer *57*:6–11, 1986.
29. Cohen, M.H., Creaven, P.J., Fossieck, B.E., *et al.* Intensive chemotherapy of small cell bronchogenic carcinoma. Cancer Treat. Rep. *61*:349–353, 1977.
30. Coldman, A.J. and Goldie, J.H. A model for the resistance of tumor cells to cancer chemotherapeutic agents. Math. Biosci. *65*:291–307, 1983.
31. Crafts, D., Levin, V., Edwards, M.S., *et al.* Chemotherapy of recurrent medulloblastoma with combined procarbazine, CCNU, and vincristine. J. Neurosurg. *49*:589–592, 1978.
32. Curt, G.A., Clendenin, N.J., and Chabner, B.A. Drug resistance in cancer. Cancer Treat. Rep. *68*:767–779, 1984.
33. Davignon, J.P., Trissel, L.A., Kleinman, L.M., *et al.* NCI investigational drugs pharmaceutical data. Natl. Cancer Inst., 1985.
34. de Tribolet, N., and Barrelet, L. Successful chemotherapy of pinealoma (letter). Lancet *2*: 1228–1229, 1977.
35. DeVita, V.T., Jr. The consequences of the chemotherapy of Hodgkin's disease: the 10th annual David A. Karnofsky lecture. Cancer *47*:1–13, 1981.
36. Doppman, J.L., Dedrick, R.L., Shook, D.R., *et al.* Glioblastoma: catheter techniques for isolated chemotherapy perfusion. Radiology, *159*:477–483, 1986.
37. Eagan, R.T. and Scott, M. Evaluation of prognostic factors in chemotherapy of recurrent brain tumors. J. Clin. Oncol. *1*:38–44, 1983.
38. Einhorn, L.H. Extragonadal germ cell tumors. In: *Testicular tumors: management and treatment,* edited by L.H. Einhorn, pp. 185–204. New York, Masson, 1980.
39. El-Mahdi, A.M., Phillips, E., and Lott, S. The role of radiation therapy in pinealoma. Radiology, *103*:407–412, 1972.
40. Ertel, I., Boesal, C., Evans, A., *et al.* Adjuvant chemotherapy of high-grade astrocytomas in children: radiation therapy with or without CCNU, vincristine, and prednisone. Proc. Am. Soc. Clin. Oncol. *3*:79, 1984.
41. Ervin, T. and Canellos, G.P. Successful treatment of recurrent primary central nervous system lymphoma with high-dose methotrexate. Cancer *45*:1556–1557, 1980.
42. Fenstermacher, J.D. and Cowles, A.L. Theoretic limitations of intracarotid infusions in brain tumor chemotherapy. Cancer Treat. Rep. *61*:519–526, 1977.
43. Fenstermacher, J.D. and Gazendam, J. Intraarterial infusions of drugs and hypersmotic solutions as ways of enhancing CNS chemotherapy. Cancer Treat. Rep. *65*:27–37, 1981.
44. Feun, L., Savaraj, N., Lu, K., *et al.* Disruption of the blood-brain barrier with intracarotid hydroxyurea. Proc. Am. Asso. Cancer. Res. *25*:364, 1984.
45. Feun, L.G., Lee, Y.Y., Yung, W.K., *et al.* Phase II trial of intracarotid BCNU and cisplatin in primary malignant brain tumors. Cancer Drug Deliv. *3*:147–156, 1986.
46. Firth, G.B., Oliver, A.S., and McKeran, R.O. Studies on the intracerebral injection of bleomycin free and entrapped within liposomes in the rat. J. Neurol. Neurosurg. Psychiatry *47*:585–589, 1984.
47. Foo, S.H., Choi, I.S., Berenstein, A., *et al.* Supraophthalmic intracarotid infusion of BCNU for malignant glioma. Neurology *36*:1437–1444, 1986.
48. Forbes, A.R. and Goldberg, I.D. Radiation therapy in the treatment of meningioma: The Joint Center for Radiation Therapy experience 1970 to 1982. J. Clin. Oncol. *2*:1139–1143, 1984.
49. Freeman, C.R., Berg, J.W., and Cutler, S.J. Occurrence and prognosis of extranodal lymphomas. Cancer *29*:252–260, 1972.
50. Freeman, C.R., Shustick, C., Brisson, M.L. *et al.* Primary malignant lymphoma of the central nervous system. Cancer *58*:1106–1111, 1986.
51. Frick, J.C., Hansen, R.M., Anderson, T., *et al.* Successful high-dose intravenous cytarabine treatment of parenchymal brain involvement from malignant lymphoma. Arch. Intern. Med. *146*:791–792, 1986.
52. Garfield, J. and Dayan, A.D. Postoperative intracavity chemotherapy of malignant glio-

mas: a preliminary study using methotrexate. J. Neurosurg. *39:*315–322, 1973.

53. Gilbert, M.R., Harding, B.L., and Grossman, S.A. Methotrexate neurotoxicity: in vitro studies using cerebellar explants. Cancer Res. *49:*2502–2505, 1989.

54. Goldie, J.H. and Coldman, A.J. A mathematical model for relating the drug sensitivity of tumors to the spontaneous mutation rate. Cancer Treat. Rep. *63:*1727–1733, 1979.

55. Gonzalez, D.G. and Schuster-Uitterhoeve, L.J. Primary nonHodgkin's lymphoma of the central nervous system. Results of radiotherapy in 15 cases. Cancer *51:*2048–2052, 1983.

56. Green, S.B., Byar, D.P., Walker, M.D., *et al.* Comparisons of carmustine, procarbazine, and high-dose methylprednisolone as additions to surgery and radiotherapy for the treatment of malignant glioma. Cancer Treat. Rep. *67:*121–132, 1983.

57. Greenberg, H.S., Ensminger, W.D., Chandler, W.F., *et al.* Intraarterial BCNU chemotherapy in the treatment of malignant gliomas of the central nervous system. J. Neurosurg. *61:*423–429, 1984.

58. Greenberg, H.S., Ensminger, W.D., Layton, P.B., *et al.* Phase I-II evaluation of intraarterial diaziquone for recurrent malignant astrocytomas. Cancer Treat. Rep. *70:*353–357, 1986.

59. Greig, N.H. Chemotherapy of brain metastases: current status. Cancer Treat. Rev. *11:*157–186, 1984.

60. Groothuis, D.R. and Blasberg, R.G. Rational brain tumor chemotherapy. The interaction of drug and tumor. Neurol. Clin. *3:*801–816, 1985.

61. Grossman, S.A., Sheidler, V.R., Ahn, H., *et al.* Complete and partial responses of newly diagnosed malignant astrocytomas (MA) following continuous infusion of BCNU and Cisplatin. Proc. Am. Soc. Clin. Oncol. *8:*344, 1989.

62. Grossman, S.A., Reinhard, C.S., Brem, H., *et al.* The intracerebral delivery of BCNU with surgically implanted bioerodable polymers: a quantitative autoradiographic study. Proc. Am. Soc. Clin. Oncol. *7:*84, 1988.

63. Grossman, S.A. and Burch, P.A. Quantitation of tumor response to antineoplastic therapy. Semin. Oncol. *15:*441–454, 1988.

64. Grosso, E., Geda, C., Buchi, G., *et al.* Primary brain malignant nonHodgkin's lymphoma: report of a case treated with chemotherapy in combination with radiotherapy. Tumori *72:*117–120, 1986.

65. Hayman, L.A., Evans, R.A., and Hinck, V.C. Delayed high iodine dose contrast computed tomography: cranial neoplasms. Radiology *136:*677–684, 1980.

66. Helle, T.L., Britt, R.H., and Colby, T.V. Primary lymphoma of the central nervous system. J Neurosurg. *60:*94–103, 1984.

67. Hiesiger, E.M., Voorhies, R., and Basler, G.A. Capillary permeability of experimental brain tumor and cortex after intracarotid hyperosmolar mannitol as measured by quantitative autoradiography (QAR). Neurology *33 (supp 2):*108, 1983.

68. Hiesiger, E.M., Voorhies, R., Basler, G.A., *et al.* Comparison of [^{14}C]-methotrexate [^{14}C]-MTX) delivery by intravenous vs. intracarotid (IC) route without or with IC mannitol in experimental rat brain tumors as measured by quantitative autoradiography (QAR). Proc. Am. Assoc. Cancer Res. *25:*363, 1984.

69. Hilton, J. and Sessions, R.H. Crosslinking of DNA in rat brain tumors and bone marrow by spirohydantoin mustard. Proc. Am. Assoc. Cancer Res. *18:*112, 1977.

70. Hochberg, F.H., Parker, L.M., Takvorian, T., *et al.* High-dose BCNU with autologous bone marrow rescue for recurrent glioblastoma multiforme. J. Neurosurg. *54:*455–460, 1981.

71. Hochberg, F.H., Pruitt, A.A., Beck, D., *et al.* The rationale and methodology for intraarterial chemotherapy with BCNU as treatment for glioblastoma. In: Howell, S. (ed): *Intraarterial and Intracavitary Chemotherapy,* pp. 97–109. Boston, Martinus Nijhoff, 1984.

72. Hochberg, F.H., Pruitt, A.A., Beck, D.O., *et al.* The rationale and methodology for intraarterial chemotherapy with BCNU as treatment for glioblastoma. J. Neurosurg. *63:*876–880, 1985.

73. Hoshino, T. Therapeutic implications of brain tumor cell kinetics. Modern concepts in brain tumor therapy: laboratory and clinical investigations. Natl. Cancer Inst. Monograph *46,* pp. 29–36, Dept. Health, Education and Welfare. 1977.

74. Hryniuk, W.M., Levine, M.N., and Levin, L. Analysis of dose intensity for chemotherapy in early (Stage II) and advanced breast cancer. Natl. Cancer Inst. Monograph *1:*87–94, 1986.

75. Inaba, Y., Hiratsuka, H., Komatsu, K., *et al.* Sequential delayed enhanced CT in brain tumors. Neuroradiology *16:*549–551, 1978.

76. Johnson, D.W., Parkinson, D., Wolpert, S.M., *et al.* Intracarotid chemotherapy with 1,3-bis-(2-chloroethyl)-1-nitrosourea in water in the treatment of malignant glioma. Neurosurgery *20*(4):577–583, 1987.

77. Johnson, R.K. and Goldin, A. The clinical impact of screening and other experimental tumor studies. Cancer Treat. Rev. *2:*1–131, 1975.

78. Jooma, R. and Kendall, B.E. Diagnosis and management of pineal tumors. J. Neurosurg. *58:*654–665, 1983.

79. Kapp, J.P. and Vance, R.B. Supraophthalmic carotid infusion for recurrent glioma: rationale, technique, and preliminary results for cisplatin and BCNU. J. Neurooncol. *3:*5–11, 1985.

80. Kawakami, Y., Tabuchi, K., Ohnishi, R., *et al.* Primary central nervous system lymphoma. J. Neurosurg. *62:*522–527, 1985.

81. Kikuchi, K., Watanabe, K., Miura, S., *et al.* Steroid-induced regression of primary malignant lymphoma of the brain. Surg. Neurol. *26*:291–296, 1986.
82. Kleinman, G., Hochberg, F., and Richardson, E. Systemic metastases from medulloblastoma. Cancer *48*:2296–2309, 1981.
83. Kornblith, P.L. and Walker, M. Chemotherapy for malignant gliomas. J. Neurosurg. *68*:1–17, 1988.
84. Kroin, J.S. and Penn, R.D. Intracerebral chemotherapy: chronic microinfusion of cisplatin. Neurosurgery *10*:309–354, 1982.
85. Lehane, D.E., Bryan, R.N., Horowitz, B., *et al.* Intraarterial cisplatin chemotherapy for patients with primary and metastatic brain tumors. Cancer Drug Deliv. *1*:69–77, 1983.
86. Leong, K.W., Brott, B.C., and Langer, R. Bioerodable polyanhydrides as drug-carrier matrices. I. characterization, degradation, and release characteristics. J. Biomed. Mater. Res. *19*:941–955, 1985.
87. Leong, K.W., Simonte, V., Hilton, J., *et al.* Bioerodable polyanhydrides for cancer chemotherapy. Proc. Int. Symp. Control Rel. Bioact. Mater. *12*:106–107, 1985.
88. Levin, V.A., Crafts, D.C., Norman, D.M., *et al.* Criteria for evaluating patients undergoing chemotherapy for malignant brain tumors. J. Neurosurg. *47*:329–335, 1977.
89. Levin, V.A., Kabra, P.M., and Freeman-Dove, M.A. Pharmacokinetics of intracarotid artery [^{14}C]-BCNU in the squirrel monkey. J. Neurosurg. *48*:587–593, 1978.
90. Levin, V.A., Hoffman, W.F., Pischer, T.L., *et al.* BCNU-5-fluorouracil combination therapy for recurrent malignant brain tumors. Cancer Treat. Rep. *62*:2071–2076, 1978.
91. Levin, V.A. Relationship of octanol/water partition coefficient and molecular weight to rat brain capillary permeability. J. Med. Chem. *23*:682–684, 1980.
92. Levin, V.A., Patlak, C.S., and Landahl, H.D. Heuristic modeling of drug delivery to malignant brain tumors. J. Pharmacokinet. Biopharm. *8*:257–296, 1980.
93. Levin, V.A. Chemotherapy of primary brain tumors. Neurol. Clin. *3*:855–866, 1985.
94. Loeffler, J.S., Ervin, T.J., Mauch, P., *et al.* Primary lymphomas of the central nervous system: patterns of failure and factors that influence survival. J. Clin. Oncol. *3*:490–494, 1985.
95. Lutz, R., Dedrickf, R., Boretos, J., *et al.* Mixing studies during intracarotid arterial infusion in an in vitro model. J. Neurosurg. *64*:277–283, 1986.
96. McDonell, L., Potter, P., and Leslie, R. Localized changes in blood-brain barrier permeability following the administration of antineoplastic drugs. Cancer Res. *38*:2903–2904, 1978.
97. McKeran, R.O., Firth, G., Oliver, S., *et al.* A potential application for the intracerebral injection of drugs entrapped within liposomes in the treatment of human cerebral gliomas. J. Neurol. Neurosurg. Psychiatry *48*:1213–1219, 1985.
98. Madajewicz, J.S., West, C.R., Park, H.C., *et al.* Phase II study: intraarterial BCNU therapy for metastatic brain tumors. Cancer *47*:653–657, 1981.
99. Mahaley, M.S. Jr., Whaley, R.A., Blue, M., *et al.* Central neurotoxicity following intracarotid BCNU chemotherapy for malignant gliomas. J. Neurooncol. *3*:297–314, 1986.
100. Marshall, E.K. Jr. Historical perspectives in chemotherapy. Adv. Chemother. *1*:1–8, 1964.
101. Metes, J.J., Lazo, A., Wilner, H.I., *et al.* Supraophthalmic placement of microleak balloon catheters for intracranial chemotherapy infusion: complications and results of therapy. Am. J. Neuroradiol. *6*:948–952, 1985.
102. Miller, D.F., Bay, J.W., Ledrman, R.J., *et al.* Ocular and orbital toxicity following intracarotid injection of BCNU (carmustine) and cisplatinum for malignant gliomas. Ophthalmology *92*:402–406, 1985.
103. Miraldi, F. Potential of NMR and PET for determining tumor metabolism. Int. J. Radiat. Oncol. Biol. Phys. *12*:1033–1039, 1986.
104. Mirra, S.S., Check, I.J., Porter, J.D., *et al.* Rapid evolution of central nervous system lymphoma in a renal transplant recipient. Lancet *2*:489–493, 1981.
105. Mughal, T.I., Glode, L.M., Braun, T.J., *et al.* Phase I clinical trial of intracarotid bis-chloro-ethyl-nitrosourea (BCNU) and 2'-deoxy-5-fluorouridine (FUDR) in malignant astrocytomas. J. Neurooncol. *3*:291–296, 1986.
106. Neuwelt, E.A., Howieson, J., Frenkel, E.P., *et al.* Therapeutic efficacy of multiagent chemotherapy with drug delivery enhancement by blood-brain barrier modification in glioblastoma. Neurosurgery *19*(4):573–582, 1986.
107. Neuwelt, E.A., Frenkel, E.P., Gumerlock, M.K., *et al.* Developments in the diagnosis and treatment of primary CNS lymphoma. Cancer *58*:1609–1620, 1986.
108. Norman, D., Stevens, E.A., Wings, S.D., *et al.* Quantitative aspects of contrast enhancement in cranial computed tomography. Radiology *129*:683–688, 1978.
109. Oken, M.M., Creech, R.H., Tormey, D.C., *et al.* Toxicity and response criteria of the Eastern Cooperative Oncology Group. Am. J. Clin. Oncol. *5*:649–655, 1982.
110. Oliver, S., Firth, G.B., and McKeran, R.O. Studies on the intracerebral injection of vincristine free and entrapped within liposomes in the rat. J. Neurol. Sci. *68*:25–30, 1985.
111. O'Reilly, R.J. Allogeneic bone marrow transplantation: current status and future directions. Blood *62*:941–946, 1983.
112. Pearl, G.S., Chan, W.C., Bakay, R.A.E., *et al.* Primary lymphoma of the central nervous system diagnosed by computed tomographic

scan-directed needle biopsy with a frozen section immunoperoxidase technique. Neurosurgery *16:*1–4, 1985.

113. Peng, G., Marquex, V., and Driscoll, J. Potential central nervous system antitumor agents: spirohydantoin mustard. J. Med. Chem. *18:*846–849, 1975.

114. Penn, I. Malignant lymphoma in organ transplant recipients. Transplant Proc. *13:*736–738, 1981.

115. Phillips, P.C., Dhawan, V., Strother, C., *et al.* Reduced cerebral glucose metabolism and increased brain capillary permeability following high-dose methotrexate chemotherapy: a positron emission tomographic study. Ann. Neurol. *21:*59–63, 1986.

116. Pinkel, D., Hernandez, K., Borella, L., *et al.* Drug dose and remission duration in childhood lymphocytic leukemia. Cancer *27:*247–256, 1971.

117. Pitman, S.W. and Frei, E. III. Weekly methotrexate-calcium leucovorin rescue: Effect of alkalinization on nephrotoxicity; pharmacokinetics in the CNS; and the use in CNS nonHodgkin's lymphoma. Cancer Treat. Rep. *61:*695–701, 1977.

118. Plowman, J., Lakings, D., Owens, E., *et al.* Initial studies on the penetration of spirohydantoin mustard into the cerebrospinal fluid of dogs. Pharmacology *15:*359–366, 1977.

119. Prados, M., Rodriquez, L., Seager, M., *et al.* Phase II study of spirohydantoin mustard for the treatment of recurrent malignant glioma. Cancer Treat. Rep. *71:*1105–1106, 1987.

120. Rall, D.P. and Zubrod, C.G. Mechanism of drug absorption and excretion. Passage of drugs in and out of the central nervous system. Annu. Rev. Pharmacol. *2:*109–128, 1962.

121. Rapoport, S. and Thompson, H. Osmotic opening of the blood-brain barrier in the monkey without associated neurological defects. Science *180:*971, 1973.

122. Rapoport, S., Fredericks, W., Ohno, K., *et al.* Quantitative aspects of reversible opening of the blood-brain barrier. Am. J. Physiol. *238:*421–431, 1980.

123. Roberts, M. and German, W.J. A long term study of patients with oligodendrogliomas. Follow-up of 50 cases including Dr. Harvey Cushing's series. J. Neurosurg. *24:*697–700, 1966.

124. Rosner, D., Nemoto, T., and Lane, W.W. Chemotherapy induces regression of brain metastases in breast carcinoma. Cancer *58:*832–839, 1986.

125. Rubin, R.C., Ommaya, A.K., Henderson, E.S., *et al.* Cerebrospinal fluid perfusion for central nervous system neoplasms. Neurology *16:*680–692, 1966.

126. Salcman, M., Kaplan, R.S., Ducker, T.B., *et al.* Effect of age and reoperation on survival in the combined modality treatment of malignant astrocytoma. Neurosurgery *10:*454–463, 1982.

127. Schabel, F.M. Jr. and Simpson-Herren, L. Some variables in experimental tumor systems which complicate interpretation of data from in vivo kinetic and pharamcologic studies with anticancer drugs. Antiobiot. Chemother. *23:*113–1127, 1978.

128. Sexauer, C.L., Khan, A., Burger, P.C., *et al.* Cisplatin in recurrent pediatric brain tumors. A POG Phase II study. Cancer *56:*1497–1501, 1985.

129. Shalen, P.R., Hayman, L.A., Wallace, S., *et al.* Protocol for delayed contrast enhancement in computed tomography of cerebral neoplasia. Radiology *139:*397–402, 1981.

130. Shapiro, J.R. and Shapiro, W.R. Specific karyotypic and tumorigenic changes in cloned subpopulations of human gliomas exposed to sublethal doses of BCNU. In: *Rational Basis for Chemotherapy,* edited by B.A. Chabner, pp. 45–59. New York, Alan R. Liss, 1983.

131. Shapiro, W.R. Introduction: brain tumors. Semin Oncol *13:*1–3, 1986.

132. Shapiro, W.R., Green, S.B., Burger, P.C., *et al.* A randomized comparison of intraarterial (IA) vs. intravenous BCNU for patients with malignant glioma: interim analysis demonstrating lack of efficacy for IA BCNU. Proc. Am. Soc. Clin. Oncol. *6:*69, 1987.

133. Shoemaker, D.D., O'Dwyer, P.J., Marsoni, S., *et al.* Spiromustine: a new agent entering clinical trials. Invest. New Drugs *1:*303–308, 1983.

134. Sigman, L.M., VanEcho, D.A., Egorin, M.J., *et al.* Phase I trial of Spiromustine (NSC 172112) Proc. Am. Soc. Clin. Oncol. *3:*31, 1984.

135. Simon, S., McSherry, J.W., Krakoff, I.H., *et al.* Spiromustine: A phase I trial. Proc. Am. Soc. Clin. Oncol. *3:*29, 1984.

136. Skarin, A.T., Zuckerman, K.J., Pitman, S.W., *et al.* High-dose methotrexate with folinic acid rescue in the treatment of advanced non-Hodgkin's lymphoma including CNS involvement. Blood *50:*1039–1047, 1977.

137. Skipper, H.E., Schabel, F.M. Jr., and Wilcox, W.S. Experimental evaluation of potential anticancer agents. XVII. On the criteria and kinetics associated with "curability" of experimental leukemia. Cancer Chemother. Rep. *35:*1–111, 1964.

138. Skipper, H.E. and Schabel, F.M. Jr. Quantitative and cytokinetic studies in experimental tumor models. In: *Cancer Medicine,* edited by J. F. Holland and E. Frei, III, pp. 629–650. Philadelphia, Lea & Febiger, 1973.

139. Skipper, H.E. Reasons for success and failure in treatment of murine leukemias with the drugs now employed in treating human leukemias. Cancer Chemotherapy, Ann Arbor, MI, University Microfilms International *1:*1–166, 1978.

140. Snider, W.D., Simpson, D.M., Aronyk, K.E., *et al.* Primary lymphoma of the nervous system associated with acquired immunodeficiency syndrome. N. Engl. J. Med. *308:*45, 1983.

141. Solero, C.L., Monfardini, S., Brambilla, C., *et al.* Controlled study with BCNU vs CCNU as adjuvant chemotherapy following surgery plus radiotherapy for glioblastoma multiforme. Cancer Clin. Trials *2:*43–48, 1979.
142. Stewart, D.J., Wallace, S., Feun, L., *et al.* A Phase I study of intracarotid artery infusion of cis-diaminedichloroplatinum (II) in patients with recurrent malignant intracerebral tumors. Cancer Res. *42:*2059–2062, 1982.
143. Sung, D.I., Harisiadis, L., and Chang, C.H. Midline pineal tumors and suprasellar germinomas: highly curable by irradiation. Radiology *128:*745–751, 1978.
144. Takeda, N., Tanaka, R., Nakai, O., *et al.* Dynamics of contrast enhancement in delayed computed tomography of brain tumors: tissue-blood ratio and differential diagnosis. Radiology *142:*663–668, 1982.
145. Tamargo, R.J., Myseros, J.S., and Brem, H. Growth inhibition of the 9L gliosarcoma by the local sustained release of BCNU: a comparison of systemic versus regional chemotherapy. American Association of Neurological Surgeons. Toronto, Canada, pp. 212–214, 1988.
146. Thomas, E.D. Marrow transplantation for malignant diseases (Karnofsky Memorial Lecture). J. Clin. Oncol. *1:*517–531, 1983.
147. Todd, F.D., Miller, C.A., Yates, A.J., *et al.* Steroid-induced remission in primary malignant lymphoma of the central nervous system. Surg. Neurol. *26:*79–84, 1986.
148. Tyler, J.L., Diksic, M., Evans, A.C., *et al.* Metabolic and hemodynamic evaluation of gliomas using positron emission tomography. J. Nucl. Med. 28(7):1123–1133, 1987.
149. Vance, R.B. and Kapp, J.P. Supraophthalmic carotid infusion with low dose cisplatin and BCNU for malignant glioma. J. Neurooncol. *3:*287–290, 1986.
150. Varadachari, C., Palutke, M., Climie, A.R.W., *et al.* Immunoblastic sarcoma (histiocytic lymphoma) of the brain with B cell markers. J. Neurosurg. *49:*889–892, 1978.
151. Vick, A., Khandekar, J.D., and Bigner, D.D. Chemotherapy of brain tumors: the blood-brain barrier is not a factor. Arch. Neurol. *34:*523–526, 1977.
152. Walker, M.D. and Hurwitz, B.S. BCNU 1,3-bis(2-chloroethyl)-1-nitrosourea (NSC-409962) in the treatment of malignant brain tumor—a preliminary report. Cancer Chemother. Rep. *54:*263–271, 1970.
153. Walker, M.D., Alexander, E., Jr., Hunt, W.E., *et al.* Evaluation of mithramycin in the treatment of anaplastic gliomas. J. Neurosurg. *44:*655–667, 1976.
154. Walker, M.D., Alexander, E. Jr., Hunt, W.E., *et al.* Evaluation of BCNU and/or radiotherapy in the treatment of anaplastic gliomas: a co-operative clinical trial. J. Neurosurg. *49:*333–343, 1978.
155. Walker, M.D., Strike, T.A., and Sheline, G.E. An analysis of dose-effect relationship in the radiotherapy of malignant gliomas. Int. J. Radiat. Oncol. Biol. Phys. *5:*1725–1931, 1979.
156. Walker, M.D., Green, S.B., Byar, D.P., *et al.* Randomized comparisons of radiotherapy and nitrosoureas for the treatment of malignant glioma after surgery. N. Engl. J. Med. *303:* 1323–1329, 1980.
157. Walker, R. and Allen, J. Cisplatin in the treatment of recurrent childhood brain tumors. J. Clin. Oncol. *6:*62–66, 1988.
158. Wara, W.M., Jenkin, R.D.T., Evans, A., *et al.* Tumors of the pineal and suprasellar region: children's cancer study group treatment results 1960–1975. Cancer *43:*698–701, 1979.
159. Weiss, S.R. and Raskind, R. Treatment of malignant brain tumors by local methotrexate: a preliminary report. Int. Surg. *51:*149–155, 1969.
160. Weissman, D.W. and Grossman, S.A. A model for quantitation of peritumoral brain edema. J. Neurosci. Methods *15:*441–454, 1988.
161. Wilson, C.B., Boldrey, E.B., and Enot, K.J. 1,3-*bis*(2-chloroethyl)-1-nitrosourea (NSC 409962) in the treatment of brain tumors. Cancer Chemother. Rep. *54:*273–281, 1970.
162. Wilson, C.B., Crafts, D., and Levin, V. Brain Tumors: criteria of response and definition of recurrence. Natl. Cancer Inst. Monogr. *46:*197–203, 1977.
163. Yunis, J. The chromosomal basis of human neoplasia. Science *221:*227–236, 1983.

CHAPTER 19

Photoradiation Therapy of Brain Tumors

ROBERT E. WHAREN, JR., M.D., ROBERT E. ANDERSON, B.S., and EDWARD R. LAWS, JR., M.D.

BASIC CONCEPTS

The concept of photoradiation therapy (PRT) is based on the ability of certain substances known as photosensitizers to concentrate preferentially in malignant tissue. These photosensitizers then have the capability to selectively destroy malignant tissue when activated by light of the appropriate wavelength and intensity in the presence of oxygen. Phototherapy, photodynamic therapy, and photochemotherapy are all terms which have been used to refer to this phenomenon of photoradiation therapy.

The action of a photosensitizer is produced by the absorption of photons of a wavelength sufficient to promote electrons within the sensitizer to an excited triplet state. This excited molecule may then interact either directly with substrates within the cell or indirectly with those substrates through the production of singlet oxygen. The various photochemical reactions that are excited by light are subsequently capable of killing cells through multiple interactions with the cell membrane, cytoplasm, nuclear membrane, and nucleus. In vivo, a major reaction is destruction of the tumor vasculature through damage to the endothelium.

An ideal photosensitizer should have a number of properties: (*a*) it should be selectively absorbed or retained by all neoplastic or dysplastic cells; (*b*) it must be efficient in killing malignant cells following application of light at a wavelength capable of significant tissue penetration; (*c*) it must be nontoxic to normal tissue; and (*d*) it should have some characteristic, such as fluorescence, that makes it easily detectable.

The search for an ideal photosensitizer is currently being pursued. Although far from ideal, the photosensitizer that has received the most extensive investigation in both the laboratory and the clinic is hematoporphyrin derivative (HPD). A review of the present status of this new modality of photoradiation therapy and its current and potential applications in the field of neurosurgery are the subject of this chapter.

HISTORY OF PHOTOIRRADIATION THERAPY

At the turn of the century Raab (115) first observed that acridine orange was toxic to paramecia upon exposure to sunlight. In 1903 Tappeiner (130) showed that enzymes such as diastases, invertase, and pepsin were inactivated by illumination in the presence of eosin, and Tappeiner and Jesionek (129) similarly described the photosensitizing effect of eosin and light on superficial tumors in man. In 1905 it was observed (66) that molecular oxygen was required for this process of killing cells by illumination in the presence of certain dyes.

Hausmann (59–61) in 1909 first demonstrated that hematoporphyrin was a photosensitizer when he showed that hematoporphyrin was fatal to paramecia in the presence of light and that large doses of hematoporphyrin were lethal to mice upon exposure to light. In 1913 Meyer-Betz (96) sensitized himself to light by injecting hematoporphyrin intravenously. He remained sensitive to sunlight for 2 months after the injection, with edema and pigmentation resulting from exposure to light.

Interest in hematoporphyrin increased after Policard (110) in 1924 described the appearance of porphyrin fluorescence in some tumors of both animals and man while no fluorescence was observed in other tissues. Auler and Banzer (4) in 1942 reported a characteristic red porphyrin fluorescence in rat tumor but not in normal tissues following systemic injections of hematoporphyrin. A number of investigators (47–49, 94, 116) have subsequently demonstrated that hematoporphyrin accumulates in neoplastic, embryonic, traumatized, and lymphatic tissue, and that its presence can be detected by a bright red fluorescence under near-ultraviolet light.

The first application of hematoporphyrin to the management of brain tumors took place in the 1950s at Johns Hopkins (91). A series of experiments were performed to evaluate hematoporphyrin fluorescence for the detection of brain tumors at the time of surgery. In this report, a patient with an olfactory-groove meningioma received 500 mg of hematoporphyrin intravenously 12 hours before surgery. At surgery, the tumor was observed to fluoresce a brilliant red color. However, they also described a patient with an ependymoma of the cervical cord who received 500 mg of hematoporphyrin and in whom no fluorescence was observed.

In 1961 Lipson introduced hematoporphyrin derivative (HPD), a material prepared by an acetic acid-sulfuric acid treatment of hematoporphyrin and demonstrated that this derivative had a superior ability to localize in tumors compared to hematoporphyrin (89–91).

Subsequent reports demonstrated a good correlation between tumor fluorescence and biopsy specimens in patients with bronchogenic tumors (57,88). Fluorescence was limited not only to neoplastic tissue but included areas of cervical atypism as well (87). Thus the possibility arose that the fluorescence of hematoporphyrin derivative might make it possible to recognize cells in the process of becoming malignant.

The ability of HPD to detect malignancy has currently been investigated and utilized most thoroughly by Benson *et al.* (5) for the detection and localization of in situ carcinoma of the bladder. Results indicated that intravesically administered HPD was selectively retained in neoplastic and dysplastic transitional cells, that it identified all involved areas, and that these areas could be detected during cystoscopy with the proper detection device.

Despite the use of HPD for the detection of malignant neoplasms, the use of photosensitization for the treatment of tumors received scant attention until the 1970s. The first studies to suggest that photoactivation of hematoporphyrin might be cytotoxic to brain tumors were by Diamond *et al.* in 1972 (29,56). Using a glioma tumor model induced by methylnitrosourea in rats, they found that hematoporphyrin photoactivated by white light from fluorescent lamps was cytotoxic to glioma cells both in vitro and in vivo. Systemic hematoporphyrin caused extensive tumor necrosis in subcutaneously implanted gliomas when exposed to light, whereas neither light alone nor hematoporphyrin alone had any effect.

Dougherty *et al.* in 1975 (34) described instances of eradication of experimental tumors using HPD and red light. Red light delivered 24 hours after drug administration prevented recurrences for at least 90 days in nearly half of a group of mice with subcutaneous mammary tumors. The use of red light at 630 nm provided much better tissue penetration when compared with violet light and resulted in a useful degree of tumor destruction.

The first reports of HPD photoradiation of human tumors appeared in 1976 (36) and 1979 (37) when Dougherty and coworkers found that cutaneous metastases of breast cancer and malignant melanoma could be selectively ablated by PRT (photoradiation therapy) with HPD and red light. Since these initial reports, the concepts of HPD PRT have been applied to the treatment of a number of malignant neoplasms, including lung cancer (25,31,33) bladder cancer (5,63,75) head and neck tumors (18,137,138) ocular tumors (126) and brain tumors (73,85, 95,102,104,107,108, 126,131–134) with some success. The report by Hayata *et al.* (64) of the primary treatment of bronchial carcinoma with complete removal of small early lesions and a 3-year tumor-free survival is very encouraging and has been confirmed by Doiron (31). Photoradiation therapy is now an established treatment for carcinoma in situ of the bladder (38,114).

The application of PRT in neurosurgery was initially very encouraging. A number of investigators have reported the capability of HPD selectively to kill glioma cells both in vitro (2,29,56,131,132,136) and in vivo (22,26,29,52,56,85,95,107,108,132). More recent reports have described initial attempts in the use of PRT for the treatment of malignant brain tumors (52, 73,85,95,104,107,131,132,134). Although the results are equivocal, it is evident that, despite major differences in the protocols by various investigators, HPD PRT is capable of tumor cell destruction in man. Rounds *et al.* (118) and others (8,21), however, have warned that hematoporphyrin is not entirely contained within neoplastic tissue and some HPD accumulates in brain tissue. This small amount of HPD within normal brain tissue can produce significant morbidity and mortality in experimental animals on application of a sufficient dose of light. The challenge is thus to determine parameters that produce effective cytotoxicity while minimizing any effect on normal brain. Current efforts are being directed towards an understanding of the fundamental principles and scientific application of this modality of photoradiation therapy. This has been stimulated by the desire to develop a treatment which may open new possibilities for therapy of both benign and malignant brain tumors.

CURRENT STATUS OF PHOTORADIATION THERAPY

Analysis of the Photoactive Drug

Hematoporphyrin is a naturally occurring compound similar to the heme of hemoglobin without the iron ligand. Since the observation of Lipson (88–90) in 1960 that a derivative of hematoporphyrin (HPD) had superior tumor localizing characteristics when compared to hematoporphyrin, all subsequent clinical studies have used HPD.

Hematoporphyrin derivative (HPD) is prepared by dissolving crude hematoporphyrin in a 19:1 mixture of glacial acetic acid and concentrated sulfuric acid. This solution is then neutralized with a 3% sodium acetate solution resulting in precipitation of an acetylated derivative. The derivative is then dissolved in saline solution made alkaline by the addition of 0.1 NaOH and the final pH adjusted to 7.4 with 0.1 N HCl. The final concentration of the HPD solution is 5 mg/ml. The term HPD is usually applied to the final end product following alkaline hydrolysis. HPD is thus a complex mixture of porphyrins (7) and uncontrollable variation in its components can result during synthesis (6). There has been some attempt to standardize the preparation of HPD, and indeed the product has been marketed as Photofrin I and subsequently Photofrin II (Photofrin Medical Inc., Cheektoyyaga, NY).

HPD is usually administered clinically following sterilization as a piggy-back infusion at a dose of 3–5 mg/kg (85). Thus far there has been no toxicity associated with the administration of HPD in this manner. A significant problem with HPD, however, is that it remains in the skin for 4–6 weeks. This requires that patients remain out of direct sunlight during this period to avoid sunburn.

The absorption spectrum of HPD consists of five bands extending from the near ultraviolet (uv) to the red (10,37,80). The maximum absorption band, the soret band, occurs in the near-uv around 405 nm with minor absorption bands in the visible region. The smallest of the absorption peaks at 624 nm or red light is the wavelength most commonly used in the clinical application of photoradiation therapy, because red light penetrates tissue far better than any of the other absorption peaks at shorter wavelengths. Activation of porphyrins by light at 405 nm produces a reddish fluorescence with a broad spectrum emission of multiple peaks varying from 589 nm to 740 nm (9).

There has been extensive investigation of HPD attempting to identify which components localize in tumors, which components are the photosensitizing agents, which components produce fluorescence, and whether the tumor-localizing components are different from those that persist in the skin and cause skin photosensitivity (67). There is some evidence that the sensitizing component and the fluorescent component are not identical (46). The tumor-localizing components are postulated to be dimers, either dihematoporphyrin ether (DHE) or dihematoporphyrin ester (14,15,40,76,77). Photofrin II has been claimed to be a better sensitizer than HPD with less skin photosensitivity (71). Although Photofrin II may contain a slightly higher concentration of DHE, it is also a poorly characterized mixture of porphyrins (71).

Despite the well established property of HPD to localize within tumors, the mechanisms of its uptake and retention in malignant tissue have not yet been clearly established. Initial reports suggesting the preferential uptake of porphyrin by tumor cells (19,103) have been substantially refuted (20). Dougherty (36,37) suggested that a more rapid clearance of HPD from normal tissue than from malignant tissue provided the basis for the preferential localization of HPD. This differential clearance of HPD was considered a property of the microenvironment of a tumor where increased vascular permeability and inadequate lymphatic drainage resulted in trapping of protein-bound HPD (64,105,125) in the interstitial fluid for longer periods than in normal tissue (54,109).

Because tumors appear to accumulate mainly porphyrin aggregates, Moan (100) thought the preferential accumulation of HPD in tumors was not a property of the tumor cells, but rather was related to other factors in the tumors such as vascular permeability and lymphatic drainage as proposed previously by Dougherty (41). In addition, the high concentration of HPD noted in stromal and reticuloendothelial areas of tumors, notably in macrophages, suggested that phagocytosis may participate in the accumulation of porphyrin aggregates (100,105). Doughtery has proposed that the aggregates are retained in tumors and serve as a reservoir for monomeric porphyrins subsequently diffusing into cells (41).

Christensen *et al.* (23) have also observed that in tissue cultures, the photodynamic effects of HPD varied depending upon the stage of the cell cycle with cells in interphase being the most susceptible while cells in the early G1 phase were the least susceptible.

Studies of tumor fluorescence have not conclusively indicated the exact location of the porphyrins within the tumor. Variations in fluorescence have been noted in different portions of the tumor, with the more vascular regions usually having the greatest fluorescence (79). HPD administered intravenously is bound to albumin (99) and also to serum lipoproteins (19,117). High concentrations of HPD develop in tissues with high levels of lipoprotein receptors. How the binding of HPD to albumin or lipoproteins leads to tumor retention is unclear.

Thus, although the active components of HPD have been studied and even isolated (39) the mechanism of the localization of HPD in neoplastic tissue remains obscure. Indeed, some of the difficulty has been the complex and variable nature of the HPD mixture of porphyrins. Many authors have suggested the advantages of working with a pure substance rather than a mixture. El-Far and Pimstone (43) have reported the efficacy of uroporphyrin-I as a selective tumor localizer. This is a pure compound which when compared to HPD has a 7- to 20-fold greater tumor localizing ability with exceedingly small amounts accumulating in normal tissues. Recently, porphyrin C has been shown to selectively localize in the C6 intracerebral tumor model with a tumor/brain ratio of 1000:1 (71). Phthalocyanines (91) have also demonstrated photosensitizing properties against human glioblastoma. Further work with these and similar compounds are in progress.

The actual concentration of HPD achieved in human tumors has been quantitated by Wharen *et al.* (134) using a microfluorescence assay. HPD concentrations of 1.7 to 2.5 μg/ml were obtained in two cases of malignant gliomas 24 hours following the IV administration of 5 mg/kg of HPD, while simultaneous biopsies of surrounding normal brain tissue yielded values of 0.1 to 0.4 μg/ml and HPD tumor/brain ratios of 6 to 17. Clearly, it appears that a small amount of HPD does cross the blood-brain barrier into normal tissue (139). Whether this small amount of HPD can be damaging to normal cells during photoradiation therapy has recently been investigated (118). Under the appropriate experimental conditions in mice significant morbidity and mortality was produced upon application of light to the brain following HPD administration. This phototoxicity was considered a result of oxygen deprivation in brain tissue resulting from mitochondrial damage, as HPD is reported to concentrate in mitochondria (9), the first organelle to show damage from light exposure (24). The extrapolation of this observation to the human brain is difficult, but does reveal that the use of HPD in its present form may not be free from potential toxicity and further studies are certainly needed.

The optimum time to administer photoradiation therapy following drug administration would be when the HPD concentration in tumor versus normal brain is maximum, provided that the absolute amount in normal brain is low enough to be nontoxic. Although Wharen *et al.* (134) noted a ratio approximately two-fold higher at 4 hours compared to 24 hours after drug administration. Boggan *et al.* (12) found maximal ratios at 24 hours with a patchy uptake of HPD into the 9L gliosarcoma rat model, as only 40% of the tumor area was fluorescent. In the C6 glioma model, however, maximum fluorescence which was uniform throughout the tumor occurred at 6 hours (72). Clearly, HPD localization is dependent upon the HPD preparation and the tumor and further drug development is necessary before the timing of photoradiation therapy after drug administration can be optimized.

The toxicity of HPD in clinical applications has thus far been limited primarily to skin sensitization. Patients must remain out of bright sunlight for approximately 4 weeks following drug administration (102,133). Although carotene containing substances might theoretically diminish skin sensitization, there are no clinical reports supporting their use. McCulloch *et al.* (33) have also reported one patient who developed cerebral edema following the administration of 150 joules/cm^2 of red light 48 hours after the injection of 5 mg/kg of HPD. However, in general, cerebral edema has not been a problem in most clinical series.

There has been concern regarding the possible interaction of postoperative radiotherapy with a porphyrin sensitizer. Early studies suggested that HPD may be a radiosensitizer (83,92,119). Wharen *et al.* (135) studied the in vitro interaction between x-irradiation and HPD in 9L rat glioma cells using both trypan blue exclusion and a colony formation assay. Only at high HPD concentrations (10 to 200 μg/ml) and large x-irradiation fraction sizes (250 rads) was a potentiation of radiosensitivity observed. Kaye *et al.* (71) have not observed side effects in 15 patients treated with conventional radiotherapy (45 Gy in 20 divided doses) 4 weeks following photoradiation therapy. They do recommend, however, delaying radiotherapy for 4 weeks following phototherapy because of the potential toxicity.

Analysis of Drug-Light Interactions

The active mechanism in photoradiation therapy and in dye-sensitized photooxidation reactions for both in vitro and in vivo systems, with few exceptions, proceeds by way of a triplet sensitizer (51,65,70, 111,122). The excited triplet state (^3S) of the sensitizer (S) is produced by the absorption of a photon of light with an energy sufficient to raise the sensitizer to an excited single state (^1S). Subsequent intersystem crossing results in the transformation of an excited singlet state (^1S), as the direct excitation of the triplet state (^3S) of the sensitizer (S) is a forbidden process.

The excited triplet sensitizer (^3S) can then react with biological substrates by two major mechanisms: either directly with the substrate (Type I) by electron or hydrogen-ion transfer or indirectly with the substrate (Type II) through the production of singlet molecular oxygen.

The transfer of energy from the excited triplet state of the sensitizer (^3S) to oxygen proceeds by a process of electronic resonance energy transfer, which is a diffusion controlled process (17,69,74). The $^10_2$ producing ability of photoexcited porphyrins and hence their photosensitizing efficiency is directly related to the lifetime or the decay rate of the porphyrin triplet state (17). For this transfer of energy to occur, there must be a close overlap of the oxygen absorption peak with the energy spectrum of the excited triplet state. O_2 has multiple absorption peaks within the visible spectrum between 400 to 800 nm, including one peak at 630 nm (44,74), a wave length frequently used in photoradiation therapy. Additional peaks occur also in the near-infrared region between 1 to 2 μm and Evans (44) has reported the efficient production of $^1O_2$ and subsequent photooxidation reactions occurring at near-infrared wave lengths.

Doughtery *et al.* (35) proposed in 1976 that singlet oxygen ($^1O_2$) was the cytotoxic agent responsible for the in vitro inactivation of TA-3 mouse mammary carcinoma cells exposed to HPD photoradiation using red light therapy. $^1O_2$ was produced by the transfer of energy from an excited triplet state of hematoporphyrin to oxygen with a quantum yield for $^1O_2$ of 0.16 within the TA-e cells. Further work has demonstrated that although most porphyrin-sensitized reactions occur via a Type II mechanism involving $^1O_2$ (11, 50,123) other Type I mechanisms involving electron transfer may be important (30,58,68). Thus, although the use of $^1O_2$ quenchers such as β-carotene, ascorbic acid, and N_3, plus the enhancing effect of D_2O on the production of $^1O_2$ have clearly demonstrated the participation of $^1O_2$ in reactions in vivo, no photodynamic action so far investigated in vivo is solely explained by the $^1O_2$ mechanism.

Wharen *et al.* (136) have investigated the effect of tissue oxygenation on the HPD photocytoxicity of human glioblastoma in cell culture. Cytotoxicity was directly related to O_2 tension from 12 to 400 torr with a slight but consistent increase in cell kill at O_2 tensions from 7 to 12 torr using red light at a density of 100 mW/cm^2. The enhancement of cellular killing efficiency by increased oxygen availability to the cell was approximately fivefold between 84 and 490 mm Hg. However, at very low PO_2 values, below 12 mm Hg, there was a slight but consistent increase in killing efficiency that was not due simply to cellular hypoxia, as the survival of control cells was 100% at a PO_2 of 7 mm Hg. The direct relationship between cytotoxicity and PO_2 from 12 to 490 mm Hg suggests that reactive oxygen species are involved in the phototoxic process and the HPD photocytotoxicity of human glioma cells can be enhanced by increasing the oxygen availability to the cell. Cytotoxicity does occur, however, even at low oxygen concentrations. Lee *et al.* (86) have suggested that the oxygen present in the system can be reused to generate the toxic species because prolonged irradiation at low oxygen concentration can increase phototoxicity to an extent approaching the cytotoxicity achieved under atmospheric conditions.

Further studies (136) have demonstrated that HPD phototoxicity can be effectively quenched by β-carotene, an efficient quencher of singlet oxygen. This quenching effect of β-carotene is most evident at the higher PO_2 values. Mannitol, a quencher of free hydroxyl ion radicals, however, had no effect on the cellular killing efficiency for PO_2 values from 30 to 490 mm Hg. This supports the hypothesis that the preferred mechanism of the cytotoxic effect of HPD is by singlet oxygen and not free radical formation. However, the consistent increase in cytotoxicity at PO_2 values less than 12 mm Hg suggests that at very low PO_2, cytotoxicity may occur through other mechanisms. Indeed, Foote (51) has stated that the relative efficiency of type I and type II reactions depends on the various concentrations of oxygen substates and triplet sensitizer as well as the rate constant for each reaction and the rate for the spontaneous decay of the excited triplet state. Apparently, at very low PO_2 values, cytotoxicity either began to occur via mechanisms other than singlet oxygen or the cell for some reason became more sensitive to singlet oxygen destruction. Regardless of the mechanism, however, it is apparent that HPD phototoxicity of human glioma cells can be effective even under hypoxic conditions.

The mechanisms responsible for the loss of cell viability in photoradiation therapy are difficult to characterize because of the multiplicity of damaging reactions that occur. Photoradiation of porphyrin-loaded cells results in inhibition of membrane transport functions (42,78) and membrane damage (93); effects which may occur from photodynamic cross-linking of membrane proteins (53,78,82,84). Photodynamic damage to DNA (45–55,98) and to lysosomes (120) also occurs.

Proteins, nucleic acids, unsaturated lipids, NADH, NADPH, hyaluronic acid and other biomolecules are photooxidized with porphyrins as sensitizers (123). The predominant susceptible sites on proteins are the unprotonated thiol group of cysteine, the unprotonated imidazole ring of histidine, the thioether group of methionine, the indole ring of tryptophan, and the phenolate anion of tyrosine. Photooxidation of these sites on proteins results in the loss of enzymatic (121) and hormonal activity (106), loss of toxic properties of snake venoms and bacterial toxins (16), loss of antigenic properties (128), and loss of antibody reactivity (127). Unsaturated lipids and cholesterol are converted to hydroperoxides. Nucleic acids are photooxidized by porphyrins predominantly at guanine residues, and both single and double strand breaks can be produced in DNA (123).

Inactivation of cells by photoradiation can be classified into three major modes of action (65,123). First, the porphyrin remains either outside the cell or within the cell membrane. In this case, the cell membrane would be expected to be the major site of photodamage. Membrane damage would result from the photooxidation of membrane lipids, structural proteins and enzymes with resultant inhibition of transport processes, alterations of receptors, changes in permeability, or cross-linking of proteins in the membrane. Second, the porphyrin penetrates into the cytoplasm resulting in photodamage to mitochondria, lysosomes, ribosomes, and proteins. Cell death would then occur from uncoupling or inhibition of oxidative phosphorylation, leakage of hydrolyses from lysosomes into the cytoplasm and inhibition of microsomal activity. Third, the porphyrin penetrates the nucleus to sensitize the nucleic acids and chromosomes with resulting chromosomal breaks. As yet, no chromosomal breaks have been demonstrated in mammalian cells. Currently, the modes of action of porphyrin photosensitized reactions are considered to be multifactorial involving predominantly the cell membrane and cytoplasm.

In tissue, however, whether the cells damaged first are the tumor cells or the endothelial cells is unclear. The studies of Henderson *et al.* (62) suggest that blood vessels are damaged initially and the tumor then undergoes ischemic changes.

Optimization of the parameters of photoradiation therapy involves not only considerations of the uptake, distribution, and action mechanisms of the dye, but also considerations of the wavelength, quantity, and energy density of light necessary to achieve cell kill. The action spectrum for porphyrin sensitized cytotoxicity corresponds closely to the absorption spectrum of the porphyrin (123). Kinsey *et al.* (80) found that the cytotoxic action of HPD was directly proportional to the number of light quanta absorbed by HPD in the cell. For thin layers of cells, the Soret band at 405 nm had 12 to 30 times the cytotoxicity of red light.

Investigations of the parameters of HPD photocytotoxicity of human glioma cells in cell culture have been performed (2, 131,134). The action spectrum of human glioma cell HPD photocytotoxicity corresponds with the absorption spectrum of HPD and is consistent with reports of action spectra of different human cell lines (2,80,97). The relative killing efficiency of violet light compared with red light irradiation was approximately 12:1 and reflects the relatively poor absorption of HPD for red light. Red light is used in PRT, however, because it provides maximal tissue penetration of visible light through normal brain by approximately 1000-fold compared with violet light (113). For red light, a twofold increase in cellular killing efficiency was observed at higher power densities of 160 mW/cm^2 compared to lower power densities of 40 mW/cm^2. This phenomenon of decreased killing efficiency of red light at low power densities has also been observed by Dougherty who attributed it to a partial repair process occurring during exposure.

Not only the wavelength and power density but also the type of light appears to affect the cellular killing efficiency of HPD-photoradiation therapy. Cowled *et al.* (27) observed no difference in the HPD cell killing efficiency of a continuous wave argon pumped dye laser using Rhodamine B with a wavelength of 625–635 nm compared to a pulsed-wave Gold vapor laser at a pulse frequency of 10–14 kHz having a wavelength of 627.8 nm. Wharen *et al.* (unpublished data) found a markedly decreased cellular killing efficiency for pulsed red light (625–645 nm) produced from a tunable flash pumped dye laser at a repetition rate of 1–6 seconds compared to continuous wave red light (625 to 635 nm) from a filtered xenon arc lamp. In addition, Andreoni *et al.* (3) have reported that pulsed light from a nitrogen laser with a wavelength of 332 nm and a repetition rate of 30 Hz had a HPD cellular killing efficiency greater than a continuous light from an argon ion laser with a wavelength of 334 nm. They attributed this to a mechanism of two photon absorption and production of cytotoxic radicals of HPD. It appears that not only the wavelength of light but also the form of the light (pulsed vs. continuous) and the repetition rate, pulse width, and peak pulse power are all important variables in need of further study.

After all the drug and light parameters have been maximized in HPD photoradiation therapy, the limiting factor in its clinical application may remain the penetration of light through brain and tumor tissue. Light penetration into tissue is determined by the optical characteristics of the tissue, the wavelength of the light, and the concentration of the photosensitizer that has been used. Photons are either absorbed or scattered and the ultimate penetration of light is both wavelength and tissue dependent in an exponential manner (32). A useful concept is the penetration distance defined as the distance at which the light intensity has fallen to 1/e or 37% of its initial valve. In cadaveric human brain, the light penetrance is 0.3 mm at 488 nm, 1.2–1.6 mm at 660 nm, and 1.5–1.7 mm at 710 nm (124). In living rat brain, light from an intracerebral emitting point is attenuated by 99% at a distance of 3.8 mm at 448 nm and 4.9 mm at 633 nm (112). Dougherty (41) has stated that the useful penetration of visible light in adult brain at 630 nm is on the order of 1–1.5 mm. If that is the case, then the depth of penetration of light at 630 nm represents a significant limiting factor for the use of photoradiation therapy in brain and brain tumors. It is known, however, that the penetration of light through tissue continues to improve by several orders of magnitude as the wavelength increases from approximately 600 nm to 1.1 μm (114). Thus, the possibility exists that photoradiation therapy at these wavelengths might provide a more effective depth of tissue penetration. The search for a photosensitizer that absorbs light in the near-infrared spectral range is currently being pursued.

CLINICAL STUDIES

Clinical experience (Table 19.1) has expanded slowly. The majority of patients have had recurrent malignant tumors, predominately gliomas, and have failed prior attempts at therapy. The mean survival for those patients who died after surgery was 11.6 months. There have been three cases of metastasis and five cases involving posterior fossa tumors. In two cases (one medulloblastoma and one ependymoma), PRT was administered at the time of the initial resection.

TABLE 19.1.
HPD PRT of Brain Tumors

Pathology	No. of Cases
Glioma	21
Metastasis	3
Ependymoma	3
Medulloblastoma	2
Craniopharyngioma	1
Rhabdomyosarcoma	1

Photoradiation therapy has thus far been applied by three modalities. For inoperable deep tumors, the stereotactic implantation of one or more quartz fibers to provide argon-dye laser photoradiation (500–1000 J) has been utilized, in conjunction with prior intravenous administration of HPD. For recurrent tumors which can be resected, PRT of the tumor bed has been utilized after intravenous, and in some cases, additional topical administration of HPD. The light delivery system has consisted of a filtered high-intensity xenon-arc lamp and a fiberoptic cable with a Lucite tip. The latter is inserted into a diffusion medium (0.1% Liposol in saline) which fills the tumor bed, and also may be used to cool the operative field. A dose of 150 to 200 J is used. A third mechanism of PRT is employed for cystic or cavitary lesions. After intravenous and/or topical administration of HPD, the cyst or cavity is filled with a diffusion medium and illuminated either with the laser-quartz fiber system or the high intensity xenon arc-lamp fiberoptic system. An example of the latter was the case of a multiply recurrent cystic craniopharyngioma in which HPD was placed stereotactically into the cyst. After 15 minutes, a quartz fiber was stereotactically placed into the cyst and PRT administered.

Hematoporphyrin derivative is usually administered (following sterile preparation) as a piggyback infusion at a dose of 3–5 mg/kg over 5–10 minutes into a freely running intravenous line of D_5 0.2% normal saline. Thus far, there has been no toxicity associated with the administration of HPD in this manner.

Thirty-one patients have received HPD PRT. The initial six patients had deep-seated lesions treated with argon-pumped dye laser by stereotactic insertion of a quartz fiber, whereas the other 25 patients have received xenon arc-lamp (red light) irradiation of the tumor bed following resection. Initially, patients received PRT approximately 24 hours after administration of the drug. After the laboratory studies suggested that higher tumor levels of HPD were achieved at a shorter time interval, PRT has been applied approximately 6 hours after HPD administration. In seven patients, a light diffusion medium was used by filling the cavity of the tumor bed with the medium to disperse the light evenly across the tumor bed.

Results of the six early cases of patients treated with interstitial PRT for recurrent malignant gliomas (Table 19.2) reveals a median survival of approximately 10 months following HPD PRT. There have certainly been no cures and whether the therapy has been of benefit to these patients is difficult to know. These cases do demonstrate, however, both the feasibility of the technique and the fact that the technique is capable of tumor cell destruction. It now appears that the major problem with this technique is the limited penetration of light through brain tissue (32,112,124) and because of this HPD PRT has little if any potential for killing off large volumes of tumor.

Because HPD PRT is effective in killing glioma cells but limited by the ability of

TABLE 19.2.
Results of Interstitial HPD PRT of Recurrent Astrocytomas

		630-nm Laser Technique		
Patient No.	Pathology	Density (mW/cm²)	Duration (min)	Results
1	Grade 3 right frontal	300	30	Alive, 15 months
2	Grade 4 left frontal	400	60	Dead, 5 months
3	Grade 3 left temporal	325	45	Dead, 4 years
4	Grade 3 right frontal	400	60	Dead, 4 months
5	Grade 4 right frontal	250	30	Alive, 19 months

light to penetrate tissue, we thought that the technique could be applied most effectively by delivering the PRT to the tumor bed after resection of the tumor. In this situation, the remaining tumor cells might be within the depth of light penetration. Twenty-five patients have now received PRT administration to the tumor bed following resection of the tumor, 16 of whom had recurrent malignant gliomas. Results thus far in these 16 patients reveal a mean survival of 11 months for the eight patients who have died. Two patients are alive with recurrence and the longest survival without recurrence is 4 years. All have received red light at 50 to 100 mW/cm^2 for 30 to 60 minutes from a filtered xenon arc-lamp. Our results with malignant gliomas are similar to those reported by McCulloch *et al.* (95) who found that patients with gross total removal of their tumors followed by PRT of the tumor bed had the best results. However, in contrast to the patients described by McCulloch *et al.* with malignant gliomas, none of our patients has received PRT at the time of the initial resection.

The most encouraging cases thus far have involved the application of PRT to the tumor bed following gross total resections of posterior fossa tumors (Table 19.3). In two cases (one medulloblastoma and one ependymoma), PRT was applied at the time of the initial resection. The 10-year-old boy with a medulloblastoma is now alive without recurrence at 40 months. One patient died of disseminated intravascular coagulation. Otherwise, in this group in which PRT was administered to the region of the fourth ventricle and brain stem, there have been no complications. Three patients with metastatic tumors have received HPD PRT (Table 19.4) and thus far have done well. Two are alive without recurrence at 6 and 18 months, whereas the third is alive with recurrence at 30 months following treatment.

The patient with the multiply recurrent left orbit rhabdomyosarcoma in an enucleated globe was treated early in our series and died 2 months after therapy. In this case, PRT was applied at 12, 24, and 36 hours after HPD administration and at each treatment approximately one centimeter of tumor sloughed. Unfortunately, the patient with the multiply recurrent craniopharyngioma who received PRT stereotactically into the cyst died 4 months following treatment from a pulmonary embolus.

Overall, the technical aspects of these clinical trials in brain tumor patients have been quite satisfactory. There have been no adverse effects related to either intravenous or topical administration of HPD. The light delivery systems have functioned well, but the importance of temperature monitoring should be emphasized. Power densities greater than 200 mW of red light through a 0.6-mm quartz fiber will produce significant heating of tissue. There is less significant heating when light is delivered through a large diameter (>5.0 mm) fiberoptic system. Because hyperthermia has its own cytotoxic effects and because heat interferes with the photodynamic effect, it is essential to monitor this parameter and to avoid any significant thermal effects while delivering photoradiation.

TABLE 19.3.
HPD PRT of Posterior Fossa Lesions

Patient No.	Pathology	Postresection Xenon Arc Technique: Wavelength (nm)	Density (mW/cm^2)	Duration (min)	Results
1	Medulloblastoma	White	100	30	Alive, 40 mo
2[a]	Medulloblastoma (recurrent)	620	50	30	Alive, 22 mo
3	Ependymoma	630	100	20	Alive, 6 mo
4[a]	Ependymoma	630	50	40	Alive, 17 mo
5	Ependymoma	405	10	40	Died, DIC[b]

[a]A diffusion medium was used.
[b]Disseminated intravascular coagulation.

TABLE 19.4.
HPD PRT of Metastatic Lesions[a]

Patient No.	Pathology	Postresection Technique Density (mW/cm²)	Duration (min)	Results
1[a]	Left parietal adenocarcinoma (lung)	20	60	Alive with recurrence, 20 months
2[a]	Left frontal melanoma	10	60	Alive, 18 months
3	Right frontal adenocarcinoma (colon)	100	30	Alive, 6 months

[a]Xenon arc laser (630 nm) was used.
[b]A diffusion medium was used.

If tissue heating is avoided, we have not recognized any significant degree of post-therapy cerebral edema in any of these patients, all of whom had CT scans within 48 hours of treatment. Two patients had new neurologic signs related either to surgery or PRT, but they were transient in both. All patients were managed with pre- and post-operative corticosteroid therapy. Two patients developed postoperative wound infections which were not surprising in light of the extensive prior therapy both had received. Both responded to antibiotic therapy. One patient died postoperatively of disseminated intravascular coagulopathy (DIC) and one late death occurred at 3 months from a pulmonary embolus. Two patients developed symptoms and signs of cutaneous photosensitivity as a result of disregarding advice to protect themselves from direct sunlight.

As mentioned earlier, the analysis of this series of brain tumor patients treated by PRT with HPD does not permit any conclusions as to the effectiveness of the method. The results, however, are encouraging for several reasons. The theoretical basis of PRT for brain tumors still appears to be sound. The administration of effective amounts of HPD is relatively well-tolerated by these patients. The light delivery systems are practical in use. At least some of these patients appear to have derived some benefit from PRT. These conclusions have been supported by the work of others. As basic knowledge with regard to PRT and malignant brain tumors increases and further laboratory work in cell culture and animal model systems progresses, it should be possible to improve the efficiency and the efficacy of PRT.

CONCLUSIONS AND FUTURE CONSIDERATIONS

Currently, the application of PRT to recurrent malignant gliomas has not resulted in substantial benefit. This is not surprising considering the limited penetration depth of the technique and the biology of this malignant tumor. The greatest promise at present for this technique would be its application in the treatment of such tumors as recurrent cystic craniopharyngiomas, or meningiomas involving dura which are unresectable such as those along the posterior portion of the sagittal sinus. For cystic craniopharyngiomas, PRT can be administered stereotactically into the cyst. Since the light will be effectively attenuated by the cyst wall, there is minimal danger to surrounding structures, a danger inherent with current methods of treatment such as intracavitary radionuclide administration. In the case of meningiomas, PRT can selectively kill tumor cells within dura, and could possibly be an effective treatment for the dural base of a meningioma when the dura cannot be resected.

The future of photoradiation therapy may well involve more effective drug-light combinations operating at longer wavelengths which have a much greater penetration through brain tissue. The development of other photosensitizers with improved tumor specificity activated by light in the near-infrared spectrum is currently being pursued. A timely understanding of the nature of tumor-specific binding of an ideal photosensitizer by malignant cells may provide some clues to the etiology of carcinogenesis.

If an effective technique of photoradiation therapy could be developed it might be applicable for the management of presumably all primary brain tumors, for brain tumors metastatic to the brain from other sites, and presumably for the unusual malignant tumor appearing primarily in the brain such as the medulloblastoma of childhood, malignant meningioma, or hemangiopericytoma. Using CT-guided stereotactic techniques, it is conceivable that tumors anywhere within the brain could at least theoretically be treated by photoradiation. At this time, however, photoradiation therapy is a promising technique which may eventually become an effective therapy, and it is certainly deserving of further investigation.

ACKNOWLEDGMENTS

The authors are grateful to Ms. Jill Nicklas and Ms. Michelle Cooper for their assistance in the preparation of this manuscript. Portions of this manuscript and its accompanying tables have been published elsewhere (42,43,52,56,58,94,99).

REFERENCES

1. Abernathy, C.D., Anderson, R.E., Kooistra, K.L., *et al.* Activity of phthalocyanine photosensitizers against human glioblastoma in vitro. Neurosurgery, *21*:468–473, 1987.
2. Anderson, R.E., Wharen, R.E., Jones, C.A. *et al.* Parameters of hematoporphyrin derivative tumor cell killing efficiency: decomposition of hematoporphyrin derivative at high power densities. In: *Porphyrin Localization and Treatment of Tumors,* edited by D.R. Doiron and C.J. Gomer, pp. 483–500. New York, Alan R. Liss, 1984.
3. Andreoni, A., Cabeddu, R., DeDilvestri, S., *et al.* Two step laser activation of hematoporphyrin derivative. Chem. Phys. Lett. *88*:293–299, 1983.
4. Auler, H., and Banzer, G., Untersuchungen uber die Rolle der Porphine bei geschwulstkranken Menschen und Tieren. Z. Krebstroch, *53*:65–68, 1942.
5. Benson, R.C., Farrow, G.M., and Kinsey, J.H. Detection and localization of in situ carcinoma of the bladder with hematoporphyrin derivative. Mayo Clin. Proc., *57*:548–555, 1982.
6. Berenbaum, M.C., Akande, S.L., Bennett, R., *et al.* Meso-tetra (hydroxyphenyl) porphyrins, a new class of potent tumour photosensitizers with favourable selectivity. Br. J. Cancer, *54*:717–725, 1986.
7. Berenbaum, M.C., Bonnett, R., and Scourides, P.A. In vivo biological activity of the components of haematoporphyrin derivative. Br. J. Cancer, *45*:571–581, 1982.
8. Berenbaum, M.C., Hall, G.W., and Hoyes, A.P. Cerebral photosensitization by hematoporphyrin derivative: evidence for an endothelial site of action. Br. J. Cancer, *53*:81–89, 1986.
9. Berns, M.W., Dahlman, A., Johnson, F.M., *et al.* In vitro cellular effects of hematoporphyrin derivative. Cancer Res., *42*:2325–2329, 1982.
10. Blum, H.F. *Photodynamic Action and Diseases Caused by Light,* pp. 211–237. New York, Rheinhold, 1941.
11. Bodaness, R.S. and Chan, P.C. Singlet oxygen as a mediator in the hematoporphyrin catalyzed photooxidation of NADPH+ to NADP+ in deuterium oxide. J. Biol. Chem., *252*:8554–8560, 1977.
12. Boggan, J.E., Berns, M., and Edwards, M. Uptake, distribution, and retention of hematoporphyrin derivative in metastatic and intrinsic rat tumor models. In: *The Clayton Foundation Symposium on Porphyrin Localization and Treatment of Tumors,* edited by D. Doiron. Santa Barbara, CA, April 24–28, 1983. New York, Alan R. Liss, 1983.
13. Bonnett, R. and Berenbaum, M.C. HPD—A study of its components and their properties. In: *Porphyrin Photosensitization,* edited by D. Kessel and T. Dougherty, pp. 241–260. New York, Plenum, 1983.
14. Bonnett, R., Berenbaum, M.C., and Kaur, H. Chemical and biological studies on hematoporphyrin dose time: an unexpected photosensitization in brain. In: *Porphyrins in Tumor Phototherapy,* edited by D.R. Doiron and C.J. Gomer, pp. 67–87. New York, Plenum Press, 1984.
15. Bonnett, R., Ridge, R.J., Scourides, P.A., *et al.* On the nature of haematoporphyrin derivative. J. Chem. Soc. (Perkin Transactions I):3135–3139, 1981.
16. Boroff, D.A. and DasGupta, B.R. Study of the toxin of Clostridium botulinum. J. Biol. Chem., *239*:3694–3698, 1964.
17. Cannistrado, S., Van de Vorst, A., and Jori, G. EPR studies on singlet oxygen production by porphyrins. Photochem. Photobiol., *28*:257–259, 1978.
18. Carpenter, R.J. III, Neel, H.B. III, Ryan, R.J., *et al.* Tumor fluorescence with hematoporphyrin derivative. Ann. Otol. Rhinol. Laryngol., *86*:661–666, 1977.
19. Carrano, C.J., Tsatsui, M., and McConnell, S. Tumor localizing agents: The transport of meso-tetra (P-sulfurphenyl) porphine by Vero and HEp-2 cells in vitro. Chem. Biol. Interact. *21*:233–248, 1975.
20. Chang, C. and Dougherty, T.J. Photoradiation therapy: kinetics and thermodynamics of porphyrin uptake and loss in normal and malignant cells in culture. Abstr. Radiat. Res. Soc. *74*:498–499, 1978.

21. Cheng, M.K., McKean, J., Boisvert, D., *et al.* Effects of photoradiation therapy on normal rat brain. Neurosurgery *15:*804–810, 1984.
22. Cheng, M.K., McKean, J., Mielke, B., *et al.* Photoradiation therapy of 9L-gliosarcoma in rats: hematoporphyrin derivative (types I and II) followed by laser energy. J. Neurooncol. *3:*217–288, 1985.
23. Christensen, T., and Moan, J., *et al.* Photodynamic effect of hematoporphyrin throughout the cell cycle of the human cell line NHIK 3025 cultivated in vitro. Br. J. Cancer *34:*64, 1979.
24. Coppola, A., Viggiani, E., Salzarulo, L., *et al.* Ultrastructural changes in lymphoma cells treated with hematoporphyrin and light. Am. J. Pathol. *99:*175–181, 1980.
25. Cortese, D.A. and Kinsey, J.H. Hematoporphyrin derivative phototherapy for local treatment of cancer of the tracheobronchial tree. Ann. Otol. Rhinol. Laryngol. *91:*652–655, 1982.
26. Cowled, P.A., Grace, J.R., and Forbes, I.J. Comparison of the efficacy of pulsed and continuous-wave red laser light in induction of photocytotoxicity by haematoporphyrin derivative. Photochem. Photobiol., *39:*115–117, 1984.
27. Cowled, P.A., MacKenzie, L., and Forbes, I.J. Potentiation of photodynamic therapy with hematoporphyrin derivatives of glucocorticoids. Cancer Lett. *29:*107–114, 1985.
28. Dahlman, A., Wile, A.G., and Berns, M.W. Laser photoradiation therapy of cancer. Cancer Res. *43:*430–434, 1983.
29. Diamond, I., Granelli, S.G., McDonagh, A.F., *et al.* Photodynamic therapy of malignant tumors. Lancet *2:*1175–1177, 1972.
30. Dixit, R., Mulchtar, H., and Bickers, D.R. Destruction of microsomal cytochrome P-450 by reactive oxygen species generated during photosensitization of hematoporphyrin derivative. Photochem. Photobiol. *37:*173–176, 1983.
31. Doiron, D.R. and Balcham, O. PRT for treatment of lung cancer. In: *Porphyrin Localization and Treatment of Tumors,* edited by D.P. Doiron and C.J. Gomer, p. 78. New York, Alan R. Liss, 1984.
32. Doiron, D.R. Photophysics and Instrumentation. In: *The Clayton Foundation Symposium on Porphyrin Localization and Treatment of Tumors,* edited by D.R. Doiron, pp. 41–73. Santa Barbara, CA, April 24–28, 1983. New York, Alan R. Liss, 1984.
33. Doiron, D.R., Svaasand, C.O., and Profio, A.E. Light dosimetry in tissue application to photoradiation therapy. Adv. Exp. Med. Biol. *160:*63–76, 1981.
34. Dougherty, T.J., Dridey, G.B., Fiel, R., *et al.* Photoradiation therapy. II. Cure of animal tumors with hematoporphyrin and light. J. Natl. Cancer Inst. *55:*115–119, 1975.
35. Dougherty, T.J., Gomer, C.J., and Weishaupt, K.R. Energetics and efficiency of photoinactivation of murine tumor cells containing hematoporphyrin. Cancer Res. *36:*2330–2333, 1976.
36. Dougherty, T.J., Kaufman, J.E., Goldfarb, A., *et al.* Photoradiation therapy for the treatment of malignant tumors. Cancer Res. *38:*2628–2635, 1978.
37. Dougherty, T.J., Lawrence, G., Kaufman, J.H., *et al.* Photoradiation in the treatment of recurrent breast carcinoma. J. Natl. Cancer Inst. *62:*231–237, 1979.
38. Dougherty, T.J. Photoradiation therapy. Urology *23(suppl):*61–64, 1984.
39. Dougherty, T.J. and Potter, W.R. Structure and properties of HPD active component. In: *The Clayton Foundation Symposium on Porphyrin Localization and Treatment of Tumors,* edited by D. Doiron, Santa Barbara, CA, April 24–28, 1983. New York, Alan R. Liss, 1984.
40. Dougherty, T.J., Potter, W.R., and Weishaupt, K.R. The structure of the active component of hematoporphyrin derivative, In: *Porphyrin Localization and Treatment of Tumors,* edited by D.R. Doiron and C.J. Gomer, pp. 301–314. New York, Alan R. Liss, 1984.
41. Dougherty, T.J. Recent advances in photoradiation therapy (PRT). In: *The Clayton Foundation Symposium on Porphyrin Localization and Treatment of Tumors,* edited by D.R. Doiron, Santa Barbara, CA, April 24–28, 1983. New York, Alan R. Liss, 1984.
42. Dubbleman, T.M.A.R., deGoeij, A.F.P.M., and Stevenick, J. Protoporphyrin-induced photodynamic effects of transport processes across the membrane of human erythrocytes. Biochem. Biophys. Res. Commun., *595:*133–139, 1980.
43. El-Far, M.A. and Dimstone, N.R. Superiority of uroporphyrin I over other porphyrins in selective tumor localization. In: *The Clayton Foundation Symposium on Porphyrin Localization and Treatment of Tumors,* edited by D. Doiron, Santa Barbara, CA, April 24–28, 1983. New York, Alan R. Liss, 1984.
44. Evans, D.F. Oxidation by photochemically produced singlet states of oxygen. J. Chem. Soc., *8:*367–368, 1969.
45. Evenson, J.F. and Moan, J. Photodynamic action and chromosomal damage: a comparison of haematoporphyrin derivative (HPD) and light with x-irradiation. Br. J. Cancer *45:*456–465, 1982.
46. Evensen, J.F., Sommer, S., Moan, J., *et al.* Tumor localizing and photosensitizing properties of the main components of hematoporphyrin derivative. Cancer Res. *44:*482–486, 1984.
47. Figge, F.H.J., Diehl, J., Peck, W.K. *et al.* Evaluation of the use of intravenous hematoporphyrin injections to improve surgical and radiation therapy of cancer of human subjects

(Abstr.). Proc. Am. Assoc. Cancer Res. *2*:105, 1956.
48. Figge, F.H.J., Mack, H.P., Peck, G.C., *et al.* Use of red fluorescent porphyrins to delineate normal and abnormal anatomical structures and neoplastic tissues in human subjects (abstr.). Anat. Rec. *121*:292, 1955.
49. Figge, F.H.J., Weiland, G.S., and Manganiello, L.O.J. Cancer detection and therapy. Affinity of neoplastic, embryonic, and traumatized tissues for porphyrins and metalloporphyrins. Proc. Soc. Exp. Biol. Med. *68*:640–641, 1948.
50. Foote, C.S. Mechanisms of photooxygenation. In: *The Clayton Foundation Symposium on Porphyrin Localization and Treatment of Tumors,* edited by D. Doiron. Santa Barbara, CA, April 24–28, 1983. New York, Alan R. Liss, in press, 1990.
51. Foote, C.S. Mechanisms of photosensitized oxidations. Science, *162*:963–970, 1968.
52. Forbes, I.J., Cowled, P.A., Leong, A.S., *et al.* Phototherapy of human tumors using hematoporphyrin derivative. Med. J. Aust. *2*:489–493, 1980.
53. Girotti, A. Photodynamic effect of protoporphyrin IV on human erythrocytes: cross-linking of membrane proteins. Biochem. Biophys. Res. Commun. *72*:1367–1374, 1976.
54. Goldacre, R.J. and Sylven, B. On the access of blood-borne dyes to various tumor regions. Br. J. Cancer *16*:306–322, 1962.
55. Gomer, C.J. DNA damage and repair in CHO cells following hematoporphyrin photoradiation. Cancer Lett. *11*:161–167, 1980.
56. Granelli, S.G., Diamond, I., McDonagh, A.F., *et al.* Photochemotherapy of glioma cells by visible light and hematoporphyrin. Cancer Res. *35*:2567–2570, 1975.
57. Gregorie, H.B., Horger, E.O., Ward, J.L., *et al.* Hematoporphyrin derivative fluorescence in malignant neoplasms. Ann. Surg. *167*:820–828, 1968.
58. Grossweiner, L.I., Patel, A.S., and Grossweiner, J.B. Type I and Type II mechanisms in the photosensitized lysis of phosphatidylcholine liposomes by hematoporphyrin. Photochem. Photobiol. *36*:159–167, 1982.
59. Hausmann, W. Die sensibilisierende Wirkung des Porphyrins. Biochem. Z. *30*:276–316, 1911.
60. Hausmann, W. Uber die giftige Wirkung des Hematoporphyrins aut Wambluter bei Belichtung. Wien Klin. Wochenschr. *22*:1820–1821, 1909.
61. Hausmann, W. Uber die sensibilisierende Wirkung des Prophyrins. Biochem. Z. *67*:309–317, 1914.
62. Henderson, B.W., Dougherty, T.J., and Malone, P.B. Studies on the mechanism of tumor destruction by photoradiation therapy. In: *Porphyrin Localization and Treatment of Tumors,* edited by D.R. Doiron and C.J. Gomer, pp. 601–612. New York, Alan R. Liss, 1984.
63. Hisazumi, H., Misaki, T., and Miyoshi, N. Photoradiation therapy of bladder tumors. J. Urol. *130*:685–687, 1983.
64. Hyata, Y., Kato, H., and Konaka, C. Hematoporphyrin derivative and laser photoradiation in the treatment of lung cancer. Chest *81*:269–277, 1982.
65. Ito, T. Cellular and subcellular mechanisms of photodynamic action: the $^1O_2$ hypothesis as a driving force in recent research. Photochem. Photobiol. *28*:493–508, 1978.
66. Jodlbaur, A.H. and Von Tappeiner, H. Dtsch. Arch. Klin. Med. *82*:520–546, 1905.
67. Jori, G.,Cozzani, I., Reddi, E., *et al.* In vitro and in vivo studies on the interaction of hematoporphyrin and its dimethylester with normal and malignant cells. In: *Porphyrin Localization and Treatment of Tumors,* edited by D.R. Doiron and C.J. Gomer, pp. 471–482. New York, Alan R. Liss, 1984.
68. Jori, G., Reddi, E., Tomio, L., *et al.* Factors governing the mechanism and efficiency of porphyrin—sensitized photooxidations in homogenous solutions and organized media. In: *Porphyrin Photosensitization,* edited by D. Kessel and D.H. Dougherty, pp. 193–212. New York, Plenum Press, 1983.
69. Karreman, G. and Steele, R.H. On the possibility of long distance energy transfer by resonance in biology. Biochim. Biophys. Acta *25*:280–291, 1957.
70. Kasha, M. and Khan, A.V. The physics, chemistry, and biology of singlet molecular oxygen. Ann. N.Y. Acad. Sci. *171*:5–23, 1970.
71. Kaye, A.H., Morstyn, G., and Apuzzo, M.L.J. Photoradiation therapy and its potential in the management of neurological tumors. J. Neurosurg. *69*:1–14, 1988.
72. Kaye, A.H., Morstyn, G., and Ashcroft, R.G. Uptake and retention of hematoporphyrin derivative in an in vivo/in vitro model of cerebral glioma. Neurosurgery *17*:883–890, 1985.
73. Kaye, A.H., Morstyn, G., and Brownbill, D. Adjuvant high dose photoradiation therapy in the treatment of cerebral glioma: a Phase 1–2 study. J. Neurosurg. *67*:500–505, 1987.
74. Kearns, D. Physical and chemical properties of singlet molecular oxygen. Chem. Rev. *71*:395–427, 1971.
75. Kelly, J., Snell, M.E., and Berenbaum, M.C. Photodynamic destruction of human bladder carcinoma. Br. J. Cancer *31*:237–244, 1975.
76. Kessel, D., Chang, C.K., and Musselman, B. Chemical biologic and biophysical studies on "hematoporphyrin derivative." In: *Methods in Porphyrin Photosensitization,* edited by D. Kessel, pp. 213–227. New York, Plenum Press, 1985.
77. Kessel, D. and Cheng, M.L. On the preparation and properties of dihematoporphyrin ether, the tumor-localizing component of HPD.

Photochem. Photobiol. *41*:277-282, 1985.

78. Kessel, D. Effects of photoactivated porphyrins at the cell surface of leukemia LIZIO cells. Biochemistry *16*:3443-3449, 1977.
79. Kessel, D. In vivo fluorescence of tumors after treatment with derivatives of hematoporphyrin. Photochem. Photobiol. *44*:107-108, 1986.
80. Kinsey, J.H., Cortese, D.A., Moses, H.L., *et al.* Photodynamic effect of hematoporphyrin derivative as a function of optical spectrum and incident energy density. Cancer Res., *41*:5020-5026, 1981.
81. Kocholaty, W. Detoxification of Russell's viper (Vipera russellii) venoms by photooxidation. Toxicon *3*:187-94, 1966.
82. Kohn, K. and Kessel, D. On the mode of cytotoxic action of photoactivated porphyrins. Biochem. Pharmacol. *28*:2465-2470, 1979.
83. Kostron, H., Swartz, M.R., Miller, D.C., *et al.* The interaction of hematoporphyrin derivative, light, and ionizing radiation in a rat glioma model. Cancer *57*:964-970, 1986.
84. Lamola, A.A. and Doleiden, F.H. Cross-linking of membrane proteins and protoporphyrin-sensitized hemolysis. Photochem. Photobiol. *31*:597-601, 1980.
85. Laws, E.R., Cortese, D.A., Kinsey, J.H., *et al.* Photoradiation therapy in the treatment of malignant brain tumors: a phase I (feasibility) study. Neurosurgery *9*:672-678, 1981.
86. Lee See, K., Forbes, W., and Betts, W.H. Oxygen dependency of photocytoxicity with hematoporphyrin derivative. Photochem. Photobiol. *39*:631-634, 1984.
87. Lipson, R.L., Baldes, E.J., and Gray, M.S. Hematoporphyrin derivative for detection and management of cancer. Cancer *20*:2255-2257, 1967.
88. Lipson, R.L., Baldes, E.J., and Olsen, A.M. A further evaluation of the use of hematoporphyrin derivative as a new aid for the endoscopic detection of malignant disease. Dis. Chest *46*:676-679, 1964.
89. Lipson, R.L., Baldes, E.J., and Olsen, A.M. The use of a derivative of hematoporphyrin in tumor detection. J. Natl. Cancer Inst. *26*:1-8, 1961.
90. Lipson, R.L. and Baldes, E.J. Photosensitivity and heat. Arch. Dermatol. *82*:517-520, 1960.
91. Lipson, R.L. and Baldes, E.J. The photodynamic properties of a particular hematoporphyrin derivative. Arch. Dermatol., *82*:517-520, 1960.
92. Loken, M.K. Porphyrins as modifiers of the effects of roentgen rays. Radiology *69*:201-203, 1957.
93. Malik, Z. and Djaldetti, M. Destruction of erythroleukemia, myelocytic leukemia, and Burkett lymphoma cells by photoactivated protoporphyrin. Int. J. Cancer *26*:495-500, 1980.
94. Manganiello, L.O.S. and Figge, G.H.J. Cancer detection and therapy II. Methods of preparation and biological effects of metalloporphyrins. Bull. Univ. Maryland School Med. *36*:3-7, 1951.
95. McCulloch, G.A.J., Forbes, I.J., Lee See, K., *et al.* Phototherapy in malignant brain tumors. In: *Porphyrin Localization and Treatment of Tumors,* edited by D.R. Doiron and C. J. Gomer, pp. 709-718. New York, Alan R. Liss, 1984.
96. Meyer-Betz, F. Untersuchungen uber die biologische (photodynamische) Wirkung des Hamatoporphyrins und anderer Derivate des Blut-und Gallen-tarbstotts. Dtsch. Arch. Klin. Med. *112*:476-503, 1913.
97. Moan, J., Christiansen, T., and Jacobsen, P.B. Porphyrin-sensitized photoirradiation of cells in vitro. In: *Porphyrin Localization and Treatment of Tumors,* edited by D.R. Doiron and C.J. Gomer, pp. 419-442. New York, Alan R. Liss, 1984.
98. Moan, J. and Christiansen, T. Photodynamic effects on human cells exposed to light in the presence of hematoporphyrin. Localization of the active dye. Cancer Lett. *11*:209-214, 1982.
99. Moan, J., Rimington, C., Evensen, F., *et al.* Binding of porphyrins to serum proteins. In: *Porphyrin Photosensitization,* edited by D. Kessel, pp. 193-205. New York, Plenum Press, 1985.
100. Moan, J. and Sommer, S. Uptake of the components of hematoporphyrin derivative by cells and tumors. Cancer Lett. *21*:167-174, 1983.
101. Morgan, W.T. and Muller-Eberhard, U. Interactions of porphyrins with rabbit hemopexin. J. Biol. Chem. *247*:7181-7182, 1972.
102. Morstyn, G., Kaye, A.H., Thomas, R., *et al.* High dose photoirradiation therapy of human tumours using the gold metal vapor laser. Photochem. Photobiol. *46*:945-998, 1987.
103. Mossman, B.T., Gray, M.J., and Silberman, L. Identification of neoplastic versus normal cells in human cervical cell culture. Obstet. Gynecol. *43*:635-639, 1974.
104. Muller, P.J. and Wilson, B.C. Photodynamic therapy: cavitary photoillumination of malignant cerebral tumours using a laser coupled inflatable balloon. Can. J. Neurol. Sci. *12*:371-373, 1985.
105. Muller-Eberhard, U. and Morgan, W.T. Porphyrin-binding proteins in serum. Ann. N.Y. Acad. Sci. *244*:624-650, 1975.
106. Paiva, A.C.M. and Paiva, T.B. The photooxidative inactivation of angiotensinamide. Biochem. Biophys. Acta *48*:412-414, 1961.
107. Perria, C., Capuzzo, T., and Cavagnaro, G. First attempts at the photodynamic treatment of human gliomas. J. Neurosurg. Sci. *24*:119-129, 1980.
108. Perria, C. Photodynamic therapy of human gliomas by hematoporphyrin and He-Ne laser. IRCS Med. Sci. Cancer *9*:57-58, 1981.

109. Peterson, H.I. and Applegren, K.L. Experimental studies in the uptake and retention of labelled proteins in a rat tumor. Eur. J. Cancer, *9:*543–547, 1973.
110. Policard, A. Etudes sur les aspects offerts par des tumeurs experimentales examinees a la lumiere de Woods. Compt. Rend. Soc. Biol. *91:*1423–1424, 1924.
111. Politzer, I.R., Griffin, G.W., and Laseter, J.L. Singlet oxygen and biological systems. Chem. Biol. Interact. *3:*73–93, 1971.
112. Powers, S.K. and Brown, J.T. Light dosimetry in brain tissue: an in vivo model application to photodynamic therapy. Lasers Surg.Med. *6:*1986.
113. Preass, L.E., Bolin, F.P., and Cain, B.W. Tissue as a medium for laser light transport implications for photoradiation therapy. Lasers Surg. Med., (Proc SPIE), *357:*77–84, 1982.
114. Prout, G.R., Lin, C., Benson, R.C., *et al.* Photodynamic therapy with hematoporphyrin derivative in the management of superficial papillary transitional cell carcinoma of the bladder. N. Engl. J. Med. *317:*1251–1255, 1987.
115. Raab, O. Ue ber die Wirking fluorescirender stoffe auf Intusorien Z. Biol. *39:*524–546, 1900.
116. Rassmussen-Tasdel, D.S., Ward, G.E., and Figge, G.H.J. Fluorescence of human lymphatic and cancer tissue following high doses of intravenous hematoporphyrin. Cancer *8:*78–81, 1955.
117. Reyftmann, J.P., Morliere, P., Goldstein, S., *et al.* Interaction of human serum low density lipoproteins with porphyrins: a spectroscopic and photochemical study. Photochem. Photobiol. *40:*721–729, 1984.
118. Rounds, D.E., Jacques, S., and Shelden, C.H. Development of a protocol for photoradiation therapy of malignant tumors. I. Photosensitization of normal brain tissue with hematoporphyrin derivative. Neurosurgery *11:*500–505, 1982.
119. Schwartz, S.K., Absolon, K., and Vermund, H. Some relationships of porphyrins, x-rays and tumors. Univ. Minn. Med. Bull. *27:*7–8, 1955.
120. Slater, T.F. and Riley, P.A. Photosensitization and lysosomal damage. Nature *209:*151–154, 1966.
121. Spikes, J.D. and Livingston, R. Molecular biology of photodynamic action: sensitized photoautoxidations in biological systems. Adv. Radiat. Biol. *3:*29–35, 1969.
122. Spikes, J.D. and MacKnight, M.L. Dye-sensitized photooxidation of proteins. Ann. NY Acad. Sci. *171:*149–161, 1971.
123. Spikes, J.D. Photobiology of porphyrins. In: *The Clayton Foundation Symposium on Porphyrin Localization and Treatment of Tumors,* edited by D. Doiron. Santa Barbara, CA, April 24–28, 1983. New York, Alan R. Liss, 1984.
124. Svasand, L.O. and Ellinger, R. Optical properties of human brain. Photochem. Photobiol. *38:*293–299, 1983.
125. Tipping, E., Ketterer, B., and Koskelo, P. The binding of porphyrins by ligandin. Biochem. J. *169:*509–516, 1978.
126. Tse, P.T. Photoradiation therapy in the management of intraocular, orbital, and periocular tumors. Read before the First International Conference on the Clinical Applications of Photosensitization for Diagnosis and Treatment, Tokyo, April 30–May 2, 1986.
127. Tyler, A. Analphylactic properties of photooxidized rabbit antisera (vs. sheep erythrocytes and pneumococci) and horse antiserum (vs. diptherial toxin) containing univalent antibodies. J. Immunol. *51:*329–337, 1945.
128. Vodrazka, Z. Photooxidation of proteins. Chem. List, *53:*829–836, 1959.
129. Von Tappeiner, H. and Jesionek, A. Therapeutische Versuche mit fluoreszieranden stoffen. Munch. Med. Wochenschr. *47:*2042–2044, 1903.
130. Von Tappeiner, H. Berl. Dtsch. Chem. Ges. *36:*3035, 1903.
131. Wharen, R.E., Anderson, R.E., and Laws, E.R. Laboratory and clinical investigations of HPD photoradiation therapy of malignant brain tumors: technique and results in 31 patients. Read before the First International Conference on the Clinical Applications of Photosensitization for Diagnosis and Treatment, Tokyo, April 30–May 2, 1986.
132. Wharen, R.E., Anderson, R.E., and Laws, E.R. Photoradiation therapy of malignant brain tumors. In: *Application of Lasers in Neurosurgery,* edited by L.J. Cerullo, pp. 156–171. Chicago, Year Book Medical Publishers, 1988.
133. Wharen, R.E., Anderson, R.E., and Laws, E.R. Photoradiation therapy with hematoporphyrin derivative in the management of brain tumors. In: *Advanced Intraoperative Technologies in Neurosurgery,* edited by V.A. Fasano, pp. 211–227. New York, Springer-Verlag, 1986.
134. Wharen, R.E., Anderson, R.E., and Laws, E.R. Quantitation of hematoporphyrin derivative in human gliomas, experimental central nervous system tumors, and normal tissue. Neurosurgery *12:*446–450, 1983.
135. Wharen, R.E., Kristofik, M.P., Randall, M.S., *et al.* The interaction of ionizing radiation and hematoporphyrin derivative, an effective radiation sensitizer. In: *Porphyrin Localization and Treatment of Tumors 2,* edited by D.R. Doiron and C.J. Gomer. New York, Alan R. Liss, in press, 1988.
136. Wharen, R.E., So, S., Anderson, R.E., *et al.* Hematoporphyrin derivative (HPD) photocytotoxicity of human glioblastoma in cell culture. Neurosurgery *19:*495–501, 1986.
137. Wile, A.G., Dahlman, A., and Burns, M.W. Laser photoradiation therapy of recurrent

human breast cancer and cancer of the head and neck. In: *Porphyrin Photosensitization,* edited by D. Kessel and T.J. Dougherty, pp. 47–52. New York, Plenum, 1983.
138. Wile, A.G., Novatry, J., Mason, G.R., *et al.* Photoradiation therapy of head and neck cancer. Am. J. Clin. Oncol. *6*:39–43, 1984.
139. Wise, B.L. and Taxdal, D.R. Studies of the blood brain barrier utilizing hematoporphyrin: short communication. Brain Res. *4*:387–389, 1967.

CHAPTER 20

Hyperthermia

MICHAEL SALCMAN, M.D.

Since at least the time of the ancient Greeks, man has dreamed of using heat against malignant tumors. Gradually, the concept of employing mildly elevated temperatures (i.e., hyperthermia) came to replace the crude desire of applying simple cautery. In the late 19th century, anecdotal reports appeared in which human cancers spontaneously regressed in the face of fevers associated with concomitant infections. In the early 20th century, Coley used intravenous toxins to stimulate systemic fever in order to treat tumors (4). Unfortunately, it has never been possible to determine whether the immunologic response to the toxins or the fever per se was responsible for Coley's results. Less than 20 years later, radiation therapists began to combine the use of local hyperthermia and external irradiation to treat tumors in the abdomen and thorax (52). Crile later provided dramatic experimental evidence in support of this policy; tumors implanted in the feet of mice that were subjected to hyperthermia (40 to 42°C by water bath) were cured by less than half the dose of radiation usually required for their eradication (8). Contemporary interest in the use of hyperthermia began with the perfusion of limbs by heated solutions for the treatment of melanoma and the production of whole-body hyperthermia in man by immersion in wax baths or by encasement in special NASA space suits (49,50). These clinical experiences demonstrated the selective vulnerability of hepatocytes and neurons to relatively low temperatures (41 to 42°C) and the mortal risks posed by unsuspected intracranial metastases. For these and other reasons, the production of local or regional hyperthermia rather than whole body heating has assumed increasing importance in both clinical and experimental research. Capacitive and resistive electromagnetic systems, implanted ferromagnetic seeds, external and internal microwave antennas, and focused ultrasound have all been used to produce local heating. The combined use of internal radiation and interstitial hyperthermia is actively being explored for a variety of human solid tumors (6,26).

HEAT AS A THERAPEUTIC AGENT

The general advantages and disadvantages of heat as an antineoplastic agent are listed in Table 20.1. The biological effects of hyperthermia are directly related to the magnitude of the temperature achieved and the duration of application (57). For a wide variety of experimental and naturally occurring neoplasms, it can be shown that

TABLE 20.1.
Advantages and Disadvantages of Hyperthermia

Advantages	Disadvantages
1. Active in hypoxic and undervascularized tissue.	1. Thermal tolerance on repeated exposure.
2. Active against S-phase and G_0 (noncycling) cells.	2. Possible metastatic spread at low temp.
3. Potentiates cell-killing of ionizing radiation.	3. Difficult to heat deep targets.
4. Potentiates chemotherapy (esp. BCNU and cis-Pt)	4. Narrow therapeutic index.
5. No cumulative toxicity.	

the duration of application can be decreased by 50% for each additional degree of temperature elevation above 41°C (15) (Fig. 20.1). The cellular locus of thermal injury is unknown but may include enzyme inactivation, nuclear damage, and osmotic changes in the plasma membrane. Hyperthermal potentiation of the cell-killing effects of ionizing radiation and chemotherapy can be dramatic and is largely based on inhibition of the repair of sub-lethal damage produced by the other agents in the

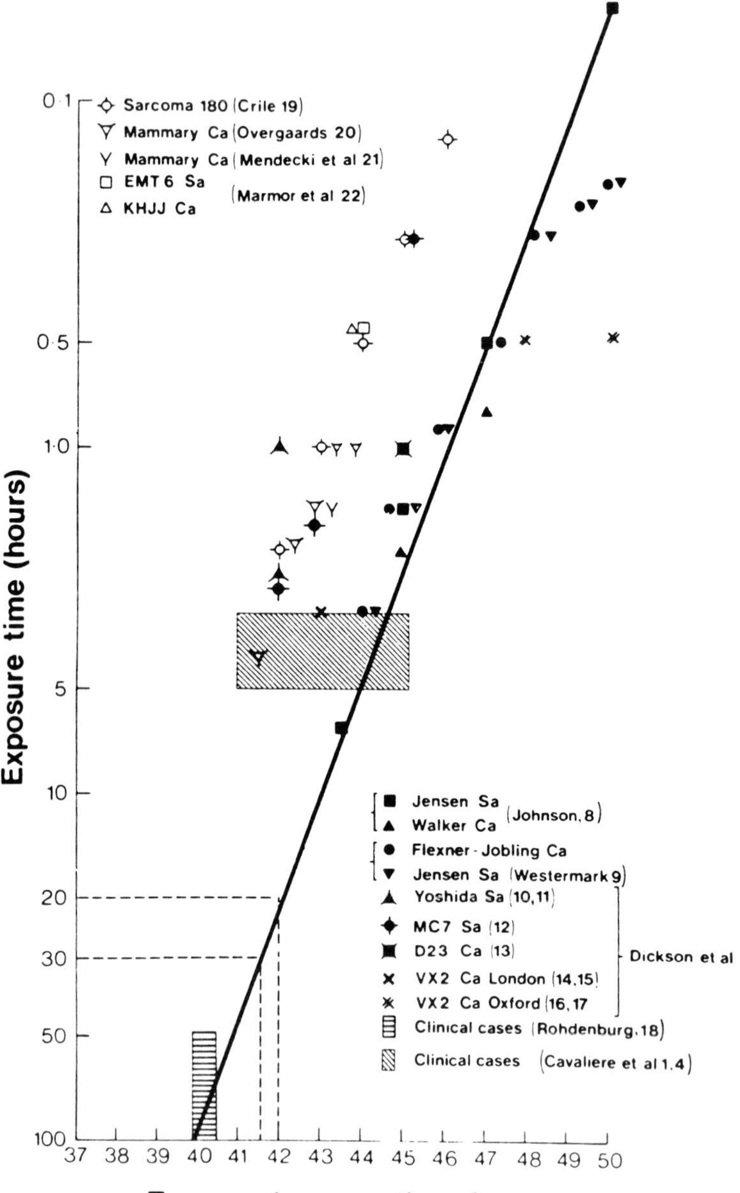

Figure 20.1. Thermal death times for animal and human cancers determined in vivo. For a wide variety of naturally occurring and experimental tumors, the exposure time required to achieve equal cell kill in vitro is halved for each degree of temperature elevation above 43°C. A similar relationship is seen in vivo for treatments required to cure 50 to 100 percent of the tumors. Note the clustering of points at 45°C for 1 hour. (Reprinted with permission from Dickson, J. A. and Calderwood, S. K. Temperature range and selective sensitivity of tumors to hyperthermia: a critical review. Ann. NY Acad. Sci., *335:*180–205, 1980.)

nucleus (3,12,13,29,30,40,44). Both direct cell killing by heat and the hyperthermal potentiation of other agents depends on the minimal temperature produced in the target; some inhomogeneity in the thermal field is acceptable if a minimum threshold temperature is otherwise exceeded (14,25). Those portions of the cell cycle most susceptible to hyperthermia are usually the least sensitive to the effects of ionizing radiation; the effects of hyperthermia are actually increased in acidic and poorly oxygenated tissues (24,78). Direct cell killing by heat can also be increased under hyperglycemic conditions (74). Maximum potentiation of radiation in experimental systems is seen when hyperthermia closely precedes the application of radiation, especially when the latter is employed at relatively slow dose rates of 100 rads/hour (23,31,32).

Hyperthermal potentiation of chemotherapeutic agents is most pronounced when the two modalities are used simultaneously (3,29,43). Nucleophilic drugs with a prominent alkylating mode of action, especially nitrosoureas and the platinum compounds, are the most effective agents used in concert with hyperthermia. Doses of nitrosourea and hyperthermia that are sublethal when used separately are curative for model tumors when used together (10) (Fig. 20.2.). Direct thermal cell killing can also occur in those noncycling and undervascularized portions of a tumor that are inherently the most resistant to chemotherapy. In some situations, hyperthermia increases cellular and subcellular access to the active moiety of the drug, inhibits the repair of sublethal drug damage in the nucleus, and disrupts enzymatic degradation of chemotherapeutic agents. The interaction of hyperthermia with photochemotherapy is presently under investigation as are the possible immunologic consequences of hyperthermia.

Although some normal tissues are inherently more sensitive to the effects of heat than others, the reputed selective vulnerability of tumor cells in comparison to nonneoplastic cells is very slight. In the brain, the therapeutic index for hyperthermia is

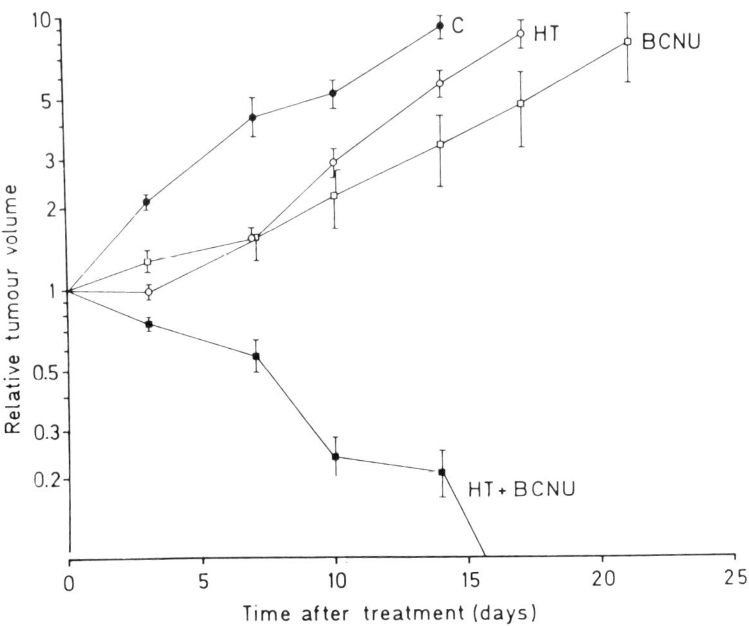

Figure 20.2. Potentiation of chemotherapy by hyperthermia. When 20 mg/kg of BNCU or 1 hour at 44°C of hyperthermia (HT) are used individually to treat this experimental rat tumor, the growth in the volume of the tumor over time is similar to that for the untreated or control (C) animals. However, when the same doses of BCNU and HT are used together, the tumor is cured. (Reprinted with permission from Dahl, O. and Mella, O. Enhanced effect of combined hyperthermia and chemotherapy in a neurogenic rat tumor in vivo. Anticancer Res., *2*:359–364, 1982.

quite narrow and only 0.5 to 1.0°C may separate the threshold of damage for tumor cells and for neurons (28,59). This situation is further complicated by the fact that tumor cells can rapidly develop thermal tolerance if they are heated too frequently at too low a temperature (46,47). The growth of some tumors can even be accelerated by low-level heating, perhaps through a generalized stimulation of enzyme systems by the Arrhenius effect (16). Therapeutic temperatures are not only lethal to neurons (Fig. 20.3) but can also disrupt the normal functioning of the blood brain barrier (11) (See Chapter 13). Slightly lower temperatures produce conduction block in axons and disturbances of spontaneous and evoked electrical activity (33). Although low-level heating can increase blood flow, therapeutic temperatures produce vascular stasis; these effects have been observed in the systemic circulation, in the brain and in model tumors (18,19,67,75). The combination of cellular swelling, blood-brain barrier disruption and vascular engorgement can produce uncontrollable cerebral swelling. This has been observed in clinical heat stroke, in experimental whole-body hyperthermia and when hyperthermal fields and instrumentation are too large for the mass of cerebral tissue to which they are applied (Fig. 20.4). The approximate threshold for thermal damage in the brain is 30 to 60 minutes at 42°C.

Safe and effective use of hyperthermia therefore requires that a minimum desired temperature be precisely produced in the target volume of interest without creating undue temperature elevations in immediately adjacent normal tissues outside the target. Modern microwave technology lends itself well to this goal by virtue of its

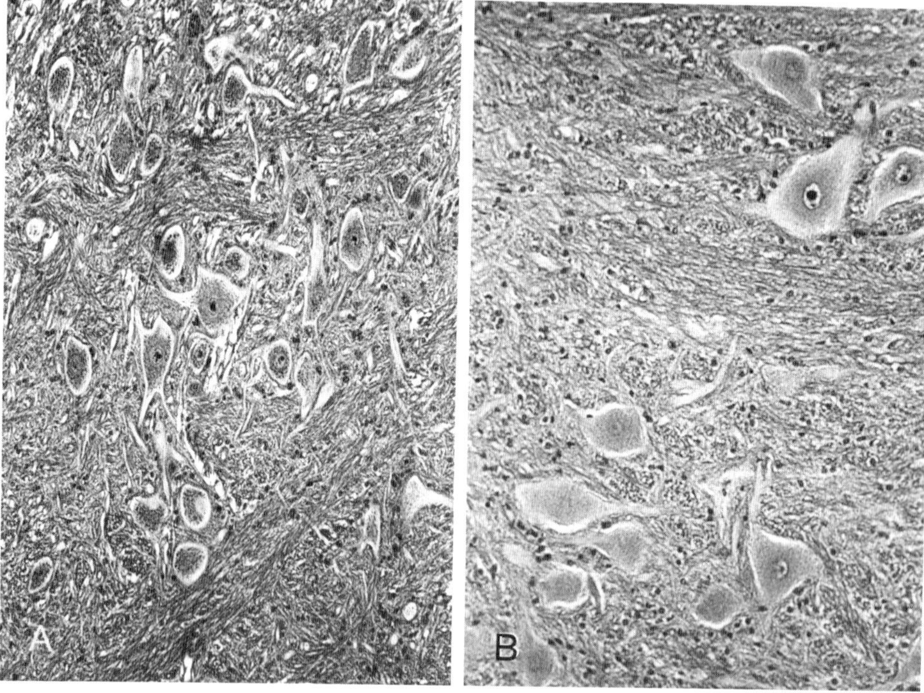

Figure 20.3. Effect of whole body hyperthermia on the dentate nucleus. Cats were anesthetized with barbiturates to paralyze thermoregulation and immersed in a precision waterbath. Brain hyperthermia at 43° for 60 minutes (*B*) resulted in clearing of the perikarya beneath the plasma membrane (degranulation) and ballooning of the cells; compare with dentate nucleus from control animal treated at 37°C for 60 minutes (*A*). (Reprinted with permission from Salcman, M., Samaras, G. M., Mena, H., *et al.* Whole body hyperthermia: potential hazards in its application to glioblastoma. In: *Multi-disciplinary Aspects of Brain Tumor Therapy,* edited by Paoletti, P., Walker, M. D., Butti, G., and Knerich, L. R., pp. 351–356. Amsterdam, Elsevier/North Holland, Biomedical Press, 1979.)

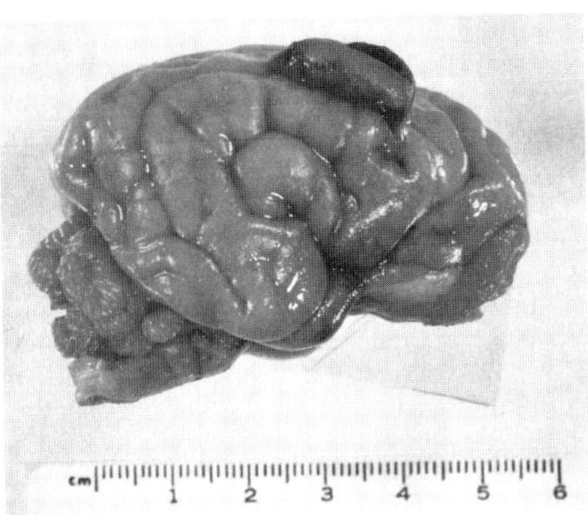

Figure 20.4. Brain swelling produced by hyperthermia. Note herniation of cerebral gyri at craniectomy site in small canine brain implanted with an improperly scaled 2450-MHz microwave antenna after too large a volume of the hemisphere was heated to 43°C.

control capability but shares with many other modalities the difficulty of heating deep targets without excessive heating of the surface. Indeed, the limited penetration of microwave energy virtually precludes the use of microwave sources external to the scalp. Hence, the necessity of invasive techniques for delivering microwaves into the brain.

INTERSTITIAL MICROWAVE HYPERTHERMIA

Interstitial implantation of a microwave radiator or antenna has the potential for sharply localizing hyperthermia to a small target volume and for facilitating useful interactions with radiation and chemotherapy in a restricted portion of the organism (53). Microwaves exist in that portion of the electromagnetic spectrum immediately adjacent to radiowaves and produce their purely thermal effects through rotational and frictional changes in molecular orientation and movement. Like all forms of electromagnetic energy, the depth of penetration in tissue is quite limited and the absorbed energy falls off exponentially with distance (Fig. 20.5). The absorbed power at any point in the microwave field is related to both the strength of the field at that point and the dielectric constant of the medium or tissue into which it is deposited. Since it is not possible to alter the dielectric

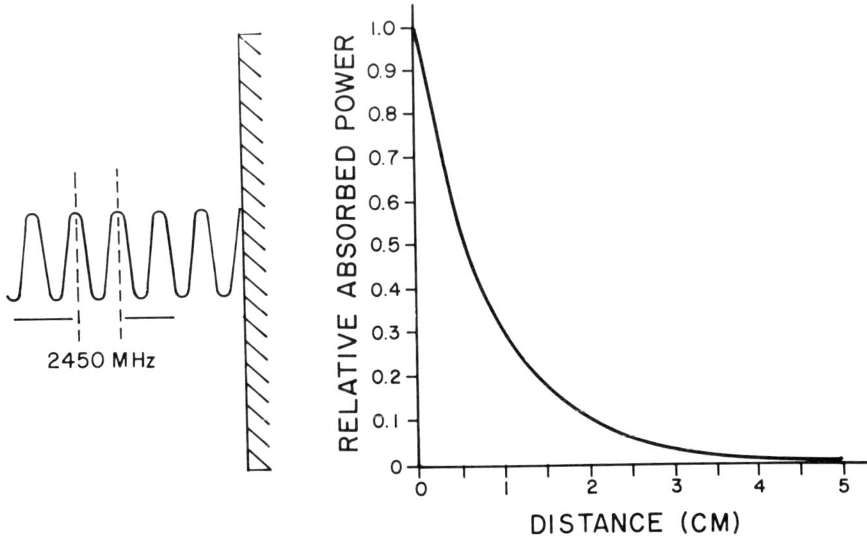

Figure 20.5. Relative absorbed power versus depth in tissue. The relative absorbed power of a 2450-MHz microwave plane wave incident at a surface is plotted against the perpendicular distance into the depth of the tissue in centimeters. Note that 50% of the power is absorbed in the first 0.5 cm and that the 1/e point is approximately 0.85 cm. (Reprinted with permission from Salcman, M. Feasibility of microwave hyperthermia for brain tumor therapy. Prog. Exp. Tumor Res., *28:*220–231, 1984.)

properties of the tissue, increased power deposition at a point can only be produced by increasing the depth of penetration from the microwave source. The depth of penetration of a microwave is inversely related to its frequency (Table 20.2) and nearly doubles when the frequency is lowered from 2450 to 915 MHz. It would seem a simple matter to treat a brain tumor 5 cm in diameter by making microwave antennas that function at lower and lower frequencies. As we shall see, however, this is not a trivial problem and it has, until recently, posed a technological barrier to the practical implementation of interstitial hyperthermia within the special confines of the intracranial cavity.

THERMAL FIELDS AND BLOOD FLOW

As we have seen, the temperature produced at any point in a microwave field depends on the amount of energy absorbed at that point. In a field that is otherwise uniform, absorption will vary based on local electrical properties such as conductivity and the dielectric constant. In a biologic tissue, electrical properties are inhomogeneous and their local values depend on water content, protein concentration, and the presence of mobile charges. Fortunately, differences in the magnitude of electrical properties from one region of the brain to another are small (21), although differences between gray and white matter values can be significant.

Once the microwave energy is absorbed and heat is produced, the thermal and blood flow properties of tissue are responsible for far greater variations in the distribution of temperatures across the target volume (3,21,67,68). Since the hyperthermal field exists at a higher temperature than the surrounding tissue, heat must flow from areas of high temperature to low. In addition, the blood entering the heated volume is cooler than the surrounding tissue and has the capacity for carrying heat away and dumping it into the systemic circulation. The first process, the passive flow of heat across the tissue, depends upon the thermal properties of the brain and is termed conduction; the second process, the active flow of heat carried by a fluid, is critically dependent on blood flow and is termed convection. In addition to the heat injected by the microwave antenna, a much smaller amount of heat is produced by the metabolic processes of the brain cells. The interaction of these four factors varies over time and distance to produce a spatial variation of temperature with time ($\delta T/\delta t$). This interaction can be described by a variety of heat balance equations (7).

Under certain conditions, the primacy of some of these factors becomes intuitively obvious. For example, the heat injected by metabolic work is negligibly small in comparison to the heat produced by an external source such as a microwave antenna. In addition, rapid and efficient cooling of tissue is more easily produced by convection than by conduction. Furthermore, the heterogeneity of blood flow within the tissue and between brain and tumor is greater than the heterogeneity of thermal constants in the tissue (5). In this regard, one should be careful not to confuse vascular engorgement with blood flow since increased blood volumes are not necessarily indicative of efficient blood flow in the tissue at the microcirculatory level. For example, PET

TABLE 20.2.
Microwave Frequency, Tissue Penetration, and Antenna Size

Frequency (f, MHz)	Wavelength (λ, cm)	Tissue Penetration (cm)	Antenna Half-length (cm)	
			e_1[a]	e_2[b]
300	100.0	3.89	3.57	17.7
433	69.3	3.57	2.47	12.2
915	32.8	3.04	1.17	5.8
2450	12.24	1.70	0.44	2.16

[a] e_1 = 50, the dielectric constant of the brain.
[b] e_2 = 2, the dielectric constant of a plastic catheter.

scanning has confirmed the presence of increased blood volumes in brain tumors which also demonstrate decreased blood flow and reduced metabolic rates for oxygen and glucose. Inefficient blood flow in brain tumors is consistent with the clinical and experimental observation that thermal fields are larger in the tumor than in the normal brain and that thermal cooling is slower in the tumor than in normal tissue (57,58).

The importance of blood flow in shaping the thermal field is illustrated in Figures 20.6 and 20.7. In Figure 20.6, two miniature microwave antennas have been implanted perpendicularly to the surface of the brain and 20 mm apart. The thermal field peaks near each antenna and has a valley of lower temperatures at the midpoint plane between them; furthermore, individual temperature points vary irregularly in the long axis of the antenna. In Figure 20.7, cerebral blood flow has been eliminated and the thermal field has become much more regular in shape. The valley has disappeared and uniform temperatures are maintained parallel to the long axis of the antenna. In the absence of cerebral blood flow (CBF), heat flow within the field and between the field and the surrounding brain is smoothed out by the thermal constants of the tissue. Although the presence of heterogeneous flow within the tumor can be expected to create difficulties in the creation of a uniform thermal field within the target volume, the differences between the tumor and the surrounding brain should increase the safety factor at the margin of

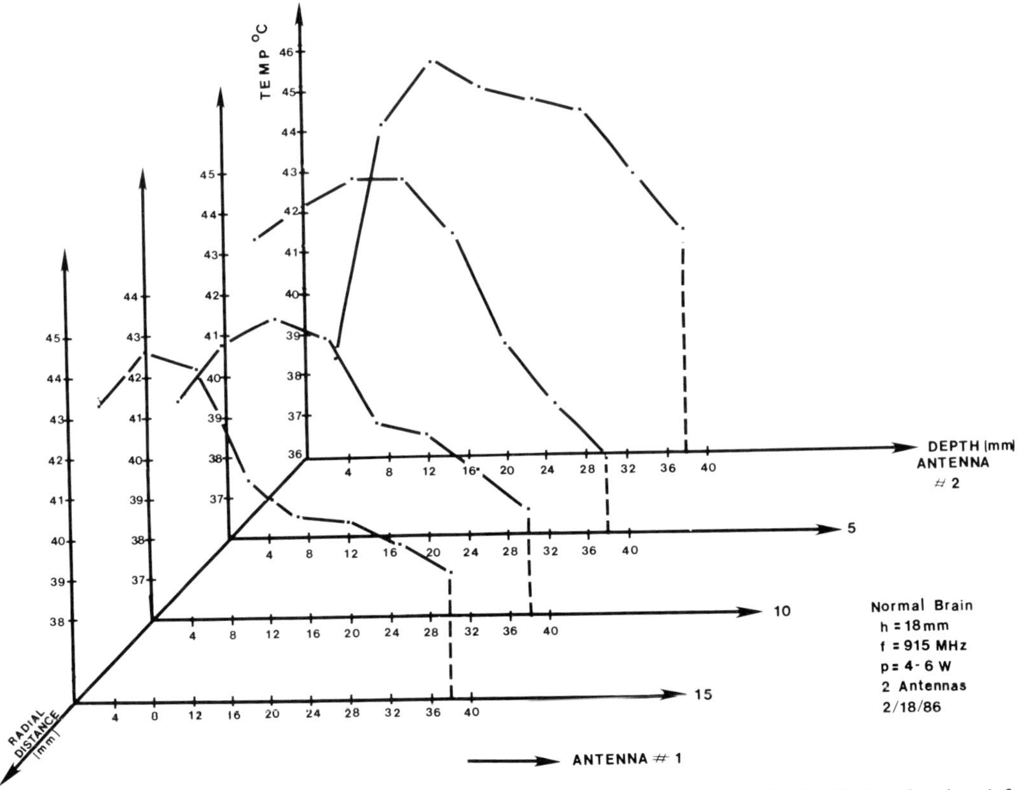

Figure 20.6. Thermal field plot for two miniature microwave antennas in canine brain. Cortical surface is at left, depth into the brain is to the right. The two 915-MHz antennas were implanted parallel to one another, 20 mm apart, with the temperature of each held at 45°C. Temperatures were measured along each antenna and in planes at 5 mm radial increments between the antennas. Note that although there is a drop in the field at the center plane (i.e., 10 mm), the temperature is still about 43°C from 8 to 20 mm into the brain. Note also the irregular shape of the field.

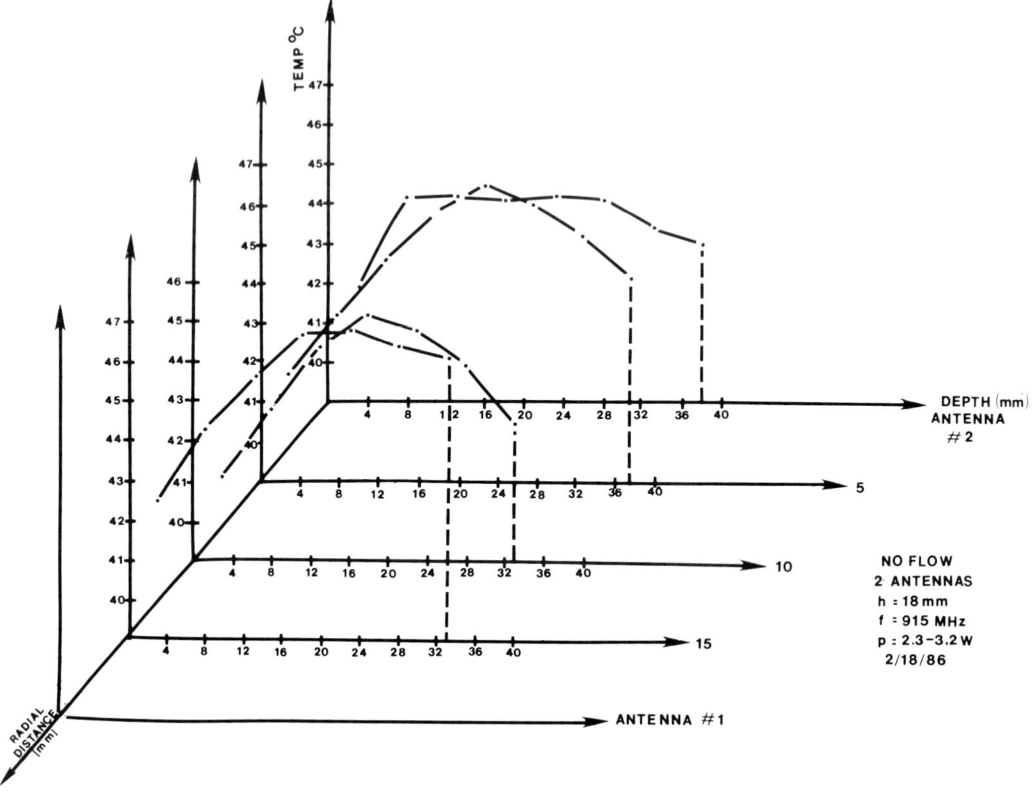

Figure 20.7. Thermal field plot for two miniature microwave antennas in the absence of blood flow. Same experiment and orientation as in Figure 20.6 with measurements carried out after animal was euthanized. Note that temperature plots are now rectangular and regular in shape (compare with Figure 20.6) with no evidence of a central dip between the two antennas. The shape of the thermal field now depends only on the passive thermal properties of the brain (conduction) without heat being carried away by cerebral blood flow (convection).

the lesion by accentuating differences in the temperature elevations produced in the normal and neoplastic tissue (27). Heat can also be used to "drive" the CBF in the normal brain, with the increase in blood flow proportional to the degree of temperature elevation (Fig. 20.8).

THE THERMAL SENSITIVITY OF GLIOMA CELLS

Impetus for the use of hyperthermia in the treatment of malignant glioma is based on a number of theoretical advantages derived from studies carried out on other tumors; despite the growing number of clinical trials employing this therapeutic modality, relatively little information is available on the heat sensitivity of glioma cells. A number of model neuroectodermal tumors have been employed including the murine ependymoblastoma (71), the rat 9L gliosarcoma (37), the BT_4A rat tumor (10, 43), and the Rous sarcoma virus-induced mouse glioma (38); only four studies have been carried out on cultured human glioma cells (17, 24, 61, 65). Whole-body hyperthermia at 40°C given for 120 minutes on 4 separate days had no effect when administered alone to mice bearing intracerebral ependymoblastoma, a tumor known to be sensitive to CCNU alone (71). When the two modalities were used in concert, microscopic evidence of accelerated tumor destruction was apparent within 24 hours of drug administration, and the percent of 60-day survivors was significantly increased at the $p<0.001$ level over that seen with drug alone. The critical level of CCNU was 8 to 16 mg/kg. In another study, subcutaneous

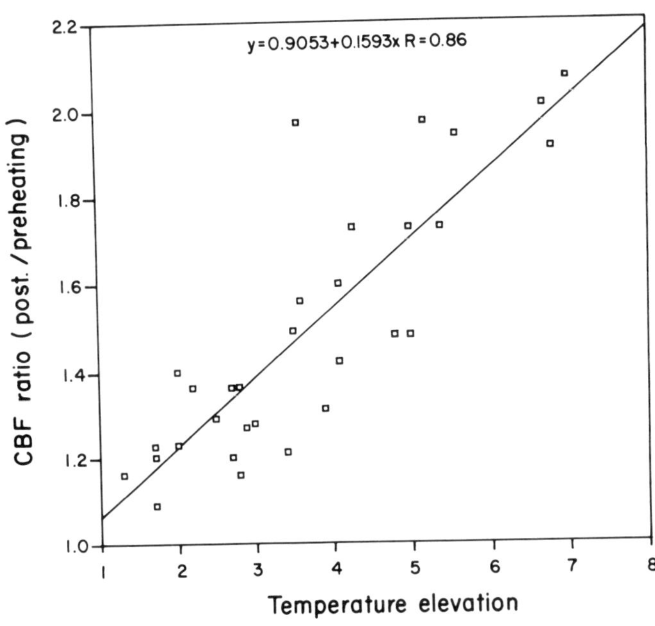

Figure 20.8. Ability of heat to drive CBF in normal brain. Correlation of change in cerebral blood flow (CBF) and temperature elevation. The change in CBF is plotted as the ratio of the value measured after heating to the value measured before heating versus the degree of temperature elevation for 31 paired observations. The linear correlation coefficient (r) = 0.86. The CBFs in this plot were obtained by the hydrogen clearance method. (Reprinted with permission from Salcman, M., Corradino, G., Moriyama, E., *et al.* Cerebral blood flow and the thermal properties of the brain: a preliminary analysis. J. Neurosurg., *70:* 592–598, 1989.)

9L tumors were locally exposed to 2450 MHz microwaves and heated at 42.5 to 45.0°C for durations of 0 to 180 minutes (76). An in vivo to in vitro colony formation technique was used to determine cell survival, and the latter was found to be an exponential function of temperature; a direct correlation between time at 44°C and percentage of in vivo tumor cures was also observed. When BCNU chemotherapy is combined with hyperthermia in the treatment of 9L cells in vitro, the amount of DNA interstrand cross-linking produced by the BCNU is dramatically increased (72). The same relative order for cell survival was found in respect to time at 42°C as for DNA cross-linking. A companion study comparing the effects of hyperthermia and BCNU on drug-sensitive and drug-resistant 9L cell lines demonstrated higher dose enhancement ratios in the resistant cells (66). Hyperthermia was thought to increase the concentration of reactive species produced by hydrolysis of BCNU at higher temperatures and an increase in cross-links through the effect of hyperthermia on DNA chromatin structure and the deactivation of repair enzymes.

The effect of combined hyperthermia and chemotherapy has been studied in vivo on the BT_4A tumor implanted in the hind leg of the rat when exposed to water bath heating at 44°C for 60 minutes (10,43). Tumor volumes that could not be controlled by either heat or drug alone were eradicated when the two modalities were combined for either bleomycin (20 mg/kg) or BCNU (20 mg/kg); these effects were significant at the $p < 0.01$ level (10). A follow-up timing study indicated that the combined effect was greatest when the administration of either BCNU or *cis*-platinum (DDP) immediately preceded the application of hyperthermia (43). In addition to drug activation and DNA sensitization, hyperthermia also has effects on tumor vascularity. Within a few days of magnetic induction hyperthemia on an intradermally implanted T9 gliosarcoma, the tumor demonstrated hemorrhage and vascular engorgement (37). The use of hyperthermia may also change the native immunologic response to neurogenic tumors and the effectiveness of biologic response modifiers. For example, hyperthermia at 40°C increases the in vitro antiproliferative activity of recombinant beta interferon, as well as its in vivo antitumor effect, when injected into the Rous sarcoma mouse glioma (38).

In vitro studies on human cell lines and tumor explants indicate that glioblastomas manifest decreased proliferation and prolonged DNA synthesis times when incubated at 40 or 42°C (61). Nevertheless, human glioblastoma cells appear to be more resistant than other types of tumor studied in vitro and may develop thermal tolerance when treated < 44°C (24); above this temperature, the rate of cell killing doubles for each 1° increase at a pH of 7.4. A pH sensitizing effect could be demonstrated below 7.0 and was more pronounced at lower temperatures; the change in the inactivation rate with a drop in pH can range between 1.25- and 2.5-fold. Recently, an in vitro study evaluated the interaction of hyperthermia and chemotherapy in the cell killing of the U-87MG glioma line (65). Drug dose enhancement ratios of 1.6, 2.8, 2.0, and 1.1 were observed for BCNU, AZQ, *cis*-DDP, and spirohydantoin mustard (SHM), respectively. The treating temperature was 42°C for 60 minutes, and each drug was used at a concentration of 1 mg/ml.

The first experiments to study the interactions of hyperthermia, chemotherapy, and radiation on human glioblastoma cells have recently been carried out in our laboratories (17). The response of human U-87MG cells to each modality used alone and in combinaton with each of the others was tested and compared with the response of our model canine glioma. Both tumors demonstrated increased sensitivity to hyperthermia at higher temperatures with an approximate halving in exposure time for each 1° elevation above 43°C to achieve the same cell kill. The effectiveness of radiation therapy (RT) (500 rads), BCNU, and *cis*-DDP given individually was potentiated by hyperthermia for each cell line. Hyperthermia and RT were more effective than hyperthermia and BCNU, but the triple combination was marginally the most effective of all. Similar findings have been observed for the threefold combination in Ehrlich ascites cells (36). Finally, the canine glioma appears to be an excellent test system since its spectrum of sensitivities parallels that of the human U-87MG.

CLINICAL EXPERIENCE

Tumors in and about the head and neck were among the first neoplasms in the body to be exposed to combinations of hyperthermia and radiation (52). The initial approach to the use of hyperthermia specifically for brain tumors was very similar to that employed in contemporaneous trials in the treatment of malignant melanoma of the extremities i.e., regional infusion of heated solutions that often contained chemotherapeutic agents. Woodhall and Mahaley utilized regional perfusion, presumably delivered to the distribution of the middle cerebral artery, to administer cyclophosphamide and nitrogen mustard at moderate levels of hyperthermia; no prolonged survivals were obtained in the eight glioblastoma patients treated in this manner (80). Anecdotal reports have been published of heated solutions at 42°C delivered into the carotid artery with subsequent neurological improvement (9); unfortunately, no long-term evaluaton of these patients has been reported, and virtually none of the early studies carried out direct thermometry within the brain or brain tumor. Noninvasive hyperthermia for brain tumors has also been delivered by the magnetic loop induction technique, wherein the patient's head is placed inside a large RF-induction coil. One chordoma and one glioma have been treated by this method in combination with simultaneous BCNU infusion (63). Temperature measurements are available only for the glioma patient and indicate that the tumor reached a temperature of 42 to 42.5°C at at least one point; the intracranial pressure was noted to be greater than 20 cm H_20 in five of the six treatment sessions. As indicated by our experimental evidence and the anecdotal clinical experience of others, regional or whole-body methods of hyperthermia that result in holohemispheric heating can be expected to produce elevations in intracranial pressure and brain swelling, especially when these methods are employed without a preceding surgical reduction in tumor mass (59, 64).

Sutton pioneered the use of invasive methods for the delivery of hyperthermia into the intracranial cavity (69). His original method consisted of a large RF probe that produced hyperthermia by resistive heating. Liquefaction necrosis of a glioblastoma was demonstrated in vivo after two

6-hour sessions of localized heating carried out at 42°C (69). Specimens obtained from several other patients confirmed this finding as well as vascular engorgement of the tumor and relatively little peritumoral swelling; unfortunately, these important observations were clouded by the fact that all of the patients received simultaneous chemotherapy with 5-fluorouracil. Interstitial microwave hyperthermia for recurrent malignant astrocytoma was first carried out in 1980 and initially reported as a feasibility study in three patients in 1981 (57). Each patient was implanted with a single radiator and sensor that functioned at 2450 MHz; the terminal diameter of the microwave antenna was less than 1.5 mm and was formed by stripping away the outer layers of a flexible coaxial cable. This device had undergone several years of testing in experimental animals and was known to produce a relatively restricted thermal field (radius < 1 cm) in normal feline brain. When implanted in human brain tumors, however, the thermal field expanded to an effective diameter of 4 cm (57). In addition, thermal cooling in the brain tumor was noticeably slower than that observed in normal brain; these findings were felt to be the result of relatively inhomogeneous and inefficient blood flow in the tumors. It was also felt that this factor should provide an extra margin of safety at the interface between the tumor and the rapidly self-cooling brain. In the initial series of patients, manual control of the power delivered to the antenna was based on the operator's visual feedback of the temperature recorded at the center of the antenna. In a subsequent series of three additional patients, automatic power control was achieved by a computer-based system utilizing a three-level algorithm for tracking the recorded temperatures (58). The antennas were implanted at open craniotomy and all patients were also implanted with subarachnoid intracranial pressure (ICP) monitors over the contralateral hemisphere. The two postoperative treatments were given at 45°C for 60 minutes on the night of surgery and 2 days later. No patient was aware of power on/off; there were no permanent neurologic sequelae; and there was no significant change in the ICP. Subsequent investigators have confirmed the feasibility and safety of interstitial microwave hyperthermia by both stereotactic and open techniques (41, 77, 79).

More recently, Roberts and co-workers reported on the safety and feasibility of combined interstitial microwave irradiation and interstitial iridium implants in a series of six patients (51), and we have initiated two protocols at 915 MHz, utilizing combined interstitial radiation (60) and hyperthermia in one and combined hyperthermia and systemic BCNU chemotherapy in the other (34). To date, seven implants have been carried out in our second series and a 10-year follow-up is available on the six patients from the first clinical trial (see Table 20.3). Two of the latter patients are alive at 9 and 10 years following single microwave antenna implants for recurrent tumor. The 10-year survivor also received simultaneous BCNU intravenously. In the second series, systemic and neurologic complications have been unusual, and some dramatic radiographic regressions have been observed (Fig. 20.9). Minor discomfort from surface heating of the scalp can be minimized by proper antenna design and local cooling techniques (45, 62).

Other investigators have employed ferromagnetic seeds with fixed Curie-points to produce hyperthermia by magnetic induction, capacitive plates applied to the head to produce RF heating, and ultrasonic hyperthermia (2, 37, 70). These techniques appear less attractive than microwave-induced hyperthermia because of unusual requirements for multiple implants, permanent craniotomy, or unusually complex control units required for the generation of the hyperthermal field. The temperature distributions produced by different interstitial technologies are roughly equivalent (42).

FUTURE DEVELOPMENTS

Since safe and effective hyperthermia depends on the production of a sharply delineated temperature field that everywhere exceeds some possibly critical threshold (e.g., 43 to 45°C), a premium is placed on decreasing the number and size of the antennas required to produce such a field in

TABLE 20.3.
Initial Microwave Hyperthermia Series

Case	Age/Sex	Location	Date	Protocol	Complications	Status
			Hyperthermia Alone			
1	29/M	R. Frontotemporal	6/80		Hygroma	LFU[a] (12/81)
2	30/F	R. Frontoparietal	7/80	BCNU	None	Well (3/90)
3	58/M	L. Frontoparietal	8/80		Transient dysphasia	Died (4/81)
4	46/M	R. Frontotemporal	4/81		CSF leak	Died (11/82)
5	27/F	L. Parietooccipital	6/81		None	Recurrence (7/88)
6	54/F	L. Parietal	9/81		None	Died (3/82)
		Combination Hyperthermia with BCNU or Interstitial Radiation				
7	32/M	R. Frontoparietal	8/87	BCNU	None	Died (4/88)
8	39/M	R. Temporal	8/88	RT	None	Well (3/90)
9	35/F	L. Frontal	10/88	RT	Thermal skin changes Technical failure	 Hospice (3/90)
10	68/F	R. Occipital	11/88	RT	Thermal skin changes	Died (7/89)
11	63/F	R. Frontoparietal	a)11/88 b) 2/89	BCNU	CSF leak Transient edema Hemiparesis	Died (4/89)
12	22/M	R. Frontal	12/88	RT	CSF leak Meningitis Technical failure	 Died (10/89)
13[b]	42/M	R. Frontal	10/89	BCNU	None	Died (3/90)

[a]Lost to follow-up.
[b]Case 13 was melanoma; all other cases were glioblastoma multiforme.

the intracranial cavity (53). Conventional antenna and radiation catheter design results in electrical mismatches between the antenna and the brain and requires antennas of impractical length (i.e., 10–12 cm) to produce the required field at 915 MHz (56, 73). Swept frequency measurements carried out in the canine brain indicate that small antennas can be built (2–4 cm) if ceramic catheters are employed and antenna design ignores the theoretical optimum dimension imposed by classical formulae (20, 56). Such small antennas can be used to produce near-uniform heating over 4 cm fields in small arrays and together with fluorooptical thermometry, they can be used to measure CBF in small regions of the brain by thermal washout (54). A proper understanding of the interaction of heat with CBF is also essential to the production of well-behaved thermal fields. The recent in vitro results on human and canine glioma cells as well as the safety and feasibility demonstrated in our thermochemotherapy and thermoradiotherapy trials clearly indicate the desirability of initiating

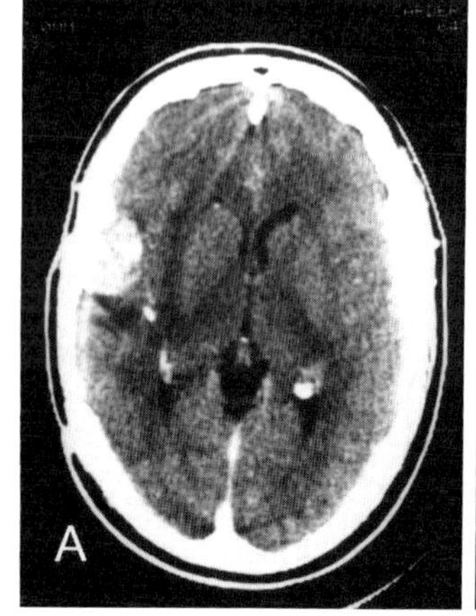

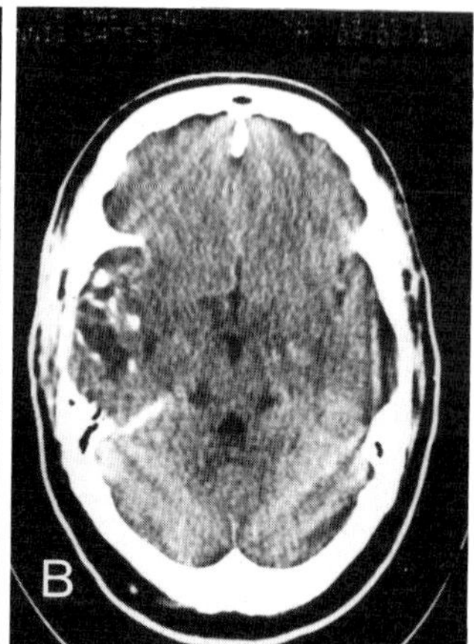

Figure 20.9. Radiographic response of grade 3 astrocytoma to combined interstitial radiation and hyperthermia. Forty-year-old male with Grade 3 astrocytoma as seen on preimplant CT scan (*A*). Massive tumor necrosis and clearing of scan is seen 60 days after 8 catheter implant (*B*). Patient remains clinically well but with radiographic recurrence 24 months after implant.

a clinical trial in which all three modalities are used in concert. The discovery that thermotolerance is produced through the activation of genes coding for heat shock proteins raises the possibility of monoclonal antibodies or other immunologicals being used to potentiate hyperthermia through the inhibition of the cell's protective mechanisms (35). Other possible means for increasing thermosensitivity may include the induction of hyperglycemia and lactic acidosis or the depletion of intracellular polyamines (22). It may even be possible to employ NMR imaging to noninvasively measure temperature and guide therapy (48). The observation that subpopulations of cells from single solid tumors vary in their thermosensitivity and the known variability of heat sensitivity between different tumor types (15, 39) clearly indicates that hyperthermia must be used in concert with other therapeutic modalities. This conclusion is consistent with the view that glioblastoma multiforme and other solid tumors represent complex and heterogeneous entities for which true multimodality therapy is the most likely ultimate solution (1, 55).

ACKNOWLEDGMENT

This research was supported in part by the Mildred Mindell Cancer Foundation and the Neuro-Oncology Research Fund at the University of Maryland.

REFERENCES

1. Bigner, D.D. Biology of gliomas: potential clinical implications of glioma cellular heterogeneity. Neurosurgery, *9*:320–326, 1981.
2. Britt, R.H., Lyons, B.E., Pounds, D.W., *et al.* Feasibility of ultrasound hyperthermia in the treatment of malignant brain tumors. Med. Instrum., *17*:172–177, 1983.
3. Bull, J.M. An update on the anticancer effects of a combination of chemotherapy and hyperthermia. Cancer Res. (Suppl.), *44*:4853–4956, 1984.
4. Coley, W.B. The treatment of malignant tumors by repeated inoculation of erypsipelas: with a report of 10 original cases. Am. J. Med. Sci., *105*:487–511, 1983.
5. Cooper, T.E. and Trezek, G.J. A probe technique for determining the thermal conductivity of tissue. J. Heat Transfer, *94*(2):133–140, 1972.
6. Cosset, J.M., Dutreix, J., Dufour, J., *et al.* Combined interstitial hyperthermia and brachytherapy: Institute Gustave Roussy technique and preliminary results. Int. J. Radiat. Oncol. Biol. Phys., *10*:307–312, 1984.
7. Cravalho, E.G., Fox, L.R., and Kan, J.C. The application of the bioheat equation to the design of thermal protocols for local hyperthermia. Ann. NY Acad. Sci., *335*:86–97, 1980.
8. Crile, G. Jr. The effects of heat and radiation on cancers implanted on the feet of mice. Cancer Res., *23*:373–380, 1963.
9. Cummins, B., Macintosh, I., Cooper, R., *et al.* Selective hyperthermia in the treatment of malignant glioma. J. Neurol. Neurosurg. Psychiatry, *40*:1028, 1977.
10. Dahl, O. and Mella, O. Enhanced effect of combined hyperthermia and chemotherapy (bleomycin, BCNU) in a neurogenic rat tumor (BT_4A) in vivo. Anticancer Res., *2*:359–364, 1982.
11. Deswal, K. and Chohan, I.S. Effects of hyperthermia on enzymes and electrolytes in blood and cerebrospinal fluid in dogs. Int. J. Biometeorol., *25*:227–233, 1981.
12. Dewey, W.C. Interaction of heat with radiation and chemotherapy. Cancer Res. (Suppl), *44*: 4714–4720, 1984.
13. Dewey, W.C., Hopwood, L.E., Sapareto, S.A. *et al.* Cellular responses to combinations of hyperthermia and radiation. Radiology, *123*:463–474, 1977.
14. Dewhirst, M.W., Sim, D.A., Sapareto, S. *et al.* Importance of minimum tumor temperature in determining early and long-term responses of spontaneous canine and feline tumors to heat and radiation. Cancer Res., *44*:43–50, 1984.
15. Dickson, J.A. and Calderwood, S.K. Temperature range and selective sensitivity of tumors to hyperthermia: a critical review. Ann. NY Acad. Sci., *335*:180–205, 1980.
16. Dickson, J.A. and Ellis, H.A. Stimulation of tumour cell dissemination by raised temperature (42°C) in rats with transplanted Yoshida tumours. Nature, *248*:180–205, 1974.
17. Ebert, P. and Salcman, M. In vitro response of human glioblastoma and canine glioma cells to hyperthermia, radiation and chemotherapy, in preparation, 1990.
18. Eddy, H.A. and Chmielewski, G. Effect of hyperthermia, radiation and adriamycin combinations on tumor vascular function. Int. J. Radiat. Oncol. Biol. Phys., *8*:1167–1175, 1982.
19. Emami, B., Nussbaum, G.H., Hahn, N., *et al.* Histopathological study on the effects of hyperthermia on microvasculature. Int. J. Radiat. Oncol. Biol. Phys., *7*:343–348, 1981.
20. Ferraro, F.T., Salcman, M., Broadwell, R.D., *et al.* Alumina ceramic as a biomaterial for use in afterloading radiaton catheters for hyperthermia. Neurosurgery, *25*:209–213, 1989.
21. Foster, K.R., Schepps, J.L., Stoy, R.D. *et al.* Dielectric properties of brain tissue between 0.01 and 10 GHz. Phys. Med. Biol., *24*:1177–1187, 1979.
22. Fuller, D.J. and Gerner, E.W. Delayed sensitization to heat by inhibitors of polyamine-biosynthetic enzymes. Cancer Res., *42*:5046–5049, 1982.
23. Gerner, E.W., Oval, J.H., Manning, M.R., *et al.*

Dose-rate dependence of heat radiosensitization. Int. J. Radiat. Oncol. Biol. Phys., *9:*1401–1404, 1983.

24. Gerweck, L.E. and Richards, B. Influence of pH on the thermal sensitivity of cultured human glioblastoma cells. Cancer Res., *41:*845–849, 1981.
25. Gibbs, F.A., Peck, J.W., and Dethlefsen, L.A. The importance of intratumor temperature uniformity in the study of radiosensitizing effects of hyperthermia in vivo. Radiat. Res., *87:*187–197, 1981.
26. Grady, E.D., McLaren, J., Auda, S.P. *et al.* Combination of internal radiation therapy and hyperthermia to treat liver cancer. South. Med. J., *76:*1101–1105, 1983.
27. Gullino, P.M., Jain, R.K., and Grantham, F.H. Temperature gradients and local perfusion in a mammary carcinoma. J. Natl. Cancer Inst., *68:*519–531, 1982.
28. Gwozdz, B., Dyduch, A., Grzybek, H., *et al.* Structural changes in brain mitochondria of mice subjected to hyperthermia. Exp. Pathol., *15:*124–126, 1978.
29. Hahn, G.M. Hyperthermia for the engineer: a short biological primer. IEEE Trans. Biomed. Eng., *31:*3–8, 1984.
30. Hahn, G.M., Braun, J., Har-Kedar, I. Thermochemotherapy: Synergism between hyperthermia (42–43°) and adriamycin (or bleomycin) in mammalian cell inactivation. Proc. Natl. Acad. Sci. USA, *72:*937–940, 1975.
31. Harisidias, L., Hall, E.J., Kraljevic, U., *et al.* Hyperthermia: biological studies at the cellular level. Radiology, *117:*447–452, 1975.
32. Harisidias, L., Sung, D., Kessaris, N. *et al.* Hyperthermia and low-dose rate irradiation. Radiology, *129:*195–198, 1978.
33. Harris, A.B., Erickson, L., Kendig, J.H., *et al.* Observations on selective brain heating in dogs. J. Neurosurg., *19:*514–521, 1962.
34. Huhn, S., Salcman, M., Amin, P., *et al.* Combined Interstitial Hyperthermia and Either Interstitial Radiation or Chemotherapy for Malignant Glioma, (abstract). *Neurosurgery, 24:*947, 1989.
35. Johnston, R.N. and Kucey, B.L. Competitive inhibition of hsp 70 gene expression causes thermosensitivity. Science, *242:*1551–1554, 1988.
36. Kai, H., Matsufuji, H., Sugimachi, K., *et al.* Combined effects of hyperthermia, bleomycin and x-rays on Ehrlich ascites tumor. J. Surg. Res., *41:*503–509, 1986.
37. Kobayashi, T., Kida, Y., Tanaka, T., *et al.* Magnetic induction hyperthermia for brain tumor using ferromagnetic implant with low Curie temperature. 1. Experimental study. J. Neuro. Oncol., *4:*175–181, 1986.
38. Kuroki, M., Tanaka, R., and Hondo, H. Antitumor effect of interferon combined with hyperthermia against experimental brain tumor. Int. J. Hyperthermia, *3:*527–534, 1987.
39. Leith, J.T., Heyman, P., Dewngaert, J.K., *et al.* Survival responses of cell subpopulations isolated from a heterogeneous human colon tumour after combinations of hyperthermia and x-irradiation. Int. J. Radiat. Biol., *43:*303–311, 1983.
40. Li, G.C., Evans, R.G., and Hahn, G.M. Modification and inhibition of repair of potentially lethal x-ray damage by hyperthermia. Radiat. Res., *67:*491–501, 1976.
41. Lindhold, C.E., Kjellen, E., Landberg, T., *et al.* Local ionizing radiation with and without microwave induced hyperthermia in superficial malignant tumors in brain. Adv. Exp. Med. Biol., *157:*145–146, 1982.
42. Mechling, J.A. and Strohbehn, J.W. A theoretical comparison of the temperature distributions produced by three interstitial hyperthermia systems. Int. J. Radiat. Oncol. Biol. Phys., *12:*2137–2149, 1986.
43. Mella, O. and Dahl, O. Timing of combined hyperthermia and 1,3-bis (2-chloroethyl)-1-nitrosourea or cis-diaminedichloroplatinum in BD IX rats with BT_4A tumours. Anticancer Res., *5:*259–264, 1985.
44. Mills, M.D. and Meyn, R.E. Hyperthermic potentiation of unrejoined DNA strand breaks following irradiation. Radiat. Res., *95:*327–338, 1983.
45. Moriyama, E., Matsumi, N., Shiraishi, T., *et al.* Hyperthermia for brain tumors: improved delivery with a new cooling system. Neurosurgery, *23:*189–195, 1988.
46. Nielsen, O.S., Overgaard, J., and Kamura, T. Influence of thermotolerance on the interaction between hyperthermia and radiation in a solid tumour in vivo. Br. J. Radiol., *56:*267–273, 1983.
47. Overgaard, J. and Nielsen, O.S. The importance of thermotolerance for the clinical treatment with hyperthermia. Radiother. Oncol., *2:*343–366, 1984.
48. Parker, D.L. Applications of NMR imaging in hyperthermia: an evaluation of the potential for localized tissue heating and non-invasive temperature monitoring. IEEE Trans. Biomed. Eng., *31:*161–167, 1984.
49. Pettigrew, R.T., Galt, J.M., Ludgate, C.M., *et al.* Circulatory and biochemical effects of whole body hyperthermia. Br. J. Surg., *61:* 727–730, 1974.
50. Pettigrew, R.T., Galt, J.M., Ludgate, C.M., *et al.* Clinical effects of whole-body hyperthermia in advanced malignancy. Br. Med. J., *4:*679–682, 1974.
51. Roberts, D.W., Coughlin, C.T., Wong, T.Z., *et al.* Interstitial hyperthermia and iridium brachytherapy in treatment of malignant glioma: a Phase I clinical trial. J. Neurosurg., *64:*581–587, 1985.
52. Rohdenburg, G.L. and Prime, F. The effect of combined radiation and heat on neoplasms. Arch. Surg., *2:*116–129, 1921.
53. Salcman, M. Feasibility of microwave hyperthermia for brain tumor therapy. Prog. Exp. Tumor. Res., *28:*220–231, 1984.

54. Salcman, M., Corradino, G., Moriyama, E., *et al.* Cerebral blood flow and the thermal properties of the brain: a preliminary analysis. J. Neurosurg., *70:*592–598, 1989.
55. Salcman, M., Kaplan, R.S., Samaras, G.M., *et al.* Aggressive multimodality therapy based on a multicompartmental model of glioblastoma. Surgery, *92:*250–259, 1982.
56. Salcman, M., Neuberth, G., Nudelman, R.W., *et al.* Swept frequency measurements of microwave antennas in feline and canine brain. IEEE MTT-S Int. Microwave Symp. Dig., pp.771–774, 1986.
57. Salcman, M. and Samaras, G.M. Hyperthermia for brain tumors: biophysical rationale. Neurosurgery, *9:*327–335, 1981.
58. Salcman, M. and Samaras, G.M. Interstitial microwave hyperthermia for brain tumors. Results of a phase-1 clinical trial. J. Neurooncol., *1:*225–236, 1983.
59. Salcman, M., Samaras, G.M., Mena, H., *et al.* Whole body hyperthermia: potential hazards in its application to glioblastoma. In: *Multidisciplinary Aspects of Brain Tumor Therapy,* edited by P. Paoletti, M. D. Walker, G. Butti, and R. Knerich, pp. 351–356, Amsterdam, Elsevier/North Holland Biomedical Press, 1979.
60. Salcman, M., Sewchand, W., Amin, P.P., *et al.* Technique and preliminary results of interstitial irradiation for primary brain tumors. J. Neurooncol., *4:*141–149, 1986.
61. Schiffer, L.M., Braunschwieger, P.G., and Selker, R.G. Glioblastoma cell kinetics and effects of in vitro hyperthermia. Proc. AACR and ASCO abstract C-31, p.300, 1979.
62. de Sieyes, D.C., Couple, E.B., Strohbehm, J.W. *et al.* Some aspects of optimization of an invasive microwave antenna for local hyperthermia treatment of cancer. Med. Phys., *8:*174–183, 1981.
63. Silberman, A.W., Morgan, D.F., Storm, K.F., *et al.* Combination radiofrequency hyperthermia and chemotherapy (BCNU) for brain malignancy. Animal experience and two case reports. J. Neuro Oncol., *2:*19–28, 1984.
64. Silberman, A.W., Rand, R.W., Krag, D.N., *et al.* Effect of localized magnetic-induction hyperthermia on the brain. Temperature versus intracranial pressure. Cancer, *57:*1401–1404, 1986.
65. da Silva, V.F., Raaphorst, G.P., Goyal, R., *et al.* Drug cytotoxicity at elevated temperature. In vitro study on the U-87MG glioma cell line. J. Neurosurg., *67:*885–888, 1987.
66. da Silva, V.F., Tofilon, P.J., Gutin, P.H., *et al.* Effects of hyperthermia on DNA interstrand crosslinking after treatment with BCNU in 9L rat brain tumor cells. Radiat. Res., *103:*373–382, 1985.
67. Song, C.W., Lokshina, A., Rhee, J.G., *et al.* Implications of blood flow in hyperthermic treatment of tumors. IEEE Trans. Biomed. Eng. *31:*9–16, 1984.
68. Strohbehn, J.W., Trembly, B.S., and Douple, E. B. Blood flow effects on the temperature distributions from an invasive microwave antenna array used in cancer therapy. IEEE Trans. Biomed. Eng., *29:*649–661, 1982.
69. Sutton, C.H. Tumor hyperthermia in the treatment of malignant gliomas of the brain. Trans. Am. Neurol. Asso., *96:*195–199, 1971.
70. Tanaka, R., Kim, C.H., Yamada, N. *et al.* Radiofrequency hyperthermia for malignant brain tumors: preliminary results of clinical trials. Neurosurgery, *21:*478–483, 1987.
71. Thuning, C.A., Bakir, N.A., and Warren, J. Synergistic effect of combined hyperthermia and a nitrosourea in treatment of a murine ependymoblastoma. Cancer Res., *40:*2726–2729, 1980.
72. Tofilon, P.J., da Silva, V., Gutin, P.H., *et al.* Effects of hyperthermia on DNA interstrand crosslinking after treatment with BCNU in 9L rat brain tumor cells. Radiat. Res., *103:*373–382, 1985.
73. Trembly, R.S. The effects of driving frequency and antenna length on power deposition within a microwave antenna array used for hyperthermia. IEEE Trans. Biomed. Eng., *32:* 152–157, 1985.
74. Urano, M., Montoya, V., and Booth, A. Effect of hyperglycemia on the thermal response of murine normal and tumor tissues. Cancer Res., *43:*453–455, 1983.
75. Vaupel, P. and Kallinowski, F. Physiological effects of hyperthermia. Recent Results Cancer Res., *104:*71–109, 1987.
76. Wallen, C.A., Michaelson, S.M., and Wheeler, K.T. Cell survival as a determinant of tumor cure for rat 9L subcutaneous tumors following microwave-induced hyperthermia. Eur. J. Cancer Clin., *18*(1):37–44, 1982.
77. Wen, H.L., Dahele, J.S., Mehal, Z.D., *et al.* Application of invasive microwave hyperthermia for the treatment of gliomas. J. Neurooncol., *6:*93–101, 1988.
78. Wike-Hooley, J.L., Haveman, J., and Reihnold, J.S. The relevance of tumour pH to the treatment of malignant disease. Radiother. Oncol., *1:*167–178, 1983.
79. Winter, A., Laing, J., Paglione, R., *et al.* Microwave hyperthermia for brain tumors. Neurosurgery, *17:*387–399, 1985.
80. Woodhall, B. and Mahaley, M.S. Isolated perfusion in treatment of advanced carcinoma: brain and face tumors. Am. J. Surg., *105:*624–627, 1963.

Index

Page numbers in *italics* denote figures; those followed by *t* denote tables.

Aberrant differentiation, 36–37
Accelerated fractionation, 304–305
Acoustic neuromas
  bilateral, 56
  in NF-2, 57, 59
Acromegaly, 313
ACTH-secreting adenomas, 289
Adenomas, pituitary, 288–289
  radiation response of, 313
Adrenalectomy, and BBB alteration, 241
Adriamycin, 244
Adult tumors, versus embryonal tumors, 35–36
Aklylation, DNA damage with, 67–69
Alkylated bases, 67–68
Alkylating anticancer agents, DNA damage with, 57–59
Alkylnitrosoureas, brain tumors with, 68
Allogenic bone marrow cell infusion, 219
Aminoisobutyric acid, and BBB alteration, 240–241
Anaplasia, 104
  in astrocytomas, *105, 107*
  change in tumor cell kinetics with, 106
  definition of, 21
  with genetic modifications, 108
  histological findings with, 108
Anaplastic gliomas
  clinical features of, 276
  prognosis of, 276–277
  survival factors in, 277–278
Angioblastomas, 117
Angiogenenin, 111
Angiogenetic factors, 111
Angiography, of gliomas, 265
Animal brain tumor models, 174–176
Antibody response, cytotoxic, 213
Antibromodeoxyuridine monoclonal antibody, 149–154
Antigen-antibody complexes
  formation of, 222
  T-suppressor cells and, 214
Antigens
  glioma-specific, 213, 215–216
  probes, 186
Anti-GFAP monoclonal antibodies, 193–194
Antigloma response, humoral, 213
Antineoplastic agents, properties of, 321–322
Anti-NF antibodies, 193–194
Antioncogene. *See* Tumor suppressor gene
Antisera, 186
Arachidonic acid
  and BBB alteration, 250–251
  lipoxygenase metabolism of, 240
Astroblastomas
  cell of origin of, 42–43
  narrow window of vulnerability in, 42–43
Astrocytes
  in BAT, *126–127*
  lack of GFAP-positive in tumors, 95–98
  marker of differentiation of, 106
  mature, 44
  oligodendrocytes and, 93
  proliferation of in MS plaque, 79
  transformed, 46
  vimentin-positive reactive, *99*
Astrocytic differentiation, 42
Astrocytomas, *106*
  anaplastic, 21, 22, 104, *105, 107*
    labeling index, growth fraction and cell cycle time in, 154*t*
  astrocytic gliomas, intracranial, 10
  cell lines from, 163
  cerebellar, radiation response of, 311–312
  classification of, 19
    and nomenclature of, 29
  in cortex, *104*
    low-grade, 278
  grading of, 20, 22
  high-grade, chemotherapeutic results in, 326–327
  intercellular chondroid matrix in, 37
  low-grade, 56, 58, 278
    chemotherapeutic results in, 327
    radiation response of, 309–310
  narrow window of vulnerability of, 44–46
  in NF-2, 59–60
  papovavirus-induced, 79
  prognosis of, 278
  proliferation patterns of, 156
Autoradiographic study, 147–148
Avian sarcoma virus (ASV), and BBB permeability, 237

BAT (brain adjacent to tumor), 123–127
  astrocytes in, *126–127*
  in glioblastomas, 127
  permeability of, 237
  vascular glomeruli and endothelial buds in, *125*
B cells, immunoglobulin-secreting, 216
BCNU chemotherapy, 218
  autologous bone marrow rescue and, 330
  DNA damage with, 69
  effects on medulloblastomas, 328
  for ENU tumors, 102

BCNU chemotherapy—*continued*
in high-grade astrocytomas, 326
intraarterial, 330–331
with radiotherapy, 315
resistance to, 329
serum half-life of, 176
subtherapeutic doses of, 329
thermal sensitivity and, 367–369
topical, 334
BCNU sensitive cells, 69
Bergmann's fibers, 91
Bifunctional alkylating agents, DNA damage with, 69
Biological markers
cell type specific, 187–201
of glial and primitive tumors, 185–201
ideal, 185
Bleomycin, neurotoxicity of, 244
Blood-brain barrier, 214, 229
alteration of in disease, 235–236
in brain tumors, 270–271
breakdown of, 238
and chemotherapy, 324–326
definition of, 229–235
disruption of, 270–271, 325
with chemotherapy, 331–332
increased permeability of, 235–236, 239
modification of, 238–243
in brain tumor therapy, 243–245
permeability of, effects of chemical and biological agents on, 239–241
in tumors, 236–238
Blood-brain barrier endothelium
abluminal plasma membranes of, *234*
abluminal surface of, 235
blood-borne macromolecules absorbed through, 234–235
characteristics of, 232–233
Blood flow. *See also* Cerebral blood flow
in brain tumors, 268–269
thermal fields and, 364–366
Bone marrow rescue, autologous, 330
Brain. *See also* Brain tumor
glioma following injury to, 46
immunologic privilege of, 214–215
radiation acute and late effects on, 307–308
Brain-specific drug carrier system, *333*
Brain stem gliomas
prognostic factors in, 280–281
radiation response of, 312
Brain tissue transplantation, and BBB alteration, 241–242, 245
Brain tumor. *See also specific types*
angiogenesis of, 111
biological markers of, 185–201
and blood-brain barrier, 236–238, 270–271
modification of in therapy for, 243–245
blood flow and oxygen utilization in, 268–269
bordering IV ventricle, *125*
cell kinetics of, 145–146
cell lines of, experimental applications of, 170–174
chemotherapy for, 321–335
classification of, 19–30, 145
unresolved issues in, 25–30
clinical evaluation of metabolism of, 252–253
and CNS trauma, 75–78, 82
demyelinating disease and, 78–82
diagnosis of type and degree of malignancy of, 262
ENU-induced, 238
transplacental, 85–102
future of immunotherapy for, 222–223
glucose metabolism in, 269–270
grading of, 22–25
growth fraction and cell cycle time in, 154–155
growth pattern and secondary transformation of, 117–123
heterogenity of, 275
immunotherapy for, 216–223
in vitro growth of, 163–176
in vivo estimates of kinetic parameters of, 259–271
labeling index of, 147–154
markers for, 167–170
metabolic studies of
correlation of basic and clinical data in, 256–257
in vivo, 251–257
quantitative results of, 253–258
necrosis and vasculature of, 109–111
pathogenesis of, 23–24
permeability of capillaries in, 237
photoradiation therapy of, 341–352
prognostic factors for, 275–291
proliferative centers in, *88*
radiation dose-response of, 307
resistance of to chemotherapeutic agents, 322–324
in septum pellucidum, *124*
studies of glucose metabolism in, 251
trauma and demyelination as etiologic factors in, 73–82
undifferentiated, 28
vascular glomeruli and endothelial buds in BAT, *125*
visual appearance of, 253
Brain Tumor Study Group, 309
interstitial irradiation trial of, 301
results of, 326
Breast cancer, metastasis of to brain, 5
Bromodeoxyuridine (BrdU), 108
cytokinetic studies using, 30
labeling indices, of neuroectodermal tumors, 153*t*
labeling techniques, 150–151, 156
prolonged administration of, 149–150
and radiotherapy, 316
Bronchogenic carcinoma, metastasis of to brain, 5

C-6 cell line, 174–175
Cafe-au-lait marks
in NF-1, 54, 55
in NF-2, 57
Cancer cells, differentiation deficiency in, 137
Carboanhydrase C, in normal vs. tumorous oligodendrocytes, 98–100
Carbonic anhydrase isoenzymes, 190
Carcinogenesis
augmenting factors in, 73
concept of, 82
DNA in, 63–70
general concepts of, 73
inhibition of, 73
non-CNS, 74
as two-stage process, 73–74

Carcinogens, 73
  with cocarcinogenic agents, 73–74
Carcinomas, in long-standing scars, 74–75
Carmustine, effectiveness of, 172
Case-control study, 11–13
CCNU chemotherapy, 218
  effects on medulloblastomas, 328
  for ENU tumors, 102
  in high-grade astrocytomas, 326–327
  sensitivity, 170
  and thermal sensitivity, 366–367
  topical, 334
Cell cycle time, 146
  growth fraction and, 154–155
Cell death, postmitotic, 307
Cell differentiation
  in diagnosis and clinical management of gliomas, 137–142
  divergent versus aberrant, 36–37
  neoplastic versus normal, 37
Cell killing, 303
  by chemotherapy, 321
  oxygen dependence of, 315
  thermal, 361
Cell kinetics. *See also* Tumor cell kinetics
  basic concepts of, 145–147
  of brain tumors, 259–262
Cell lines. *See also* astrocytoma, C-6 cell line, D283 Med Cell Line, D341 Med Cell Line, EpA cell line, Ep cell line, GL261 cell lines, Glioma cell lines, 9L cell line, RG2 cell lines
  animal brain tumor models of, 174–176
  development of, 163–164
  experimental applications of, 170–174
  initial culture of, 166
  long-term, 164–165
  morphology and cytogenetics of, 168–170
Cell loss factor, 146–147, 260
  variation in, 262
Cell-mediated cytotoxicity, 214
Cell-mediated immune mechanisms, 212
Cell renewal systems, 145–146
Cell type identification, 28
Cell typing, 19
  difficulties of, 20
Cellular gliosis, production of, 47–48
Cellular proliferation patterns, 155–156
Central nervous system. *See also* Central nervous system tumors
  embryonal and adult tumors of, 35–36
  lymphomas, chemotherapeutic results in, 328–329
  markers for cell types in, 167–168
  myelin, composition of, 189–190
  neoplasms of
    classification of, 4, 5*t*
    clinical pattern of, 4–5
    epidemiologic studies of, 4
    seeding of, 5
    sites of origin of, 5
  oligodendrocytes in remyelination of, 45
  trauma to and brain tumor, 75–78, 82
  two-stage carcinogenesis in, 74
Central nervous system tumors
  biological markers of, 185–201
  cell kinetics of, 145
  chemotherapeutic agents for, 332
  growth fraction in, 24
  WHO histological classification of, 26–27*t*
  window of vulnerability of, 39
    narrow, 39–43
    wide, 43–46
c-erb B-2 oncogene, 174
Cerebellar astrocytomas, radiation response of, 311–312
Cerebellar gliomas, prognostic factors in, 281–282
Cerebellar medulloblastoma, 43–44
Cerebral arteriography, preirradiation, 313
Cerebral artery occlusion, and BBB permeability, 236
Cerebral blood flow
  in brain tumors, 268–269
  heat and, 370
  thermal fields and, 365–366
Cerebral blood volume, in brain tumors, 268–269
Cerebral glioblastoma multiforme, clinical outcome of, 137
Cerebral medulloepithelioma, 39–41
Cerebral medullomyoblastomas, 38
Cerebral neuroblastomas, 41
Cerebrospinal fluid (CSF)
  substances in, 229
  tumor cells spread through, 120
Chang Staging System, 285*t*
Chemical agents, DNA damage with, 66–69
Chemically defined (CD) media, 166–167
Chemodectoma, multicentric CNS, 10
Chemosensitivity, 170, 172
Chemotherapy, 170
  agents for, 321–324
  for anaplastic gliomas, 277
  basic principles of, 321–324
  for CNS malignancies, 332
  continuous infusion, 332–334
  doses and schedules for, 324
  effectiveness of, 172
  experimental approaches to delivery of, 329–334
  future uses of, 334–335
  high dose, 330
  hyperthermia-enhanced, 370
  intraarterial, 330–331, 334
  mechanisms of action of, 321–322
    and sites of, *323*
  molecular weight and lipid solubility of, 325*t*
  potentiation of by hyperthermia, 361
  for primitive neuroectodermal tumors, 287
  principles of combination of, 324
  with radiotherapy, 314–315
  resistance to, 322–324
  results of, 326–329
  special opportunities of, 325–326
  special problems of, 324–325
  thermal sensitivity and, 366–368
  topical, 333–334
Chiasmatic gliomas, prognostic factors in, 279–280
Children's Cancer Study Group, 327, 328
Cholera toxin, 188
  receptors for, 188–189
Choroid plexus papillomas, 37
  GFA protein in, 37
  growth of, 117

Chromatin bodies, extrachromosomal double-minute, 24
Chromogranin A, 191
Chromophobe adenoma, 9
Chromosomal abnormalities, 24
  structural, 109
Chromosomal analysis, 25
Chromosome 17, loss of segments of, 60
Chromosome 22
  inactivation of genes on, 60
  long arm of, 59–60
  in NF-2, 58, 59
cis-Platinum
  neurotoxicity of, 244
  and thermal sensitivity, 367
Classification, biological, 19
Clostridium tetani endotoxin, 189
Cobalt-60 gamma photons, 299
Cocarcinogenic agents, 73
Computerized tomography (CT)
  for brain tumors, 223
  dynamic, 264
  and gliomas, 262–265
  in kinetic parameter studies, 262
  in meningioma diagnosis, 77
  for radiation dosimetry, 301
  xenon enhanced, 264
Connecticut Tumor Registry data, 7, 8
  survival rates in, 9
Copper, in brain tumor cells, 111
Cortical anaplastic gliomas
  chemotherapy for, 277
  clinical features of, 276
  grading of, 277
  prognosis of, 276–277
  radiation therapy for, 277
  study of, 276
  survival factors in, 277–278
Corticosteroids
  autologous bone marrow rescue and, 330
  and BBB alteration, 241
  postoperative, 351
Craniopharyngiomas
  photoradiation therapy for, 351
  prognostic factors in, 290–291
  radiation response of, 313–314
  surgical resection and outcome with, 290–291
Craniotomy
  for gliomas, 218
  and radiotherapy, 301
Cultures
  general techniques of, 164–166
  isolation of purified populations in, 166–167
  of newly explanted cell lines, 167
Cyclophosphamide, effectiveness of, 172
Cytogenetic abnormalities, 24
Cytogenetics, 163
  for brain tumor cell lines, 168–170
Cytokeratins, 23
Cytokines, manufactured, 219
Cytokinetic studies, 30

D283 Med cell line, 164
  NF expression in, 201
  study of, 200–201
D341 Med cell line, 164
DBcAMP, study of effects of, 138–141
Delayed hypersensitivity reaction (DHRs)
  with active nonspecific immunotherapy, 219
  with active specific immunotherapy, 217, 218
  cell-mediated immune mechanisms and, 212
Demyelinating disease, brain tumors and, 78–82
Demyelination
  in multiple sclerosis, 47
  with radiation, 303
Desmoplastic infantile ganglioglioma, 41–42
Diagnosis, 19
Diaziquone, effectiveness of, 172
Differentiating agents
  clinical efficacy of, 137–138
  study of effects of, 138–141
Differentiation, definition of, 21
Dimethyl sulfoxide (DMSO)
  and BBB alteration, 240
  effectiveness with cytotoxic agents, 141–142
Disease
  community patterns of, 3
  magnitude of in community, 4
Divergent differentiation, 36
DMF, study of effects of, 138–142
DNA, 63
  alkylation products from, 40
  cellular distribution, 150
  cytometry, 25
  damage to
    by chemical agents, 66–69
    by physical agents, 64–66
    with radiation, 302–304
  double helix, 64
  fingerprinting, 163, 164, 168
  flow cytometry in measuring of, 148–149
  monoadducts formation, 64
  mutagen-induced modification to, 64*t*
  repair mechanisms of, 62–70
  spontaneous damage of, 63–64
  synthesis of, 93, 147
DNA analysis
  in NF-2, 58, 59
  of tumor cell kinetics, 260–261
DNA cross-linking agent, 304, 332
DNA cross-link repair, 69
DNA replication
  errors in, 64
  faulty template for, 66
Doubling time, 146
Drug-light interactions, 345–348

Eagle's Minimal Essential Medium (MEM), 166
Eastern Cooperative Oncology Group criteria, 335
Edema, in BAT, 123–127
EGFR gene amplification, 173–174
Electron dense tracers, 229
Electron microscopy, 19
Embryonal central neuroepithelial tumors, classification of, 25–29
Embryonal tumors
  versus adult tumors, 35–36
  heteroplastic differentiation in, 38–39
  nomenclature issues of, 28

Endocytosis, 231–232
Endothelial cell growth factor (ECGF), 111
Endothelial proliferation, in malignant gliomas, 109–111
Enolase, neuron-specific and nonneuronal, 188
EpA cell line, 174–175
Ep cell line, 174–175
Ependymoblastomas, 42
Ependymomas
  association of with nervous system neoplasms, 10
  chemotherapeutic results in, 328
  growth pattern of, 117
  histologic features of, 283
  intracranial, 10
  malignant, 22
  multicentric CNS, 10
  in NF-2, 60
  prognostic factors in, 283–284
  radiation response of, 310–311
  spread of, 120
  surgical resection and outcome of, 283–284
  in von Hippel-Lindau disease, 10
Epidemiologic indices, common, 4*t*
Epidemiologic studies, of primary intracranial neoplasms, 3–14
  special problems of, 4–5
Epidermal growth factor (EGF), 25, 109, 166–167
  studies of role in glioma growth, 172–173
Epithelial neuroendocrine tumors, 191
Erb B oncogene, 25
Erythrocythemia, 10
Ethylnitrosourea (ENU)
  decreasing oncogenic effect of, 94
  effects of in conjunction with head trauma, 77–78
  and neurocytogenesis, 40
  O-alkylation effect of, 94
  target of, 90
  transplacental induction of brain tumor with, 85–102
Ethylnitrosourea-induced tumors, 238
  clinical latency period in, 85
  cell characteristics of, 95–100
  cyst in, *101*
  microtumor development in, 85
  spreading of, 102, *103*
  therapeutic studies of, 102
  transformation process in, 85–95
  vasculature of, 100–102
Extracellular matrix (ECM), 166

Factor VII/RAg
  in glioblastoma, *116*
  in gliosarcomas, 115
Fenestrated junctions, in CNS, 109
Fibroblastic growth factor (FGF), 111
Fibronectin, 36
FITC-conjugated anti-BrdU MAb, 150
Fleurettes, in pineoblastomas, 38
Flexner rosettes, in pineoblastomas, 38
Flow cytometry, 148–149
  DNA analysis by, 25
Fludarabine, effectiveness of, 172
Fluorescein isothiocyanate (FITC), 149
5-Fluorouracil, neurotoxicity of, 244
Foreign body tumorigenesis, 74
Fractionation, 304–306
  acute effects of, 308

Galactocerebroside (GalC), 189–190
Gamma photons, 299–301
Gangliogliomas, desmoplastic infantile, 41–42
Ganglioneuroma
  association of with nervous system neoplasms, 10
  multicentric CNS, 10
  of nervous system, 10
Gastrointestinal carcinoma, metastasis of to brain, 5
Gene expression, altered, 24
Genetic factors, for intracranial neoplasm, 9–10
Gene transcription, tissue-specific, 24
Germ cell tumors
  chemotherapeutic results in, 329
  prognostic factors in, 287–288
Germinomas, radiation response of, 311
Giant-cell astrocytoma, 29
Giant cell glioblastomas, 115
GL261 cell line, 174–175
Glial cells
  cultured, 163
  division of, *92*
  germinal cells of, 91
  migration of, 90–91
  neoplastic, 42
  neoplastic vulnerability of in relation to postnatal life events, 46–47
  production of, 91
  turnover of, 35
Glial fibrillary acidic protein (GFAP), 23, 36, 37, 189–190
  antibodies to, 193, 201
  expression of, 98, 106, 108, 194–197, 200
    in nonastrocytomas, 198–199
  immunoreactive cells, 199
  monoclonal antibodies, 168
  in oligodendrocytes, 45
  positive radial glia, 44
  presence of, 42
Glial fibrillary acidic protein-positive network, 199–200
Glial filaments, 194–196
Glial maturation factor (GMF), 141
Glial tumor
  cell type specific biological markers for, 187–201
  classification of, 276
  composition of, 275
  examination of, 275–276
  head trauma and, 82
  innovations in evaluation of, 185–186
  multiple sclerosis and, 79
Glioblastoma, *107*
  association of with nervous system neoplasms, 10
  autoradiographic study of, 147–148
  BAT in, 127
  cell lines from, 163
  characteristic proliferation patterns in, 155–156
  difficulty in grading of, 24–25
  endothelial buds in, *112*
  endothelial proliferations in, *112*
  filling lateral ventricle, *119*

Glioblastoma—*continued*
giant cell, 115
glial component of, *116*
head trauma as risk factors for, 76
invading corpus callosum, *122*
labeling index, growth fraction and cell cycle time in, 154*t*
multicentric CNS, 10
multiforme, 22
necrosis of, 109, *110, 113*
one-year survival and radiation fractionation, 305*t*
primary vs. secondary, 108
radiation response of, 308–309
relative frequency of, 7
spread of, 120
transition to, 108
vascular glomeruli in, *116*, 123
vasculature of, *113, 114*
Gliocytogenesis, normal, 45
Gliogenesis, 93
Glioma cell line-induced xenografts, 175–176
Glioma cell lines, morphology and cytogenetics of, 168–170
Glioma cells
cultured, 163
methods for differentiation study of, 138
morphologic effects of differentiating agents in, *140–141*
morphology of, *139*
regulating differentiated phenotype in cultured, 138–142
Glioma-mesenchymal matrix glycoprotein, extracellular, 36–37
Gliomas
of adult-cell type, 44
anaplastic and low-grade
characteristic proliferation patterns in, 155–156
blood-brain barrier in, 270–271
blood flow and oxygen utilization of, 268–269
brain stem, 280–281
radiation response of, 312
cell kinetics of, 260–261
cerebellar, 281–282
chiasmatic, 279–280
classification of, 155, 259
cortical anaplastic, 276–278
CT scanning of, 262–265
cytogenetic studies of, 61
cytogeny and differentiation of, 35–48
demyelinating disease and, 82
development and malignant phenotypes of, 102–127
differentiation and phenotypic expression in, 137–142
following brain injury, 46
and glial cell neoplastic vulnerability, 46–47
glucose metabolism in, 269–270
grading of, 263
growth by infiltration of, 117–118
growth fraction in, 24
growth pattern, spreading and secondary transformation of cerebral, 117–123
histopathological diagnosis and grading of, 145
of hypothalamus, 278–279
immunocompetence in, 211–223
immunotherapy for, 215–223
isotope scanning of, 265
labeling index and median survival times with, 148*t*
MRI scanning of, 265–267
multicentric growth of, 123
optic nerve, radiation response of, 312–313
particular aspects of, 109–116
peritumoral tissue of, 123–127
persistence of after irradiation, 302–303
PET scanning of, 267–268
photoradiation therapy for, 351
plain skull x-ray and angiography of, 265
polymorphic, *89*
prognostic factors in, 276–283
radiation-induced, 47
simulating multiple sclerosis, 78
S phase duration in, 154
spread of, 120
thalamic, 278–279
radiation response of, 312
thermal sensitivity of cells in, 366–368
thrombosis and endothelial proliferation in, 109–111
transformation process of, 102–109
trials to study value of misonidazole for, 317*t*
vascularization of, *243*
well-circumscribed, 42
Glioma-specific antigens, 215–216
identification of, 215–216
studies of using heteroantisera, 216
Gliosarcomas, 115
cells of origin of, 45
Glucocorticoids, effects on CNS lymphomas, 329
Glucose
cerebral utilization of, 269–270
metabolism of
in brain tumors, 251, 269–270
and tumor grade, 252, 257
Glycolipids, myelin associated, 189
Glycolysis rate, 37
Glycosaminoglycans (GAGs), accumulation of, 95
in oligodendroglioma, *96*
Grading systems, 21–25
Growth factors. *See also* Endothelial cell growth factor (ECGF), Transforming growth factor (TGF), TGF-beta, Epidermal growth factor (EGF), Fibroplastic growth factor (FGF), Platelet derived growth factor (PDGF)
in glioma growth, 173–174
studies of role in glioma growth, 172
Growth fraction, 146
and cell cycle time, 154–155
in gliomas, 156
kinetics and, 259–260
variation in, 62
Gunshot injuries, glioma following, 46

Halogenated pyrimadines, with radiotherapy, 316
Hansson's cobalt-phosphate method, 190
Head trauma, brain tumor and, 73–82
Heat. *See also* Hyperthermia
as therapeutic agent, 359–363
variability in sensitivity to, 371
Hemangioblastoma, multicentric CNS, 10
Hemangiomas, 30

Hematoporphyrin, 341–342
  increased interest in, 342
Hematoporphyrin derivative (HPD)
  absorption spectrum of, 343
  accumulation of in tumors, 344–345
  analysis of, 343–345
  experimental use of, 342
  interactions of with light, 345–348
  introduction of, 342
  photoradiation therapy, 349–351
  phototoxicity of, 346–347
  preferential accumulation of in tumors, 344
  selectivity of, 343
Hemerogenes, 109
Hemangioblastomas, 10
Heparin, 111
Heteroplasia, 36–37
Heteroplastic differentiation, frequency of in embryonal tumors, 38–39
Histiocytes, adventitial, 115
Histology, in diagnosis, 19
Homogeneously stained regions (HSR), 24
Horseradish peroxidase
  blockade of at blood-brain barrier, 229, *231*, 231–232
  entry of into brain, 238
Humoral immune mechanisms, 212
Humoral immune responses, 213, 221–222
Hybridoma technology, 216
Hydroxyurea, with radiotherapy, 314–315
Hyperbaric oxygen, with radiotherapy, 315
Hyperfractionation, 305–306
Hyperthermia, 359
  advantages and disadvantages of, 359*t*
  and BBB alteration, 238–240, 244–245
  clinical experience with, 368–369
  future developments in, 369–371
  and glioma cells, 366–368
  and heat as therapeutic agent, 359–363
  interstitial microwave, 363–364
  microwave, 369, 370*t*
  safe and effective use of, 362–363
  and thermal fields and blood flow, 364–366
Hypothalamic tumors, prognostic factors in, 278–729
Hypoxic cell radiosensitizers, 315–316

IgG, binding of, 213
Imaging methods, in diagnosis of tumor and degree of malignancy, 262
Immune mechanisms
  cell-mediated, 212
  humoral, 212
Immune responses, humoral, 213, 221–222
Immunochemical methods, 186
Immunocompetence
  general in malignant glioma patients, 211–214
  of malignant glioma patients, 211–223
  suppressor factors in, 212
Immunocytochemistry
  cell-specific markers in, 167–168
  using antibromodeoxyuridine monoclonal antibody, 149–154
Immunodeficiency diseases, malignancy with, 211
Immunohistochemical methods, 24–25, 186
Immunological surveillance concept, 211–212
Immunostaining, 24
Immunosuppressive factors, 212
Immunosuppressive therapy, malignancy with, 211
Immunotherapy
  active nonspecific, 218–219
  active specific, 216–218
  adoptive, 219
  biologics in, 219–221
  future of for brain tumors, 222–223
  for malignant gliomas, 216–223
  passive, 221–222
Indifferent cells, 91
Interferon
  mechanism of antitumor action of, 219–220
  in recombinant form, 219–220
Interferon-alpha
  in glioma immunotherapy, 220
  manufactured, 219
Interferon-beta, 220
Interferon-gamma, 220
Interleukin–2
  in glioma immunotherapy, 220
  insufficient, 212
  manufactured, 219
Intermediate filament (IF) antibodies
  in cell line study of primitive brain tumors, 200–201
  in glial and primitive brain tumor studies, 197–200
Intermediate filament (IF) proteins, 186, 192–201
  antibodies to, 193
  types of, 192–193
Intermediate filaments (IF), 23, 187
  vimentin, 196
International Society of Pediatric Oncology, 328
Interstitial irradiation, 301
Interstitial microwave hyperthermia, 363–364
Intracranial neoplasms
  disease magnitude and distribution studies for, 6–14
  identification of high-risk persons for
    analytic studies in, 10–14
    genetic factors in, 9–10
    multicentric primary nervous system neoplasms and, 10
  morbidity data on, 7–9
  mortality data on, 6–7
  primary, epidemiology of, 3–14
  prospective survival studies on, 9
  risk factors of, documentation of, 10–14
Intraendothelial transfer vesicles, 230
Intraspinal neoplasms, 9
In vitro clonogenic cell assays, 302
In vitro culture, 164–166
  cell growth in, 165–166
  with short- or long-term assays, 170
Iododeoxyuridine (IUdR), 316
Ionizing radiation
  acute and late effects of, 307–308
  biological interactions with, 302–304
  chemical additives and, 314–315
  DNA damage with, 65–66
  fractionation of, 304–306
  physical and chemical modifiers and, 315–316

Ionizing radiation—*continued*
  response of tumors to, 308–314
  value of, 299
  volume and dose of, 306–307
Iphosphamide, 172
Isotope scanning, 265

Karyotypes
  of biopsy of D245 MG cell line, *171*
  of medulloblastomas, 168–170
  of sporadic meningiomas, 58
Karyotyping, 164, 168
Keimzellen, 91
Ki-67
  correlation of with BrdU labeling index, 155
  immunostaining for, 24
  index, 24
    antiserum, 25
  reaction with nuclear antigen, 108
Ki-67 labeling methods, cytokinetic studies using, 30
Kidney carcinoma, metastasis of to brain, 5
Kinetic parameters
  in vivo estimates of, 259–271
  tumor size and, 259–262
Knock on protons, 302

Labeling index, 108, 147–154
  and median survival time, 148*t*
Lamins, 192
9L cell line, 174–175
Lectins
  to characterize tumors, 187–188
  transcytosis of, 230
Leptomeninges, tumor growth to, 120
Leukemia, CNS malignancies following cure of, 47
Light microscopy, 19
Lymphocytes, cytotoxic, 213
Lymphokine-activated killer (LAK) cells
  in glioma immunotherapy, 220–221
  inhibition of activity of, 223

Magnetic resonance imaging, 265–267
Malignant gliomas
  cytogenetic abnormalities of, 24
  immunocompetence in, 211–223
  immunotherapy for, 211
  prognosis of, 211
  trials to study value of misonidazole for, 317*t*
Malignant melanoma, metastasis of to brain, 5
Malignant transformation, phenotype of, 93
Malignancy, 21–22
Markers, 23. *See also* Biological markers
  for brain tumors
    cell types in CNS, 167–168
    morphology and cytogenetics of, 168–170
  interpretation of studies with, 186–187
Medulloblastomas
  bipotential differentiating capacity of, 44
  cell lines from, 163–164
    chemosensitivity of, 170–172
  cerebellar, narrow window of vulnerability of, 43–44
  chemotherapeutic results in, 328
  karyotypes of, 168, 170
  prognostic factors in, 284–287
  radiation response of, 310
  spread of, 120
Medullomyoblastomas, 38
Melanin-containing cells, 29
Melanin macroglobule (MMG), in CAL biopsies, 55
Melanocyte, diffuse meningeal proliferation of, 10
Melphalan, 172
Meningiomas
  biologic behavior of, 30
  BrdU stained, *153*
  chemotherapeutic results in, 327–328
  classification and nomenclature of, 29–30
  cytokinetic studies, 30
  head trauma and, 76–77, 82
  histology of, 290
  incidence rates for, 8
  intracranial, 10
  location of, 290
  multicentric CNS, 10
  in NF-2, 57–58, 59
  photoradiation therapy for, 351
  prognostic factors in, 289–290
  radiation response of, 314
  relative frequency of, 7
  study of, 151
  suprasellar, 289–290
  WHO definition of, 29
Meningitis, BBB alteration with, 236
Metabolic studies
  evaluation and correlation of data from, 252
  methods for, 251–252
Metaplasia, 36–37
Metastasis, 21–22
Methotrexate, topical, 334
Methylnitrosourea (MNU), 85
  and cerebral neuroblastoma development, 41
Metronidazole, 316
Microcysts, 22
Microcytophotometry, 148, 150
Microtumors, ENU-induced, 85, *86–87*
Microwave energy, 364
Microwave hyperthermia, 369
  interstitial, 363–364
  series, 370*t*
Microwaves, 363
Misonidazole
  and radiotherapy, 316
  trials to study value of, 317*t*
Mitotic index, 108
Moc-antibodies, 191–192
Molecular genetic studies, of neurofibromatosis-2 tumors, 58–61
Molecular pathology methods, 24
Monoclonal antibodies, 186
  application of, 186
  immunoreactivity to, 43
  limitations in application of, 23
  in study of glioma-specific antigens, 216
  for vimentin, 197
Mononuclear cells, in peripheral blood, 213
MOPP, 328
Mortality statistics, underlying cause of death in, 6
Moya-Moya disease, 313
Multiple sclerosis

brain tumor and, 79
and glial cell neoplastic vulnerability, 46–47
plaque of as focal point of cerebral mass lesion, 78
Mutagenesis
DNA repair mechanisms and, 63–70
process of, 63
Myelin forming cells, 190
Myelin proteins, 189–190
Myelosuppression, 330

N-alkylnitrosoureas, neurooncogenic potential of, 63
Nasopharynx malignant tumors, metastasis of to CNS, 5
Natural killer (NK) cells, 221
Necrosis
in glioblastoma, *110*
types of in tumors, 109
Neoplasia
diagnosis of, 19
phenotypic expression of, 40
principles in differentiation of, 37
Neoplasms. *See also* Tumors
growth of, 146
primary intracranial, 3–14
systematic classification of, 20
Neoplastic cells, flexibility of adaptation in, 37
Neoplastic proliferations, early (ENPs), 85, *86*
transition from hyperplasia to, 95
Neoplastic transformation
of malignant gliomas, 102–109
research on mechanism of, 23–24
Neoplastic vulnerability
glioma cytogeny and differentiation viewed through, 35–48
window of, 102–104
Nerve sheath tumors, of CNS, 10
Nervous system. *See also* Central nervous system
neoplasms of
multicentric primary, 10
multiple primary tumors and genetic syndromes of, 11*t*
neurofibromatosis as tumor formation model in, 53–61
polymorphic cell composition of, 90
neu oncogene, 174
Neural carcinogens, susceptibility to in demyelinated areas, 82
Neural tumors, papovavirus-induced, 79
Neurinomas
cell growth in, 90
ENU-induced, 85–90
Neuroblastomas, cerebral, 41
Neurocytogenesis
final stages of, 91
neoplastic transformation during, 98
normal stages of in forebrain and window of vulnerability, 39–41
Neuroectodermal tumors, BrdU labeling indices of, 153*t*
Neuroendocrine cells
dispersed, 188, 191
link of to nervous system, 192
Neuroendocrine markers, 191–192
Neuroendocrine system
diffuse, 188
epithelial tumors of, 191
Neuroepidemiology
case selection in, 5–6
contributions of, 3
definition of, 3
descriptive studies in, 6–14
design of studies in, 3–4
Neuroepithelial cells
neoplastic vulnerability of, 47–48
primitive, 28
Neuroepithelial-mesodermal tumors, 111
nosography of, 115
Neuroepithelial tumors
central, 35–36
spreading capacity of, 118
Neurofibromas
multiple cutaneous, 54
plexiform, 55–56
spinal nerve root, 56
Neurofibromatosis, 53
benign neurologic tumors in, 55–56
clinical features of, 54–57
forms of, 10, 53–54
molecular genetic studies of tumors in, 58–61
neurologic tumors in, 57–58
as tumor formation model, 53–61
Neurofibrosarcomas, studies of development of, 60–61
Neurofilament (NF) proteins, 187
antibodies to, 201
tumor expression of, 194
Neurofilaments, 23
in PNET studies, 200
types of, 194, 197–198
Neuroglial mitosis, 94
Neurologic tumors, in NF-2, 57–58
Neuromyelitis, 79
Neurons
germinal cells of, 91
migration of, 90
production of, 91–93
Neuron-specific enolase, 188
Neuropeptides, 192
NF-2 gene, 61
Nitroimidazoles, 315
Nitrosourea derivatives, 85. *See also* Ethylnitrosourea (ENU); Methylnitrosourea (MNU)
for ENU tumors, 102
N-nitroso compounds
study of, 63
susceptibility to in demyelinated areas, 82
Nomenclature, 19
issues of for brain tumors, 25–30
Nonneuronal enolase, 188

O-alkylation, 94
Oligodendroglia
astrocytes and, 93
carboanhydrase C in, 98–100
degeneration of in MS plaque, 79
GFA protein in, 45
role of in remyelination of CNS, 45
in cerebral cortex, *87*

Oligodendroglia—*continued*
markers for, 98–100
neoplastic, 36
Oligodendroglioma
CAC-negative and-positive cells in, *101*
chemotherapeutic results in, 327
following trauma, 75
GAG accumulation in, *96*
growth and spread of, *118–119*
histologic features of, 283
isomorphic, in white matter, *88–89*
narrow window of vulnerability of, 44–46
perineuronal satellitosis in, *121*
prognostic factors in, 282–283
radiation response of, 310
tumor proliferation of, *121*, *122*
Oncogenes, 24, 25. *See also* c-erb oncogene, Erb B oncogene, neu oncogene, N-F 2 gene, proto-oncogenes
in brain tumor growth, 174
contribution of to tumor progression, 100, 109
in tumor cells, 53
Optic nerve gliomas
multicentric CNS, 10
radiation response of, 312–313
Organ culture, 165
Oxygen utilization, in brain tumors, 268

Papovaviruses, 79
Parasitic disease, intracranial masses due to, 5
Parkinson's disease, BBB alteration with treatment of, 242
Pathogenesis, 23–24
PCNU, effectiveness of, 172
Peripheral blood lymphocytes (PBL), blastogenic responses to, 212
Peripheral nervous system, biological markers of, 185
Peritumoral angiogenesis, 100–102
Peritumoral tissue, 123–127
Perivascular rosettes, 22
Phakomatoses, 10
Phenotypic expression, 20
Pheochromocytoma
multicentric CNS, 10
in von Hippel-Lindau disease, 10
Photoactive drug, analysis of, 343–345
Photoradiation therapy
clinical studies of, 348–351
concepts of, 341
current status of, 343–348
and drug-light interactions, 345–348
future considerations in, 351–352
history of, 341–343
loss of cell viability in, 347
optimization of parameters of, 347–348
Photosensitizer action, 341
pH sensitizing effect, 368
Pineal region tumors
chemotherapeutic results in, 329
classification and nomenclature of, 29
growth of, 118–120
radiation response of, 311
Pineoblastomas, Flexner rosettes and fleurettes in, 38
Pineocytomas, 39
Pinocytosis, in brain tumors, 109
Pituitary adenomas
incidence rates for, 8–9
prognostic factors in, 288–289
radiation response of, 313
Plain skull x-rays, 265
Plasmalemma
of blood-brain barrier endothelia, 233
energy-dependent pumps of, 231
Platelet-derived growth factor (PDGF)
B chain gene of, 111
expression of by tumor cells, 109
studies of role in glioma growth, 172
study of, 173
in transformed glioma cells, 100
Plexiform neurofibromas, 55–56
Population doubling time, 146
Positron emission tomography (PET)
consistency in, 253
culture methodology and, 256–257
development of, 251
of gliomas, 267–268
quantitative results of, 253–257
in study of brain tumor and BBB alteration, 238
tumor visual appearance on, 253
PPD injections, 218
Primitive brain tumors
cell line studies with antibodies to IF, 200–201
cell type specific biological markers for, 187–201
innovations in evaluation of, 185–186
Primitive neuroctodermal tumors (PNETs). *See also* Medulloblastoma, 25–28, 191.
cellular differentiation in, 286
chemotherapy for, 287
detection of, 192
dissemination of, 285–286
double-fluorescence in, *199*
histological features of, 286
immunoperoxidase studies of, *194–195*
immunoreactivity of, 200
location of, 284–285
neural markers in, 198*t*
neuronally differentiated, 198–199
and patient age, 284
prognostic factors in, 284–287
staging of, 285
studies of, 197
surgical resection and outcome of, 286–287
Procarbazine, 172
Prognosis
factors in, 275–291
statistical data gathering for, 23
Progressive multifocal leukoencephalopathy (PML), 46
brain tumor and, 78–79
Prolactin-secreting tumors, 288–289
Prospective study, 11
Prostaglandins, in brain tumor cells, 111
Proteins, structural vs. soluble, 23
Proto-oncogenes, 24
Psammomatous hemangiomas, 30

Radial glia, 91
Radiation
DNA damage with, 65–66

ionizing, 299–317
Radiation beams, 300
Radiation cell survival curves, 303
Radiation dosimetry, 301
Radiation-induced gliomas, 47
Radiation therapy, 218
for anaplastic gliomas, 277
of ENU tumors, 102
for ependymonas, 284
for gliomas of thalamus and hypothalamus, 278–289
implantation procedure for, 301–302
modalities of, 299–302
value of, 299
Radiobiologic effect (RBE), 303–304
Radioiodinated serum albumin (RISA), in brain tumor diagnosis, 236–237
Radiotherapy. *See* Radiation therapy
Recombinant DNA technology, 24, 219
Regression, 299
Restriction fragment length polymorphism (RFLP) studies, 24
Retinoblastoma, 38–39
mechanism of, 60
multicentric CNS, 10
RG-2 cell line, 174–175
Risk factors
for intracranial neoplasms, 10–14
putative, 12–13
RNA retroviruses, 24
Rochester Tumor Registry data, 8

Sarcomas, classification of, 20
Scandinavian Glioblastoma Study Group, 309
Schwann cells, 29
Schwann cell tumors, 55–56
in NF-2, 57
Schwannoma, multicentric CNS, 10
Skin tumors, 73–74
Sodium butyrate, 138–141
Soluble proteins, 23
S phase
DNA synthesis during, 147
duration of in gliomas, 154
fractions, 151
Spheroid culture system, 165–166
Spinal nerve root neurofibromas, 56
in NF-2, 57
Spongioblasts, 91
Stem cells, in myelination glia, 93–94
Structural proteins, 23
Subarachnoid hemorrhage, BBB alteration after, 236
Subarachnoid space, tumor spreading in, *103*
Subarachnoid spinal seeding, 310
Subependymal plate, dividing cells in, *93*
Suprasellar germinoma, 311
Surgical trauma, tumors following, 75
Synaptophysin, 191
Syringomyelia, 10

Tanycyte, structure of, 42
T-cell deficiency states, malignancies with, 211
Teratoma, multicentric CNS, 10
Tetanus toxin receptors, 189
Thalamic gliomas, 312
Thalamic tumors, prognostic factors in, 278–279
Thermal death times, *360*
Thermal fields, 364–366
Thermochemotherapy, 370
Thermoradiotherapy, 370–371
Thermosensitivity, variability in, 371
Thermotolerance, 370–371
Thiotepa, 172
Thrombosis, 109–111
[^{3}H]-Thymidine autoradiographic study, 147–148
Tight junctional complex
and blood-borne macromolecules, 229
endothelial, abnormalities in, 237
T-lymphocytes
circulating, 212
cytotoxic, 222
blocking of, 214
Transcytosis
process of through blood-brain barrier, 233
receptor-mediated, 231
Transdifferentiation, 38
Transfer vesicles, intraendothelial, 230
Transforming growth factor (TGF), 111
Transforming growth factor-beta, 173, 212
Transplacental ENU model
cell characteristics of tumors in, 95–100
therapeutic studies in, 102
transformation process in, 85–95
tumor spreading in, 102
vasculature of tumors in, 100–102
Trauma
in brain tumor etiology, 73–82
CNS, 75–78
and glial cell neoplastic vulnerability, 46
in non-CNS carcinogenesis, 74
Trilateral retinoblastoma, 38
T-suppressor lymphocytes, 213
antigen-antibody complexes and, 214
Tuberculosis, intracranial masses due to, 5
Tuberous sclerosis, 10
Tumor cell kinetics
concepts of, 145–147
measurement of, 147–156
in vivo measurement of, 259–262
ways to measure, 108
Tumor classification
definitions in, 21
difficulties with, 23
grading systems in, 21–25
history of, 20–21
Tumorigenic phenotype, reversibility of, 137
Tumor nomenclature system, 19–20
Tumors
benign vs. malignant, 21–22
capillaries of, 19
cell loss in, 146–147
definition of, 19, 21
differentiated vs. undifferentiated, 21
grading of, 20–25
histologic characteristics of, 20
patterns of growth of, 85–127
regression of, 299
Tumor suppressor gene, 53
Typing. *See* Cell typing; Grading systems

Ultraviolet photoradiation, 65
Undifferented tumor, 21

Vasculature
  of brain tumors, 109–111
  of ENU tumors, 100–102
  of glioblastomas, *113–114*
Vesicle-crowned lamellae, 38
Vesicle-crowned rodlets, 38
Vibrio cholerae, endotoxin of, 188–189
Vimentin, 23, 196–197
  distribution of in ENU tumors, 98, *99*
Vincristine, in astrocytomas, 327
VM/Dk strain mouse, 174
von Hippel-Lindau disease, 10
  hemangioblastomas in, 30
von Recklinghausen's neurofibromatosis, 313. *See also* Neurofibromatosis
  forms of, 10

Wilms tumor, mechanism of, 60
Window of vulnerability, 47–48
  in CNS tumors, 39
    narrow, 39–43
    wide, 43–46
  in gliomas, 102–104
World Health Organization classification of CNS tumors, 21, 25, 26–27*t*

Xenogeneic transplantation, 36, 38
Xenon arc-lamp irradiation, 349
X-rays, 299–300
  biological interaction of, 302